Brain Tumors

Contemporary Cancer Research

Jac A. Nickoloff, SERIES EDITOR

Brain Tumors

Edited by

Francis Ali-Osman, DSC

Department of Surgery, Comprehensive Cancer Center,
Duke University Medical Center, Durham, NC

HUMANA PRESS ✳ TOTOWA, NEW JERSEY

Production Editor: Mark J. Breaugh.

Cover design by Patricia F. Cleary.

Cover illustration: MRI of a child with medulloblastoma. *See* Fig. 1 on p. 128.

For additional copies, pricing for bulk purchases, and/or information about other Humana titles, contact Humana at the above address or at any of the following numbers: Tel: 973-256-1699; Fax: 973-256-8341; E-mail: humana@humanapr.com, or visit our Website: http://humanapress.com

Printed in the United States of America. 10 9 8 7 6 5 4 3 2 1

e-ISBN: 1-59259-843-9

Library of Congress Cataloging in Publication Data

Brain tumors / edited by Francis Ali-Osman.
    p. ; cm. -- (Contemporary cancer research)
  Includes bibliographical references and index.
  ISBN 1-58829-042-5 (alk. paper)
  1. Brain--Tumors.
  [DNLM: 1. Brain Neoplasms. WL 358 B813465 2005] I. Ali-Osman, Francis.
II. Series.
  RC280.B7B7232 2005
  616.99'481--dc22
                                    2004017417

Preface

Exciting new developments and discoveries of the last two decades are beginning to shed light on the complex biology of brain tumors and are advancing our understanding of the cellular and molecular processes involved in their initiation, progression, and clinical and biological behavior. The disease process in brain tumors is quite complex and the resulting tumors are characterized by a high degree of biological and clinical diversity. Thus, despite the advances of the last two decades, prognosis for patients with malignant brain tumors remains abysmal. Significant progress in the diagnosis, treatment and, ultimately, prevention of these tumors will require both the timely harnessing of the advances in basic and clinical brain tumor research, and a continuing concerted effort at increasing our understanding of brain tumor biology, in particular, the molecular genetic changes and perturbations of cellular pathways involved in brain oncogenesis and which drive the biological and clinical behavior of the tumors. Brain tumor diagnosis and prognosis, which is still largely based on histopathology and other clinical criteria, will, in the future, acquire a significant molecular component, with the incorporation of knowledge of genes that are mutated, over-expressed, deleted, silenced, or functionally altered in the tumors. Treatment strategies for brain tumors, rather than being empirical, will be rationally developed based on an understanding of the cellular and molecular mechanisms and targets that have been activated, suppressed, or otherwise altered. The discovery of new therapeutics will employ novel paradigms of rational drug discovery that incorporate structural biology, genomics, proteomics, computational chemistry and high throughput approaches. Advances in genetic epidemiology and neuro-oncogenesis will lead to the definition of high risk genotypes and phenotypes and provide the basis for genetic counseling of individuals and populations at risk for brain tumors, and facilitate the development of brain tumor prevention strategies.

The goal of *Brain Tumors* is to bring together the major scientific advances and developments in important areas of brain tumor research of the last two decades. The explosion of knowledge in the neurosciences and in neuro-oncology that has marked this period make this a timely and much needed undertaking. The chapters, organized into three main sections, emphasize recent research advances, rather than a review of established knowledge. The first section is devoted to the molecular biology, genetics, epidemiology, and pathology of brain tumors, and includes chapters on molecular profiling, molecular pathology and classification, in vitro and in vivo brain tumor models, brain metastasis and progenitor cell biology. The second section focuses on the cellular and genetic pathways involved in brain oncogenesis, malignant progression, and therapeutic response. Individual chapters cover oncogenes and tumor suppressor genes, DNA damage and repair, invasion and migration, cell cycle, growth factors, signaling, apoptosis, and developmental biology. The final section covers areas relevant to brain tumor therapy, with chapters focusing on advances in pharmacological concepts, therapeutic modalities, novel therapeutic targets, rational drug design, gene and viral therapy, drug delivery, and the blood–brain barrier, immunotherapy, and brain imaging. *Brain Tumors* provides for the established brain tumor scientist and clinician, as well as, for the new investigator, graduate, or undergraduate student, a comprehensive, up-to-date guide to the critical research topics in the rapidly evolving area of neuro-oncology. The contributors of the chapters in this volume are all leaders at the frontiers of basic and clinical neuro-oncology research and practice whose work over the years has helped define the field. To each of them, I express my deepest thanks for a scholarly contribution that has resulted in a volume that is a major effort to better understand and ultimately eradicate, or at least minimize, human suffering from brain tumors.

Francis Ali-Osman, DSC

Contents

Contributors

FRANCIS ALI-OSMAN, DSC • *Department of Surgery and the Comprehensive Cancer Center, Duke University Medical Center, Durham, NC*

GAMIL R. ANTOUN, PhD • *Department of Neurosurgery, The University of Texas M. D. Anderson Cancer Center, Houston, TX*

MARTIN BEGEMANN, MD • *Department of Human Molecular Genetics, Max Planck Institute for Molecular Genetics, Berlin, Germany*

DARELL D. BIGNER, MD, PhD • *Department of Pathology, Duke University Medical Center, Durham, NC*

MELISSA BONDY, PhD • *Department of Epidemiology, The University of Texas M. D. Anderson Cancer Center, Houston, TX*

HENRY BREM, MD • *Department of Neurological Surgery, The Johns Hopkins Hospital, Baltimore, MD*

JOHN K. BUOLAMWINI, PhD • *Department of Pharmaceutical Sciences, College of Pharmacy, University of Tennessee Health Science Center, Memphis, TN*

J. GREGORY CAIRNCROSS, MD • *Department of Clinical Neurosciences, Foothills Medical Centre and University of Calgary, Calgary, Alberta, Canada*

CHARLES A. CONRAD, MD • *Department of Neuro-Oncology, The University of Texas M.D. Anderson Cancer Center, Houston, TX*

HELGA E. DE VRIES • *Departments of Molecular Cell Biology and Pathology, Vrije Universiteit University Medical Center, Amsterdam*

DENNIS F. DEEN, PhD • *Brain Tumor Research Center, Departments of Neurosurgery and Radiation Oncology, University of California, San Francisco, CA*

JOERG DIETRICH, MD • *Department of Biomedical Genetics, University of Rochester Medical Center, Rochester, NY*

CHRISTINE D. DIJKSTRA • *Departments of Molecular Cell Biology and Pathology, Vrije Universiteit University Medical Center, Amsterdam*

M. EILEEN DOLAN, PhD • *Section of Hematology/Oncology, Department of Medicine, The Cancer Research Center, The University of Chicago, Chicago, IL*

RANDA EL-ZEIN, MD, PhD • *Department of Epidemiology, The University of Texas M. D. Anderson Cancer Center, Houston, TX*

ISAIAH J. FIDLER, DVM, PhD • *Department of Cancer Biology, The University of Texas M. D. Anderson Cancer Center, Houston, TX*

JOHN R. FIKE, PhD • *Brain Tumor Research Center, Departments of Neurosurgery and Radiation Oncology, University of California, San Francisco, CA*

JAMES FRAZIER, BA • *Department of Neurological Surgery, The Johns Hopkins Hospital, Baltimore, MD*

HENRY S. FRIEDMAN, MD • *Departments of Surgery, Pathology, Medicine, and Neuro-Oncology, Duke University Medical Center, Durham, NC*

JUAN FUEYO, MD • *Department of Neuro-Oncology, The University of Texas M. D. Anderson Cancer Center, Houston, TX*

TAKAMITSU FUJIMAKI, MD, DMSC • *Department of Cancer Biology, The University of Texas M. D. Anderson Cancer Center, Houston, TX*

GREGORY N. FULLER, MD, PhD • *Department of Pathology, The University of Texas M. D. Anderson Cancer Center, Houston, TX*

CANDELARIA GOMEZ-MANZANO, MD • *Department of Neuro-Oncology, The University of Texas M.D. Anderson Cancer Center, Houston, TX*

NALIN GUPTA, MD, PhD • *Brain Tumor Research Center, Department of Neurosurgery, University of California, San Francisco, CA*

FADI HANBALI, MD • *Department of Neurosurgery, The University of Texas M. D. Anderson Cancer Center, Houston, TX*

AMY B. HEIMBERGER, MD • *Department of Surgery (Neurosurgery), Duke University Medical Center, Durham, NC*

JOHN R. HILL, MD, PhD • *Department of Pediatrics, Norris Cotton Cancer Center, Dartmouth Medical School, Lebanon, NH*

ERIC C. HOLLAND, MD, PhD • *Departments of Surgery (Neurosurgery), Neurology, and Cancer Biology and Genetics, Memorial Sloan Kettering Cancer Center, New York, NY*

MARK A. ISRAEL, MD • *Departments of Pediatrics and Genetics, Norris Cotton Cancer Center, Dartmouth-Hitchcock Medical Center, Dartmouth Medical School, Lebanon, NH*

C. DAVID JAMES, PhD • *Division of Experimental Pathology, Mayo Clinic and Medical School, Rochester, MN*

MINSOO KANG, MD • *Department of Cancer Biology, The University of Texas M. D. Anderson Cancer Center, Houston, TX*

PAUL KLEIHUES • *International Agency for Research on Cancer, World Health Organization, Lyon, France*

LOIS A. LAMPSON, PhD • *Department of Neurosurgery, Brigham and Women's Hospital, Harvard Medical School, Boston, MA*

MACIEJ S. LESNIAK, MD • *Department of Neurological Surgery, The Johns Hopkins Hospital, Baltimore, MD*

DAVID N. LOUIS, MD • *Molecular Neuro-Oncology and Molecular Pathology Laboratories, Massachusetts General Hospital, Harvard Medical School, Boston, MA*

TIMOTHY J. MCDONNELL, MD, PhD • *Department of Molecular Pathology, The University of Texas M.D. Anderson Cancer Center, Houston, TX*

SANJEEVA MOHANAM, PhD • *Program of Cancer Biology, Department of Biomedical and Therapeutic Sciences, University of Illinois College of Medicine, Peoria, IL*

LISETTE MONTAGNE • *Departments of Molecular Cell Biology and Pathology, Vrije Universiteit University Medical Center, Amsterdam*

MARK NOBLE, PhD • *Department of Biomedical Genetics, University of Rochester Medical Center, Rochester, NY*

CATHERINE L. NUTT, PhD • *Molecular Neuro-Oncology and Molecular Pathology Laboratories, Massachusetts General Hospital, Harvard Medical School, Boston, MA*

HIROKO OHGAKI • *International Agency for Research on Cancer, World Health Organization, Lyon, France*

SHOICHIRO OHTA • *Department of Protective Bioregulation, Saga Medical School, Saga, Japan*

VINAGOLU K. RAJASEKHAR • *Department of Developmental and Cell Biology, University of California, Irvine, CA*

JASTI S. RAO, PhD • *Program of Cancer Biology, Departments of Biomedical and Therapeutic Sciences and Neurosurgery, University of Illinois College of Medicine, Peoria, IL*

DAVID A. REARDON, MD • *Neuro-Oncology Program, Department of Surgery (Neurosurgery), Duke University Medical Center, Durham, NC*

JOHN H. SAMPSON, MD, PhD • *Department of Surgery (Neurosurgery), Duke University Medical Center, Durham, NC*

RAYMOND SAWAYA, MD • *Department of Neurosurgery, The University of Texas M. D. Anderson Cancer Center, Houston, TX*

PENNY K. SNEED, MD • *Department of Radiation Oncology, University of California, San Francisco, CA*

ANAT O. STEMMER-RACHAMIMOV, MD • *Molecular Neuro-Oncology and Molecular Pathology Laboratories, Massachusetts General Hospital, Harvard Medical School, Boston, MA*

PHILIP J. TOFILON, PhD • *Molecular Radiation Therapeutics Branch, National Cancer Institute, Bethesda, MD*

PAUL VAN DER VALK • *Departments of Molecular Cell Biology and Pathology, Vrije Universiteit University Medical Center, Amsterdam*

MARGARET WRENSCH, PhD, MPH • *Department of Epidemiology and Biostatistics, School of Medicine, University of California, San Francisco, CA*

SEIJI YANO, MD, PhD • *Department of Cancer Biology, The University of Texas M. D. Anderson Cancer Center, Houston, TX*

W. K. ALFRED YUNG, MD • *Department of Neuro-Oncology, The University of Texas M.D. Anderson Cancer Center, Houston, TX*

I Epidemiology, Biology, Genetics, and Pathology

1

Epidemiology of Brain Tumors

Randa El-Zein, Melissa Bondy, and Margaret Wrensch

1. INCIDENCE AND RESEARCH INITIATIVES

1.1. Epidemiology

Brain cancer accounts for approx 1.4% of all cancers and 2.3% of all cancer-related deaths. The incidence of primary cerebral malignancies varies between 4 and 10/100,000 in the general population. This incidence tends to increase with age (4/100,000 up to the age of 12 yr; 6/100,000 up to the age of 35 yr; 18/100,000 up to the age of 55 yr; 70/100,000 up to the age of 75 yr).

In 2002, over 35,000 (approx 6 per 100,000) Americans were diagnosed with brain tumors *(84)*. The annual death rate from the group of conditions so classified is some 13,000/yr. Currently, in part, owing to improved diagnostic methods, approx 16,800 brain tumor cases are diagnosed each year as malignant, with poor prognosis *(3)*. However, even those cases that are classified as benign and are treatable, are significantly interfered with normal brain function that is essential for a normal life *(3)*. The continuing grim outlook for patients, the often devastating impact of even treatable low grade pediatric cancers and other benign disorders, as well as breakthroughs in genetic research, have given new impetus to brain cancer research.

Two types of epidemiologic studies, descriptive and analytical, have figured prominently in the notable recent increase in research effort in brain tumors. Descriptive studies characterize incidence, mortality, and survival rates associated with brain tumors by category of histologic tumor type and patient demography, such as age, sex, and geographic region. Analytic epidemiologic studies compare, in cohorts the ri sk of brain tumors in people with and without certain characteristics and histories, explore risk factors that can be implicated in the development of cancer.

A wide variety of risk factors, including diet, smoking, alcohol, occupation exposures, radiation, infections, allergies, head trauma, and family history are being intensively investigated for their role in brain tumors. In recent years, a greater focus is being directed at inherited polymorphisms in genes related to carcinogen metabolism, and DNA repair, as well as, gene environment interactions. The relative rarity of brain tumors makes the assembly of large cohort studies difficult and, therefore, most commonly these analytic studies use the case-control approach.

Though increasingly illuminating, epidemiologic studies of brain cancer lack consensus on the nature and weight of individual risk factors. Variations in study designs, population and information sources, measurement, and classification together cloud the research. Studies differ in methodologies such as those for selection of study subjects and determination of whether the subjects are representative, and the definition and selection of control groups. Studies vary in their reliance on proxy and historical information and the standards of precision and fullness that these must meet. They also face basic classification problems arising from the heterogeneity of primary brain tumors; inconsistencies

From: *Contemporary Cancer Research: Brain Tumors*
Edited by: F. Ali-Osman © Humana Press Inc., Totowa, NJ

in histologic diagnoses, definitions, and groupings. In 1993, the World Health Organization (WHO) tumor classification was last updated but is not in universal use. This complexity is further compounded by difficulties in verifying past exposures.

1.1.1. Age and Sex of Patients

The likelihood of different histologic types of brain tumor having different etiologic factors is suggested by age distribution and differences in site and histology of the tumors. For all primary brain tumors, although patient average age at onset is about 54 yr, there is a significant variation for each histological category. For example, the average age of onset for glioblastoma and meningiomas is 62 yr *(84)*. In meningioma, the incidence increases with age, except for a slight decline in those 85 yr or older. In contrast, astrocytoma and glioblastoma peak in incidence at age 65 to 74 yr, whereas oligodendroglioma peaks at age 35 to 44 yr. Some of this variation may reflect differing diagnostic practices and access to diagnosis in different age groups. Much of the age-related tumor incidence increase may be accounted for by the duration of exposure required for malignant transformation, the number of genetic alterations required to produce clinical disease, or poorer immune surveillance with advancing age. An intriguing and incompletely explained feature of brain tumors is a peak in incidence in young children, which is not completely attributable to tumors of primitive neuroectodermal origin, which are primarily pediatric tumors.

In general, men experience higher rates of primary brain tumors than women, with the exceptions of meningiomas, which affect 80% more females than males, and tumors of cranial and spinal nerves, and the sellar region, which affect males and females almost equally *(110)*. Gliomas affect about 40% more males than females *(110)*. A New York State study showed that gender differences in glioblastoma appeared around the age of menarche, peaked near the age of menopause, and decreased thereafter, suggesting a protective effect of female hormones *(85)*. Any comprehensive theory of the distribution and causes of brain tumors needs to include an explanation for the consistently observed age and gender differences.

As the incidence has become more accurately described a result of better and more consistent diagnosis and study designs approaching congruity, dramatic progress in the molecular classification of tumors opens the possibility of identifying etiologically homogeneous subsets of tumors. The accelerating characterization of potentially relevant genes has also created an opportunity to determine which of them might enhance susceptibility or resistance to brain tumors or etiologic environmental agents. Of special interest in carcinogenesis are *proto-oncogenes*, which initiate carcinogenesis by activating cell division, and *suppressor genes* that inhibit tumor growth and progression *(120)*. Because such genes play a role in disease progression and sensitivity (or resistance) to radiation or drug treatments, knowledge from their study may result in feasible prevention strategies.

1.2. Histology and Molecular Genetics of Brain Tumor Types

Primary brain tumors are currently classified by histology and location. However, this classification is complicated by the potential ability of any of the cells of the nervous system to become cancerous, resulting in a mixture of cell types often seen in many brain tumors. Brain tumors have been further categorized by the WHO on the basis of their invasiveness or malignancy. The more invasive forms, which often show more frequent gene mutations, are given higher numbers. The relevant research findings on the individual brain tumors are summarized below.

1.2.1. Gliomas

Gliomas arise from the glial component of the nervous system and their cells provide an interface between neurons and brain fluids. They are the most common primary brain tumor and account for more than 40% of all central nervous system neoplasms with a peak incidence around age 60 yr *(61)*. Despite the fact that gliomas are derived from astrocytes, oligodendrocytes, or ependymal cells, significant variations exist between them that may reflect the genes involved in their genesis *(62)*. In general, glial tumors are named after their putative cell type of their origin: viz., astrocytomas, oligo-dendrogliomas, and ependymomas.

1.2.1.1. ASTROCYTOMAS

Astrocytomas account for the majority of brain tumors, with an incidence in children of about 700 annually for low-grade forms, and approx 100 high-grade cases affecting the ubiquitous star-shaped cells that provide extensive structural and physiological support of neurons in the central nervous system (CNS). Astrocytic tumors comprise a wide range of neoplasms that differ in their location within the CNS, age and gender distribution, growth potential, extent of invasiveness, morphological features, tendency for progression, and clinical course. There is increasing evidence that these differences reflect the type and sequence of genetic alterations acquired during the process of transformation. The WHO has distinguished the following clinicopathological subtypes of astrocytomas:

a. WHO grade I, or pilocytic astrocytoma, the most common brain tumor in children and primarily a pediatric tumor, rarely undergoes neoplastic transformation. Even though the most benign of the astrocytomas, depending on location, they can interfere with vital sensory functions and often recur after apparentlycomplete resection.

b. WHO grade II, or fibrillary astrocytomas account for 25% of all gliomas and are infiltrative in nature. Despite their r⁻ ⁻ᵛe lack of aggressive histologic features, low-grade astrocytomas in adults are fatal in the great maj⁻ ⁻ients.

c. WHO grade⁻ ⁻ malignant astrocytomas, are highly malignant gliomas and have an increased tendency ⁻ ⁻na.

d. WHO g⁻ ⁻r glioblastoma multiforme, is a highly malignant brain tumor and typical⁻ ⁻ has poor prognosis, in part, because the poorly defined tumor rapid⁻ ⁻e are the most common intracranial neoplasm and account for⁻

Th⁻ ⁻as has led to the recognition that the nonran-dom⁻ ⁻gnancy and clinical grade *(49)*. Several com-me⁻ ⁻at are associated with changes in the expression ⁻ ⁻utations in the *p53* gene on chromosome 17p have⁻ ⁻rades. These mutations occur primarily in gliomas ⁻er gene whose loss or alteration occurs rarely in low-⁻e cyclin-dependent kinase N2 (*CDKN2*) or *p16*. Dele-⁻hromosome 9p is common in high-grade astrocytomas ⁻nts in the p16 gene have also been reported. Deletions of ⁻al tumor suppressor genes) *(56)*, commonly occurs in ⁻heterozygosity at 10q23 has been reported in approx 70% of

gli⁻ ⁻ gene, *MMAC1* or phosphatase tensin homolog (*PTEN*), on
10q is ⁻. ⁻omas, but rarely mutated in low-grade gliomas. As a result,
MMAC1 has ⁻ ⁻y an important role in progression from low-grade to high-grade gliomas *(8)*.

Some chromosoma⁻ ⁻s in gliomas often include both loss of tumor suppressor genes and activation of oncogenes, resulting in altered, often increased cell proliferation. The epidermal growth factor receptor (EGFR) gene is the gene most frequently amplified in malignant astrocytomas. The EGFR protein is a receptor for epidermal growth factor, an important proliferative stimulant for astrocytes. Amplification of a mutated EGFR allele has been found in approximately one-third of glioblastomas but absent in low-grade astrocytomas *(55)*.

1.2.1.2. OLIGODENDROGLIOMAS

Oligodendroglioma develops from oligodendrocytes, which are cells that produce the lipid covering of the axons of nerve cells. This type of tumor occurs normally in the cerebrum, particularly in the frontal or temporal lobes, and is more common in adults than in children and in men more than women. Oligodendrogliomas constitute 5–12% of all glial tumors and 5–7% of all intracranial tumors. They tend to grow slowly and demonstrate characteristic calcifications both in histological as well as on computed tomography and X-ray examinations. Although, clinically less aggressive than astrocytomas, oligodendrogliomas are invasive and can traverse into the cerebral spinal fluid (CSF). Oligodendrogliomas are capable of metastasizing and are often more difficult to remove surgically; however, they generally have a better prognosis and survival outlook than do other gliomas. Like other gliomas, oligodendrogliomas are graded between 1 and 4 depending on their malignancy and rate of growth.

Oligodendrogliomas characteristically exhibit loss of chromosomal regions on 1p and 19q13 and, less frequently, on 9q and 22 *(97)*. Hoang-Xuan et al. *(51)* examined the molecular profile of 26 oligodendrogliomas (10 grade II and 16 grade III) and found that the most frequent alterations were loss of heterozygosity on 1p and 19q. These two alterations were closely associated, suggesting that the two loci may be involved in the same pathway of tumorigenesis. This study also showed that a combination of homozygous deletion of the *P16/CDKN2A* tumor suppressor gene, loss of heterozygosity (LOH) on chromosome 10, and amplification of the *EGFR* oncogene was present at a higher rate than previously reported *(52)*. A statistically significant exclusion was noted between these three genetic alterations and the LOH on 1p/19q, suggesting that there are at least two distinct genetic subsets of oligodendroglioma. *EGFR* amplification and LOH on 10q were significant predictors of shorter progression-free survival (PFS), thus characterize a more aggressive form of tumor whereas LOH on 1p was associated with longer PFS.

1.2.1.3. EPENDYMOMAS

These tumors develop from ependymal cells, which line the *ventricles of the brain* and the central canal of the spinal cord. Ependymomas may spread from the brain to the spinal cord via the CSF causing notable swelling of the ventricle or hydrocephalus. Ependymomas account for 4–6% of all brain tumors and occur mainly up to the age of 20 yr. In children, 30% of ependymomas appear before the age of 3 yr and are more aggressive than in adults. Nearly 90% of pediatric ependymomas are intracranial: they occur in supratentorial or posterior fossa locations, and only 10% are intraspinal. In contrast to the earlier mentioned tumors, low-grade ependymomas (grade I/II) develop metastases along the neuroaxis. The most commonly described genetic alterations in ependymomas are deletions of 17p and monosomy 22 *(49)*.

1.2.2. Meningiomas

Meningiomas are regarded as benign tumors originating from endothelial cover cells of the meninges surrounding the brain. They account for 10–19% of all brain tumors. Meningiomas constitute a large proportion of tumors of the cranial base, so that the term "anatomic malignancy" is used in this region to denote meningiomas (in contrast to biologic malignancy). Age distribution of meningiomas is homogeneous; however the disease occurs in less than 2% of children. At least 3000 new cases of meningiomas are diagnosed each year in the United States with a 2:1 predominance in women over men. The tumors occur over all age groups but generally peak at midlife. High-grade or malignant meningiomas are associated with deletions of loci on chromosome 1 and, to a lesser extent deletions on 6p, 9q, and 17p *(49)*. Mutations in the *p53* gene have also been reported in malignant meningioma.

1.2.3. Medulloblastomas

Medulloblastomas are malignant tumors originating from primitive or poorly developed cells, constitute 3–5% of all brain tumors, but as much as 25% of all brain tumors in childhood. The disease most commonly occurs between the ages of 3 and 8 yr, although occasionally, medulloblastoma are also observed in adults. Because of the median location of these lesions and their association with the fourth ventricle they are frequently accompanied by metastases to the ventricular system and the neuroaxis

(25–45%), usually via the CSF. In 5% of cases, metastases are already present at the time of diagnosis. Although medulloblastoma is one of the most common pediatric malignancies, little is known of the outcome of long-term survivors of childhood medulloblastoma. Treatment of medulloblastoma with radiation has been implicated in the development of secondary malignancies. Chromosome 17p is a frequent site of deletions in medulloblastomas. Other, less frequent sites of deletions are 2p, 6q 10q, 11p, 11q, and 16q *(49)*.

1.2.4. Ganglioglioma

Gangliogliomas are tumors that contain both neurons and glial cells and usually occur in the temporal lobes and cerebral hemispheres. They are highly curable by surgery alone or by surgery combined with radiation therapy. Central gangliomas occur in 0.4–8% of children and 1% of adults and show no higher incidence either by sex or race. Most gangliogliomas are observed in patients younger than 30 yr. In 75–100% of cases gangliomas are manifested by epileptic seizures that h occur long before alterations are seen on computed tomography (CT) or magnetic resonance imagining (MRI) *(92)*. Among genetic alterations observed in ganglioglioma is loss of genetic material on the short arm of chromosome 9 and over-representation of partial or the whole chromosome 7. It has been recently reported that polymorphism in the tuberous sclerosis 2 (TSC2) gene may predispose to the development of sporadic gangliogliomas.

1.2.5. Schwannomas (Neurilemomas)

Schwannomas, usually benign tumors, arise from Schwann cells and often form near the cerebellum and in the cranial nerves responsible for hearing and balance *(47)*. These benign tumors are twice as common in women as in men, and are most often diagnosed in patients between the ages 30 to 60 yr. Intracranial schwannomas account for approx 8% of primary brain tumors. The most common schwannoma is the acoustic neuroma, a tumor of the eighth cranial nerve, but these tumors can also occur on other cranial nerves. Malignant schwannomas originate from peripheral nerves and have a malignant course with recurrent disease and metastases developing early. Losses on 1p and gains on 11q have been detected in a few schwannomas, but no single consistent genetic alteration associated with schwannomas, other than a loss on 22q, has been found to date. Such changes have not been systematically searched previously.

1.2.6. Chordomas

Chordomas are relatively rare neoplasms arising from embryonic notochordal remnants and comprise less than 1% of intracranial neoplasms. They typically occur along the neuraxis, especially at the developmentally more active cranial and caudal ends, notably in the spheno-occipital, sacro-coccygeal, and vertebral locations. Twenty-five to 40% of chordomas occur in the skull base region. These tumors occur predominately in the 30 to 50 yr age range and show a slight predominance in men. They are amenable to treatment but stubbornly recur over a span of 10 to 20 yr. Genetic research into this disorder is underway. One study has detected chromosomal imbalances in chordomas and produced data suggesting that tumor suppressor genes or mismatch repair genes (located at 1p31 and 3p14) and oncogenes (located in 7q36) might be involved in chordoma genesis *(101)*.

1.3. Heritable Syndromes Associated With Central Nervous System Tumors

Original studies of CNS tumor associated syndromes and hereditary conditions associated with CNS tumors parallel in method and implication the studies of other congenital anomalies. These and follow-up studies associate astrocytoma with arteriovenous malformation of the overlying meninges, glioblastoma multiforme with adjacent arteriovenous angiomatous malformation and pulmonary arteriovenous fistula, congenital medulloblastoma with gastrointestinal and genitourinary system anomalies, and congenital ependymoma with multisystem anomalies *(88)*.

CNS tumors commonly occur in association with Down's syndrome, a disorder involving trisomy 21 and gliomatous tumors with syringomyelia *(88)*. Mental retardation and brain cancer may also be associated, becausechildren with astrocytomas had a mentally retarded sibling three times more frequently than controls (*p* {lt} 0.05), and mentally retarded siblings, nieces, and nephews in families of adult males with brain tumors were seen 4.8 times more than in families of controls *(64)*. The most frequently identified hereditary syndromes co-occuring with CNS tumors are described here.

1.3.1. Tuberous Sclerosis

Tuberous sclerosis (TSC), or Bourneville's disease, is an autosomal dominantly inherited progressive disorder occurring in 1 per 6,000 live births. It is characterized by hamartomas of the skin, CNS, and kidneys *(41,45)*, and results in sebaceous adenomas of the skin, muscle and retinal tumors, epileptic seizures, mental retardation, and nodes of abnormal glial fibers and ganglion cells in the brain *(40)*. Its association with CNS tumors is anecdotal, although one hospital study reported 7 CNS tumors in 48 cases (15%) of TSC *(59)*, another found 22 cases of subependymal giant-cell astrocytoma in 345 patients (6.4%) with tuberous sclerosis *(2)*. Astrocytoma, ependymoma, and glioblastoma multiforme have been associated with tuberous sclerosis in up to 5% of cases *(103,104,111)*. *TSC* displays genetic heterogeneity with two genes being linked to this condition, the first in 1993 is *TSC2* mapping to 16p13 (The European TSC Consortium) and the second, *TSC1* was mapped to 9q34 in 1997 *(116)*. *TSC2* is a large gene with at least 41 exons spanning approx 45 kb of genomic DNA and encodes the protein tuberin. *TSC1* contains 23 exons spanning approx 40 kb of genomic DNA and encodes the protein hamartin *(21)*. The majority (98% in *TSC1* and 77% in *TSC2*) of mutations seen in both *TSC1* and *TSC2* are of a nature predicted to truncate the proteins, suggesting that these genes function as tumor suppressor genes *(21)*. Further, loss of heterozygosity (LOH) at both the *TSC1* and *TSC2* loci have been observed in TSC hamartomas, suggestive of Knudson's "second-hit." Of interest, intellectual disability has been more frequently associated with de novo mutation of *TSC2* than *TSC1* *(58)*. Mosaicism has been reported, having important implications for molecular diagnostics.

1.3.2. Neurofibromatosis

Neurofibromatosis (NF-1), or von Recklinghausen's disease, occurring in 1 of 3000 live births *(27)* has an autosomal dominant pattern of inheritance and is regarded by some as among the most common single-gene disorders. Paternal origin of the mutation was found in one study in 12 of 14 families *(57)*, but single-gene etiology has yet to be firmly established, because the spontaneous mutation rate of large populations has been put at 50% *(99)*. NF-1 constitutes 90% of all cases of neurofibromatosis and is manifested within the first 5 yr of life. It is characterized by cutaneous pigmentation (cafe-au-lait spots), multiple neurofibromas involving the skin and possibly deeper peripheral nerves and neural roots. The majority of NF-1 patients (94%) present with Lisch nodules or pigmented iris hamartomas *(95)* and experience optic nerve gliomas, astrocytomas, ependymomas, acoustic neuromas, neurilemmomas, meningiomas, and neurofibromas. Of NF-1 patients, 4–45% experience brain tumors *(8,53,106)*. We recently reported that females with NF-1 are at a higher risk of developing neoplasia than males with NF-1 *(1)*. We also found no elevated cancer risk in unaffected first-degree relatives, regardless of whether the proband had cancer or not. Our data suggested that the malignancy in the proband is not the result of a modifying gene that has a significant impact on general cancer risk *(1)*. Within the past few years, the gene causing NF-1 has been identified and the protein encoded by this gene, neurofibromin, has been the subject of detailed investigation. Studies of tumors from NF-1 patients with homozygous deletions in the NF1 gene suggest a role for NF-1 as a tumor suppressor *(118)*.

1.3.3. Neurofibromatosis Type 2

Neurofibromatosis type 2 (NF-2), or bilateral acoustic neurofibromatosis, occurs with one-tenth the frequency of NF-1. NF-2 is regarded as the central form of NF, occurring in 1 out of 50,000 persons and accounting for 10% of all NF. It is also an autosomal dominant inherited disease. In terms of molecular biology, there is a defect on chromosome 22. Meningiomas associated with NF-2 occur in 25% of cases. NF-2 presents the clinical characteristics of multiple tumors, usually schwannomas of the cranial and spinal nerve roots. Multiple ependymomas, meningiomas developing from arachnoidal cells in the cranial cavity and spinal canal, and spinal cord or brain stem astrocytic gliomas occur in individuals with NF-2. These are often low-grade malignancy but with devastating neurological effects *(83)*. NF-2 is caused by a deletion in the long arm of chromosome 22 associated with meningiomas, gliomas, and spinal neurofibromas *(102,122)*.

1.3.4. Nevoid Basal Cell Carcinoma Syndrome

Nevoid basal cell carcinoma syndrome (Gorlin syndrome), an autosomal dominant disorder, presents with multiple basal cell carcinomas arising early in life, jaw cysts, characteristic facies, skeletal anomalies, intracranial calcifications of the falx, and ovarian fibromas. The syndrome is associated with medulloblastoma *(42)*. One in 200 patients with basal cell carcinomas (one or more) had the syndrome, but the proportion is much higher (one in five) among those in whom a basal cell carcinoma develops before age 19 yr. Only a few of the nevi grow and become locally invasive, and basal cell carcinomas do not develop at all in about 15% of affected persons. Radiation treatment can result in fresh crops of aggressive basal cell carcinomas and can lead to severe disfigurement. By linkage analysis it has been shown that the gene is located on chromosome 9q22.3-q31 *(34)*. LOH at the chromosomal location examined, particularly in hereditary tumors, implies that the gene normally functions as a tumor suppressor andis homozygously inactivated *(34,38)*.

1.3.5. Turcot's Syndrome, Gardner's Syndrome, and Familial Polyposis

Turcot's syndrome, Gardner's syndrome, and familial polyposis are characterized by adenomatous polyps, have been associated with medulloblastoma and glioblastoma *(24,70)*. Because of their marked similarity, some authorities consider Turcot's syndrome, Gardner's syndrome, and classical adenomatous polyposis variations of a single genetic defect. Investigators associate chromosome 5q with these three syndromes *(9,25,70)*. Familial adenomatous polyposis (FAP) is an autosomal dominant disorder that typically presents with colorectal cancer in early adult life secondary to extensive adenomatous polyps of the colon. Polyps also develop in the upper gastrointestinal tract and malignancies may occur in other sites including the brain and the thyroid. Helpful diagnostic features include pigmented retinal lesions known as congenital hypertrophy of the retinal pigment, jaw cysts, sebaceous cysts, and osteomata.

1.3.6. Sturge-Weber Syndrome

Sturge-Weber Syndrome (SWS) is an inherited neurocutaneous syndrome characterized by sporadic occurrence; distribution of lesions in an asymmetrical pattern; variable extent of involvement; lack of diffuse involvement of entire body and or an organ; almost equal sex ratio; facial and leptomeningeal angiomas; and, frequently, facial and optical port-wine lesions. The true prevalence of this disease is unknown. One in 200 individuals are born with a Port Wine Stain (PWS) in the United States. The incidence of SWS is thought to be 8–15% in live births with an associated PWS. The sporadic occurrence of SWS and distribution of lesions in a scattered or asymmetrical pattern suggests the occurrence of a somatic mutation in an otherwise essential gene, leading to mosaicism for the mutation. Computer-assisted tomography and MRI of SWS cases show cerebral lobar atrophy, brain calcification, choroid plexus enlargement, and venous abnormalities *(82)*.

1.3.7. Von Hippel-Lindau Disease

Von Hippel-Lindau disease (VHL), an autosomal dominant multi-system disorder, involves cerebellar hemangioblastoma of the CNS and visceral organs, retinal angiomatosis, pancreatic cysts, and benign and malignant renal lesions *(69)*. VHL genetic research indicates that it is underdiagnosed, i.e., more common than previously thought and possibly one of the most common of the familial cancers. Age at onset of diagnosis varies from early childhood up through the eighth decade of life. Affected individuals will have one or more manifestations including hemangioblastomas of brain (especially cerebellum) and spinal cord; endolymphatic sac tumors, retinal angiomas, renal cell carcinomas and cystic masses, pheochromocytomas, epididymal cystadenomas, pancreatic islet cell tumors, cystadenomas and cysts; and an adenocarcinoma of the pancreas has been reported. Angioma pressure in the brain or spinal cord may press on nerve or brain tissue and cause symptoms such as headaches and may weaken the walls of blood vessels causing damage to surrounding tissues. Blood leakage from angiomas in the retina can interfere with vision. Cysts and tumors, benign or cancerous, may also grow around angiomas, occurring beyond the CNS in the kidney, pancreas, liver, or adrenal glands. Several studies link VHL disease to the short arm of chromosome 3. This arm has two commonly deleted sites 3p13-14.3 and 3p25-26 *(29,102,125)*. Genetic heterogeneity has not been observed in VHL and a single gene for this syndrome was identified in 1993 using positional cloning strategies *(67)*. Loss of the wild-type allele in VHL component tumors has been reported, and is consistent with a tumor suppressor gene function *(26)*. A wide spectrum of germline mutations have been identified in VHL patients including missense and nonsense point mutations, microdeletions, micro-insertions, splice site, complex rearrangements (including inversions), whole gene and gross deletion *(109)*. Mutations are scattered along the entire gene and "hotspots" have been reported, most because of *de novo* events in unrelated families at hypermutable sequences such as CpG dinucleotides *(96)*. Founder mutations have also been reported *(15)*. Given the heterogeneity of mutation type, it has recently been reported that by using a combination of molecular techniques mutations can be identified in nearly 100% of VHL families *(109)*.

1.4. Familial Associations of Brain Tumors

In addition to the association of hereditary syndromes with CNS tumors, investigation of brain cancer etiology focuses on families of CNS tumor patients aggregating CNS and other cancers *(35,71–74,112)*. Tumors of patients and their relatives in these "cancer families" are histologically and biologically similar and well documented, though the precise relationship between genetics and CNS neoplasms remains unknown *(111)*. Methodologic constraints unfortunately limit the authority of many of these studies. They are also obscured by the confounding factor of common familial exposure to environmental agents potentially contributing to neoplasia induction, but they consistently report the presence of similar brain or other tumors in siblings *(31,35,87)*, and the cancer family syndrome *(71–74,76–77)*. With regard to etiology, two possible explanations of family occurrence emerge: (1) a genetic factor may in itself cause family clustering of CNS tumors, or (2) a hereditary vulnerability to exposures may produce the clusters.

1.4.1. CNS Tumors Among Twins

A challenge to studies of heritability of brain tumors is the lack of concordance CNS tumors in twins. Neither increased risk nor histological congruence has been proven in twin studies *(46,63,87)*. Norris and Jackson *(90)* found 54 solid tumors and 21 brain cancers in a review of 145,708 twins and singletons born between 1940 and 1964, but no evidence of concordance of CNS neoplasms in these twins. Results from a study of 556 twins with cancer suggest that there is not in general a strong constitutional genetic component for childhood cancers other than retinoblastoma *(16)*. In another study, data on 44,788 pairs of twins listed in the Swedish, Danish, and Finnish twin registries were analyzed in order to assess the risks of cancer at 28 anatomical sites for the twins of persons with cancer. Results indicate that inherited genetic factors make a minor contribution to susceptibility to most types of neoplasms and that the environment has the principal role in causing sporadic cancer *(91)*.

1.4.2. CNS Tumors Among Siblings

Seeking epidemiological information, investigators have long collected information on siblings of cancer patients, and from the first, this information has indicated sibling's higher risk of cancer from genes. Early surveys finding sibling concordance for brain tumors or siblings with different types of cancer were challenged because of small numbers *(73,87)* although larger studies have supported a genetic hypothesis. Farwell and Flannery *(35)* traced the cancer histories of relatives of 643 patients in the Connecticut Tumor Registry matching them with sex, age, and birthplace, and discovered a significantly higher risk of brain cancer in case siblings. Another large study *(31)* reviewed over 20,000 cases from the Marie Curie/Oxford Survey of Childhood Cancers in England, Scotland, and Wales, and identified 11 sibling pairs with brain tumors and 21 sibling pairs with dissimilar cancers.

1.4.3. CNS Tumors and Cancer Family Syndrome

In addition to studies of twins and siblings, the results of other studies of family pedigrees of brain and other tumor patients have been consistent with a dominantly inherited disorder *(73)*. Li et al. *(75)* described this cancer family syndrome in 24 kindred that had both childhood and adult onset cancers of diverse sites. Fourteen (9%) of the 151 cancers that occurred before age 45 yr were brain tumors. The Li-Fraumeni Syndrome has since been linked to a *p53* mutation on chromosome 17p in some families *(79)*.

Additional evidence for a brain tumor family syndrome comes from many epidemiologic comparisons of family medical histories of brain tumor cases with those of controls. These reports show a relative risk of 1–1.8 for any cancer in families of brain tumor cases and a relative risk of brain tumors in these families of 1–9 *(13,17,23,31,46,64,87,94,100,124)*. Two case-control studies further suggest that risks for other types of cancer may be elevated in family members of brain cancer patients. One study found elevated risk of leukemia and liver cancers and another observed elevated breast and respiratory tract cancer *(17,124)*. Relatives of children with brain tumors have also been reported to be at increased risk for colon cancer, whereas families with colon polyposis experience elevated frequencies of gliomas *(13,24,77,117)*. Also of interest are reports of familial clustering of brain tumors with Hodgkin's disease *(5)*.

1.4.3.1. FAMILIAL AGGREGATION

A multigenerational history of disease in a family could suggest, aside from genetics, the possibility of common environmental exposures. This possibility is further indicated by the variable findings of familial aggregation where studies report ranges of brain tumors in relatives of cases from nearly one to ten *(11,48,80,123)*. Although sibling and twin studies cast doubt on the hypothesis of a simple genetic etiology, that aggregation was not only because of chance and was the result of a set of factors, as shown in a family study of 250 children with brain tumors *(11)*. Segregation analysis found aggregation as a result of multifactorial inheritance. A polygenic model best explained occurrence patterns of brain tumors in another study employing segregation analyses of more than 600 adult glioma patients' families *(28)*. Segregation analyses of 2141 first degree relatives of 297 glioma families did not reject a multifactorial model, but an autosomal recessive model provided the best fit *(81)*. The study estimated that 5% of all glioma cases were familial. Grosman et al. *(44)* showed brain tumors can occur in families without a known predisposing hereditary disease and that the pattern of occurrence in many families suggest environmental causes.

Discovery that some families with the hereditary Li-Fraumeni cancer family syndrome inherited mutated *p53* led to studies revealing the importance of *p53* in many human cancers including brain tumors *(89)*. Li et al. *(74)* reported in a population-based study of adults who had developed glioma, that more cases with *p53* mutant tumors than controls had first-degree relatives with cancer (58% vs 42%), and more cases had a previous cancer (17% vs 8%). Germ-line *p53* mutations occur more often in patients with multifocal glioma, glioma, and another primary malignancy, or in those with a family history of cancer than in patients with other brain tumors *(65)*. Currently, research in this area is focused on determining the frequency of *p53* mutations in tumors and on correlation between specific *p53* mutations and specific exposures. Alterations in other important cell-cycle regulators in tumors, such as *p16*, Rb, and MDM2 are also being evaluated. One study designed to identify germ-line mutations in genes mutated, deleted, or amplified in sporadic gliomas showed no evidence of germ-line mutations of *CDK4, p16,* and *p15 (39)*.

1.4.3.2. Metabolic Susceptibility: Polymorphisms (Common Variations)
in Genes Relevant to Cancer Causation or Prevention

Because evidence suggests that inherited rare mutations are a factor in only a small proportion of primary brain tumors, investigators are turning their attention to common polymorphisms in genes that, in concert with environmental exposures, might influence susceptibility to brain tumors or make the tumors more aggressive. Alterations conferring susceptibility to brain and other tumors could occur in genes that affect oxidative metabolism, detoxification of carcinogens, DNA stability and repair, or immune response. Genetic polymorphisms' influence on susceptibility to carcinogenic exposures has been studied primarily in relation to tobacco smoking, but recent advances in genetic technology permit the epidemiologic evaluation of polymorphisms potentially relevant to other cancers.

Elexpuru-Camiruaga et al. *(33)* first showed that cytochrome p450 2D6 (*CYP2D6*) and glutathione transferase theta (*GSTT1*) were significantly associated with an increased risk of brain tumor. Kelsey et al. (60 found that *GSTT1* null genotype was associated only with an increased risk of oligodendroglioma. Trizna et al. *(114)* found no statistically significant associations between the null genotypes of *GSTM1*, *GSTT1*, and *CYP1A1* and risk of gliomas in adults, but observed a nearly two-fold increased risk for rapid *N*-acetyltransferase acetylation and a 30% increased risk for intermediate acetylation. However, that finding was not confirmed in another case-control study of adults with glioma *(93)*. Chen et al. *(22)* showed that patients with oligoastrocytoma were 4.6 times (95% CI 1.6–13.2) as likely as controls to have AA or AC vs CC genotype in nucleotide 8092 of *ERCC1 (22)*. However, the odds ratio of those genotypes was about the same in patients with glioblastoma and controls. Although this variant is a silent polymorphism (i.e., does not lead to an amino acid change), it might affect *ERCC1* messenger ribonucleic acid (mRNA) stability, and the same polymorphism leads to an amino acid substitution of lysine to glutamine in a nucleolar protein and T-cell receptor complex subunit. Using the same populations as those reported by *(20,22)* Caggana et al. found the AA genotype (C to A polymorphism [R156R]) of *ERCC2* to be statistically significantly more common than the CC or CA genotypes in patients with glioblastoma, astrocytoma, or oligoastrocytoma than in controls. This variant is also a silent polymorphism, suggesting that another gene linked to it may account for the associations observed. Moreover, as genotyping data from blood tests were not available for those patients with the poorest survival in this population-based study of gliomas, it is not certain whether these polymorphisms were related to survival or to etiology. Further work is clearly warranted to confirm or refute these provocative findings. Larger studies may be needed as chance can play a role in falsely identifying or failing to identify associations especially when sample sizes are small.

1.4.4. Mutagen Sensitivity

Cytogenetic assays of peripheral blood lymphocytes have been extensively used to determine response to genotoxic agents. The basis for these cytogenetic assays is that genetic damage reflects critical events in carcinogenesis in the affected tissue. To test this hypothesis Hsu et al. *(54)* developed a mutagen sensitivity assay in which the frequency of in vitro bleomycin-induced breaks in short-term lymphocyte cultures is used to measure genetic susceptibility. We have modified the assay by using γ-radiation to induce chromosome breaks because radiation is a risk factor for brain tumors and can produce double-stranded DNA breaks and mutations *(12)*. It is believed that mutagen sensitivity indirectly assesses the effectiveness of one or more DNA repair mechanisms. The following observations support this hypothesis. First, the relationship between chromosome instability syndromes and cancer susceptibility is well-established *(19)*. Patients with these syndromes also have defective DNA repair systems *(119)*. Furthermore, patients with ataxia telangiectasia, who are extremely sensitive to the clastogenic effects of X-irradiation and bleomycin, differ from normal people in the speed with which aberrations induced by these agents are repaired but not in the number of aberrations produced *(50)*.

γ-Radiation induced mutagen sensitivity is one of the few significant independent risk factors for brain tumors *(12)*. DNA repair capability and predisposition to cancer are hallmarks of rare chromosome instability syndromes, and are related to differences in radiosensitivity. An in vitro study showed that individuals vary in lymphocyte radiosensitivity, which correlates with DNA repair capacity *(12)*. Therefore, it is biologically plausible that increased sensitivity to γ-radiation results in increased risk of developing brain tumors because of an individual's inability to repair radiation damage. Bondy et al. *(12,14)* have shown that lymphocyte mutagen sensitivity to γ-radiation is significantly associated with a risk of glioma. The mutagen sensitivity assay has also been shown to be a risk factor for other cancers such as head and neck and lung cancers suggesting that sensitivity to the mutagen is constitutional *(50)*, especially that the breaks are not affected by smoking status or dietary factors (micronutrients) *(108)*.

1.4.5. Chromosome Instability

A number of chromosomal loci have been reported to play a role in brain tumorigenesis because of the numerous gains and losses in those loci. For example, Bigner et al. *(7)* reported gain of chromosome 7 and loss of chromosome 10 in malignant gliomas and structural abnormalities involving chromosomes 1, 6p, 9p, and 19q; Bello et al. *(4)* reported involvement of chromosome 1 in oligodendrogliomas and meningiomas; and Magnani et al. *(78)* demonstrated involvement of chromosomes 1, 7, 10, and 19 in anaplastic gliomas and glioblastomas. Loss of heterozygosity for loci on chromosome 17p *(37)* and 11p15 *(105)* have also been reported.

There is little data on chromosomal alterations in the peripheral blood lymphocytes of brain tumor patients. Information on such changes might shed light on premalignant changes that lead to tumor development. We demonstrated that compared with controls, glioma cases have less efficient DNA repair, measured by increased chromosome sensitivity to gamma radiation in stimulated peripheral blood lymphocytes *(12)*. This inefficiency was shown to be an independent risk factor for glioma *(12)*. Recently, we investigated whether glioma patients have increased chromosomal instability that could account for their increased susceptibility to cancer *(32)*. Using fluorescent *in situ* hybridization methods, background instability in these patients was measured at hyperbreakable regions in the genome. Reports indicate that the human heterochromatin regions are frequently involved in stable chromosome rearrangements *(30,66)*. Smith and Grosovsky *(107)* and Grosovsky et al. *(43)* reported that breakage affecting the centromeric and pericentromeric heterochromatin regions of human chromosomes can lead to mutations and chromosomal rearrangements and increase genomic instability. Our study demonstrated that individuals with a significantly higher level of background chromosomal instability have a 15-fold increased risk of development of gliomas *(32)*. A significantly higher level of hyperdiploidy was also detected. Chromosome instability leading to aneuploidy has been observed in many cancer types *(68)*. Although previous studies have demonstrated the presence of chromosomal instability in brain tumor tissues *(86,98,121)*, our study was the first to investigate the role of background chromosomal instability in the peripheral blood lymphocytes of patients with gliomas *(32)*. This suggests that accumulated chromosomal damage in peripheral blood lymphocytes may be an important biomarker for identifying individuals at risk of developing gliomas.

2. DIRECTIONS FOR FUTURE STUDIES

Primary malignant brain tumors clearly represent a heterogeneous group of diseases. Therefore, a workable consensus on classification and increased use of molecular tumor markers in concert with improved surveillance and registration are necessary to characterize homogeneous subgroups of the many heterogeneous categories of primary brain tumors. For example, the recently elucidated distinction between de novo and "progressive" glioblastomas has significant implications for epidemiologic research *(61)*. This concept and others reinforce the notion that glioblastoma multiforme is not one but probably many diseases that must be distinguished if progress is to be made in determining etiology.

Molecular characterization of tumors may help to disentangle causes of subtypes of glioma by enabling researchers to group tumors with similar molecular lesions. Use of rapidly developing technology to examine arrays of either gene or protein expression may help enormously to categorize tumors into more homogeneous groups with regard to lesions of etiologic or prognostic importance. A major challenge to interpreting this information will be deciphering which alterations represent early changes of potential etiologic significance, and which represent later changes that may have serious prognostic consequences. Genetic and molecular epidemiologic methods to collect and define pertinent subject data from well-defined source populationsand to follow-up subjects for recurrence and survival, might help to make sense of the complex information about tumor molecular alterations.

The descriptive epidemiology of brain tumors suggests that a major task is to formulate and evaluate explanations for the consistently observed gender and ethnic differences for glioma and meningioma. Among the most provocative clue to the etiology of primary brain tumors in adults is the characteristic gender difference, with glioma being more prevalent among men and meningioma among women. The glaring absence of analytic epidemiologic research into risk factors for meningioma provides little information to hypothesize reasons for the female preponderance other than the probable importance of hormonal factors (10). Furthermore, very few studies of glioma have shed any light on gender and ethnic differences in occurrence of these tumors, despite the extensive research of gliomas (22,85).

Further analytic studies of environmental factors (viruses, radiation, and carcinogenic or protective chemical exposures through diet, workplace, or other sources), when combined with incorporation of potentially relevant polymorphisms that might influence susceptibility, may help us understand this devastating collection of diseases. Multicenter studies or sharing of data between ongoing studies might be needed to obtain sufficient numbers of cases to compare subgroups of subjects with specific molecularly defined tumor types. Studies of potentially relevant polymorphisms, viral factors, other infectious agents, and immunologic factors are promising understudied areas for further etiologic research. Moreover, as currently established or suggested risk factors probably account for a small proportion of cases, novel concepts of neurocarcinogenesis may be required before we are able to discover a more comprehensive picture of the natural history and pathogenesis of brain tumors. With the rapid pace of discovery of meaningful tumor markers and susceptibility genes, this is an ideal time for neurosurgeons, oncologists, pathologists, and epidemiologists to forge new collaborations within and between their institutions and professional organizations to design and conduct meaningful epidemiologic research into the causes of primary brain tumors.

To conclude, primary brain tumors probably stem from multiple exogenous and endogenous events. To date, the few proven causes (i.e., inherited genetic syndromes, therapeutic ionizing radiation giving rise to brain lymphomas) account for only a small proportion of cases. Brain malignancies are devastating diseases, but there is hope that a continuing explication of their cause and biologic course and new concepts about neuro-oncogenesis might emerge to advance the study of brain tumor epidemiology and the possibilities for prevention and cure.

REFERENCES

1. Airewele G.E., Sigurdson A.J., Wiley K.J., Frieden B.E., Caldarera L.W., Riccardi V.M., et al. 2001. Neoplasms in neurofibromatosis 1 are related to gender but not to family history of cancer. *Genet. Epidemiol.* **20**:75–86.
2. Altermatt H.J., Shepherd C.W., Scheitauer B.W., and Gomez M.R. 1991. Subependymal giant cell astrocytoma. *Zentralbl. Pathol.* **137**:105–116.
3. American Cancer Society 2002. *Cancer Facts and Figures.* American Cancer Society, Inc.
4. Bello M.J., De Campos J.M., Kusak M.E., Sarasa J.L., Saez-Castresana J., Pestana A., et al. 1994. Molecular analysis of chromosome 1 abnormalities in human gliomas reveals frequent loss of 1p in oligodendroglial tumors. *Int. J. Cancer* **57**:172–175.
5. Bernard S.M., Cartwright R.A., Darwin C.M. et al. 1987. Hodgkin's disease: case control epidemiological study in Yorkshire. *Br. J. Cancer* **55**:85–90.
6. Biernat W., Tohma Y., Yonekawa Y., Kleihues P., Ohgaki H. 1997. Alterations of cell cycle regulatory genes in primary (de novo) and secondary glioblastomas. *Acta. Neuropathol.* **94**:303–309.

7. Bigner S.H., Mark J., Burger P.C., Mahaley M.S., Bullard D.E., Muhlbaier L.H., et al. 1988. Specific chromosomal abnormalities in malignant gliomas. *Cancer Res.* **88**:405–411.
8. Blatt J., Jaffee R., Deutsch M., et al. 1986. Neurofibromatosis and childhood tumors. *Cancer* **57**:1225–1229.
9. Bodmer W.F., Bailey C.J., Ellis A., et al. 1987. Localization of the gene for familial adenomatous polyposis on chromosome 5. *Nature* **328**:614–616.
10. Bondy M., Ligon B.L. 1996. Epidemiology and etiology of intracranial meningiomas: a review. *J. Neurooncol.* **29:** 197–205.
11. Bondy M., Wiencke J., Wrensch, M., Kyritsis, A.P. 1994. Genetics of primary brain tumors: a review. *J. Neurooncol.* **18**:69–81.
12. Bondy M.L, Kryitsis A.P., Gu J., de Andrade M., Cunningham J., Levin V.A., et al. 1996. Mutagen sensitivity and risk of gliomas: a case-control study. *Cancer Res.* **56**:1484–1486.
13. Bondy M.L., Lustbader E.D., Buffler P.A. et al. 1991. Genetic epidemiology of childhood brain tumors. *Genet. Epidemiol.* **8**:253–267.
14. Bondy M.L., Wang, L.E., El-Zein R., de Andrade, M., Selvan, M.S., Bruner, J.M., et al. 2001. Gamma-radiation sensitivity and risk of glioma. *J. Natl. Cancer Inst.* **93**:1553–1557.
15. Brauch H., Kishida T., Glavac D., Chen F., Pausch F., Hofler H., et al. 1995. Von Hippel-Lindau (VHL) disease with pheochromocytoma in the Black Forest region of Germany: evidence for a founder effect. *Hum. Genet.* **95**:551–556.
16. Buckley J.D., Buckley C.M., Breslow N.E., Draper G.J., Roberson P.K., Mack T.M. 1996. Concordance for childhood cancer in twins. *Med. Pediatr.Oncol.* **26**:223–229.
17. Burch, J.D., Craib, K.J., Choi, B.C., Miller, A.B., Risch, H.A., Howe, G.R. 1987. An exploratory case-control study of brain tumors in adults. *J. Natl. Cancer. Inst.* **78**:601–609.
18. Burk R.R. 1991. Von Hippel-Lindau disease angiomatosis of the retina and cerebellum. *J. Am. Optometry Assoc.* **62:** 382–385.
19. Busch D. 1994. Genetic susceptibility to radiation and chemotherapy injury: diagnosis and management. *Int. J. Rad. Oncol. Biol. Phys.* **30**:997–1002.
20. Caggana M., Kilgallen J., Conroy J.M., Wiencke J.K., Kelysey K.T., Mike, R., Chen P., et al. 2001. Associations Between ERCC2 Polymorphisms and Gliomas. *Cancer Epidemiology, Biomarkers and Prevention* **10**:355–360.
21. Cheadle J.P., Reeve M.P., Sampson J.R., Kwiatkowski D.J., Cheadle J.P., Reeve M.P., Sampson J.R., et al. 2000. *Hum. Genet.* **107**:97–114.
22. Chen P., Wiencke J., Aldape K., Kesler-Diaz A., Miike, R., Kelsey K., et al. 2000. Association of an ERCC1 polymorphism with adult-onset glioma. *Cancer Epidemiol. Biomarkers Prev.* **9**:843–847.
23. Choi N.W., Schuman L.M., Gullen W.H. 1970. Epidemiology of primary central nervous system neoplasms. II. Case-control study. *Am. J. Epidemiol.* **91**:467–485.
24. Chowdhary U.P., Boehme D.H., Al-Jishi M. 1985. Turcot syndrome glioma polyposis. *J. Neurosurg.* **63**:804–807.
25. Costa O.L., Silva D.M., Colnago F.A., et al. 1987. Turcot Syndrome autosomal dominant or recessive transmission? *Dis. Colon Rectum* **30**:391–394.
26. Crossey P.A., Foster K., Richards F.M., Phipps M.E., Latif F., Tory K., et al. 1994. Molecular genetic investigations of the mechanism of tumourigenesis in von Hippel-Lindau disease: analysis of allele loss in VHL tumours. *Hum. Genet.* **93**:53–58.
27. Crowe F.W., Schull W.J., Neel J.V. 1956. *A Clinical, Pathological, and Genetic Study of Multiple Neurofibromatosis.* Charles C. Thomas, Springfield, IL.
28. de Andrade, M., Barnholtz, J.S., Amos, C.I., Adatto, P., Spencer, C., Bondy, M.L. 2001. Segregation analysis of cancer in families of glioma patients. *Genet. Epidemiol.* **20**:258–270.
29. Dietrich P.Y., Droz J.P., 1992. Renal cell cancer: Oncogenes and tumor suppressor genes. *Rev. Pract.* **42**:1236–1240.
30. Doneda L., Ginelli E., Agresti A., Larizza L. 1989. In situ hybridization analysis of interstitial C-heterochromatin in marker chromosomes of two human melanomas. *Cancer Res.* **49**:433–438.
31. Draper G.J., Heaf M.M., Kinnier Wilson LM. 1977. Occurrence of childhood cancers among sibs and estimation of familial risks. *J. Med. Genet.* **14**:81–90.
32. El-Zein R., Bondy M.L., Wang L.E., de Andrade M., Sigurdson A.J., Bruner J.M., et al. 1999. Increased chromosomal instability in peripheral lymphocytes and risk of human gliomas. *Carcinogenesis.* **20**:811–815.
33. Elexpuru-Camiruaga, J., Buxton, N., Kandula, V., Dias P.S., Campbell, D., McIntosh, J., et al. 1995. Susceptibility to astrocytoma and meningioma: influence of allelism at glutathione-S-transferase (GSTT1 and GSTM1) and cytochrome P-450 (CYP2D6) loci. *Cancer Res.* **55**:4237–4239.
34. Farndon P.A., Del Mastro R.G., Evans D.G., Kilpatick M.W. 1992. Location of gene for Gorlin syndrome. *Lancet* **339**:581,582.
35. Farwell J. and Flannery J.T. 1984. Cancer in relatives of children with central nervous system neoplasms. *N. Engl. J. Med.* **311**:749–753.
36. Farwell, J.R., Dohrmann, G.J., Flannery, J.T. 1984. Medulloblastoma in childhood: an epidemiological study. *J. Neurosurg.* **61**:657–664.

37. Fults D., Tippets R.H., Thomas G.A., Nakamura Y., White R. 1989. Loss of heterozygosity for loci on chromosome 17p in human malignant astrocytoma. *Cancer Res.* **49:**6572–6577.

38. Gailani M.R., Bale S.J., Leffell D.J., et al. 1992. Developmental defects in Gorlin syndrome related to a putative tumor suppressor gene on chromsome 9. *Cell* **69:**111–117.

39. Gao, L., Liu, L., van Meyel, D., Cairncross, G., Forsyth, P., Kimmel, D., Jenkins, R.B., Lassam, N.J., Hogg, D. 1997. Lack of germ-line mutations of CDK4, p16(INK4A), and p15(INK4B) in families with glioma. *Clin. Cancer Res.* **3:**977–981.

40. Gold E.B. Epidemiology of brain tumors. 1980. *Reviews in Cancer Epidemiology* **1:**245–254.

41. Gomez MR. *Tuberous Sclerosis.* Raven Press, New York, 1988.

42. Gorlin RJ. 1987. Nevoid basal cell carcinoma syndrome. *Medicine* **66:**98–113.

43. Grosovsky A.J., Parks K.K., Giver C.R., Nelson S.L. 1996. Clonal analysis of delayed karyotypic abnormalities and gene mutations in radiation-induced genetic instability. *Mol. Cell Biol.* **16:**6252–6262.

44. Grossman S.A., Osman M., Hruban R., and Piantadosi S. 1999. Central nervous system cancers in first-degree relatives and spouse. *Cancer Investigation* **17:**299–308.

45. Haines J.L., Short M.P., Kwiatkowski D.J., et al. 1991. Localization of one gene for tuberous sclerosis within 9q32-9q34, and further evidence for heterogeneity. *Am. J. Hum. Genet.* **49:**764–772.

46. Harvald B., Hauge M. 1956. On the heredity of glioblastoma. *J˜20Natl Cancer Inst.* **17:**289–296.

47. Hass-Kogan D.A., Kogan S.S., Yount G., Hsu J., Haas M., Deen D.F., Israel M.A. 1999. P53 function influences the effect of fractionated raditherapy on glioblastoma tumors. *Int. J. Radiat. Oncol. Biol. Phys.* **43:**399–403.

48. Hemminki K., Li, Vaittinen X., Dong P., 2000. Cancers in the first degree relatives of children with brain tumors. *Br. J. Cancer* **83:**407–411.

49. Hill J.R., Kuriyama N., Kuriyama H., Israel M.A. 1999. Molecular genetics of brain tumors. *Arch. Neurol.* **56:**439-441.

50. Hittelman W.N., Sen P. Heterogeneity in chromosome damage and repair rates after bleomycin in ataxia telangiectasia cells. *Cancer Res.* **48:**276–279.

51. Hoang-Xuan K, Aguirre-Cruz L, Mokhtari K, Marie Y, Sanson M. 2002. OLIG-1 and 2 gene expression and oligodendroglial tumours. *Neuropathol. Appl. Neurobiol.* **28:**89–94.

52. Hoang-Xuan K., He J., Huguet S., Mokhtari K., Marie Y., Kujas M., et al. 2001. Molecular heterogeneity of oligodendrogliomas suggests alternative pathways in tumor progression. *Neurology* **57:**1278–1281.

53. Hope D.G., Mulvihill J.J. 1981. Malignancy in neurofibromatosis, in *Advances in Neurology Vol 29: Neurofibromatosis von Reckinghausen Disease* (Riccardi V.M., Mulvihill J.J., eds.). Raven Press, New York.

54. Hsu T.C., Johnston D.A., Cherry L.M., Ramkisson D., Schantz S.P., Jessup J.M., et al. 1989. Sensitivity to genotoxic effect of bleomycin in humans: possible relationship to environmental carcinogenesis. *Int. J. Cancer* **43:**403–409.

55. Hunter S.B., Abbot K., Varma V.A., Olson J.J., Barnett D.W., James C.D. 1995. Reliability of differential PCR for the detection of EGFR and MDM2 gene amplification in DNA extracted from FFPE glioma tissues. *J. Neuropathol. Exp. Neurol.* **54:**57–64.

56. Ichimura K., Schmidt E.E., Miyakawa A., Goike H.M., Collins V.P. 1998. Distinct patterns of deletion on 10p and 10q suggest involvement of multiple tumor suppressor genes in the development of astrocytic gliomas of different malignancy grades. *Genes Chromosomes Cancer* **22:**9–15.

57. Jadayel D., Fain P., Upadhyaya M., et al. 1990. Paternal origin of new mutations in von Recklinghausen neurofibromatosis. *Nature* **343:**558.

58. Jones A.C., Shyamsundar M.M., Thomas M.W., Maynard J., Idziaszczyk S., Tomkins S., et al. 1999. Comprehensive mutation analysis of TSC1 and TSC2-and phenotypic correlations in 150 families with tuberous sclerosis. *Am. J. Hum. Genet.* **64:**1305–1315.

59. Kapp J.P., Paulson G.W., Odom G.L. 1967. Brain tumors with tuberous sclerosis. *J. Neurosurg.* **26:**191.

60. Kelsey K.T., Wrensch M., Zuo Z.F., Miike R., Wiencke J.K. 1997. A population-based case-control study of the CYP2D6 and GSTT1 polymorphisms and malignant brain tumors. *Pharmacogenetics* **7:**463–468.

61. Kleihues P., Ohgaki H. 2000. Phenotype vs genotype in the evolution of astrocytic brain tumors. *Toxicologic Pathology* **28:**164–170.

62. Kleihues P., Soylememzoglu F., Schauble B., et al. 1995. Histopathology, classification and grading of gliomas. *Glio.* **15:**211–221

63. Koch G. 1972. Genetic aspects of phacomatoses, in *Handbook of Clinical Neurology,* Vol. 14 (Vinken P.G., Bruyn G.W., eds.). North Holland, Amsterdam.

64. Kuijten R.R., Bunin G.R., Nass C.C., et al. 1990. Gestational and familial risk factors for childhood astrocytoma: results of a case-control study. *Cancer Res.* **50:**2608–2612.

65. Kyritsis A.P., Bondy M.L., Xiao M., Berman E.L. Cunningham J.E., Lee P.S., et al. 1994. Germline p53 gene mutations in subsets of glioma patients [see comments]. *J. Natl. Cancer Inst.* **86:**344–349.

66. Larizza L., Doneda L., Ginelli E., Fossati G. 1988. C-heterochromatin vartiation and transposition in tumor progression, in *Cancer Metastasis: Biological and Biochemical Mechanisms and Clinical Aspects* (Gprodi et al. eds.), Plenum Publishing Corp., NY, pp. 309–318.

67. Latif F., Tory K., Gnarra J., Yao M., Duh F.M., Orcutt M.L., et al. 1993. Identification of the von Hippel-Lindau disease tumor suppressor gene. *Science* **260:**1317–1320.

68. Lengauer,C., Kinzler,K.W., Vogelstein,B. 1997. Genetic instability in colorectal cancers. *Nature* **386:**623–627.

69. Levine C., Skimming J., Levine E. 1992. Familial pheochromocytomas with unusual associations. *J. Pediatr. Surg.* **27:**447–451.

70. Lewis J.H., Ginsberg A.L., Toomey K.E. 1983. Turcot's syndrome: evidence for autosomal dominant inheritance. *Cancer* **51:**524–528.

71. Li F.P., Fraumeni J.F. Jr. 1982. Prospective study of a family syndrome. *J. Am. Med. Assoc.* **247:**2692–2694.

72. Li F.P., and Fraumeni J.F., Jr. 1975. Soft tissue, breast cancer and other neoplasms. *Ann. Int. Med.* **83:**833,834.

73. Li F.P., Fraumeni J.F. Jr. 1969. tissue sarcoma, breast cancer, and other neoplasms. A family syndrome? *Ann. Int. Med.* **71:**747–752.

74. Li F.P., Fraumeni J.F. Jr, Mulvihill J.J., et al. 1988. A cancer family syndrome in twenty-four kindreds. *Cancer Res.* **48:**5358–5362.

75. Li Y, Millikan, R.C., Carozza, S., Newman, B., Liu, E., Davis, R., Miike, R., Wrensch, M. 1998. p53 mutations in malignant gliomas. *Cancer Epidemiol., Biomarkers and Prevention* **7:**303–308.

76. Lynch H.T., Guirgis H.A., Lynch P.M. et al. 1977. Familial cancer syndromes. A survey. *Cancer* **39:**1867–1881.

77. Lynch H.T., Lynch J.F. 1985. Genetics and colorectal cancer, in *Familial Cancer* (Muller H., Weber W., eds.), Karger, Basel, Switzerland, p. 72.

78. Magnani I., Guerneri S., Pollo B., Cirenei N., Colombo B.M., Broggie G., et al. 1994. Increasing complexity of the karyotype in 50 human gliomas: Progressive evolution and de novo occurrence of cytogenetic alterations. *Cancer Genet. Cytogenet.* **75:**77–89.

79. Malkin D., Li F.P., Strong L.C., et al. 1990. Germ line p53 mutations in a familial syndrome of breast cancer, sarcoma, and other neoplasms. *Science* **250:**1233–1238.

80. Malmer B., Gronberg, H., Bergenheim, A.T., Lenner, P., Henriksson, R. 1999. Familial aggregation of astrocytoma in northern Sweden: an epidemiological cohort study. *Int. J. Cancer* **81:**366–370.

81. Malmer B., Iselius, L., Holmberg, E., Collins, A., Henriksson, R., Gronberg, H. 2001. Genetic epidemiology of glioma. *Br. J. Cancer* **84:**429–-434.

82. Marti-Bonmati L., Menor F., Poyatos C., Cortina H. 1992. Diagnosis of Sturge Weber syndrome: comparison of the efficacy of CT and MR imaging in 14 cases. *J. Roentgenol.* **158:**867.

83. Martuza R.L., Eldridge R. 1988. Neurofibromatosis 2: bilateral acoustic neurofibromatosis. *N. Engl. J. Med.* **318:** 684.

84. McCarthy B.J., Surawicz T., Bruner J.M., Kruchko C., Davis F. 2002. Consensus Conference on Brain Tumor Definition for registration. November 10, 2000. *Neurooncol* **2:**134–145.

85. McKinley B.P., Michalek A.M., Fenstermaker R.A., Plunkett R.J. 2000. The impact of age and sex on the incidence of glial tumors in New York state from 1976 to 1995. *J. Neurosurg.* **93:**932–939.

86. Mohapatra, G., Kim D.H., Feuerstein B.G. 1995. Detection of multiple gains and losses of genetic material in ten glioma cell lines by comparative genomic hybridization. *Genes Chromosomes Cancer* **13:**86–93.

87. Miller R.W. 1971. Deaths from childhood leukemia and solid tumors among twins and other sibs in the United States, 1960-67. *J. Natl. Cancer Inst.* **46:**203–209.

88. Mulcahy G.M., Harlan W.L. 1976. Occurrences of central nervous system tumors, with special reference to relative genetic factors, in *Cancer Genetics.* (Lynch H.T. ed.), Thomas Books, Springfield, IL.

89. Nichols K.E., Malkin D., Garber, J.E., Fraumeni, J.F., Jr., Li, F.P. 2001. Germ-line p53 mutations predispose to a wide spectrum of early-onset cancers. *Cancer Epidemiology, Biomarkers and Prevention,* **10:**83–87.

90. Norris F.D., Jackson E.W. 1970. Childhood cancer deaths in California born twins—a further report on types of cancer found. *Cancer* **25:**212–218.

91. O'Brien J.M. 2000. Environmental and heritable factors in the causation of cancer—analysis of cohorts of twins from Sweden, Denmark, and Finland. *N. Engl. J. Med.* **343:**78–85.

92. Parry L., Maynard J.H., Patel A., Hodges A.K., von Deimling A., Sampson J.R., et al. 2000. Molecular analysis of the TSC1 and TSC2 tumour suppressor genes in sporadic glial and glioneuronal tumours. *Hum. Genet.* **4:**350–356.

93. Peters E.S., Kelsey K.T., Wiencke J.K., Park S., Chen P., Miike R., Wrensch, M.R. 2001. NAT2 and NQO1 polymorphisms are not associated with adult glioma. *Cancer Epidemiology, Biomarkers and Prevention* **10:**151–152.

94. Preston-Martin S., Mack W., Henderson B.E. 1989. Risk factors for gliomas and meningiomas in males in Los Angeles County. *Cancer Res.* **49:**6137–6143.

95. Riccardi V.M. 1981. Von Recklinghausen neurofibromatosis. *N. Engl. J. Med.* **305:**1617–1627.

96. Richards F.M., Payne S.J., Zbar B., Affara N.A., Ferguson-Smith M.A., Maher ER. 1995. Molecular analysis of de novo germline mutations in the von Hippel-Lindau disease gene. *Hum. Mol. Genet.* **11:**2139–2143.

97. Ritland S.R., Ganju.V, Jenkins R.B. 1995. Region-specific loss of heterozygosity on chromosome 19 is related to the morphologic type of human glioma. *Genes Chromosomes Cancer* **12:**277–282.

98. Rosso S.M., Van Dekken H., Krishnadath K.K., Alers J.C., Kros J.M. 1997. Detection of chromosomal changes by interphase cytogenetics in biopsies of recurrent astrocytomas and oligodendrogliomas. *J. Neuropathol Exp. Neurol.* **56:**1125–1131.

99. Rubenstein A.E. Neurofibromatosis: a review of the clinical problem. 1986. *Ann. NY Acad. Sci.* **486:**1–13.

100. Ryan P., Lee M.W., North B., McMichael A.J. 1992. Risk factors for tumors of the brain and meninges: results from the Adelaide Adult Brain Tumor Study. *Intl. J. Cancer* **51**:20–27.

101. Scheil S., Bruderlein S., Liehr T., Starke H., Herms J., Schulte M., Moller P. 2001. Genome-wide analysis of sixteen chordomas by comparative genomic hybridization and cytogenetics of the first human chordoma cell line, U-CH1. *Genes Chromosomes Cancer* **3**:203–211.

102. Seizinger B.R., Smith D.I., Filling-Katz M.R., et al. 1991. Genetic flanking markers refine diagnostic criteria and provide insights into the genetics of von Hippel Lindau disease. *Proc. Natl. Acad. Sci. USA* **88**:2864–2868.

103. Shepherd C.W., Gomez M.R., Lie J.T., Crowson C.S. 1991. Causes of death in patients with tuberous sclerosis. *Mayo Clin. Proc.* **66**:792–796.

104. Shepherd C.W., Scheithauer B.W., Gomez M.R., et al. 1991. Subependymal giant cell astrocytoma: a clinical, pathological, and flow cytometric study. *Neurosurgery* **28**:864–868.

105. Sonoda Y., Iizuka M., Yasuda J., Makino R., Ono T., Kayama T., Yoshimoto T., Sekiya T. 1995. Loss of heterozygosity at 11p15 in malignant gliomas. *Cancer Res.* **55**:2166–2168.

106. Sorenson S.A., Mulvihill J.J., Nielson A., et al. 1986. Long-term follow-up of von Recklinghausen neurofibromatosis: survival and malignant neoplasms. *N Engl. J. Med.* **314**:1010–1015.

107. Smith L.E., Grosovsky A.J. 1993. Genetic instability on chromosome 16 in a B lymphoblastoid cell line. *Somat. Cell Mol. Genet.* **19**:515–527.

108. Spitz M.R., McPherson R.S., Jiang H., Hsu T.C., Trizna Z,. Lee J.J., et al. 1997. Correlates of mutagen sensitivity in patients with upper aerodigestive tract cancer. *Cancer Epidemiol. Biomarkers Prev.* **6**:687–692.

109. Stolle C., Glenn G., Zbar B., Humphrey J.S., Choyke P., Walther M., et al. 1998. Improved detection of germline mutations in the von Hippel-Lindau disease tumor suppressor gene. *Hum. Mutat.* **12**:417–423.

110. Surawicz T.S., McCarthy B.J., Kupelian V., Jukich P.J., Bruner J.M., Davis, F.G. 1999. Descriptive epidemiology of primary brain and CNS tumors: Results from the Central Brain Tumor Registry of the United States, 1990–1994. *Neurooncol.* **1**:14–25.

111. Tijssen C.C. 1985. Genetic aspects of brain tumors—tumors of neuroepithelial and meningeal tissue, in *Familial Cancer* (Muller H, Weber W eds.) Karger, Basel, Switzerland.

112. Tijssen C.C., Halprin M.R., Endtz L.J. 1982. *Familial Brain Tumours. A Commented Register.* Martinus Nijhoff, Boston, MA.

113. The European Chromosome 16 Tuberous Sclerosis Consortium. 1993. Identification and characterization of the tuberous sclerosis gene on chromosome 16. *Cell* **75**:1305–1315.

114. Trizna, Z., de Andrade, M., Kyritsis, A.P., Briggs, K., Levin, V.A., Bruner, J.M., et al. 1998. Genetic polymorphisms in glutathione S-transferase mu and theta, N-acetyltransferase, and CYP1A1 and risk of gliomas. *Cancer Epidemiol. Biomarkers Prev.* **7**:553–555.

115. Ueki K., Ono Y., Henson J.W., Efird J.T., von Deimling A., Louis D.N. 1996. CDKN2/p16 or RB alterations occur in the majority of glioblastomas and are inversly correlated. *Cancer Res.* **56**:150–153.

116. van Slegtenhorst M., de Hoogt R., Hermans C., Nellist M., Janssen B., Verhoef S., et al. 1997. Identification of the tuberous sclerosis gene TSC1 on chromosome 9q34. *Science* **277**:805–808.

117. Vieregge P., Gerhard L., and Nahser HC. 1987. Familial glioma: occurrence within the "familial cancer syndrome" and systemic malformations. *J. Neurol.* **234**:220–232.

118. von Deimling A., Krone W., and Menon A.G. 1995. Neurofibromatosis type 1: pathology, clinical features and molecular genetics. *Brain Pathol.* **5**:153–162.

119. Wei Q., Spitz M.R., Gu J., Cheng L., Xu X., Strom S.S., et al.1996. DNA repair capacity correlates with mutagen sensitivity in lymphoblastoid cell lines. *Cancer Epidemiol. Biomarkers Prev.* **5**:199–204.

120. Weinberg RA. 1991. Oncogenes, tumor suppressor genes, and cell transformation: trying to put it all together, in *Origins of Human Cancer.* (Brugge J., Curran T., Harlow E. et al. (eds.). Cold Spring Harbor Laboratory Press, Cold Spring Harbor, New York.

121. Wernicke C., Thiel G., Lozanova T., Vogel S., and Witkowski R. 1997. Numerical aberrations of chromosomes 1,2 and 7 in astrocytomas studied by interphase cytogenetics. *Genes Chromosomes Cancer* **19**:6–13.

122. Wolff R.K., Frazer K.A., Jackler R.K., et al. 1992. Analysis of chromosome 22 deletions in neurofibromatosis type 2-related tumors. *Am. J. Hum. Genet.* **51**:478–485.

123. Wrensch M., Lee M., Miike R., Newman B., Barger G., Davis R., Wiencke J., and Neuhaus J. 1997. Familial and personal medical history of cancer and nervous system conditions among adults with glioma and controls. *American Journal of Epidemiology* **145**:581–593.

124. Wrensch M.R., Barger G.R. 1990. Familial factors associated with malignant gliomas. *Genet. Epidemiol.* **7**:291–301.

125. Yamakawa K., Morita R., and Takahashi E., et al. 1991. A detailed deletion mapping of the short arm of chromosome 3 in sporadic renal cell carcinoma. *Cancer Res.* **51**:4707–4711.

2

Molecular Genetics of Tumors of the Central Nervous System

C. David James

1. INTRODUCTION

1985 marked the first reporting of a specific gene alteration in a human central nervous system (CNS) tumor: epidermal growth factor receptor (EGFR) gene amplification in glioblastoma *(43)*. Since that time, a relatively short period by most standards, neuro-oncology research has revealed many genetic abnormalities that indicate consistent genotype-phenotype associations for the various cancers that are collectively referred to as CNS tumors. This chapter reviews the established CNS tumor genotype associations, and discusses resulting molecular biologic consequences as well as the clinical implications of these genetic alterations.

2. TYPES OF GENE ALTERATIONS IN CANCER

2.1. Oncogenes

As is the case for all human cancers, the genes that are altered in CNS tumors can be grouped into two general categories: (1) oncogenes and (2) tumor suppressors *(37)*. The protein products of oncogenes promote cell proliferation and/or promote other characteristics important to tumor growth, such as invasion, angiogenesis, and resistance to apoptosis. Oncogenes can be activated by increasing the synthesis of their corresponding protein, in normal form, or by alteration of corresponding protein function through gene mutation.

In nervous system tumors, oncogene activation occurs almost entirely by gene amplification. Gene amplification causes an increase in number of a specific gene within a cell, and invariably results in a corresponding increased expression of the gene's encoded protein. In nearly all instances, CNS tumor gene amplifications have been revealed by Southern analysis; a technique in which DNA probes for specific genes reveal elevated gene copy number in tumor DNAs *(83)*.

2.2. Tumor Suppressor Genes

As might be suspected from their name, proteins encoded by tumor suppressor genes (TSGs) inhibit cell growth. Their identification has resulted largely through the application of two molecular genetic methods. One of these is linkage analysis that relies upon subtle DNA sequence variations (polymorphisms) between chromosome homologs that allow one to "track" the segregation pattern of a disease-predisposing gene through multiple generations of an affected family *(96)*. In a study of such families, the chromosomal proximity of a polymorphic variant to a cancer-predisposing gene is indicated by the consistency of its co-segregation with the occurrence of cancer within a family. This approach has been useful in identifying and/or associating tumor suppressor genes, such as *TP53*,

From: *Contemporary Cancer Research: Brain Tumors*
Edited by: F. Ali-Osman © Humana Press Inc., Totowa, NJ

(NF2), and (VHL), with their respective cancer syndromes: Li-Fraumeni *(TP53),* neurofibromatosis type 2 *(NF2),* and von Hippel-Lindau *(VHL)* disease *(see* Subheading 3.3).

The other approach that has been extensively used for TSG identification is deletion mapping. Deletion mapping is performed through loss of heterozygosity (LOH) analysis *(41),* in which the patterns of DNA fragments from restriction enzyme digestions or polymerase chain reactions (PCRs) are compared in a patient's normal and tumor DNAs. Loss of a restriction or PCR fragment-length allele in a tumor DNA sample indicates a genetic alteration directed at the deletion of a TSG. By applying a battery of mapped probes (markers) from a chromosome of interest, one can limit the chromosomal location of a TSG by determining the smallest common region of deletion among a panel of similar tumors. This type of analysis has been applied extensively to brain tumors and has revealed several associations between detectable chromosome losses and tumor histopathology.

3. MALIGNANT ASTROCYTOMAS: A DETAILED GENETIC DESCRIPTION

Given the combined concerns of malignant astrocytoma frequency and mortality, it is perhaps to be expected that the details of genetic alterations in these tumors would be the most extensive among the CNS cancers. Although it is likely that additional gene alterations of importance will be discovered in malignant astrocytomas, it is also possible that most and perhaps all of the high-frequency activation/inactivation targets have been identified. Regardless of the possible discovery of additional high-frequency gene alterations, there is sufficient information on hand to provide a reasonably thorough account of genetic events that promote the development of these tumors.

3.1. Oncogene Alterations in Malignant Astrocytoma: EGFR

The vast majority of CNS tumor oncogene alterations have been identified in malignant astrocytomas, and in most instances oncogene activation is accomplished through gene amplification. The most frequent oncogene alteration in CNS tumors is amplification of the, *EGFR (12,43,98). EGFR* encodes a transmembrane tyrosine kinase that is activated by its binding of epidermal growth factor (Egf), transforming growth factor alpha (TGF-α), as well as other growth factor ligands. The aforementioned discovery as well as specificity of *EGFR* amplification in glioblastoma, or grade IV astrocytoma, has stood up well over the years, although this gene alteration is also observed in grade III anaplastic astrocytoma at a lesser frequency *(12,98).* Occurrences of *EGFR* amplification in other types of CNS tumors are at best rare events, and consequently the detection of this gene alteration is predictive of high malignancy grade astrocytoma.

In approximately two-thirds of the tumors having *EGFR* amplification, amplified genes undergo intragene deletion rearrangements that result in the overexpression of mutant Egf receptors *(20).* The most common *EGFR* mutant, Egfr-vIII, is known to have constitutive, ligand-independent tyrosine kinase activity, as well as an extended half-life that stimulates cell proliferation and enhances the tumorigenicity of human glioma cells in nude mice *(13,14,54).* Furthermore, the activity of this mutant has been shown to promote tumor angiogenesis *(17),* as well as to confer tumor resistance to programmed cell death by increasing Bcl-XL expression *(51).*

EGFR amplification and/or overexpression have been evaluated as prognostic indicators in multiple glioma series, and the majority of these studies suggest that increased *EGFR* gene dosage and high level Egf receptor expression are not predictive of patient survival for glioblastoma patients *(58,92).* However, a recent report indicates that analysis of this gene alteration may be a useful if also considered in the context of patient age *(78),* whereas another study suggests that detection of Egf receptor mutants in glioblastoma may help predict their differential clinical behavior *(16).*

3.2. Other Oncogene Activations in Astrocytomas

Additional oncogenes whose amplification have been observed in patients with malignant astrocytomas include *MYCN (4), CDK4* and *MDM2 (27,67), CCND1 (27),* and *MET (19),* the latter of which, like *EGFR,* is a member of the family of tyrosine kinase growth factor receptors. The reported amplification frequency for these genes is lower than that for *EGFR*, with the highest being 10–15% for *CDK4* in anaplastic astrocytomas and glioblastomas. There is a positive correlation between amplification and increasing glial tumor malignancy grade for each of these genes.

3.3. Tumor Suppressor Gene Alterations in Malignant Astrocytomas
3.3.1. TP53

LOH analysis was of fundamental importance towards identifying the TSG whose inactivation is most frequently involved in the development of malignant astrocytomas, as well as for human cancer in total. The gene, *TP53*, is located at chromosomal region 17p13.1 and is often deleted in astrocytomas *(34)*. The remaining *TP53* copy in a cell with a *TP53* deletion is usually inactivated by a subtle mutation, most of which result in amino acid substitutions that occur in four coding sequence "hot spots" that are located in exons 5 through 8 *(29)*. CNS tumors other than those with predominant astrocytic differentiation do not have an appreciable incidence of *TP53* mutation. With regard to malignancy, studies in which large series of astrocytomas have been examined for *TP53* mutations indicate that similar mutation rates are observed in grade II and grade III tumors, whereas a decreased mutation rate occurs in the glioblastomas *(35; see* Subheading 3.4.). Although *TP53* mutations are most often observed in sporadic astrocytomas, inherited mutations of the *TP53* gene have been identified in CNS tumor patients with Li-Fraumeni syndrome, an inherited condition that confers an elevated risk for the development of several types of cancer *(47)*.

Results from a few studies support *TP53* mutation status as being of prognostic relevance to astrocytoma patients. In a study of 66 similarly treated anaplastic astrocytoma patients *(81)*, *TP53* mutation was a strong univariate predictor of increased survival. For another investigation, the analysis of p53 expression in a series of 51 astrocytic gliomas, most of which were glioblastoma, showed a statistically significant association between increased p53 expression and disease-free survival *(38)*. Although not examined in the latter study, elevated p53 immunohistochemical reacitvity is known to be highly predictive of *TP53* mutation.

3.3.2. CDKN2A

The existence of at least two more astrocytoma TSGs, in addition to *TP53*, had been predicted by results from cytogenetic and loss of heterozygosity studies conducted during the 1980s *(3,33)*, but these genes were slow to be discovered as a result of, primarily, the relative lack of available human genome sequence during that time *(see* Subheading 7.1). One of the TSGs was believed to reside on the short arm of chromosome 9 that is frequently deleted in astrocytomas. Although the 9p deletions were initially localized to a relatively large region that generally includes the centromere-proximal end of the interferon alpha gene cluster, it is now clear that the *CDKN2A* gene, which resides close to the interferon genes, represents the primary chromosome 9p deletion target *(36,56)*. However, there are two additional genes within as well as near *CDKN2A* that are also thought to have a growth-suppressive function: *CDKN2B* and *p14^ARF*. Deletion of both copies of all these genes, along with *CDKN2A*, occur in a variety of cancers, including malignant astrocytomas. Unlike *TP53*, however, for which cancer mutations are common, mutations of the three 9p TSGs have been reported in very few instances. However, a lack of *CDKN2A*-encoded protein, p16, has been shown in a significant fraction of astrocytomas having intact *CDKN2A* genes, indicating that loss of p16 expression can occur in the absence of a corresponding gene alteration. In at least some of these cases, the loss of expression appears to be associated with *CDKN2A* gene hypermethylation *(53)*. As opposed to *TP53* mutations which are observed at a decreasing frequency with increasing tumor malignancy, *CDKN2A* deletions occur more frequently with increasing glioma malignancy grade; *CDKN2A* alterations are also observed more frequently with increasing astrocytic composition of the tumor *(35)*.

3.3.3. Phosphatase Tensin Homolog (PTEN/MMAC1) Inactivation

The most recent and possibly final of the frequent TSG mutations that has been discovered in association with astrocytoma development involves the phosphatase tensin homolog *(PTEN)* gene (also referred to as *MMAC1*) *(42,85)* that resides at chromosomal location 10q23. As for *TP53*, *PTEN* inactivation is often accomplished through deletion with mutation of the remaining allele. *PTEN* has been shown to be inactivated in up to 44% of all glioblastomas, and in 60% of glioblastomas having 10q deletions *(93)*. These results are consistent with *PTEN* being the primary target of inactivation associated with chromosome 10 loss that was originally observed in glioblastoma multiforme by cytogenetic analysis and subsequently by deletion mapping *(3,33)*.

The encoded protein of *PTEN*, Tep1, has been shown to have dual-specificity phosphatase activity (tyrosine and serine) *(50)*, and recent evidence suggests that its biologically relevant targets include inositol phospholipids and proteins. Among the phospholipid substrates is phosphoinositol triphosphate *(46)*, that promotes the activity of Akt, a serine/threonine kinase that is an important regulator of cell survival and cell proliferation *(8)*. Additionally, Tep1 modulates cell migration and invasion by negatively regulating the signals generated at the focal adhesions *(87)* through the direct dephosphorylation and inhibition of focal adhesion kinase. Tep1 can also act as a negative regulator of receptor tyrosine kinase signaling through its inhibition of the adaptor protein Shc *(25)*, and in this regard the activity of Tep1 can be viewed as being antagonistic to Egf receptor function.

PTEN genetic alterations represent the TSG inactivation most highlyassociated with advanced-stage astrocytoma malignancy, and results are accumulating that suggest that the genetic status of *PTEN* is an important prognostic variable in malignant astrocytoma. Lin et al. *(44)* used LOH analysis to examine the *PTEN* locus in 110 such tumors and showed that *PTEN* LOH was a significant predictor of shorter survival. A similar conclusion was reached from the analysis of *PTEN* mutations in pediatric malignant astrocytomas *(63)*. More recently, *PTEN* status in anaplastic astrocytomas has been shown to be an important independent variable in predicting survival, with reduced survival being associated with detectable *PTEN* mutation *(81)*.

3.4. Molecular Genetics Studies Suggest Two Types of Malignant Astrocytoma

Current thinking regarding the genetic pathogenesis of malignant astrocytoma views these tumors as arising through one of two mechanisms: (1) either from a series of genetic steps, with each step conferring an additional, incremental growth advantage to a tumor becoming progressively more malignant, or (2) as a result of a key gene alteration that "spontaneously" produces a tumor of high grade malignancy *(55)*. The major genetic determinants that distinguish the two types of GBM are *EGFR* amplification and *TP53* mutation, with the first being predominantly associated with the spontaneous variant, and the latter being primarily associated with GBMs arising from astrocytoma malignant progression (Fig. 1). In one study, it was shown that the incidence of *TP53* mutations was approximately sixfold less in *de novo*, primary glioblastomas than in secondary glioblastomas that had undergone malignant progression from a lower malignacy precursor *(95)*. The significance of glioblastoma classification is related to potential differences in clinical behavior between the two glioblastoma multiforme (GBM) types, and, consequently, their genetic classification will continue to be of interest. From the cumulative data that has been published on the genetic origin of glioblastoma, it is possible to construct a model that shows the characteristic alterations giving rise to each type of this tumor (Fig. 2).

4. ONCOGENE ACTIVATIONS IN OTHER CENTRAL NERVOUS SYSTEM TUMORS

Oncogene alterations have not been shown to occur frequently in other types of CNS tumors. Although several reports have revealed *CMYC* and *MYCN* amplification in primitive neuroectodermal tumor (PNET)/medulloastoma, the cumulative data from such studies suggest that these gene alterations are infrequent, and have a combined incidence of less than 10% *(64,94)*. Presumed activating mutations of β-catenin, a regulator of T-cell-specific transcription factors (TCF)-mediated transcription, have also been shown in a minor proportion of PNET/medulloblastoma *(100)*. The only

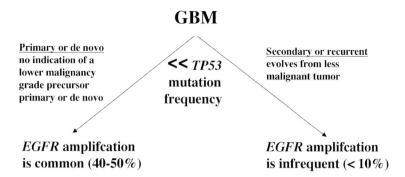

Fig. 1. Association of *EGFR* amplification and *TP53* mutation with primary *(de novo)* and secondary (recurrent) glioblastoma, respectively. *EGFR* amplifications are as much as 5 times more common in primary GBM, whereas *TP53* mutations occur much more frequently in recurrent GBM.

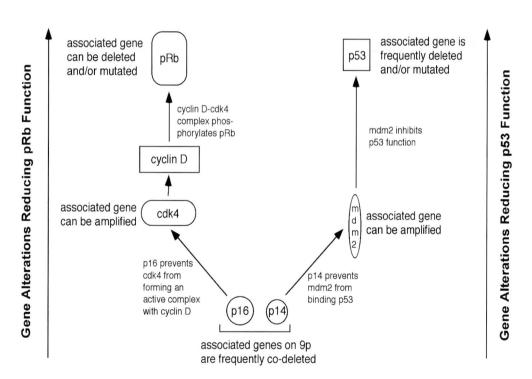

Fig. 2. Gene alterations effecting retinoblastoma (Rb) and/or p53 function. Chromosome 9p deletions occur frequently in malignant astrocytomas, and simultaneously inactivate both *CDKN2A* (encoding the p16 protein) and *p14^{ARF}* genes. *CDK4* and/or *MDM2* gene amplifications are often observed in malignant astrocytomas having intact chromosome 9p tumor suppressor genes. In malignant astrocytomas without alterations of *CDKN2A*, *p14ARF*, *CDK4*, or *MDM2*, inactivating mutations of *RB* and *TP53* are found in nearly all instances.

other gene alteration that has been suggested to be anything more than a rare event in any group of CNS tumor involves the amplification of *PDGFRA* in highly malignant oligodendrogliomas (vascularization and/or necrosis), of which some 20% may be affected *(82)*.

5. TUMOR SUPPRESSOR GENE ALTERATIONS IN OTHER CENTRAL NERVOUS SYSTEM TUMORS

5.1. PNET/Meduloblastoma

The identification of tumor suppressor genes whose inactivation are involved with the development of PNET/medulloblastoma has been an area of active research for several years, but one that has only recently yielded an accepted TSG target. The gene, patched homolog (*PTCH*), was discovered as a result of its mutation being associated with predisposition to nevoid basal cell carcinoma (NBCC) syndrome, an inherited condition in which there is occasional development of medulloblastoma as well as the more commonly occurring nevoid basal cell carcinomas *(26)*. The *PTCH* gene is thought to be inactivated in approx 20% of sporadic medulloblastoma, and mutation/deletion of *PTCH* appears to preferentially occur in the desmoplastic subtype of this tumor *(65,97)*. Additional investigations have been conducted to determine whether genes that encode Ptch-interacting proteins are mutated in medulloblastoma, but their results have yet to support this speculation *(69)*.

5.2. Oligodendroglioma

TSG alterations that are frequently or specifically associated with oligodendroglial tumors have yet to be identified, although cytogenetic and deletion mapping studies support the existence of two such genes. Allelic losses of 19q occurs in 50–80% of oligodendroglial tumors and, with rare exception, involve the entire 19q chromosomal arm *(68,91)*. The chromosome 19q deletion region has been progressively narrowed to an interval occupying a portion of 19q13.3 *(70,79)*, allowing for candidate genes within this region to be examined for mutation. The incidence of 19q deletion is not significantly different between low- and high-grade oligodendrogliomas, suggesting that this alteration is an early event in the neoplastic development of these tumors *(68)*. This finding contrasts with the 19q loss observed in astrocytic gliomas that is generally restricted to the high-grade cases *(79)*.

Deletion of chromosome 1p is another frequent event in oligodendrogliomas, occurring in 40–90% of these tumors *(2,68)*. Interestingly, nearly all cases of oligodendroglioma studied with deletion of 1p also exhibit deletion of 19q, suggesting that inactivation of one or more genes on each of these chromosomal arms is an important event in oligodendroglioma development. Data from a recent report showed two distinct deletion regions on 1p, D1S76-D1S253 at 1p36.3 and D1S482-D1S2743 at 1p34-35, and these contain several candidate TSG targets *(30)*.

Evaluation of chromosomal arms 1p and 19q are of prognostic significance for the oligodendroglioma patient. Cairncross et al. *(7)*, examined 39 anaplastic oligodendroglioma patients, 37 of which had received procarbazine, lomustine, and vincristine (PVC) chemotherapy. Allelic loss of 1p was a statistically significant predictor of chemosensitivity, and combined loss of 1p and 19q were significantly associated with both chemosensitivity and longer recurrence-free survival following chemotherapy. Moreover, Smith et al. *(80)* have demonstrated that the association of 1p and 19q loss with prolonged survival is also evident in low grade oligodendroglioma patients, but that this association may be independent of PCV chemotherapy.

5.3. Pilocytic Astrocytoma

Inheritance of a mutated *NF1* gene (chromosome location 17q11) predisposes to type 1 neurofibromatosis, a syndrome characterized by the development of neurofibromas, cafe-au-lait-spots, and an increased risk for pheochromocytomas, schwannomas, neurofibrosarcomas, and primary brain tumors such as optic gliomas and pilocytic astrocytomas *(61)*. Pilocytic astrocytomas occurring in the absence of NF1 syndrome may also be from *NF1*-inactivating mutations as deletions of this gene have been found in up to 20% of such tumors *(90)*. *NF1* encodes a GTPase-activating protein, neurofibromin, that has been shown to down-regulate the activity of ras, an important effector of receptor tyrosine kinase signaling *(49)*.

5.4. Acoustic Neuromas and Schwannomma

Frequently, acoustic neuromas and schwannomas are observed in patients with neurofibromatosis type 2, and inherited *NF2* gene (chromosomal region 22q12) defects are responsible for these tumors *(61)*. It is therefore not unexpected that somatic *NF2* gene mutations have been observed in a majority (> 60%) of sporadic schwannomas *(32,71)*. The *NF2* gene product, merlin/schwannomin, is a cytoskeleton-associated protein whose function is important to the regulation of cell adhesion *(24)*.

5.5. Hemangioblastoma

VHL syndrome is a consequence of germline *VHL* gene mutations and is characterized by predisposition to the development of hemangioblastomas of the CNS and retina, as well as to other malignancies (renal cell carcinomas, pheochromocytomas, etc.) *(9)*. In addition to its association with hemangioblastoma in VHL patients, somatic mutations of the *VHL* gene are seen in up to 40% of sporadic hemangioblastomas *(88)*. Functional analyses indicate that the *VHL* gene product is an inhibitor of transcription elongation *(11)*. In addition, the VHL protein has been implicated in controlling the expression of vascular endothelial growth factor (VEGF) *(23)*, a potent angiogenesis factor.

6. RELATIONSHIPS BETWEEN GENE ALTERATIONS IN ASTROCYTOMAS AND CELL CYCLE REGULATION

6.1. p53-mdm2-p14^{ARF}-p21

Unrestricted cell multiplication represents a hallmark feature of cancer, and this process is a result of continued cell-cycle progression. In normal cells, cell cycling is kept under control by a complex system of positive and negative regulators that constitute a series of checkpoints. One of the most important of these checkpoints consists of the p53, mdm2, p14 ^{ARF}, and p21 proteins that regulate progression of cells through the G1 cell-cycle phase.

The loss of p53 function is known to promote accelerated growth and malignant transformation of astrocytes both in vitro and in vivo *(5,99)*. In human cancer, it was initially believed that p53 protein function could only be compromised through *TP53* gene deletion or mutation. However, a considerable amount of information has emerged during the past few years that indicates that p53 function is effected by other cellular proteins. Important among these is mdm2 that binds to, destablilizes, and inactivates p53 *(57)*. Significantly, amplification of the *MDM2* gene has been demonstrated as an alternative mechanism to inactivating mutations of *TP53* in astrocytomas *(66)*. *MDM2* gene amplification has been reported in up to 10% of anaplastic astrocytomas lacking *TP53* mutations, and the combined frequency of *TP53* and *MDM2* gene alterations indicates the inactivation of p53 function in approximately one-half of these tumors *(66)*.

Mdm2-mediated destabilization of p53 is inhibited by p14^{ARF}*(62)*, the corresponding gene for which resides mostly within the coding sequence of the p16 gene, *CDKN2A (48)*. As a result of its overlapping localization with *CDKN2A*, both copies of the *p14^{ARF}*gene are often deleted in astrocytomas. Consequently, the 9p alterations, that are so common in these tumors, contribute to aberrant p53 function by promoting increased interaction between p53 and mdm2 (Fig. 3). Because of the relationships between p53, p14^{ARF} and mdm2, it can be argued that nearly all malignant astrocytomas have compromised p53 function from an alteration of one of the corresponding genes for these proteins *(22)*.

The activity of wild-type p53 is known to promote the synthesis of the universal cyclin-cdk inhibitor p21-waf1-cip1 *(15)*, and this is thought to prevent the replication of altered DNA in normal cells that have incurred DNA damage *(10)*. Because the synthesis of p21 is stimulated by wild-type p53 activity, *TP53* gene inactivation, *MDM2* amplification, or *p14^{ARF}* gene deletion can contribute to reduced p21 synthesis, and thus promote the accumulation of gene alterations in tumor cells as a result of the reduced function of a checkpoint preventing the synthesis of damaged DNA. Although reduced p21 expression appears to play an important role in tumor development, there has been no demonstration of the p21 gene itself as a mutagenic target in human cancers *(77)*.

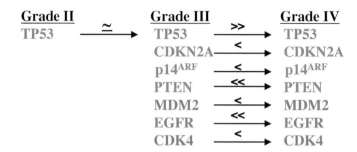

Fig. 3. Associations between gene alterations and astrocytoma malignancy grades. Similar frequencies of *TP53* mutations are observed among grade II and grade III astrocytoma, with their incidence being much higher than is observed among glioblastomas. All other astrocytoma signature gene alterations are most common among glioblastomas, with *EGFR* amplifications and *PTEN* mutations being most highly associated with grade IV malignancy.

6.2. p16-cdk4-Rb-Cyclin D

Another important G1 checkpoint is constituted by the p16, Rb, cdk4, and cyclin D proteins. The protein encoded by the *CDKN2A* gene, p16, acts as a negative regulator of cell growth and proliferation through its binding to cdk4 protein kinase and preventing it from forming an activated complex with cyclin D proteins *(75)*. The primary substrate of this complex is the retinoblastoma protein *(45)*, Rb. In its hypophosphorylated form, Rb arrests cells at the G1/S cell-cycle checkpoint. This checkpoint is abrogated when Rb is phosphorylated, and cyclin D1-cdk4 has been shown to phosphorylate most of the retinoblastoma sites in vitro that are phosphorylated in vivo during late G1.

In association with the proposed model relating the activities of these proteins, one might anticipate the existence of at least three tumor-associated mechanisms for suppression of retinoblastoma function (Fig.3): (1) inactivation of p16; (2) increased expression of cdk4; or (3) inactivation of the retinoblastoma protein. Consistent with this hypothesis, *CDK4* gene amplification and associated overexpression of cdk4 protein has been determined to occur in gliomas with intact and expressed *CDKN2A* genes *(28,73)*. Furthermore, it has been shown that loss of Rb expression, in association with inactivating *RB* gene mutations, generally occurs in glial tumors and cell lines for which there is no evidence of *CDKN2A* or *CDK4* gene alterations *(28,89)*.

It is generally thought that the function of cdk4, p16, or Rb is altered during the malignant transformation of nearly every malignant astrocytoma *(31)*. Interestingly, molecular genetic studies have shown that one and only one of the corresponding genes for these proteins is altered in each tumor, suggesting that a single alteration within the pathway is sufficient to disrupt its regulatory function. Although the prognostic significance of this checkpoint's alteration in astrocytoma is unclear, one study suggests that detection of *CDKN2A* deletions in tumors from patients with oligodendroglioma, albeit an infrequent event, is significantly associated with decreased survival, and additionally occur in tumors having intact copies of chromosomes 1 and 19 *(7)*.

Because the activity of cdk4 is dependent on its binding to D-type cyclins, one might predict that increased cyclin D synthesis would contribute towards oncogenesis by promoting the formation of active cyclin D/cdk4 complexes. Increased cyclin D1 expression in association with gene amplification has been reported in a number of cancers *(59)*, but is uncommon in gliomas. However, it has been shown that cyclin D1 expression is increased by stimulating receptor tyrosine kinase activity *(76)*, and on this basis it is reasonable to speculate that the increased receptor tyrosine kinase activity that commonly occurs in malignant gliomas, usually in association with *EGFR* gene amplification or alteration, may play an important role in promoting cyclin D expression and thereby contribute to Rb protein inactivation.

7. MOLECULAR GENETICS IN THE STUDY AND TREATMENT OF CNS TUMORS: NOW AND THE FUTURE

7.1. Microarrays

At the time of this writing, the ability to perform comprehensive analyses of gene expression patterns in human tumors is nearly at hand, and the application of this analysis, through use of microarrays *(6)*, is already generating substantial information regarding the identities of genes that are consistently overexpressed or underexpressed in specific types of cancer *(40)*.

Microarrays consist of a solid support template upon which thousands of DNAs, representing coding sequences of different genes, are placed. These arrays or "chips" are used for competitive hybridizations of normal and tumor tissue cDNA pairs. Overrepresentation of a tumor cDNA (synthesized from corresponding tumor mRNA) at a specific coordinate on the array indicates overexpression of the gene whose nucleotide sequence was spotted onto that coordinate. Hybridizations can be carried out with DNAs labeled with isotopes or with fluorochromes. From a time-cost perspective the potential efficiency of this process for providing extensive information on gene expression patterns is significant, and is allowing for the development of databases containing expression profiles for many common cancers (Cancer Genome Anatomy Project: CGAP; http://cgap.nci.nih.gov/). Microarray technology is being extended to the detection of gene sequence alterations, and a first generation model for *TP53* mutation detection has been marketed *(1)*. In addition, comprehensive genome arrays for the detection of gene amplification and gene deletion are also being developed *(84)*.

Developments in microarray technology have been largely driven by the progress and completion of the Human Genome Project (http://www.ncbi.nlm.nih.gov/genome/guide/human/). In 1989, The Department of Energy and the National Institutes of Health began funding this project whose purpose is to provide a series of linked data sets containing the genetic and physical location of all genes on each human chromosome, plus the complete nucleotide sequence of the human genome. This initiative has provided us with a complete and accurate whole genome sequence containing a genetic blueprint of the human species. With respect to its gene identification and localization objectives, more than 30,000 genes have been localized to specific chromosomal regions with a high degree of accuracy. The total gene content within our cells is not currently known, but most estimates place it near 50,000. The human genome map that currently exists can already be applied to the identification and isolation of genes that either directly cause disease, or increase susceptibility to disease. It is obvious that the information being generated by the project, when combined with emerging technologies such as the microarrays, will allow for the rapid and, in many cases, complete diagnosis of specific genetic lesions in individual brain tumors.

7.2. Fluorescence In Situ Hybridization Tissue Arrays

Recently, molecular genetic techniques have been combined with conventional cytogenetic methods to produce new procedures for identifying chromosomal alterations in cancers. The resulting molecular cytogenetic procedures have not only helped to make infrequently used archival material amenable to genetic analysis, but have also provided information leading to the identification of novel gene alterations. One method that is proving to have a significant impact in clinical genetic practices for diagnosing specific types of cancer is fluorescence *in situ* hybridization (FISH). The FISH method involves the fluorescent labeling of relatively large segments of cloned human DNA. The cloned DNA segments, each of which has been previously determined to contain known genes from specific chromosomal regions, can be hybridized to either isolated metaphase chromosomes or to intact interphase nuclei. In many instances the probes can be used to find their target sequence in cells that have been embedded and preserved in paraffin. By labeling different probes with different fluorochromes it is possible to examine multiple chromosomes for alterations. There is, in fact, a

Table 1
Signature Gene/Chromosomal Alterations Associated With CNS Tumor Subtypes

Tumor types	Genes/chromosomes	Frequency
Glioblastoma and anaplastic astrocytoma	EGFR[a,m,*]	30–40%[GBM]
		10–15%[AA]
	CDK4[a]	10–15%
	MDM2[a]	5–10%
	TP53[d,m,*]	20–30%[GBM]
		30–40%[AA]
	CDKN2A[d]	30–40%
	PTEN[d,m]	25–30%[GBM]
		10%[AA]
	RB[d,m]	10–15%
Astrocytoma	TP53[d,m]	30–40%
Oligodendroglioma	Chromosome 1p[d]	40–90%
	Chromosome 19q[d]	50–80%
Medulloblastoma/PNET	MYCN[a]	5–10%
	CMYC[a]	5–10%
	PTCH[†d,m]	10–20%
	β-catenin[†m]	5%
	Chromosome 17p[d]	30–50%
Pilocytic astrocytoma	Chromosome 17q[d]	20–30%
Schwannoma	NF2[d,m]	50–60%
Hemangioblastoma	VHL[d,m]	10–20%

Type of gene alterations: [a], amplification; [d], deletion; [m], mutation. Chromosome arms are listed in instances where the corresponding gene alteration is yet to be identified.

*Frequency in different glioblastoma series is strongly influenced by proportion of *de novo* vs secondary tumors.

[†] Observed primarily in desmoplastic variant.

derivative of FISH known as spectral karyotyping (SKY) *(74),* in which probes for each chromosome are labeled with a different fluorochrome or combination of fluorochromes, and simultaneously hybridized to normal metaphase chromosome preparations. Although yet to be extensively applied to the study of brain tumors, this technique may prove to be useful for the analysis of complex karyotypes that are typical of many nervous system malignancies.

8. DIAGANOSTIC AND THERAPEUTIC IMPLICATIONS

8.1. CNS Tumor Diagnosis

This chapter has made reference to the specificity of certain gene alterations for CNS tumor malignancy grade and cellular differentiation (Table 1). Whether molecular genetic analysis will become as efficient and cost-effective as conventional histopathologic analysis for the diagnosis of CNS tumors remains to be seen, but there are an increasing number of reports in the literature that indicate important associations between gene alterations and outcome for CNS tumor patients. Because of the increasing detail of the information that can be obtained through molecular genetic analysis, it seems likely that the accuracy of predicting clinical behavior for individual tumors will similarly increase. At a minimum, one would suppose that genetic testing of all tumor types will be viewed as a necessary component of diagnostic services.

8.2. Central Nervous System Tumor Treatment

The characterization of the genetic mechanisms associated with malignant transformation has opened the way to test novel molecular therapeutic modalities, such as the delivery of small molecules that target disrupted growth-regulatory pathways. Examples of small molecules that may be useful in targeting unbalanced pathways include cdk4 inhibitors *(72)*, farnesyltransferase inhibitors *(18)*, and inhibitors of Egf receptor-associated tyrosine kinase activity *(21)*. More recently, there have been indications that tumor cells with *PTEN* mutations show increased sensitivity to growth inhibition by rapamycin, which targets the mammalian target of rapamycin/FKBP rapamycin-associated protein (mTOR/FRAP) protein *(52,60)*. Knowing whether a tumor has a gene alteration that affects the function of a protein that is being used as a therapeutic target could be critical to determining the success of the agent. For example, it is clear that p53 function is fundamentally important to determining the manner in which cells respond to radiation-induced DNA damage *(39)*. Consequently, information regarding a tumor's *TP53* gene status may help determine a patient's response to radiation treatment: at least one report suggests this is the case for glioblastoma patients *(86)*.

The identification of specific genetic lesions, in combination with promising new therapeutic strategies that are dependent upon the knowledge of tumor genotypes, should greatly facilitate the development of effective, individualized therapies for patients with CNS tumors. It is reasonable to suspect that knowledge of tumor genotypes will soon play an important part in the clinical decision-making process for all cancer patients, and that this information will result in improved patient care.

REFERENCES

1. Ahrendt S.A., Halachmi S., Chow J.T., et al. 1999. Rapid p53 sequence analysis in primary lung cancer using an oligonucleotide probe array. *Proc. Natl. Acad. Sci. USA* **96**:7382–7387.
2. Bello M.J., Vaquero J., de Campos J.M., et al. 1994. Molecular analysis of chromosome 1 abnormalities in human gliomas reveals frequent loss of 1p in oligodendroglial tumors. *Int. J. Cancer* **57**:172–175.
3. Bigner S.H., Mark J., Burger P.C., et al. 1988. Specific chromosomal abnormalities in malignant human gliomas. *Cancer Res.* **48**:405–411.
4. Bigner S.H. Wong A.J., Mark J., et al. 1987. Relationship between gene amplification and chromosomal deviations in malignant human gliomas. *Cancer Genet. Cytogenet.* **29**:165–170.
5. Bogler O., Huang H.J., Cavenee W.K. 1995. Loss of wild-type p53 bestows a growth advantage on primary cortical astrocytes and facilitates their in vitro transformation. *Cancer Res.* **55**:2746–2751.
6. Brown P.O., Botstein D. 1999. Exploring the new world of the genome with DNA microarrays. *Nat. Genet.* **21**:33–37.
7. Cairncross J.G., Ueki K., Zlatescu M.C., et al. 1998. Specific genetic predictors of chemotherapeutic response and survival in patients with anaplastic oligodendrogliomas. *J. Natl. Cancer Inst.* **90**:1473–1479.
8. Cantley L.C., Neel B.G. 1999. New insights into tumor suppression: PTEN suppresses tumor formation by restraining the phosphoinositide 3-kinase/AKT pathway. *Proc. Natl. Acad. Sci. USA* **96**:4240–4245.
9. Decker H.J., Weidt E.J., Brieger J. 1997. The von Hippel-Lindau tumor suppressor gene. A rare and intriguing disease opening new insight into basic mechanisms of carcinogenesis. *Cancer Genet. Cytogenet.* **93**:74–83.
10. Di Leonardo A., Linke S.P., Clarkin K., Wahl G.M. 1994. DNA damage triggers a prolonged p53-dependent G1 arrest and long-term induction of Cip1 in normal human fibroblasts. *Genes Dev.* **8**:2540–2551.
11. Duan D.R., Pause A., Burgess W.H., et al. 1995. Inhibition of transcription elongation by the VHL tumor suppressor protein. *Science* **269**:1402–1406.
12. Ekstrand A.J., James C.D., Cavenee W.K., et al. 1991. Genes for epidermal growth factor receptor, transforming growth factor alpha, and epidermal growth factor and their expression in human gliomas in vivo. *Cancer Res.* **51**:2164–2172.
13. Ekstrand A.J., Liu L., He J., et al. 1995. Altered subcellular location of an activated and tumour-associated epidermal growth factor receptor. *Oncogene* **10**:1455–1460.
14. Ekstrand A.J., Longo N., Hamid M.L., et al. 1994. Functional characterization of an EGF receptor with a truncated extracellular domain expressed in glioblastomas with EGFR gene amplification. *Oncogene* **9**:2313–2320.
15. el-Deiry W.S., Harper J.W., O'Connor P.M., et al. 1994. WAF1/CIP1 is induced in p53-mediated G1 arrest and apoptosis. *Cancer Res.* **54**:1169–1174.
16. Feldkamp M.M., Lala P., Lau N., Roncari L., Guha A. 1999. Expression of activated epidermal growth factor receptors, Ras-guanosine triphosphate, and mitogen-activated protein kinase in human glioblastoma multiforme specimens. *Neurosurg.* **45**:1442–1453.
17. Feldkamp M.M., Lau N., Rak J., et al. 1999. Normoxic and hypoxic regulation of vascular endothelial growth factor (VEGF) by astrocytoma cells is mediated by Ras. *Int. J. Cancer* **81**:118–124.

18. Ferrante K., Winograd B., Canetta R. 1999. Promising new developments in cancer chemotherapy. *Cancer Chemother. Pharmacol.* **43:**S61–68.

19. Fischer U., Muller H.W., Sattler H.P., et al. 1995. Amplification of the MET gene in glioma. *Genes Chromosom. Cancer* **12:**63–65.

20. Frederick L., Wang X.Y., Eley G., James C.D. 2000. Diversity and frequency of epidermal growth factor receptor mutations in human glioblastomas. *Cancer Res.* **60:**1383–1387.

21. Fry D.W. 1999. Inhibition of the epidermal growth factor receptor family of tyrosine kinases as an approach to cancer chemotherapy: progression from reversible to irreversible inhibitors. *Pharmacol. Ther.* **82:**207–218.

22. Fulci G., Labuhn M. Maier D., et al. 2000. p53 gene mutation and ink4a-arf deletion appear to be two mutually exclusive events in human glioblastoma. Oncogene**19:**3816–3822.

23. Gnarra J.R., Zhou S., Merrill M.J., et al. 1996. Post-transcriptional regulation of vascular endothelial growth factor mRNA by the product of the VHL tumor suppressor gene. *Proc. Natl. Acad. Sci. USA* **93:**10,589–10,594.

24. Gonzalez-Agosti C., Xu L., Pinney D., et al. 1996. The merlin tumor suppressor localizes preferentially in membrane ruffles. *Oncogene* **13:**1239–1247.

25. Gu J., Tamura M., Yamada K.M. 1998. Tumor suppressor PTEN inhibits integrin- and growth factor-mediated mitogen-activated protein (MAP) kinase signaling pathways. *J. Cell. Biol.* **143:**1375–1383.

26. Hahn H., Wicking C., Zaphiropoulous P.G., et al. 1996. Mutations of the human homolog of Drosophila patched in the nevoid basal cell carcinoma syndrome. *Cell* **85:**841–851.

27. He J., Allen J.R., Collins V.P., et al. 1994. CDK4 amplification is an alternative mechanism to p16 gene homozygous deletion in glioma cell lines. *Cancer Res.* **54:**5804–5807.

28. He J., Olson J.J., James C.D. 1995. Lack of p16INK4 or retinoblastoma protein (pRb) or amplification-associated overexpression of cdk4 is observed in distinct subsets of malignant glial tumors and cell lines. *Cancer Res.* **55:**4833–4836.

29. Hollstein M., Sidransky D., Vogelstein B., Harris C.C. 1991. p53 mutations in human cancers. *Science* **253:**49–53.

30. Husemann K., Wolter M., Büschges R., et al. 1999. Identification of two distinct deleted regions on the short arm of chromosome 1 and rare mutation of the CDKN2C gene from 1p32 in oligodendroglial tumors. *J. Neuropathol. Exp. Neurol.* **58:**1041–1050.

31. Ichimura K., Schmidt E.E., Goike H.M., Collins V.P. 1996. Human glioblastomas with no alterations of the CDKN2A (p16INK4A, MTS1) and CDK4 genes have frequent mutations of the retinoblastoma gene. *Oncogene* **13:**1065–1072.

32. Irving R.M., Moffat D.A., Hardy D.G., et al. 1994. Somatic NF2 gene mutations in familial and non-familial vestibular schwannoma. *Hum. Mol. Genet.* **3:**347–350.

33. James C.D., Carlbom E., Dumanski J.P., et al. 1988. Clonal genomic alterations in glioma malignancy stages. *Cancer Res.* **48:**5546–5551.

34. James C.D., Carlbom E., Nordenskjold M., et al. 1989. Mitotic recombination of chromosome 17 in astrocytomas. *Proc. Natl. Acad. Sci. USA* **86:**2858–2862.

35. James CD, Galanis E, Frederick L, et al. 1999. Tumor suppressor gene alterations in malignant gliomas: histopathological associations and prognostic evaluation. *Int. J. Oncol.* **15:**547–553.

36. Kamb A., Gruis N.A., Weaver-Feldhaus J., et al. 1994. A cell cycle regulator potentially involved in the genesis of many tumor types. *Science* **264:**436–440.

37. Klein G. 1988. Oncogenes and tumor suppressor genes. *Acta Oncol.* **27:**427–437.

38. Korkolopoulou P., Christodoulou P., Kouzelis K., et al. 1997. MDM2 and p53 expression in gliomas: a multivariate survival analysis including proliferation markers and epidermal growth factor receptor. *Br. J. Cancer* **75:**1269–1278.

39. Kuerbitz SJ, Plunkett BS, Walsh WV, Kastan MB. 1992. Wild-type p53 is a cell cycle checkpoint determinant following irradiation. *Proc. Natl. Acad. Sci. USA* **89:**7491–7495.

40. Kuska B. 1996. Cancer genome anatomy project set for take-off. *J. Natl. Cancer Inst.* **88:**1801–1803.

41. Lasko D., Cavenee W., Nordenskjold M. 1991. Loss of constitutional heterozygosity in human cancer. *Ann. Rev. Genet.* **25:**281–314.

42. Li J., Yen C., Liaw D., et al. 1997. PTEN, a putative protein tyrosine phosphatase gene mutated in human brain, breast, and prostate cancer. *Science* **275:**1943–1947.

43. Libermann T.A., Nusbaum H.R., Razon N., et al. 1985. Amplification, enhanced expression and possible rearrangement of EGF receptor gene in primary human brain tumours of glial origin. *Nature* **313:**144–147.

44. Lin H., Bondy M.L., Langford L.A., et al. 1998. Allelic deletion analyses of MMAC/PTEN and DMBT1 loci in gliomas: relationship to prognostic significance. *Clin. Cancer Res.* **4:**2447–2454.

45. Lukas J., Parry D., Aagaard L., et al. 1995. Retinoblastoma-protein-dependent cell-cycle inhibition by the tumour suppressor p16. *Nature* **375:**503–506.

46. Maehama T., Dixon J.E. 1998. The tumor suppressor, PTEN/MMAC1, dephosphorylates the lipid second messenger, phosphatidylinositol 3,4,5-trisphosphate. *J. Biol. Chem.* **273:**13,375–13,378.

47. Malkin D. 1993. p53 and the Li-Fraumeni syndrome. *Cancer Genet. Cytogenet.* **66:**83–92.

48. Mao L., Merlo A., Bedi G., et al. 1995. A novel p16INK4A transcript. *Cancer Res.* **55:**2995–2997.

49. Martin G.A., Viskochil D., Bollag G., et al. 1990. The GAP-related domain of the neurofibromatosis type 1 gene product interacts with ras p21. *Cell* **63**:843–849.

50. Myers M.P., Stolarov J.P., Eng C., et al. 1997. P-TEN, the tumor suppressor from human chromosome 10q23, is a dual-specificity phosphatase. *Proc. Natl. Acad. Sci. USA* **94**:9052–9057.

51. Nagane M., Levitzki A., Gazit A., et al. 1998. Drug resistance of human glioblastoma cells conferred by a tumor-specific mutant epidermal growth factor receptor through modulation of Bcl-XL and caspase-3-like proteases. *Proc. Natl. Acad. Sci. USA* **95**:5724–5729.

52. Neshat M.S., Mellinghoff I.K., Tran C., et al. 2001. Enhanced sensitivity of PTEN-deficient tumors to inhibition of FRAP/mTOR. *Proc. Natl. Acad. Sci. USA* **98**:10,314–10,319.

53. Nishikawa R., Furnari F.B., Lin H., et al. 1995. Loss of p16INK4 expression is frequent in high grade gliomas. *Cancer Res.* **55**:1941–1945.

54. Nishikawa R., Ji X.D., Harmon R.C., et al. 1994. A mutant epidermal growth factor receptor common in human glioma confers enhanced tumorigenicity. *Proc. Natl. Acad. Sci. USA* **91**:7727–7731.

55. Ng H.K., Lam P.Y. 1998. The molecular genetics of central nervous system tumors. *Pathology* **30**:196–202.

56. Nobori T., Miura K., Wu D.J., Lois A, et al. 1994. Deletions of the cyclin-dependent kinase-4 inhibitor gene in multiple human cancers. *Nature* **368**:753–756.

57. Oliner J.D. Pietenpol J.A., Thiagalingam S., et al. 1993. Oncoprotein MDM2 conceals the activation domain of tumor suppressor p53. *Nature* **362**:857–860.

58. Olson J.J., Barnett D., Yang J., et al. 1998. Gene amplification as a prognostic factor in primary brain tumors. *Clin. Cancer Res.* **4**:215–222.

59. Peters G. 1994. The D-type cyclins and their role in tumorigenesis. *J. Cell. Sci. Suppl.* **18**:89–96.

60. Podsypanina K., Lee R.T., Politis C., et al. 2001. An inhibitor of mTOR reduces neoplasia and normalizes p70/S6 kinase activity in Pten+/- mice. *Proc. Natl. Acad. Sci. USA* **98**:10,320–10,325.

61. Pollack I.F., Mulvihill J.J. 1997. Neurofibromatosis 1 and 2. *Brain Pathol.* **7**:823–836.

62. Pomerantz J., Schreiber-Agus N., Liegeois N.J., et al. 1998. The Ink4a tumor suppressor gene product, p19Arf, interacts with MDM2 and neutralizes MDM2's inhibition of p53. *Cell* **92**:713–723.

63. Raffel C., Frederick L., O'Fallon J.R., et al. 1999. Analysis of oncogene and tumor suppressor gene alterations in pediatric malignant astrocytomas reveals reduced survival for patients with PTEN mutations. *Clin. Cancer Res.* **5**:4085–4090.

64. Raffel C., Gilles F.E., Weinberg K.I.. 1990. Reduction to homozygosity and gene amplification in central nervous system primitive neuroectodermal tumors of childhood. *Cancer Res.* **50**:587–591.

65. Raffel C., Jenkins R.B., Frederick L., et al. 1997. Sporadic medulloblastomas contain PTCH mutations. *Cancer Res.* **57**:842–845.

66. Reifenberger G., Liu L., Ichimura K., et al. 1993. Amplification and overexpression of the MDM2 gene in a subset of human malignant gliomas without p53 mutations. *Cancer Res.* **53**:2736–2739.

67. Reifenberger G., Reifenberger J., Ichimura K., et al. 1994. Amplification of multiple genes from chromosomal region 12q13-14 in human malignant gliomas: preliminary mapping of the amplicons shows preferential involvement of CDK4, SAS, and MDM2. *Cancer Res.* **54**:4299–4303.

68. Reifenberger J., Reifenberger G., Liu L., et al. 1994. Molecular genetic analysis of oligodendroglial tumors shows preferential allelic deletions on 19q and 1p. *Am. J. Pathol.* **145**:1175–1190.

69. Reifenberger J., Wolter M., Weber R.G., et al. 1998. Missense mutations in SMOH in sporadic basal cell carcinomas of the skin and primitive neuroectodermal tumors of the central nervous system. *Cancer Res.* **58**:1798–1803.

70. Rosenberg J.E., Lisle D.K., Burwick J.A., et al. 1996. Refined deletion mapping of the chromosome 19q glioma tumor suppressor gene to the D19S412-STD interval. *Oncogene* **13**:2483–2485.

71. Sainz J., Huynh D.P., Figueroa K., et al. 1994. Mutations of the neurofibromatosis type 2 gene and lack of the gene product in vestibular schwannomas. *Hum. Mol. Genet.* **3**:885–891.

72. Sausville E.A., Zaharevitz D., Gussio R., et al. 1999. Cyclin-dependent kinases: initial approaches to exploit a novel therapeutic target. *Pharmacol. Ther.* **82**:285–292.

73. Schmidt E.E., Ichimura K., Reifenberger G., Collins V.P. 1994. CDKN2 (p16/MTS1) gene deletion or CDK4 amplification occurs in the majority of glioblastomas. *Cancer Res.* **54**:6321–6324.

74. Schrock E., du Manoir S., Veldman T., et al. 1996. Multicolor spectral karyotyping of human chromosomes. *Science* **273**:494–497.

75. Serrano M., Hannon G.J., Beach D. 1993. A new regulatory motif in cell-cycle control causing specific inhibition of cyclin D/CDK4. *Nature* **366**:704–707.

76. Sherr CJ. 1995. D-type cyclins. *Trends Biochem. Sci.* **20**:187–190.

77. Shiohara M., el-Deiry W.S., Wada M., et al. 1994. Absence of WAF1 mutations in a variety of human malignancies. *Blood* **84**:3781–3784.

78. Simmons M.L., Lamborn K.R., Takahashi M., et al. 2001. Analysis of complex relationships between age, p53, epidermal growth factor receptor, and survival in glioblastoma patients. *Cancer Res.* **61**:1122–1128.

79. Smith J.S., Alderete B., Minn Y., et al. 1999. Localization of common deletion regions on 1p and 19q in human gliomas and their association with histological subtype. *Oncogene* **18**:4144–4152.

80. Smith J.S., Perry A., Borell T.J., et al. 2000. Alterations of chromosome arms 1p and 19q as predictors of survival in oligodendrogliomas, astrocytomas, and mixed oligoastrocytomas. *J. Clin. Oncol.* **18**:636–645.

81. Smith J.S., Tachibana I., Passe S.M., et al. 2001. PTEN mutation, EGFR amplification, and outcome in patients with anaplastic astrocytoma and glioblastoma multiforme. *J. Nat. Cancer Inst.* **93**:1246–1256.

82. Smith J.S., Wang X.Y., Qian J., et al. 2000. Amplification of the platelet-derived growth factor receptor-A (PDGFRA) gene occurs in oligodendrogliomas with grade IV anaplastic features. *J. Neuropathol. Exp. Neurol.* **59**:495–503.

83. Southern EM. 1975. Detection of specific sequences among DNA fragments separated by gel electrophoresis. *J. Mol. Biol.* **98**:503–517.

84. Snijders A.M., Nowak N., Segraves R., et al. 2001. Assembly of microarrays for genome-wide measurement of DNA copy number. *Nat. Genet.* **29**:263–264.

85. Steck P.A., Pershouse M.A., Jasser S.A., et al. 1997. Identification of a candidate tumour suppressor gene, MMAC1, at chromosome 10q23.3 that is mutated in multiple advanced cancers. *Nat. Genet.* **15**:356–362.

86. Tada M., Matsumoto R., Iggo R.D., et al. 1998. Selective sensitivity to radiation of cerebral glioblastomas harboring p53 mutations. *Cancer Res.* **58**:1793–1797.

87. Tamura M., Gu J., Matsumoto K., Aota S., Parsons R., Yamada K.M. 1998. Inhibition of cell migration, spreading, and focal adhesions by tumor suppressor PTEN. *Science* **280**:1614–1617.

88. Tse J.Y., Wong J.H., Lo K.W., et al. 1997. Molecular genetic analysis of the von Hippel-Lindau disease tumor suppressor gene in familial and sporadic cerebellar hemangioblastomas. *Am. J. Clin. Pathol.* **107**:459–466.

89. Ueki K. Ono Y., Henson J.W., et al. 1996. CDKN2/p16 or RB alterations occur in the majority of glioblastomas and are inversely correlated. *Cancer Res.* **56**:150–153.

90. von Deimling A., Louis D.N., Menon A.G. et al. 1993. Deletions on the long arm of chromosome 17 in pilocytic astrocytoma. *Acta Neuropathol.* **86**:81–85.

91. von Deimling A., Louis D.N., von Ammon K., et al. 1992. Evidence for a tumor suppressor gene on chromosome 19q associated with human astrocytomas, oligodendrogliomas, and mixed gliomas. *Cancer Res.* **52**:4277–4279.

92. Waha A., Baumann A., Wolf H.K., et al. 1996. Lack of prognostic relevance of alterations in the epidermal growth factor receptor-transforming growth factor-alpha pathway in human astrocytic gliomas. *J. Neurosurg.* **85**:634–641.

93. Wang S.I., Puc J., Li J., et al. 1997. Somatic mutations of PTEN in glioblastoma multiforme. *Cancer Res.* **57**:4183–4186.

94. Wasson J.C., Saylors R.L. III, Zeltzer P., et al. 1990. Oncogene amplification in pediatric brain tumors. *Cancer Res.* **50**:2987–2990.

95. Watanabe K., Tachibana O., Sata K., et al. 1996. Overexpression of the EGF receptor and p53 mutations are mutually exclusive in the evolution of primary and secondary glioblastomas. *Brain Pathol.* **6**:217–223.

96. White R, Lalouel JM. 1988. Chromosome mapping with DNA markers. *Sci. Am.* **258**:40–48.

97. Wolter M., Reifenberger J., Sommer C, et al. 1997. Mutations in the human homologue of the Drosophila segment polarity gene patched (PTCH) in sporadic basal cell carcinomas of the skin and primitive neuroectodermal tumors of the central nervous system. *Cancer Res.* **57**:2581–2585.

98. Wong A.J., Bigner S.H., Bigner D.D., et al. 1987. Increased expression of the epidermal growth factor receptor gene in malignant gliomas is invariably associated with gene amplification. *Proc. Natl. Acad. Sci. USA* **84**:6899–6903.

99. Yahamada A.M., Bruner J.M., Donehower L.A., Morrison R.S. 1995. Astrocytes derived from p53-deficient mice provide a multistep in vitro model for development of malignant gliomas. *Mol. Cell. Biol.* **15**:4249–4259.

100. Zurawel R.H., Chiappa S.A., Allen C., Raffel C. 1998. Sporadic medulloblastomas contain oncogenic beta-catenin mutations. *Cancer Res.* **58**:896–899.

3

Molecular Pathology of Nervous System Tumors

Catherine L. Nutt, Anat O. Stemmer-Rachamimov, J. Gregory Cairncross, and David N. Louis

1. INTRODUCTION

In modern clinical neuro-oncology, no variable affects therapeutic decisions and prognostic estimation more than tumor classification. The most widely used method of brain tumor classification is that of the World Health Organization (WHO), most recently revised in 2000 *(51)*, which is based on microscopic examination of tissue by a pathologist. The WHO classification divides nervous system tumors into many nosological entities (Table 1) and assigns a grade of I to IV, grade I being benign and grade IV being highly malignant. Although, in the majority of cases, the assignment of tumors in the WHO classification system is relevant and appropriate, unfortunately there are many situations in which this classification is problematic, primarily because pathological diagnosis remains quite subjective *(67)*. For example, some brain tumors are difficult to place neatly into one of the categories. For others, the histological diagnosis and corresponding predicted clinical behavior do not concur with the actual clinical course. Finally, it is doubtful that the current histopathological system alone will accurately predict patient response to targeted therapies once available. As such, information capable of augmenting the WHO system could result in marked improvements in the current approach to brain tumor classification.

Inquiries into the genetic basis of gliomas have yielded much information on specific genetic events that underlie brain tumorigenesis. Significant advances in molecular genetics have begun to provide pertinent clinical information, aiding in both the classification and the management of brain tumors. This chapter reviews the current molecular pathology and classification of primary neoplasms of the nervous system.

2. DIFFUSE GLIOMAS

Gliomas are the most common of primary brain tumors and comprise the bulk of adult tumors in neuro-oncology practice. Glial neoplasms are extremely heterogeneous and, from a practical point of view, the most important initial distinction is to separate diffuse from circumscribed gliomas. The infiltrative growth pattern of diffuse gliomas essentially prevents surgical cure and the majority of these tumors are resistant to standard radiotherapeutic and chemotherapeutic approaches. Nonetheless, some subtypes of diffuse glioma respond to therapy, highlighting the importance of proper classification and grading of glial tumors. The 2000 WHO system divides diffuse gliomas into astrocytomas, oligodendrogliomas, and oligoastrocytomas. Using standard histological criteria, these tumors are then graded into degrees of malignancy. For oligodendrogliomas and

From: *Contemporary Cancer Research: Brain Tumors*
Edited by: F. Ali-Osman © Humana Press Inc., Totowa, NJ

Table 1
Classification of Tumors of the Nervous System

Tumors of neuroepithelial tissue
    Astrocytic tumors
    Oligodendroglial tumors
    Mixed gliomas
    Ependymal tumors
    Choroid plexus tumors
    Glial tumors of uncertain origin
    Neuronal and mixed neuronal-glial tumors
    Neuroblastic tumors
    Pineal parenchymal tumors
    Embryonal tumors
Tumors of peripheral nerves
    Schwannoma
    Neurofibroma
    Perineurioma
    Malignant peripheral nerve sheath tumor
Tumors of the meninges
    Tumors of meningothelial cells
    Mesenchymal, non-meningothelial tumors
    Primary melanocytic lesions
    Tumors of uncertain histogenesis
Lymphomas and hemopoietic neoplasms
Germ cell tumors
Tumors of the sellar region
Metastatic tumors

oligoastrocytomas, there are grade II (low-grade) and anaplastic, grade III lesions. For diffuse astrocytomas, there are grade II, grade III, and grade IV lesions, with grade IV also known as glioblastoma.

2.1. Diffuse Astrocytomas, Including Glioblastoma

2.1.1. Standard Pathology

Diffuse, fibrillary astrocytomas, including glioblastoma, the most malignant form, are the most common type of brain tumor in adults. Grade II fibrillary astrocytomas are characterized histologically by cells with moderately pleomorphic nuclei and cellular processes that form a glial fibrillary background. In addition to fibrillary astrocytomas, there exist gemistocytic astrocytomas, featuring cells with prominent and copious eosinophilic cytoplasm and shorT-cellular processes, as well as protoplasmic astrocytomas characterized by inconspicuous cytoplasm and cellular processes. Most astrocytic tumors display immunohistological positivity for glial fibrillary acidic protein (GFAP). Mitotic activity is not present in grade II astrocytomas and the presence of a single mitosis in a small biopsy is sufficient to upgrade the tumor to an anaplastic, grade III astrocytoma. In addition to mitotic activity, grade III astrocytomas are more densely cellular and have more pleomorphic nuclei than grade II tumors. Many gemistocytic astrocytomas conform to grade III. Glioblastoma is the most malignant grade of astrocytoma. In addition to the dense cellularity and high proliferation indices characteristic of high-grade tumors, the diagnosis of glioblastoma requires the presence of microvascular proliferation and/or necrosis.

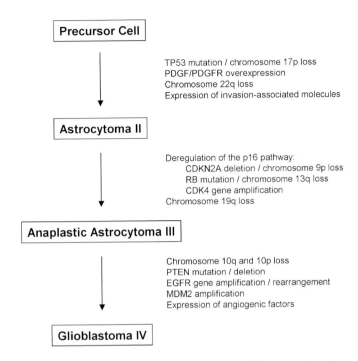

Fig. 1. Molecular genetic alterations characteristic of different grades of astrocytoma.

2.1.2. Molecular Pathology (Fig. 1)

WHO grade II astrocytomas are best characterized by inactivating mutations of the *TP53* tumor suppressor gene on chromosome 17p, as well as overexpression of the platelet-derived growth factor (PDGF) A chain, and the PDGF α-receptor *(66)*. Interestingly, loss of chromosome 17p in the region of the *TP53* gene is closely correlated with PDGF α-receptor overexpression *(38)*, suggesting that *TP53* mutations may have an oncogenic effect only in the presence of PDGF α-receptor overexpression. This interdependence is supported by observations that mouse astrocytes without functional p53 become transformed only in the presence of specific growth factors *(10)*.

Allelic loss of chromosome 17p and *TP53* mutations have been observed in at least one-third of adult astrocytomas, irrespective of tumor grade *(65)*. An integral role for p53 in the early stages of astrocytoma tumorigenesis is further evidenced by so-called secondary glioblastomas; it has been demonstrated that grade IV lesions with homogeneous *TP53* mutations evolve clonally from subpopulations of similarly mutated cells present in the initial, grade II astrocytic tumors *(119)*. Functional studies have recapitulated a role for p53 inactivation in the early stages of astrocytoma formation. For example, cortical astrocytes from mice that lack a functional p53 become immortalized when grown in vitro and rapidly acquire a transformed phenotype. In addition, although cortical astrocytes from mice with one copy of a functional p53 behave in a manner comparable to wild type astrocytes, subsequent loss of the one functional copy renders these cells immortal and transformation can ensue *(10,148)*. Interestingly, those cells without functional p53 become markedly aneuploid *(148)*, confirming prior reports that p53 loss results in genomic instability and that human astrocytomas with mutant *TP53* are often aneuploid *(133)*. Thus, the abrogation of astrocytic p53 function appears to facilitate conditions conducive to neoplastic transformation, setting the stage for subsequent malignant progression.

The transition from WHO grade II astrocytoma to WHO grade III anaplastic astrocytoma is accompanied by a number of molecular abnormalities. Studies suggest that most of these alterations converge on one critical cell-cycle regulatory complex that includes the p16, retinoblastoma (Rb), cyclin-dependent kinase 4 (cdk4), cdk6, and cyclin D1 proteins. Individual members of this pathway are altered in up to 50% of anaplastic astrocytomas and in the vast majority, if not all, glioblastomas. Loss of chromosome 9p primarily affects the region of the *CDKN2A* gene and occurs in approx 50% of anaplastic astrocytomas and glioblastomas *(131)*. The *CDKN2A* gene encodes the p16 and p14[alternate open reading frame (ARF)] proteins and expression of these proteins is most commonly altered by homozygous deletion of the *CDKN2A* gene, although point mutations and hypermethylation of *CDKN2A* have also been found to alter p16 and p14[ARF] expression *(12,74,79)*. Chromosome 13q loss occurs in one-third to one-half of high-grade astrocytomas, with the *RB* gene preferentially targeted by losses and inactivating mutations *(37)*. Analyses of the loss of chromosome 13q, *RB* gene mutations, and Rb protein expression suggest that the *RB* gene is inactivated in approx 20% of anaplastic astrocytomas and 35% of glioblastomas *(12,37)*. Interestingly, *RB* and *CDKN2A* aberrations are inversely correlated in gliomas, rarely occurring together in the same tumor *(131)*. Located on chromosome 12q13-14, *CDK4* is amplified in approx 15% of malignant gliomas *(98)*. This amplification frequency may be higher among gliomas without *CDKN2A* loss, perhaps reaching 50% of glioblastomas with intact p16 expression *(113)*. CDK4 amplification and cyclin D1 overexpression appear to represent alternative events to *CDKN2A* deletions in glioblastomas because these genetic changes only rarely occur in the same tumor *(34,113)*. Within this pathway, CDK6 amplification also occurs, although not as commonly as CDK4 amplification *(19)*.

Progression to glioblastoma is characterized by the loss of chromosome 10; although occurring far less commonly in anaplastic astrocytomas, this alteration can be found in 60–95% of glioblastomas *(44,136)*. At least two tumor suppressor loci are implicated on the long arm of chromosome 10, as well as one potential locus on the short arm. The phosphatase and tensin homolog (*PTEN*)/ mutated in multiple advanced cancers 1 (*MMAC1*)/ TGF β-regulated and epithelial cell-enriched phosphatase 1 (*TEP-1*) gene at 10q23.3 is one example of a tumor suppressor gene that has been studied, with *PTEN* mutations identified in approx 20% of glioblastomas *(22,62,124)*. Moreover, introduction of wild-type *PTEN* into glioma cells with mutant *PTEN* leads to growth suppression *(26)*. Nonetheless, given the remarkably high frequency of chromosome 10 loss in glioblastoma, glioma tumor suppressor genes other than *PTEN* likely reside on this chromosome.

The epidermal growth factor receptor (*EGFR*) gene is the most frequently amplified oncogene in astrocytic tumors *(24)* and is characteristic of so-called *de novo* glioblastomas. Although *EGFR* is amplified in few anaplastic astrocytomas *(23)*, approx 40% of glioblastomas display amplification *(136)*. *EGFR* amplification in glioblastomas is almost always accompanied by loss of genetic material on chromosome 10 *(136)* and these tumors often exhibit *CDKN2A* deletions *(33)*. Glioblastomas with *EGFR* gene amplification display overexpression of *EGFR* at both the messenger ribonucleic acid (mRNA) and protein levels, stressing the importance of this growth signal pathway to glioblastomas *(23,147)*. Approximately one-third of glioblastomas with *EGFR* gene amplification also display *EGFR* gene rearrangements that produce truncated proteins similar to the *v-erbB* oncogene *(17)*. These truncated receptors are capable of conferring dramatically enhanced tumorigenicity to these tumors *(80)*.

EGFR amplification and *TP53* mutations appear to be mutually exclusive genetic aberrations in glioblastomas. One-third of glioblastomas have *TP53*/chromosome 17p alterations, one-third display EGFR gene amplification, and one-third have neither change *(138)*. Experimental data supports this distinction by showing that cells lacking functional p53 are not transformed when cultured in the presence of epidermal growth factor (EGF) but are transformed in the presence of other growth factors *(10)*; glioblastomas with *TP53* mutations may therefore not be expected to acquire *EGFR* gene amplification if activation of the EGF-EGFR pathway does not produce a increased growth advantage in such cells.

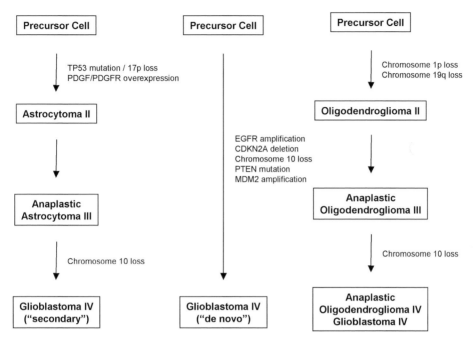

Fig. 2. Molecular genetic subsets of glioblastoma.

A number of additional molecular alterations occur in astrocytic gliomas for which little functional information is known. Less common genomic alterations associated with low-grade astrocytomas include loss of chromosome 22q, suggesting the presence of a chromosome 22q glioma tumor suppressor gene *(43)*, and gains of chromosome 7q *(117)*. In anaplastic astrocytomas and glioblastomas, allelic loss on 19q is quite common, being observed in up to 40% of these tumors and suggestive of a putative tumor suppressor gene *(137)*. In addition to confirming the genetic alterations discussed in this section, comparative genomic hybridization (CGH) studies have identified numerous other amplifications and deletions in astrocytic gliomas *(56,75,81,112,144)*. Moreover, the recent implementation of array-based CGH has enabled the identification of amplicons with single gene resolution in these lesions *(41)*. Further exploration with this technique should allow for the development of a more comprehensive overview of the genetic aberrations found in astrocytic tumors.

2.1.3. Molecular Diagnostics and Prognostics

As discussed in Subheading 2.1.2., *TP53* mutations and *EGFR* gene amplification often appear to be mutually exclusive genetic aberrations in glioblastomas. These two distinct alterations provide additional information for the classification of glioblastomas (Fig. 2). The genetic pathway involving *TP53* mutations usually involves malignant progression from a lower-grade astrocytic tumor to a secondary glioblastoma *(100,138,140)*. In contrast, glioblastomas with *EGFR* gene amplification often arise *de novo*, without a clinically evident, preceding lower-grade astrocytoma *(138,140)*. Furthermore, glioblastomas with loss of chromosome 17p tend to occur in patients younger than those characterized by *EGFR* gene amplification *(69,95)*. Interestingly, initial diagnosis at a younger age has been an important prognostic parameter among patients with glioblastoma, with younger patients faring better than older patients. These genetic alterations may therefore reflect the age-based difference in prognosis, suggesting that genetic analysis may begin to explain the clinical observations concerning age differences in astrocytic lesions.

Although convincing differences in prognosis have not been observed in earlier studies of either *TP53* or *EGFR* alterations in astrocytic gliomas, recent studies suggest that the relationship between age, p53, EGFR, and survival may be more complex than originally anticipated in patients with glioblastoma. In one study, when glioblastoma patients were initially differentiated based on length of survival, nuclear expression of p53 was significantly more frequent in long-term survivors and EGFR overexpression appeared slightly more frequent in short-term survivors *(13)*. However, when glioblastoma patients were initially differentiated based on age, EGFR overexpression indicated worse prognosis in younger glioblastoma patients but better prognosis in older patients *(120,122)*. Furthermore, within the subgroup of glioblastoma patients younger than the median age, EGFR overexpression has been negatively associated with survival in p53 wild-type cases, but not in tumors positive for p53 immunohistochemistry *(120)*. The complexity of these results suggests that prognostic estimation in patients with glioblastoma may require analysis of subgroups that incorporate information for both age and specific genetic alterations.

In addition to the diagnostic and prognostic information provided by p53 and EGFR status, other genetic alterations have been implicated as prognostic indicators in astrocytic lesions. Gains of 7p and 7q have been associated with shorter patient survival in anaplastic astrocytomas, independent of age *(56)*. Furthermore, 10q loss of heterozygosity (LOH) *(127)* and *PTEN* mutations *(122)* have been significantly associated with shorter survival in astrocytic tumors. Recently, genetic alterations have also been correlated with therapeutic response in astrocytic tumors; relative radio-resistance of some glioblastomas may be associated with EGFR overexpression *(2)*. Taken together, these studies provide strong evidence for molecular genetic subgroups of astrocytic gliomas that vary in treatment response and prognostic outcome.

2.2. Oligodendroglioma

2.2.1. Standard Pathology

Oligodendrogliomas appear moderately cellular and are characterized histologically by cells with round nuclei and perinuclear halos ("fried egg" appearance). These tumors often display delicate, branching vessels ("chickenwire" vasculature) and calcification. GFAP staining of neoplastic cells is sparse in most oligodendrogliomas (with the exception of so-called microgemistocytes), although reactive astrocytes within the tumor are often positive for GFAP. The presence of additional histological features of malignancy can result in the diagnosis of an anaplastic, WHO grade III oligodendroglioma. These features include brisk mitotic activity, vascular proliferation, and necrosis.

2.2.2. Molecular Pathology

The most common allelic losses in oligodendrogliomas occur on chromosomes 1p and 19q, affecting 40–80% of the tumors *(55,99,137)*. Mapping of the 1p chromosome locus has implicated the telomeric region of 1p *(55,121)*. Similar mapping of chromosome 19q has demonstrated that the gene resides in the same vicinity as the putative astrocytoma 19q gene and is likely the same gene *(106,121)*. Interestingly, chromosome 1p and 19q losses are closely correlated, suggesting that the two putative tumor suppressor genes may be involved in biologically distinct pathways *(55,99)*. The frequent loss of these loci appears to be independent of tumor grade and, as such, is probably important in the initial stages of oligodendroglioma tumorigenesis. Anaplastic oligodendrogliomas may display allelic losses of chromosome 9, involving the *CDKN2A* gene, and chromosome 10 *(15,99)*. Disruption of the RB1/CDK4/p16INK4a/p15INK4b and the TP53/p14[ARF]/ MDM2 pathways appears frequently in anaplastic oligodendrogliomas *(141,146)*, with simultaneous disruption of both pathways occurring in 45% of lesions in one study *(141)*. In particular, hypermethylation appears to be an important epigenetic mechanism by which oligodendroglial tumors may escape cell-cycle control *(21,141,146)*. Oncogene amplification has only rarely been demonstrated in oligodendroglial tumors *(24,99)*.

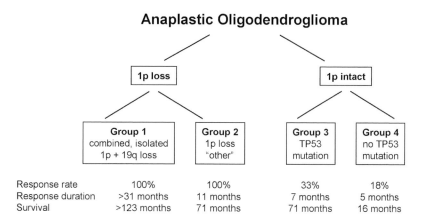

Fig. 3. Molecular genetic subsets of oligodendrogliomas. "Other" is defined as tumors that display 1p loss, but either do not have 19q loss or have other genetic alterations such as *TP53* mutation, *PTEN* mutation, 10q loss, *CDKN2A* deletion, or *EGFR* amplification.

2.2.3. Molecular Diagnostics and Prognostics

The value of molecular genetic analysis in modern clinical neuro-oncology is best exemplified by anaplastic oligodendrogliomas; these are the first brain tumors for which molecular genetic analysis has provided practical clinical ramifications. Anaplastic oligodendrogliomas that have 1p loss are sensitive to procarbazine, CCNU and vincristine (PCV) chemotherapy, with approx 50% of these tumors demonstrating a complete neuroradiological response *(15)*. In contrast, anaplastic oligodendrogliomas with an intact 1p are only PCV-sensitive in approx 25% of cases and rarely exhibit a complete neuroradiological response. Furthermore, patients whose anaplastic oligodendrogliomas have 1p and 19q loss have a median survival of approx 10 yr compared with a median survival of about 2 yr for patients whose tumors lack these genetic alterations *(15)*. Subsequently, it has been shown that anaplastic oligodendrogliomas can be divided genetically into four therapeutically and prognostically relevant subgroups (Fig. 3) *(42)*. Moreover, studies have demonstrated that the molecular subtypes of anaplastic oligodendroglioma may arise preferentially in particular lobes of the brain and have differential patterns of growth, providing additional information pertinent to clinical patient management *(155)*.

Because a diagnosis of oligodendroglioma affects both therapeutic decisions and prognostic estimation, the ability to recognize oligodendroglial tumors has become extremely important. Recently, in an attempt not to overlook patients with a better prognosis and who might benefit from chemotherapeutic treatment, an increase in oligodendroglioma diagnoses has been noted. To provide a more objective method of classifying oligodendrogliomas, a number of current studies have investigated the correlation between tumor morphology and molecular genetic profile. In a study of glioblastomas with an oligodendroglial component, evidence was provided for a subgroup of glioblastomas of oligodendroglial origin; these lesions displayed the genetic aberrations of a "standard" glioblastoma but differed by having a higher incidence of 1p and 19q LOH *(35)*. Similarly, a report by Ueki et al. *(130)* displayed a set of glioblastomas with 1p and 19q LOH, and these lesions were distinguished from 1p/ 19q LOH oligodendrogliomas by the presence of 10q LOH; these results suggest the presence of a subgroup of glioblastomas of oligodendroglial origin where 10q LOH may be characteristic of progression. Interestingly, one study of low-grade gliomas suggests that histological appearance correctly predicts genotype in approx 80% of these lesions and that neuropathologists can be "trained" to recognize the particular histopathological features responsible for an accurate diagnosis *(110)*.

However, it should be noted that even "trained" neuropathologists do not achieve 100% accuracy and the incorporation of objective molecular genetic analyses is still warranted *(110)*.

2.3. Oligoastrocytoma

2.3.1. Standard Pathology

Diffuse gliomas with an oligodendroglial component can be divided into oligodendrogliomas and oligoastrocytomas. However, most oligodendroglial tumors include astrocytic cells and the percentage of astrocytoma required to diagnose oligoastrocytoma remains controversial *(97)*. The diagnosis of oligoastrocytoma is most safely made when distinct oligodendroglial and astroglial regions are present.

2.3.2. Molecular Pathology

Many oligoastrocytomas, like oligodendrogliomas, display allelic losses on chromosomes 1p and 19q *(55,99,137)*, as well as losses on chromosomes 9 and 10 *(15,99)*. However, other oligoastrocytomas display *TP53* mutations and 17p loss, more akin to the genotype of astrocytoma *(71)*. In a recent study by Ueki et al. *(130)*, *TP53* mutation was inversely related to 1p LOH in gliomas, providing further evidence of two distinct lineages. Interestingly, although oligoastrocytomas display the histological features of both oligodendrogliomas and astrocytomas, microdissection of the oligodendroglial and astrocytic components has demonstrated that, despite histological differences, the molecular alterations are identical in the two components *(55)*.

3. OTHER GLIOMAS

3.1. "Circumscribed" Astrocytomas

3.1.1. Standard Pathology

The major types of circumscribed astrocytomas are pilocytic astrocytomas, pleomorphic xanthoastrocytomas (PXAs), and subependymal giant cell astrocytomas (SEGAs). These are generally WHO grade I lesions. Pilocytic astrocytomas are most often childhood tumors, although adult cases do occur. They are well-demarcated tumors, often with a gliotic margin, and frequently present as mural nodules within a cyst. Histologically, these lesions are characterized by elongated piloid ("hair-like") cells with long, tapering bipolar cellular processes. Pilocytic astrocytomas may have a biphasic appearance, where fibrillary regions alternate with microcystic areas. Rosenthal fibers and granular bodies are also characteristic of these lesions. Invasion of the subarachnoid space, although common, does not imply malignant behavior in these tumors. Similarly, mitotic activity, vascular proliferation, and necrosis, if present, do not necessarily indicate a more ominous prognosis as seen in diffuse gliomas. A distinguishing feature of PXAs is the presence of enlarged cells with lipidized cytoplasm. Inflammation is also characteristic of these tumors. Some PXAs may recur as glioblastomas. SEGAs, on the other hand, are usually associated with tuberous sclerosis (TS) and are histologically identical to the so-called "candle-gutterings" that line the ventricles of TS patients. These lesions are characterized by giant cells with extensive glassy, eosinophilic cytoplasm. These cells may have a neuronal appearance, with vesicular nuclei and large nucleoli, and sometimes stain positive for neuronal as well as glial immunohistochemical markers.

3.1.2. Molecular Pathology

3.1.2.1. PILOCYTIC ASTROCYTOMA

Pilocytic astrocytomas do not display the same genomic alterations as diffuse, fibrillary astrocytomas. Because pilocytic astrocytomas frequently affect patients with neurofibromatosis 1 (NF1), *NF1* on chromosome 17q would be a strong candidate tumor suppressor gene for these lesions. In fact, allelic loss occurs on chromosome 17q in 25% of these tumors *(135)*, with loss of the *NF1* allele being much more frequent in NF1-associated pilocytic astrocytomas than in sporadic cases *(52)*.

Unfortunately, owing to the large size of this gene, detailed mutational analysis of the NF1 gene in pilocytic astrocytomas has not yet been performed. One recent study screened pilocytic astrocytomas for mutations of the TS tumor suppressor genes tuberous sclerosis complex (*TSC*)*1* and *TSC2*; of 11 tumors informative for both loci, two pilocytic astrocytomas exhibited LOH *(87)*. All coding exons of the *TSC1* and *TSC2* genes were screened in the two LOH cases but no mutations were detected, suggesting that the *TSC* genes do not play a major role in pilocytic astrocytoma tumorigenesis *(87)*.

3.1.2.2. PLEOMORPHIC XANTHOASTROCYTOMA

The genetic events that underlie PXA formation and progression differ from those responsible for diffuse astrocytoma tumorigenesis *(88)*. Although p53 mutations have been found in PXAs, the few documented cases have displayed mutations somewhat different from those usually found in diffuse, fibrillary astrocytomas *(27,88)*. EGFR gene amplification does not occur in PXAs, although glioblastomas that arise from PXAs may display EGFR amplification *(88,150)*. In addition, allelic losses of chromosomes 9, 10, and 19q have not been observed in PXAs. One recent study utilized comparative genomic hybridization and demonstrated gain on chromosome 7 and loss on 8p in two out of three PXAs *(150)*.

3.1.2.3. SUBEPENDYMAL GIANT CELL ASTROCYTOMA

Because SEGAs are associated with TS, it is reasonable to hypothesize that the TS genes, *TSC1* on chromosome 9q and *TSC2* on chromosome 16p, are involved in SEGA formation. In fact, LOH studies have shown allelic loss of chromosome 9q and 16p loci in some SEGAs, particularly of the *TSC2* locus on 16p, suggesting that the TS genes act as tumor suppressors *(30,31,36)*. Detailed mutation analysis for these genes has not been completed to date in SEGA lesions, although one survey of TS hamartomas revealed a SEGA with a mutation in *TSC2* and corresponding LOH *(78)*. Kim et al. *(50)* performed an immunohistochemical study of seven SEGAs and found typically low p53 expression; one tumor was focally positive for tuberin, the protein encoded by the *TSC2* gene, providing evidence for *TSC2*, and not *TP53*, being a tumor suppressor gene in SEGAs.

3.2. Ependymoma

3.2.1. Standard Pathology

Ependymomas are a clinically diverse group of glial tumors that range from aggressive intraventricular tumors in children to benign spinal cord tumors of adults. Consequently, pathological parameters can be less predictive of biological behavior than in other glial tumors. Ependymal tumors are commonly divided into ependymomas and anaplastic ependymomas, with two benign subtypes being subependymomas and myxopapillary ependymomas. Histologically, ependymomas display moderate cellularity with oval- to carrot-shaped cells containing a dense, speckled nucleus and tapering eosinophilic cytoplasm. Some tumors exhibit a glial appearance with a prominent fibrillary background, whereas others display more epithelioid features. One distinguishing characteristic of ependymomas is the often observed perivascular pseudorosette. Less commonly, ependymoma cells are arranged into true rosettes surrounding a true lumen. Like astrocytomas, ependymomas are often GFAP positive. Anaplastic lesions have additional features of malignancy, including pleomorphic nuclei, mitotic activity, and necrosis.

3.2.2. Molecular Pathology

Chromosome 22q loss is a common genetic alteration in ependymomas *(45,94,139)*. A candidate glioma tumor suppressor gene on chromosome 22q is the neurofibromatosis 2 (*NF2*) gene, because NF2 patients have a higher incidence of gliomas, particularly spinal ependymomas, as well as schwannomas and meningiomas. Mutations of the *NF2* gene have been documented in spinal ependymoma, confirming a role for *NF2* alterations in these lesions *(8,105)*. For cerebral ependymomas, the paucity of *NF2* mutations suggests that another, as yet unidentified, chromosome 22q gene may be responsible in the genesis of these tumors. In addition to 22q alterations, comparative genomic hybridization analysis has demonstrated gain of 1q and losses on 6q, 9, 13, and X in intracranial ependymomas, whereas gain on chromosome 7 was found almost exclusively in spinal cord lesions *(39)*. In a fine mapping study utilizing 384 microsatellite markers, chromosomal losses were detected on 1p, 6q, 16p, 16q, 17q, 19q, 20q, and 22q as well as the loss of whole chromosomes 13, 16, 19, and 20 *(129)*. Lamszus et al. *(58)* demonstrated that 11q loss was significantly inversely correlated with 22q loss in ependymomas and that approximately half of the tumors displaying 11q loss had a mutation in the multiple endocrine neoplasia-1 (*MEN1*) gene. Although mutations of the *TP53* gene do not appear to play a role in ependymoma tumorigenesis *(82)*, disruption of the p53 pathway may be affected through MDM2 *(126)* or p14^{ARF} *(54)*.

4. CHOROID PLEXUS TUMORS

4.1. Standard Pathology

Choroid plexus tumors are another varied group of lesions ranging from aggressive supratentorial intraventricular tumors of childhood to benign cerebellopontine angle tumors of adults. Histologically, the degree to which choroid plexus papillomas recapitulate the structure of the normal choroid plexus generally makes identification unequivocal. These tumors consist of papillae with fronds of columnar or cuboidal epithelium supported by a stroma of vascularized connective tissue. Mitotic figures and pleomorphism are rare in choroid plexus papillomas. When present, these tumors are often infiltrative and diagnosis is upgraded to choroid plexus carcinoma.

4.2. Molecular Pathology

Choroid plexus tumors have been reported occasionally in patients with von Hippel-Lindau (VHL) disease and Li-Fraumeni syndrome, raising the possibility that the *VHL* gene on chromosome 3p or the *TP53* gene on chromosome 17p, responsible for Li Fraumeni syndrome, is involved in choroid plexus tumorigenesis. Despite these findings, studies of human choroid plexus tumors have shown neither *VHL* nor *TP53* mutations, and it is possible that the VHL tumors were actually the papillary middle ear tumors typical of VHL *(48)*. However, choroid plexus neoplasms may be induced in transgenic mice by disrupting p53 and pRB function *(132)*. In addition, one study identified sequences similar to simian virus (SV40) virus, an oncogenic virus with the ability to inactivate both the p53 and Rb proteins, in human choroid plexus papillomas and ependymomas *(3)*. This was an intriguing observation because SV40 has been implicated as an oncogenic factor in transgenic models of choroid plexus tumors *(132)*. Although the presence of SV40 sequences has since been documented in additional studies, the role of oncogenic viruses in these tumors remains unclear and controversial *(40,59,72,83,154)*.

5. EMBRYONAL TUMORS

5.1. Standard Pathology

Embryonal tumors are malignant, poorly differentiated or "primitive" neoplasms that may show neuroectodermal and/or mesenchymal differentiation. These lesions occur most frequently in young children and histologically, are described as "small round blue cell tumors of the CNS." As such, classification of these tumors remains controversial. Some pathologists consider all such lesions under the general classification of "primitive neuroectodermal tumor" (PNET), stressing their similarities. Others highlight unique clinicopathological features and classify these lesions on the basis of differentiation or tumor location. Embryonal tumors classified on the basis of differentiation include neuroblastoma and ependymoblastoma; embryonal tumors classified on the basis of location include medulloblastoma, pineoblastoma, and retinoblastoma.

The most common embryonal tumor is the medulloblastoma. Histologically, medulloblastomas are densely cellular lesions composed of cells with scant cytoplasm and hyperchromatic, oval- to carrot-shaped nuclei. Prominent mitotic activity and single-cell necrosis are common. Some medulloblastomas feature undifferentiated cells, whereas others display architectural or immunohistochemical features of differentiation along neuronal, glial, or mesenchymal cell lines. Although medulloblastomas must be distinguished from other histologically similar tumors that do not respond similarly to current therapies, of particular significance are the atypical teratoid/rhabdoid (AT/RT) tumors. AT/RTs are highly malignant, therapy-resistant tumors of children that are distinguished from medulloblastomas based on the presence of "rhabdoid" cells in a PNET-like background.

5.2. Molecular Pathology

5.2.1. Medulloblastoma

Cytogenetic analysis of medulloblastomas has demonstrated that one-third to one-half of tumors have an isochromosome 17q *(7)*, whereas molecular genetic analysis has shown allelic loss of 17p *(18,128)*. TP53 mutations, however, are relatively uncommon in medulloblastomas compared to gliomas *(82,111)*. Furthermore, the most common regions of 17p loss are telomeric to the *TP53* gene *(4,18)*, suggesting the presence of a second, more distal chromosome 17p tumor suppressor gene. Other genetic alterations frequently noted in these tumors include allelic losses of chromosomes 6q, 10q, 11, and 16q *(128,151)*, as well as genomic losses on chromosomes 10q, 11, 16q, 17p, and 8p *(96)*. In contrast to many gliomas, deletions of the *CDKN2A* gene are rare in medulloblastomas *(93)*. Although oncogene amplification has not been a common finding in medulloblastomas, comparative genomic hybridization studies have demonstrated amplification of chromosome bands 5p15.3 and 11q22.3 and gains of chromosomes 17q and 7 *(96)*. The oncogene v-myc myelocytomatosis viral oncogene homologue *(MYCC)*/(avian) is amplified in a significant number of cases, however this alteration appears more frequently in medulloblastoma cell lines than in primary tumors *(7)*.

Two hereditary syndromes have provided insight into genetic pathways involved in medulloblastoma tumorigenesis. Turcot syndrome, characterized by a higher incidence of colonic and brain tumors, has been linked to medulloblastomas. Patients with adenomatous polyposis often display mutations of the adenomatosis polyposis coli *(APC)* gene on chromosome 5q and may develop medulloblastomas *(32)*. Although loss of chromosome 5q and *APC* gene mutations are infrequent in sporadic medulloblastomas *(53,152)*, rare mutations of β-catenin, a protein that functions in a common molecular pathway, have been noted *(53,156)*. Koch et al. *(53)* demonstrated that mutations affected the phosphorylation sites of the degradation targeting box of β-catenin and resulted in nuclear β-catenin protein accumulation, suggesting that inappropriate activation of the wingless-type mouse mammary tumor virus integration site family, member 1 (WNT)/wingless signaling pathway may contribute to the pathogenesis of these lesions. Additional insight into medulloblastoma tumorigenesis has been gained through the study of Gorlin syndrome. This condition is characterized by multiple basal cell carcinomas, bone cysts, dysmorphic features, and medulloblastomas. Gorlin syndrome has been shown to arise from defects in the patched *(PTCH)* gene, a homolog of the Drosophila patched gene, located on chromosome 9q. Medulloblastomas, particularly, the nodular desmoplastic forms characteristic of Gorlin disease, can display allelic loss of chromosome 9q and PTCH mutations *(89,92,116)*. Sporadic medulloblastomas have also demonstrated rare mutations in the smoothened *(SMO)* gene *(101)*; both the PTCH and SMO proteins function in a molecular pathway regulated by the Sonic hedgehog protein. Although likely, it remains to be determined whether additional genes involved in these two pathways may by implicated in medulloblastoma tumorigenesis.

5.2.2. Atypical Teratoid/Rhabdoid Tumors

Abnormalities of chromosome 22 distinguish (AT/RTs) from other PNETs *(104)*. Cytogenetic and molecular analysis mapped a candidate tumor suppressor region to 22q11.2 and, subsequently, homozygous deletions and mutations of the homology of yeast sucrose nonfermenting 5 *(hSNF5)*/integrase interactor 1 *(INI1)* gene have been identified *(5,6,134)*. Alterations of the *hSNF5/INI1* gene, which encodes a member of the chromatin-remodeling switching (SWI)/SNF multiprotein complex, were demonstrated in sporadic tumors and as germ-line mutations. Interestingly, in addition to rhabdoid tumors of the brain, this tumor suppressor gene appears to be involved in rhabdoid tumors of the kidney and other extrarenal sites.

5.3. Molecular Diagnostics and Prognostics

Recent advances in gene expression analysis have significantly advanced our understanding of the biology of medulloblastomas. Original studies provided evidence that the level of expression of the neurotrophin-3 receptor (trkC) related to prognosis, with high trkC expression correlating with a more favorable outcome *(118)*. More recently, it has been suggested that expression levels of the ErbB2 receptor may also act as a prognostic factor *(28)*. Deoxyribonucleic acid (DNA) microarray expression profiling has provided vast quantities of new information. This type of analysis has demonstrated that medulloblastomas are molecularly distinct from PNETs and AT/RTs; that medulloblastomas may be derived from cerebellar granule cells through activation of the Sonic hedgehog pathway; and that the clinical outcome of this disease is highly predictable on the basis of gene expression profiles *(91)*. Furthermore, a comparison between metastatic and nonmetastatic medulloblastomas has identified 85 genes that are differentially expressed between these two classes; notably, PDGFR-α and members of the rat sarcoma oncogene (RAS)/mitogen-activated protein kinase (MAPK) signal transduction pathway are upregulated in metastatic lesions *(70)*.

6. MENINGIOMA

6.1. Standard Pathology

Meningiomas are common intracranial tumors that arise in the meninges, often compressing the underlying brain. Despite the fact that most meningiomas are benign, grade I lesions, some "atypical" meningiomas exhibit a greater chance of local recurrence and some lesions present as malignant tumors. Meningiomas are tumors composed of neoplastic meningothelial cells. Although these tumors are typically associated with the dura mater, they are generally considered to arise from arachnoidal cells. Histological features of meningiomas include cellular whorls, psammoma bodies, and intranuclear pseudo-inclusions. Immunohistochemically, these lesions are characteristically positive for epithelial membrane antigen and vimentin. Ultrastructurally, many display extraordinarily complex interdigitating cell processes and numerous desmosomes and vimentin intermediate filaments. "Atypical" meningiomas, WHO grade II, are diagnosed when a combination of the following features are noted: hypercellularity, pleomorphism, moderate mitotic activity, focal necrosis, and a lack of either a whorling, fascicular or lobular architectural pattern. Anaplastic meningiomas, WHO grade III, are characterized by malignant histological features and sometimes metastasis to systemic sites.

6.2. Molecular Pathology

The best characterized genetic alterations in meningiomas involve chromosome 22. Monosomy 22 is common in meningiomas and mutations of the *NF2* gene on chromosome 22q are found frequently, clearly implicating a role for NF2 in meningioma tumorigenesis *(61,107,145)*. In sporadic meningiomas, allelic loss of chromosome 22q and *NF2* mutations are more common in fibroblastic and transitional forms than in meningothelial lesions *(145)*. A few meningiomas have been described with loss of portions of chromosome 22q that do not include the *NF2* gene, suggesting that a second meningioma locus might be found on chromosome 22q *(108)*. One recent study demonstrated a potential mutation hotspot in exon 9 of the *hSNF5/INI1* gene in a small number of meningiomas, raising the possibility that *hSNF5/INI1* may be a second tumor suppressor gene on chromosome 22 in these lesions *(114)*.

Approximately 40% of meningiomas display neither *NF2* gene mutations nor chromosome 22q allelic loss and, as such, it is likely that additional meningioma tumor suppressor genes exist. One study has suggested the possibility of alternative meningioma genes on chromosomes 1p and 3p *(16)*. Moreover, allelic losses in meningiomas have been demonstrated on a number of chromosomes, including 1p, 3p, 5p, 5q, 11, 13, and 17p *(115,143)*.

Atypical meningiomas often exhibit allelic losses 1p, 6q, 9q, 10q, 14q, 17p, and 18q, implicating these loci in tumor progression *(57,63,102,143)*. Furthermore, more frequent losses of 6q, 9p, 10, and 14q are seen in anaplastic meningiomas *(86,143)*. Bostrom et al. *(11)* have suggested that the majority of anaplastic meningiomas display genetic alterations of *CDKN2A*, p14^{ARF}, and *CDKN2B*, indicating that inactivation of cell-cycle control is an important aberration in these lesions. In addition to chromosomal losses, higher-grade meningiomas have also demonstrated chromosomal gains, with gains of 20q, 12q, 15q, 1q, 9q, and 17q being the most common *(86,143)*. Overexpression of PDGF B chain and the PDGF β-receptor has also been demonstrated in meningiomas and appears to correlate with tumor grade *(149)*.

6.3. Molecular Diagnostics and Prognostics

Molecular genetic analysis has aided the diagnosis of meningioma by further defining the markers of malignancy. Although invasion into the surrounding brain was once an indicator of malignancy in meningioma, molecular studies have shown that histologically benign lesions that invade the brain do not display the genetic alterations indicative of a higher-grade meningioma *(143)*; in particular, chromosomal 10 loss has been associated with lesions designated as malignant on the basis of morphological features, but not those meningiomas thought to be malignant from the presence of brain invasion *(102)*. In the search for prognostic indicators, both 1p and 14q deletions have been implicated in the ability to predict tumor recurrence *(14,49)*.

7. PERIPHERAL NERVE SHEATH TUMORS

7.1. Standard Pathology

Peripheral nerve sheath tumors (PNSTs) are a diverse group of neoplasms with distinct clinico-pathological profiles. Although these tumors arise from peripheral nerve, their significance to the CNS can be seen in their ability to compress the CNS when they occur on cranial nerves or in paraspinal locations. The three major forms of PNST are schwannomas, neurofibromas, and malignant peripheral nerve sheath tumors (MPNSTs).

Schwannomas are benign tumors of the peripheral nerve, although they may arise on cranial nerves. Histologically, these lesions typically demonstrate two distinct architectural patterns: 1. "Antoni A" areas contain densely packed cells in fascicles and focally forming Verocay bodies and 2. "Antoni B" areas are looser in texture, with microcystic changes. Schwannoma cells are elongated, sometimes with blunt nuclei, and commonly display considerable pleomorphism. Immunohistochemically, these tumors stain strongly for the S-100 protein. Malignant transformation of schwannomas is rare.

Neurofibromas are also benign tumors that may arise within peripheral nerves. These tumors are characterized by delicate, wavy spindle cells in a prominent myxoid matrix, often with scattered mast cells. MPNSTs are highly malignant sarcomas, many of which arise in the setting of a preexisting plexiform neurofibroma, lesions characteristic of NF1. MPNSTs are densely cellular spindle tumors in which highly anaplastic, mitotically active cells form fascicles. Some MPNSTs exhibit divergent differentiation with epithelial, glandular, and skeletal muscle elements admixed.

7.2. Molecular Pathology

NF2 patients are defined by the presence of bilateral vestibular schwannomas *(68)*, in contrast to unilateral vestibular schwannomas, which are common in the general population. Schwannomas, like meningiomas, occur frequently in NF2 patients, frequently have loss of chromosome 22q, and harbor *NF2* gene mutations in at least 50% of cases *(68)*. Loss of merlin, the *NF2* encoded protein, occurs in all schwannomas, consistent with an integral and universal role for *NF2* inactivation in both inherited and sporadic forms of schwannoma *(125)*.

Analogous to schwannomas, multiple neurofibromas are associated with NF1, suggesting that the *NF1* gene on chromosome 17q is involved in the formation of these benign lesions. Unfortunately, the large size of the *NF1* gene has precluded extensive mutation analysis in these tumors. Neurofibromas, particularly the NF1-associated plexiform variants, can undergo malignant progression to MPNSTs, a transition that can be accompanied by genetic alterations including inactivation of the *NF1*, *TP53*, and *CDKN2A* genes *(60,73,77)*. However, although *CDKN2A* inactivation appears to occur almost equally in NF1-associated and sporadic MPNSTs, alterations to p53 expression are more restricted to sporadic MPNSTs *(9)*. These findings and other cytogenetic studies *(90)* suggest that NF1-associated and sporadic MPNSTs may exploit different oncogenetic pathways.

8. MISCELLANEOUS TUMORS

8.1. Hemangioblastoma

8.1.1. Standard Pathology

Hemangioblastomas are benign, well-circumscribed, and often cystic tumors. These lesions are neoplasms of uncertain origin and are composed of stromal cells, endothelial cells, and pericytes. Stromal cells feature a lipid-laden, vacuolated cytoplasm, and moderately pleomorphic nucleus. Although the nuclei of the stromal cells may be hyperchromatic, neither the stromal cells nor the endothelial cells display anaplastic features.

8.1.2. Molecular Pathology

Multiple hemangioblastomas are characteristic of VHL disease, an inherited tumor syndrome in which patients may develop a variety of lesions, including hemangioblastomas, retinal angiomas, renal cell carcinomas, and pheochromocytomas *(76)*. Allelic loss has been demonstrated in hemangioblastomas in the region of the *VHL* gene on chromosome 3 *(20)*, and the *VHL* gene is mutated in sporadic hemangioblastomas *(47)*. These observations suggest that *VHL* acts as a classical tumor suppressor gene and is involved in both familial and sporadic hemangioblastomas. The biological function of the VHL protein appears complex, with evidence suggesting it may stabilize mRNA of angiogenic compounds, such as vascular endothelial growth factor (VEGF) *(29)*, as well as extracellular matrix components such as fibronectin *(84)*. Moreover, VHL complexes have been shown to target the ubiquitination of hypoxia-inducible factor (HIF)-1α *(1)*, and expression of HIF1-α has been demonstrated in stromal cells throughout hemangioblastomas *(153)*.These actions of VHL provide a possible explanation for the highly vascular nature of hemangioblastomas. Comparative genomic hybridization in 10 cerebellar hemangioblastomas revealed common losses of chromosomes 3, 6, 9, and 18q and a gain of chromosome 19 *(123)*.

8.2. Hemangiopericytoma

8.2.1. Standard Pathology

Hemangiopericytomas (HPCs) are dural tumors that may display locally aggressive behavior and may metastasize. The classification of HPCs has been controversial, with some pathologists describing the lesion as a distinct entity and others classifying it as a subtype of meningioma. HPC cells are often homogeneously dense and are sometimes arranged in lobules. Neoplastic cells contain very little cytoplasm and have nuclei that may appear spindled and thin to oval in shape. One characteristic feature is the presence of reticulin fibers that encase individual neoplastic cells. HPCs can be subdivided into differentiated and anaplastic lesions, with anaplastic tumors displaying mitotic activity and necrosis.

8.2.2. Molecular Pathology

Homogeneous deletion of the *CDKN2A* gene is a common genetic alteration in HPCs, suggesting that the p16-mediated cell-cycle regulatory pathway may play a key tumorigenic role in some HPCs

(85). Interestingly, this alteration is not prevalent in meningiomas. Further, mutations of the *NF2* gene, common in meningiomas, are not found in HPCs implying that HPCs are genetically distinct from meningiomas *(46)*. Another common genetic alteration of HPCs is the rearrangement of chromosome 12q13, suggesting that an oncogene or tumor suppressor gene at this locus is important in HPC tumorigenesis. A number of known oncogenes reside in this region, including *MDM2*, *CDK4*, and C/EBP-homologous protein (*CHOP*)/ growth arrest- and DNA damage-inducible gene (*GADD*)*153*.

9. SUMMARY

In this chapter, we have reviewed the current classification and molecular pathology of primary neoplasms of the CNS. Molecular genetic alterations have been discussed that are characteristic of specific tumor types and stages of progression, greatly augmenting the current WHO classification system. There remain additional types of tumors that could benefit greatly from a differential diagnosis. In addition, the value of genetic profiling in clinical patient management, aiding in diagnostic and therapeutic decisions as well as prognostic estimation, has been illustrated. Of note, DNA microarray expression profiling is now providing large quantities of new information. Currently, a plethora of gene expression profiling studies are being conducted on other classes of brain tumors, in particular the diffuse gliomas *(25,64,103,109,142)*, and initial results give every indication that microarray analysis will be as informative for these lesions as it has been for medulloblastomas (Subheading 4.3.). Most importantly, as more is understood about the molecular pathways involved in brain tumorigenesis, such knowledge will likely contribute to the development of more effective treatment for these tumors.

REFERENCES

1. Aso T., Yamazaki K., Aigaki T., Kitajima S.. 2000. Drosophila von Hippel-Lindau tumor suppressor complex possesses E3 ubiquitin ligase activity. *Biochem. Biophys. Res. Commun.* **276:**355–361.
2. Barker F.G., II, Simmons M.L., Chang S.M., Prados M.D., Larson D.A., Sneed P.K., et al. 2001. EGFR overexpression and radiation response in glioblastoma multiforme. *Int. J. Radiat. Oncol. Biol. Phys.* **51:**410–418.
3. Bergsagel D.J., Finegold M.J., Butel J.S., Kupsky W.J., Garcea R.L.. 1992. DNA sequences similar to those of simian virus 40 in ependymomas and choroid plexus tumors of childhood. *N. Engl. J. Med.* **326:**988–993.
4. Biegel J. A., Burk C.D., Barr F.G., Emanuel B.S. 1992. Evidence for a 17p tumor related locus distinct from p53 in pediatric primitive neuroectodermal tumors. *Cancer Res.* **52:**3391–3395.
5. Biegel J.A., Kalpana G., Knudsen E.S., Packer R.J., Roberts C.W.M., Thiele C.J., et al. 2002. The role of INI1 and the SWI/SNF complex in the development of rhabdoid tumors: meeting summary from the Workshop on Childhood Atypical Teratoid/Rhabdoid Tumors. *Cancer Res.* **62:**323–328.
6. Biegel J.A., Zhou J.-Y., Rorke L.B., Stenstrom C., Wainwright L.M., Fogelgren B. 1999. Germ-line and acquired mutations of INI1 in atypial teratoid and rhabdoid tumors. *Cancer Res.* **59:**74–79.
7. Bigner S.H., Vogelstein B. 1990. Cytogenetics and molecular genetics of malignant gliomas and medulloblastoma. *Brain Pathol.* **1:**12–18.
8. Birch B.D., Johnson J.P., Parsa A., Desai R.D., Yoon J.T., Lycette C.A., et al. 1996. Frequent type 2 neurofibromatosis gene transcript mutations in sporadic intramedullary spinal cord ependymomas. *Neurosurgery* **39:**135–140.
9. Birindelli S., Perrone F., Oggionni M., Lavarino C., Pasini B., Vergani B., et al. 2001. Rb and TP53 pathway alterations in sporadic and NF1-related malignant peripheral nerve sheath tumors. *Lab. Invest.* **81:**833–844.
10. Bogler O., Huang H.-J.S., Cavenee W.K. 1995. Loss of wild-type p53 bestows a growth advantage on primary cortical astrocytes and facilitates their in vitro transformation. *Cancer Res.* **55:**2746–2751.
11. Bostrom J., Meyer—Puttlitz B., Wolter M., Blaschke B., Weber R.G., Lichter P., et al. 2001. Alterations of the tumor suppressor genes CDKN2A (p16(INK4a)), p14(ARF), CDKN2B (p15(INK4b)), and CDKN2C (p18(INK4c)) in atypical and anaplastic meningiomas. *Am. J. Path.* **159:**661–669.
12. Burns K.L., Ueki K., Jhung S.L., Koh J., Louis D.N. 1998. Molecular genetic correlates of p16, cdk4 and pRb immunohistochemistry in glioblastomas. *J. Neuropathol. Exp. Neurol.* **57:**122–130.
13. Burton E.C., Lamborn K.R., Forsyth P., Scott J., O'Campo J., Uyehara-Lock J., et al. 2002. Aberrant p53, mdm2, and proliferation differ in glioblastomas from long-term compared with typical survivors. *Clin. Cancer Res.* **8:**180–187.
14. Cai D.X., Banerjee R., Scheithauer B.W., Lohse C.M., Kleinschmidt-Demasters B.K., Perry A.. 2001. Chromosome 1p and 14q FISH analysis in clinicopathologic subsets of meningioma: diagnostic and prognostic implications. *J. Neuropathol. Exp. Neurol.* **60:**628–636.

15. Cairncross J.G., Ueki K., Zlatescu M.C., Lisle D.K., Finkelstein D.M., Hammond R.R., et al. 1998. Specific chromo-
    somal losses predict chemotherapeutic response and survival in patients with anaplastic oligodendrogliomas. *J. Natl.
    Cancer Inst.* **90:**1473–1479.

16. Carlson K.M., Bruder C., Nordenskjold M., Dumanski J.P.. 1997. 1p and 3p deletions in meningiomas without detect-
    able aberrations of chromosome 22 identified by comparative genomic hybridization. *Genes Chromosomes Cancer*
    20:419–424.

17. Cavenee W.K., Furnari F.B., Nagane M., Huang H.-J.S., Newcomb E.W., Bigner D.D., et al. 2000. Diffuse astrocyto-
    mas, *in Pathology and Genetics of Tumours of the Nervous System. International Agency for Research on Cancer* (P.
    Kleihues, P., Cavenee, W.K., eds.), IARC Press, Lyon, France, pp. 10–21.

18. Cogen P.H., Daneshvar L., Metzger A.K., Edwards M.S.B. 1990. Deletion mapping of the medulloblastoma locus on
    chromosome 17p. *Genomics* **8:**279–285.

19. Costello J.F., Plass C., Arap W., Chapman V.M., Held W.A., Berger M.S., et al. 1997. Cyclin-dependent kinase 6
    (CDK6) amplification in human gliomas identified using two-dimensional separation of genomic DNA. *Cancer Res.*
    57:1250–1254.

20. Crossey P.A., Foster K., Richards F.M., Phipps M.E., Latif F., Tory K., et al. 1994. Molecular genetic investigations of
    the mechanism of tumourigenesis in von Hippel-Lindau disease: analysis of allele loss in VHL tumours. *Hum. Genet.*
    93:53–58.

21. Dong S.M., Pang J.C., Poon W.S., Hu J., To K.F., Chang A.R., Ng H.K.. 2001. Concurrent hypermethylation of mul-
    tiple genes is associated with grade of oligodendroglial tumors. *J Neuropathol. Exp. Neurol.* **60:**808–816.

22. Dürr E.-M., Rollbrocker B., Hayashi Y., Peters N., Meyer-Puttlitz B., Louis D.N., et al. 1998. PTEN mutations in
    gliomas and glioneuronal gliomas. *Oncogene* **16:**2259–2264.

23. Ekstrand A.J., James C.D., Cavenee W.K., Seliger B.,Petterson R.F., Collins V.P. 1991. Genes for epidermal growth
    factor receptor, transforming growth factor α, and epidermal growth factor and their expression in human gliomas in
    vivo. *Cancer Res.* **51:**2164–2172.

24. Fuller G.N., Bigner S.H.. 1992. Amplified cellular oncogenes in neoplasms of the human central nervous system.
    Mutat. Res. **276:**299–306.

25. Fuller G.N., Hess K.R., Rhee C.H., Yung W.K.A., Sawaya R.A., Bruner J.M., Zhang W.. 2002. Molecular classifica-
    tion of human diffuse gliomas by multidimensional scaling analysis of gene expression profiles parallels morphology-
    based classification, correlates with survival, and reveals clinically-relevant novel glioma subsets. *Brain Pathol.*
    12:108–116.

26. Furnari F.B., Lin H., Huang H.S., Cavenee W.K. 1997. Growth suppression of glioma cells by PTEN requires a func-
    tional phosphatase catalytic domain. *Proc. Natl. Acad. Sci. USA* **94:**12479–12484.

27. Giannini C., Hebrink D., Scheithauer B.W., Dei Tos A.P., James C.D.. 2001. Analysis of p53 mutation and expression
    in pleomorphic xanthoastrocytomas. *Neurogenetics* **3:**159–162.

28. Gilbertson R., Wickramasinghe C., Hernan R., Balaji V., Hunt D., Jones D.- et al. 2001. Clinical and molecular strati-
    fication of disease risk in medulloblastoma. *Br. J. Cancer* **85:**705–712.

29. GnarraJ.R., Zhou S., Merrill M.J., Wagner J.R., Krumm A., Papavassiliou E., et al. 1996. Post-transcriptional regula-
    tion of vascular endothelial growth factor mRNA by the product of the VHL tumor suppressor gene. *Proc. Natl. Acad.
    Sci. USA* **93:**10589–10594.

30. Green A.J., Johnson P.H., Yates J.R. 1994. The tuberous sclerosis gene on chromosome 9q34 acts as a growth suppres-
    sor. *Hum. Mol. Genet.* **3:**1833–1834.

31. Green A.J., Smith M., Yates J.R.W. 1994. Loss of heterozygosity on chromosome 16p13.3 in hamartomas from tuber-
    ous sclerosis patients. *Nat. Genet.* **6:**193–196.

32. Hamilton S.R., Liu B., Parsons R.E., Papadopoulos N., Jen J., Powell S.M., et al.1995. The molecular basis of Turcot's
    syndrome. *N. Eng. J. Med.* **332:**839–847.

33. Hayashi Y., Ueki K., Waha A., Wiestler O.D., Louis D.N., von Deimling A.. 1997. Association of EGFR gene ampli-
    fication and CDKN2 (p16/MTS1) gene deletion in glioblastoma multiforme. *Brain Pathol.* **7:**871–875.

34. He J., Allen J.R., Collins V.P., Allalunis—Turner M.J., Godbout R., Day R.S.I., James C.D. 1994. CDK4 amplification
    is an alternative mechanism to p16 gene homozygous deletion in glioma cell lines. *Cancer Res.* **54:**5804–5807.

35. He J., Mokhtari K., Sanson M., Marie Y., Kujas M., Huguet S., et al. 2001. Glioblastomas with an oligodendroglial
    component: a pathological and molecular study. *J. Neuropathol. Exp. Neurol.* **60:**863–871.

36. Henske E.P., Scheithauer B.W., Short M.P., Wollmann R., Nahmias J., Hornigold N., et al. 1996. Allelic loss is fre-
    quent in tuberous sclerosis kidney lesions but rare in brain lesions. *Am. J. Hum. Genet.* **59:**400–406.

37. Henson J.W., Schnitker B.L., Correa K.M., von Deimling A., Fassbender F., Xu H.-J., et al. 1994. The retinoblastoma
    gene is involved in malignant progression of astrocytomas. Ann. Neurol. **36:**714–721.

38. Hermanson M., Funa K., Westermark B., Heldin C.H., Wiestler O.D., Louis D.N., et al. 1996. Association of loss of
    heterozygosity on chromosome 17p with high platelet-derived growth factor α receptor expression in human malignant
    gliomas. *Cancer Res.* **56:**164–171.

39. Hirose Y., Aldape K., Bollen A., James C.D., Brat D., Lamborn K., et al. 2001. Chromosomal abnormalities subdivide
    ependymal tumors into clinically relevant groups. *Am. J. Path.* **158:**1137–1143.

40. Huang H., Reis R., Yonekawa Y., Lopes J.M., Kleihues P., Ohgaki H. 1999. Identification in human brain tumors of DNA sequences specific for SV40 large T antigen. *Brain Pathol.* **9:**33–42.

41. Hui A.B.Y., Lo K.W., Yin X.L., Poon W.S., Ng H.K. 2001. Detection of multiple gene amplifications in glioblastoma multiforme using array-based comparative genomic hybridization. *Lab. Invest.* **81:**717–723.

42. Ino Y., Betensky R.A., Zlatescu M.C., Sasaki H., Macdonald D.R., Stemmer-Rachamimov A.O., et al. 2001. Molecular subtypes of anaplastic oligodendroglioma: implications for patient management at diagnosis. *Clin. Cancer Res.* **7:**839–845.

43. Ino Y., Silver J.S., Blazejewski L., Nishikawa R., Matsutani M., von Deimling A., Louis D.N.. 1999. Common regions of deletion on chromosome 22q12.3-13.1 and 22q13.2 in human astrocytomas appear related to malignancy grade. *J. Neuropathol. Exp. Neurol.* **58:**881–885.

44. James C.D., Carlblom E., Dumanski J.P., Hansen M., Nordenskjold M., Collins V.P., Cavenee W.K. 1988. Clonal genomic alterations in glioma malignancy stages. *Cancer Res.* **48:**5546–5551.

45. James C.D., He J., Carlbom E., Mikkelsen T., Ridderheim P.-A., Cavenee W.K., Collins V.P. 1990. Loss of genetic information in central nervous system tumors common to children and young adults. *Genes Chromosomes Cancer* **2:** 94–102.

46. Joseph J.T., Lisle D.K., Jacoby L.B., Paulus W., Barone R., Cohen M.L., et al. 1995. NF2 gene analysis distinguishes hemangiopericytoma from meningioma. *Am. J. Pathol.* **147:**1450–1455.

47. Kanno H., Kondo K., Ito S., Yamamoto I., Fujii S., Torigoe S., et al. 1994. Somatic mutations of the von Hippel-Lindau tumor suppressor gene in sporadic central nervous system hemangioblastomas. *Cancer Res.* **54:**4845–4847.

48. Kempermann G., Neumann H.P., Volk B. 1998. Endolymphatic sac tumours. *Histopathology* **33:**2–10.

49. Ketter R., Henn W., Niedermayer I., Steilen-Gimbel H., Konig J., Zang K.D., Steudel W.I.. 2001. Predictive value of progression-associated chromosomal aberrations for the prognosis of menigiomas: a retrospective study of 198 cases. *J. Neurosurg.* **95:**601–607.

50. Kim S.K., Wang K.C., Cho B.K., Jung H.W., Lee Y.J., Chung Y.S., et al. 2001. Biological behavior and tumorigenesis of subependymal giant cell astrocytomas. *J. Neurooncol.* **52:**217–225.

51. Kleihues P., Cavenee W.K.. 2000. *World Health Organization Classification of Tumours of the Nervous System.* WHO/ IARC Press, Lyon, France.

52. Kluwe L., Hagel G., Tatagiba M., Thomas S., Stavrou D., Ostertag H., et al. 2001. Loss of NF1 alleles distinguish sporadic from NF1-associated pilocytic astrocytomas. *J. Neuropathol. Exp. Neurol.* **60:**917–920.

53. Koch A.,Waha A., Tonn J.C., Sorenson N., Berthold F., Wolter M., et al. 2001. Somatic mutations of WNT/wingless signaling pathway components in primitive neuroectodermal tumors. *Int. J. Cancer* **93:**445–449.

54. Korshunov A., Golanov A., Timirgaz V. 2001. p14ARF protein (FL–132) immunoreactivity in intracranial ependymomas and its prognostic significance: an analysis of 103 cases. *Acta. Neuropathol.* **102:**271–277.

55. Kraus J.A., Koopman J., Kaskel P., Maintz D., Brandner S., Louis D.N., et al. 1995. Shared allelic losses on chromosomes 1p and 19q suggest a common origin of oligodendroglioma and oligoastrocytoma. *J. Neuropathol. Exp. Neurol.* **54:**91–95.

56. Kunwar S., Mohapatra G., Bollen A., Lamborn K., Prados M., Feuerstein B.G.. 2001. Genetic subgroups of anaplastic astrocytoma correlate with patient age and survival. *Cancer Res.* **61:**7683–7688.

57. Lamszus K., Kluwe L., Matschke J., Meissner H., Laas R., Westphal M.. 1999. Allelic losses at 1p, 9q, 10q, 14q, and 22q in the progression of aggressive meningiomas and undifferentiated meningeal sarcomas. *Cancer Genet. Cytogenet.* **110:**103–110.

58. Lamszus K., Lachenmayer L., Heinemann U., Kluwe L., Finckh U., Hoppner W., et al. 2001. Molecular genetic alterations on chromosomes 11 and 22 in ependymomas. *Int. J. Cancer* **91:**803–808.

59. Lednicky J.A., Garcea R.L., Bergsagel D.J., Butel J.S. 1995. Natural simian virus 40 strains are present in human choroid plexus and ependymoma tumors. *Virology* **212:**710–717.

60. Legius E., Marchuk D.A., Collins F.S., Glover T.W. 1993. Somatic deletion of the neurofibromatosis type 1 gene in a neurofibrosarcoma supports a tumor suppressor gene hypothesis. *Nat. Genet.* **3:**122–126.

61. Lekanne Deprez R.H., Bianchi A.B., Groen N.A., Seizinger B.R., Hagemeijer A., et al. 1994. Frequent NF2 gene transcript mutations in sporadic meningiomas and vestibular schwannomas. *Am. J. Hum. Genet.* **54:**1022–1029.

62. Li J., Yen C., Liaw D., Podsypanina K., Bose S., Wang S.I., et al. 1997. PTEN, a putative protein tyrosine phosphatase gene mutated in human brain, breast and prostate cancer. *Science* **275:**1943–1947.

63. Lindblom A., Ruttledge M., Collins V.P., Nordenskjold M., Dumanski J.P. 1994. Chromosomal deletions in anaplastic meningiomas suggest multiple regions outside chromosome 22 as important in tumor progression. *Int. J. Cancer* **56:**354–357.

64. Ljubimova J.Y., Lakhter A.J., Loksh A., Yong W.H., Riedinger M.S., Miner J.H., et al. 2001. Overexpression of $\alpha 4$ chain-containing laminins in human glial tumors identified by gene microarray analysis. *Cancer Res.* **61:**5601–5610.

65. Louis D.N. 1994. The p53 gene and protein in human brain tumors. *J. Neuropathol. Exp. Neurol.* **53:**11–21.

66. Louis D.N., Cavenee W.K. 2001. Molecular biology of central nervous system tumors, *in Cancer: Principles and Practice of Oncology*, 6 ed.(DeVita, V.T., Hellman, S., Rosenberg, S.A., eds.), Lippincott-Raven, Philadephia, PA, pp. 2013–2022.

67. Louis D.N., Holland E.C., Cairncross J.G. 2001. Glioma classification: a molecular reappraisal. *Am. J. Path.* **159:** 779–786.

68. Louis D.N., Ramesh V., Gusella J.F. 1995. Neuropathology and molecular genetics of neurofibromatosis 2 and related tumors. *Brain Pathol.* **5:**163–172.

69. Louis D.N., von Deimling A., Chung R.Y., Rubio M.-P., Whaley J.H., Ohgaki H., et al. 1993. Comparative study of p53 gene and protein alterations in human astrocytomas. *J. Neuropathol. Exp. Neurol.* **52:**31–38.

70. MacDonald T.J., Brown K.M., LaFleur B., Peterson K., Lawlor C., Chen Y., et al. 2001. Expression profiling of medulloblastoma: PDGFRA and the RAS/MAPK pathway as therapeutic targets for metastatic disease. *Nat. Genet.* **29:**143–152.

71. Maintz D., Fiedler K., Koopman J., Rollbrocker B., Nechev S., Klinkhammer M.A., et al. 1997. Molecular genetic evidence for subtypes of oligoastrocytomas. *J. Neuropathol. Exp. Neurol.* **56:**1098–1104.

72. Malkin D., Chilton-MacNeill S., Meister L.A., Sexsmith E., Diller L, Garcea R.L.. 2001. Tissue-specific expression of SV40 in tumors associated with the Li-Fraumeni syndrome. *Oncogene* **20:**4441–4449.

73. Menon A.G., Anderson K.M., Riccardi V.M., Chung R.Y., Whaley J.M., Yandell D.W., et al. 1990. Chromosome 17p deletions and p53 gene mutations associated with the formation of malignant neurofibrosarcomas in Recklinghausen neurofibromatosis. *Proc. Natl. Acad. Sci. USA* **87:**5435–5439.

74. Merlo A., Herman J.G., Mao L., Lee D.J., Gabrielson E., Burger P.C., et al. 1995. 5'CpG island methylation is associated with transcriptional silencing of the tumor suppressor p16/CDKN2/MTS1. *Nat. Med.* **1:**686–692.

75. Mohapatra G., Bollen A.W., Kim D.H., Lamborn K., Moore D.H., Prados M.D., Feuerstein B.G. 1998. Genetic analysis of glioblastoma multiforme provides evidence for subgroups within the grade. *Genes Chromosomes Cancer* **21:**195–206.

76. Neumann H.P.H., Lips C.J.M., Hsia Y.E., Zbar B. 1995. Von Hippel Lindau syndrome. *Brain Pathol.* **5:**181193.

77. Nielsen G.P., Stemmer-Rachamimov A.O., Ino Y., Møller M.B., Rosenberg A.E., Louis D.N. 1999. Malignant transformation of neurofibromas in neurofibromatosis 1 is associated with CDKN2A/p16 inactivation. *Am. J. Pathol.* **155:**1879–1884.

78. Niida Y., Stemmer-Rachamimov A.O., Logrip M., Tapon D., Perez R., Kwiatkowski D.J., et al. 2001. Survey of somatic mutations in tuberous sclerosis complex (TSC) hamartomas suggests different genetic mechanisms for pathogenesis of TSC lesions. *Am. J. Hum. Genet.* **69:**493–503.

79. Nishikawa R., Furnari F., Lin H., Arap W., Berger M.S., Cavenee W.K., Huang H.-J.S. 1995. Loss of p16[INK4] expression is frequent in high grade gliomas. *Cancer Res.* **55:**1941–1945.

80. Nishikawa R., Ji X.D., Harmon R.C., Lazar C.S., Gill G.N., Cavenee W.K., Huang H.-J.S.. 1994. A mutant epidermal growth factor receptor common in human glioma confers enhanced tumorigenicity. *Proc. Natl. Acad. Sci. USA* **91:**7727–7731.

81. Nishizaki T., Ozaki S., Harada K., Ito H., Arai H., Beppu T., Sasaki K.. 1998. Investigation of genetic alterations associated with the grade of astrocytic tumor by comparative genomic hybridization. *Genes Chromosomes Cancer* **21:** 340–346.

82. Ohgaki H., Eibl R.H., Wiestler O.D., Yasargil M.G., Newcomb E.W., Kleihues P. 1991. p53 mutations in nonastrocytic human brain tumors. *Cancer Res.* **51:**6202–5.

83. Ohgaki H., Huang H., Haltia M., Vainio H., Kleihues P. 2000. More about: cell and molecular biology of simian virus 40: implications for human infections and disease. *J. Natl. Cancer Inst.* **92:**495–497.

84. Ohh M., Yauch R.L., Lonergan K.M., Whaley J.M., Stemmer-Rachamimov A.O., et al. 1998. The von Hippel-Lindau tumor suppressor protein is required for proper assembly of extracellular fibronectin matrix. *Mol. Cell* **1:**959–968.

85. Ono Y., Ueki K., Joseph J.T., Louis D.N.. 1996. Homozygous deletions of the CDKN2/p16 gene in dural hemangiopericytomas. *Acta. Neuropathol.* **91:**221–225.

86. Ozaki S., Nishizaki T., Ito H., Sasaki H. 1999. Comparative genomic hybridization analysis of genetic alterations associated with malignant progression of meningioma. *J. Neurooncol.* **41:**167–174.

87. Parry L., Maynard J.H., Patel A., Hodges A.K., von Deimling A., Sampson J.R., Cheadle J.P. 2000. Molecular analysis of the TSC1 and TSC2 tumour suppressor genes in sporadic glial and glioneuronal tumours. *Hum. Genet.* **107:**350–356.

88. Paulus W., Lisle D.K., Tonn J.C., Roggendorf W., Wolf H.K., Reeves S.A., Louis D.N. 1996. Molecular genetic alterations in pleomorphic xanthoastrocytoma. *Acta. Neuropathol.* **91:**293–297.

89. Pietsch T., Waha A., Koch A., Kraus J., Albrecht S., Tonn J., et al. 1997. Medulloblastomas of the desmoplastic variant carry mutations of the human homologue of Drosophila patched. *Cancer Res.* **57:**2085–2088.

90. Plaat B.E., Molenaar W.M., Mastik M.F., Hoekstra H.J., te Meerman G.J., van den Berg E.. 1999. Computer-assisted cytogenetic analysis of 51 malignant peripheral-nerve-sheath tumors: sporadic vs. neurofibromatosis-type-1-associated malignant schwannomas. *Int. J. Cancer* **83:**171–178.

91. Pomeroy S.L., Tamayo P., Gaasenbeek M., Sturla L.M., Angelo M., McLaughlin M.E., et al. 2002. Prediction of central nervous system embryonal tumour outcome based on gene expression. *Nature* **415:**436–442.

92. Raffel C., Jenkins R.B., Frederick L., Hebrink D., Alderete B., Fults D.W., James C.D. 1997. Sporadic medulloblastomas contain PTCH mutations. *Cancer Res.* **57:**842–845.

93. Raffel C., Ueki K., Harsh G.R., Louis D.N. 1995. The multiple tumor suppressor 1 / cyclin dependent kinase inhibitor 2 gene (MTS1/CDKN2) in human central nervous system primitive neuroectodermal tumor. *Neurosurgery* **36:**971–974.

94. Ransom D.T., Ritland S.R., Kimmel P.J., Moertel C.A., Dahl R.J., Scheithauer R.B., Kelly P.J., Jenkins R.B. 1992. Cytogenetic and loss of heterozygosity studies in ependymomas, pilocytic astrocytomas, and oligodendrogliomas. *Genes Chromosomes Cancer* **5:**348–356.

95. Rasheed B.K.A., McLendon R.E., Herndon J.E., Friedman H.S., Friedman A.H., Bigner D.D., Bigner S.H. 1994. Alterations of the TP53 gene in human gliomas. *Cancer Res.* **54:**1324–1330.

96. Reardon D.A., Michalkiewicz E., Boyett J.M., Sublett J.E., Entrekin R.E., Ragsdale S.T., et al.1997. Extensive genomic abnormalities in childhood medulloblastoma by comparative genomic hybridization. *Cancer Res.* **57:**4042–4047.

97. Reifenberger G., Kros J.M., Burger P.C., Louis D.N., Collins V.P. 2000. Oligodendrogliomas and oligoastrocytomas, in *World Health Organization Classification of Tumours of the Central Nervous System* (Kleihues P., Cavenee W.K., eds.),. IARC/WHO, Lyon, France, pp. 55–69.

98. Reifenberger G., Reifenberger J., Ichimura K., Melzter P.S., Collins V.P. 1994. Amplification of multiple genes from chromosomal region 12q13-14 in human malignant gliomas: preliminary mapping of the amplicons shows preferential involvement of CDK4, SAS, and MDM2. *Cancer Res.* **54:**4299–4303.

99. Reifenberger J., Reifenberger G., Liu L., James C.D., Wechsler W., Collins V.P. 1994. Molecular genetic analysis of oligodendroglial tumors shows preferential allelic deletions on 19q and 1p. *Am. J. Pathol.* **145:**1175–1190.

100. Reifenberger J., Ring G.U., Gies U., Cobbers J.M.J.L., Oberstraβ J.,An H.-X, et al. 1996. Analysis of p53 mutation and epidermal growth factor receptor amplification in recurrent gliomas with malignant progression. *J. Neuropathol. Exp. Neurol.* **55:**822–831.

101. Reifenberger J., Wolter M., Weber R.G., Megahed M., Ruzicka R., Lichter P., Reifenberger G. 1998. Missense mutations in SMOH in sporadic basal cell carcinomas of the skin and primitive neuroectodermal tumors of the central nervous system. *Cancer Res.* **58:**1798–1803.

102. Rempel S.A., Schwechheimer K., Davis R.L., Cavenee W.K., Rosenblum M.L.. 1993. Loss of heterozygosity for loci on chromosome 10 is associated with morphologically malignant meningioma progression. *Cancer Res.* **53:**2387–2392.

103. Rickman D.S., Bobek M.P., Misek D.E., Kuick R., Blaivas M., Kurnit D.M., et al. 2001. Distinctive molecular profiles of high-grade and low-grade gliomas based on oligonucleotide microarray analysis. *Cancer Res.* **61:**6885–6891.

104. Rorke L.B., Packer R.J., Biegel J.A.. 1996. Central nervous system atypical teratoid/rhabdoid tumors of infancy and childhood: definition of an entity. *J. Neurosurg* **85:**56–65.

105. Rubio M.-P., Correa K.M., Ramesh V., MacCollin M.M., Jacoby L.B., von Deimling A., et al. 1994. Analysis of the neurofibromatosis 2 (NF2) gene in human ependymomas and astrocytomas. *Cancer Res.* **54:**45–47.

106. Rubio M.-P., Correa K.M., Ueki K., Mohrenweiser H.W., Gusella J.F., von Deimling A., Louis D.N. 1994. The putative glioma tumor suppressor gene on chromosome 19q maps between APOC2 and HRC. *Cancer Res.* **54:**4760–4763.

107. Ruttledge M.H., Sarrazin J., Rangaratnam S., Phelan C.M., Twist E., Merel P., et al. 1994. Evidence for the complete inactivation of the NF2 gene in the majority of sporadic meningiomas. *Nat. Genet.* **6:**180–184.

108. Ruttledge M.H., Xie Y.G., Han F.Y., Peyrard M., Collins V.P., Nordenskjold M., Dumanski J.P. 1994. Deletions on chromosome 22 in sporadic meningioma. *Genes Chromosomes Cancer* **10:**122–30.

109. Sallinen S.L., Sallinen P.K., Haapasalo H.K., Helin H.J., Helen P.T., Schraml P., et al. 2000. Identification of differentially expressed genes in human gliomas by DNA microarray and tissue chip techniques. *Cancer Res.* **60:**6617–6622.

110. Sasaki H., Zlatescu M.C., Betensky R.A., Johnk L., Cutone A., Cairncross J.G., Louis D.N.. 2002. Histopathological-molecular genetic correlations in referral pathologist-diagnosed low-grade "oligodendroglioma." *J. Neuropathol. Exp. Neurol.* **61:**58–63.

111. Saylors R.L., Sidransky D, Friedman H.S., Bigner S.H., Bigner D.D., Vogelstein B., Brodeur G.M.. 1991. Infrequent p53 gene mutations in medulloblastomas. *Cancer Res.* **51:**4721–4723.

112. Schlegel J., Scherthan H., Arens N., Stumm G., Kiessling M. 1996. Detection of complex genetic alterations in human glioblastoma multiforme using comparative genomic hybridization. *J. Neuropathol. Exp. Neurol.* **55:**81–87.

113. Schmidt E.E., Ichimura K., Reifenberger G., Collins V.P. 1994. CDKN2 (p16/MTS1) gene deletion or CDK4 amplification occurs in the majority of glioblastomas. *Cancer Res.* **54:**6321–6324.

114. Schmitz U., Mueller W., Weber M., Sevenet N., Delattre O., von Deimling A. 2001. INI1 mutations in meningiomas at a potential hotspot in exon 9. *Br. J. Cancer* **84:**199–201.

115. Schneider G., Lutz S., Henn W., Zang K.D., Blin N. 1992. Search for the putative suppressor genes in meningiomas: significance of chromosome 22. *Hum. Genet.* **53:**579–582.

116. Schofield D., West D.C., Anthony D.C., Mashal R., Sklar J. 1995. Correlation of loss of heterozygosity at chromosome 9q with histologic subtype in medulloblastomas. *Am. J. Pathol.* **146:**472–480.

117. Schrock E., Blume C., Meffert M.C., du Manoir S., Bersch W., Kiessling M., et al. 1996. Recurrent gain of chromosome arm 7q in low-grade astrocytic tumors studied by comparative genomic hybridization. *Genes Chromosomes Cancer* **15:**199–205.

118. Segal R.A., Goumnerova L.C., Kwon Y.K., Stiles C.D., Pomeroy S.L.. 1994. Co-expression of neurotrophin-3 and trkC linked to a more favorable prognosis in medulloblastoma. *Proc. Natl. Acad. Sci. USA* **91:**12,867–12,871.

119. Sidransky D., Mikkelsen T., Schwechheimer K., Rosenblum M., Cavenee W., Vogelstein B.. 1992. Clonal expansion of p53 mutant cells is associated with brain tumor progression. *Nature* **355**:846–847.

120. Simmons M.L., Lamborn K.R., Takahashi M., Chen P., Israel M.A., Berger M.S., et al. 2001. Analysis of complex relationships between age, p53, epidermal growth factor receptor, and survival in glioblastoma patients. *Cancer Res.* **61**:1122–1128.

121. Smith J.S., Alderete B., Minn Y., Borell T.J., Perry A., Mohapatra G., et al. 1999. Localization of common deletion regions on 1p and 19q in human gliomas and their association with histological subtype. *Oncogene* **18**:4144–4152.

122. Smith J.S., Tachibana I., Passe S.M., Huntley B.K., Borell T.J., Iturria N., et al. 2001. PTEN mutation, EGFR amplification, and outcome in patients with anaplastic astrocytoma and glioblastoma multiforme. *J. Natl. Cancer Inst.* **93**: 1246–1256.

123. Sprenger S.H., Gijtenbeek J.M., Wesseling P., Sciot R., van Calenbergh F., Lammens M., Jeuken J.W. 2001. Characteristic chromosomal aberrations in sporadic cerebellar hemangioblastomas revealed by comparative genomic hybridization. *J. Neurooncol.* **52**:241–247.

124. Steck P.A., Pershouse M.A., Jasser S.A., Yung W.K.A., Lin H., Ligon A.H., et al. 1997. Identification of a candidate tumour suppressor gene, MMAC1, at chromosome 10q23.3 that is mutated in multiple advanced cancers. *Nat. Genet.* **15**:356–362.

125. Stemmer-Rachamimov A.O., Xu L., Gonzalez-Agosti C., Burwick J., Pinney D., Beauchamp R., et al. 1997. Universal absence of merlin, but not other ERM family members, in schwannomas. *Am. J. Pathol.* **152**:1649–1654.

126. Suzuki S.O., Iwaki T. 2000. Amplification and overexpression of mdm2 gene in ependymomas. *Mod. Pathol.* **13**: 548–553.

127. Tada K., Shiraishi S., Kamiryo T., Nakamura H., Hirano H., Kuratsu J., et al. 2001. Analysis of loss of heterozygosity on chromosome 10 in patients with malignant astrocytic tumors: correlation with patient age and survival. *J. Neurosurg.* **95**:651–659.

128. Thomas G.A., Raffel C. 1991. Loss of heterozygosity on 6q, 16q, and 17p in human central nervous system primitive neuroectodermal tumors. *Cancer Res.* **51**:639–643.

129. Tong C.Y., Zheng P.P., Pang J.C., Poon W.S., Chang A.R., Ng H.K. 2001. Identification of novel regions of allelic loss in ependymomas by high-resolution allelotyping with 384 microsatellite markers. *J. Neurosurg.* **95**:9–14.

130. Ueki K., Nishikawa R., Nakazato Y., Hirose T., Hirato J., Funada N., et al. 2002. Correlation of histology and molecular genetic analysis of 1p, 19q, 10q, *TP53*, *EGFR*, *CDK4*, and *CDKN2A* in 91 astrocytic and oligodendroglial tumors. *Clin. Cancer Res.* **8**:196–201.

131. Ueki K., Ono Y., Henson J.W., von Deimling A., Louis D.N. 1996. CDKN2/p16 or RB alterations occur in the majority of glioblastomas and are inversely correlated. *Cancer Res.* **56**:150–153.

132. Van Dyke T.A. 1993. Tumors of the choroid plexus, in *Molecular Genetics of Nervous System Tumors* (Levine A.J., Schmidek, H.H. eds.),. WileyLiss, New York, pp. 287–301.

133. van Meyel D.J., Ramsay D.A., Casson A.G., Keeney M., Chambers A.F., Cairncross J.G. 1994. p53 mutation, expression, and DNA ploidy in evolving gliomas: evidence for two pathways of progression. *J. Natl. Cancer Inst.* **86**:1011–1017.

134. Versteege I., Sevenet N., Lange J., Rousseau-Merck M.-F., Ambros P., et al. 1998. Truncating mutations of hSNF5/INI1 in aggressive paediatric cancer. *Nature* **394**:203–206.

135. von Deimling A., Louis D.N., Menon A.G., Ellison D., Wiestler O.D., Seizinger B.R. 1993. Deletions on the long arm of chromosome 17 in pilocytic astrocytoma. *Acta. Neuropathol.* **86**:81–85.

136. von Deimling A., Louis D.N., von Ammon K., Petersen I., Hoell T., Chung R.Y., et al. 1992. Association of epidermal growth factor receptor gene amplification with loss of chromosome 10 in human glioblastoma multiforme. *J. Neurosurg.* **77**:295–301.

137. von Deimling A., Louis D.N., von Ammon K., Petersen I., Wiestler O.D., Seizinger B.R. 1992. Evidence for a tumor suppressor gene on chromosome 19q associated with human astrocytomas, oligodendrogliomas and mixed gliomas. *Cancer Res.* **52**:4277–4279.

138. von Deimling A., von Ammon K., Schoenfeld D., Wiestler O.D., Seizinger B.R., Louis D.N. 1993. Subsets of glioblastoma multiforme defined by molecular genetic analysis. *Brain Pathol.* **3**:19–26.

139. Ward S., Harding B., Wilkins P., Harkness W., Hayward R., Darling J.L., et al. 2001. Gain of 1q and loss of 22 are the most common changes detected by comparative genomic hybridisation in paediatric ependymoma. *Genes Chromosomes Cancer* **32**:59–66.

140. Watanabe K., Tachibana O., Sato K., Yonekawa Y., Kleihues P., Ohgaki H. 1996. Overexpression of the EGF receptor and p53 mutations are mutually exclusive in the evolution of primary and secondary glioblastomas. *Brain Pathol.* **6**:217–223.

141. Watanabe T., Yokoo H., Yokoo M., Yonekawa Y., Kleihues P., Ohgaki H. 2001. Concurrent inactivation of RB1 and TP53 pathways in anaplastic oligodendrogliomas. *J. Neuropathol. Exp. Neurol.* **60**:1181–1190.

142. Watson M.A., Perry A., Budhjara V., Hicks C., Shannon W.D., Rich K.M. 2001. Gene expression profiling with oligonucleotide microarrays distinguishes World Health Organization grade of oligodendrogliomas. *Cancer Res.* **61**:1825–1829.

143. Weber R.G., Bostrom J., Wolter M., Baudis M., Collins V.P., Reifenberger G., Lichter P. 1997. Analysis of genomic alterations in benign, atypical, and anaplastic meningiomas: toward a genetic model of meningioma progression. *Proc. Natl. Acad. Sci. USA* **94:**14719– 14724.

144. Weber R.G., Sabel M., Reifenberger J., Sommer C., Oberstrass J., Reifenberger G., Kiessling M., Cremer T. 1996. Characterization of genomic alterations associated with glioma progression by comparative genomic hybridization. *Oncogene* **13:**983–994.

145. Wellenreuther R., Kraus J.A., Lenartz D., Menon A.G., Schramm J., Louis D.N., et al. 1995. Analysis of the neurofibromatosis 2 gene reveals molecular variants of meningioma. *Am. J. Pathol.* **146:**827–832.

146. Wolter M., Reifenberger J., Blaschke B., Ichimura K., Schmidt E.E., Collins V.P., Reifenberger G. 2001. Oligodendroglial tumors frequently demonstrate hypermethylation of the CDKN2A (MTS1, p16INK4a), p14ARF, and CDKN2B (MTS2, p15INK4b) tumor suppressor genes. *J. Neuropathol. Exp. Neurol.* **60:**1170–1180.

147. Wong A.J., Bigner S.H., Bigner D.D., Kinzler K.W., Hamilton S.R., Vogelstein B. 1987. Increased expression of the epidermal growth factor receptor gene in malignant gliomas is invariably associated with gene amplification. *Proc. Natl. Acad. Sci. USA* **84:**6899–6903.

148. Yahanda A.M., Bruner J.M., Donehower L.A., Morrison R.S.. 1995. Astrocytes derived from p53-deficient mice provide a multistep in vitro model for development of malignant gliomas. *Mol. Cell. Biol.* **15:**4249–4259.

149. Yang S.Y., Xu G.M. 2001. Expression of PDGF and its receptor as well as their relationship to proliferating activity and apoptosis of meningiomas in human meningiomas. *J. Clin. Neurosci.* **8:**49–53.

150. Yin X.L., Hui A.B., Liong E.C., Ding M., Chang A.R., Ng H.K. 2002. Genetic imbalances in pleomorphic xanthoastrocytoma detected by comparative genomic hybridization and literature review. *Cancer Genet. Cytogenet.* **132:**14–19.

151. Yin X.L., Pang J.C., Liu Y.H., Chong E.Y., Cheng Y., Poon W.S., Ng H.K. 2001. Analysis of loss of heterozygosity on chromosomes 10q, 11, and 16 in medulloblastomas. *J. Neurosurg.* **94:**799–805.

152. Yong W.H., Raffel C., von Deimling A., Louis D.N. 1995. Lack of allelic loss at APC in sporadic medulloblastomas (Letter). *N. Eng. J. Med.* **333:**524.

153. Zagzag D., Zhong H., Scalzitti J.M., Laughner E., Simons J.W., Semenza G.L. 2000. Expression of hypoxia-inducible factor 1alpha in brain tumors: association with angiogenesis, invasion, and progression. *Cancer* **88:**2606–2618.

154. Zhen H.N., Zhang X., Bu X.Y., Zhang Z.W., Huang W.J., Zhang P., et al. 1999. Expression of the simian virus 40 large tumor antigen (Tag) and formation of Tag-p53 and Tag-pRb complexes in human brain tumors. *Cancer* **86:**2124–2132.

155. Zlatescu M.C., TehraniYazdi A., Sasaki H., Megyesi J.F., Betensky R.A., Louis D.N., Cairncross J.G. 2001. Tumor location and growth pattern correlate with genetic signature in oligodendroglial neoplasms. *Cancer Res.* **61:**6713–6715.

156. Zurawel R.H., Chiappa S.A., Allen C., Raffel C. 1998. Sporadic medulloblastomas contain oncogenic β-catenin mutations. *Cancer Res.* **58:**896–899.

4

Genetic Modeling of Glioma Formation in Mice

Martin Begemann, Vinagolu K. Rajasekhar, Gregory N. Fuller, and Eric C. Holland

1. INTRODUCTION

In humans, gliomas are the most common form of primary brain tumors. These tumors are traditionally categorized, based on their histological features, into several groups with the majority displaying either astrocytic or oligodendroglial differentiation. Both groups can appear as high-grade (malignant) or low-grade forms of tumor. In addition, tumors present that carry mixed features of oligodendroglial and astrocytic components *(159)*. To date, a wide variety of genetic and environmental factors have been found to represent a causal link in gliomagenesis. One of the best established environmental causes of human gliomas is ionizing radiation, which was demonstrated in follow-up studies of patients who received treatment for acute lymphocytic leukemia (ALL), craniopharyngioma, or pituitary adenoma during childhood *(21,293)*. Furthermore, patients with certain enzyme deficiencies are particularly susceptible to develop gliomas upon exposure to particular chemicals *(87,237)*. Patients with neurofibromatosis I and II *(137,143,159,163)*, Li-Fraumeni *(176)*, and Turcot's syndrome *(115)* are predisposed to develop high-grade astrocytoma. An increased tumor incidence, particularly lymphomas, but also gliomas and medulloblastomas were described in ataxia-teleangiectasia *(200)*. Some familial gliomas are related to mutations in *TP53* *(161,169,185)*, *CHK2* *(18,288)* or the $p16^{INK4A}/p14^{ARF}$ locus *(8,270)*; others exist in the absence of a known genetic syndrome *(108,182)*. Familial gliomas represent only a small fraction of all gliomas; the majority of gliomas are sporadic.

While the etiology of sporadic gliomas is unknown, over the last few years a number of somatic mutations have been identified that are common for each subtype of gliomas. The majority of the genes found to be mutated in gliomas, such as phosphatase and tensin homolog *(PTEN), TP53*, or $p16^{INK4A}/p14^{ARF}$, are also mutated in other cancers such as melanoma, breast, or prostate cancers and are not specific for gliomas *(5,71,81,178,179,185,187,231,295)*. Some somatic mutations found in sporadic gliomas affect the same genes as those found as germline mutations in familial gliomas. For example, mutations in *TP53*, the gene that is mutated in Li-Fraumeni syndrome *(161,185)*, are also frequently found in sporadic glioblastoma multiforme *(285,292)*. Furthermore, certain mutations are more common in some subpopulations of glioma patients. For example, the mutation spectrum and expression profile varies between histological subtypes of gliomas *(285)*, long-term and typical survivors of glioblastoma multiforme *(38)*, childhood and adult gliomas *(30,224,267)*. The association of mutations with histological features in human tumors is descriptive in nature, and does not prove that a causal role for specific mutations in tumorigenesis. Direct evidence for the role of mutations can be obtained by introduction of mutated alleles or ablation of certain genes from animals with defined genetic backgrounds.

From: *Contemporary Cancer Research: Brain Tumors*
Edited by: F. Ali-Osman © Humana Press Inc., Totowa, NJ

Table 1
Strategies Used to Model Gliomas

Strategy	Principle	Primary mutations	Cell of origin	Secondary mutations
Mutagens	DNA alkylation	Unknown	Unknown	Likely
Transplantation	Xeno- or allografts, immunodeficient animals	Unknown	Unknown	Less likely
Germline mutations	Transgene or gene targeting	Known	Unknown	Likely
Somatic gene transfer	Replication competent retrovirus	Known	Unknown	Likely
	Replication deficient retrovirus	Known	Known	Less likely

Identification of primary mutations and the cells of origin as well as secondarily acquired mutations depends on the principle employed. Somatic gene transfer employs replication competent (Moloney murine leukemia virus) or replication deficient retroviruses (RCAS). Somatic gene transfer into genetically engineered mice allows one to identify genes sufficient for glioma formation (*see* Subheadings 2 and 5 for discussion).

2. MODEL SYSTEMS

Several methods have been developed to generate brain tumors in animal models. The characteristics of these systems are summarized in Table 1 and discussed later.

2.1. Chemical Carcinogenesis

Various chemicals, predominantly alkylating agents such as nitrosurea derivatives, have been used to generate brain tumors in rodents *(63,160,269)*. The histology of these tumors is often comparable to that of human brain tumors. However, because a large number of genes are mutated in these systems it is nearly impossible to identify which mutated gene is responsible for transformation. However, subsequent advances in gene transfer technology helped to establish germline mice that could be used as murine tumor models. For a general introduction to modeling human cancer in genetically engineered mice the reader might consult recent reviews *(116,290)*.

2.2. Germline Gain-of-Function Strategies (Transgenic Mice)

Transgenic mice are generated by injection of DNA sequences in the male pronucleus of the zygote *(126)*, which is then integrated into host chromosomal DNA. Offspring from such a mouse carry a designed gene or complementary deoxyribonucleic acid (cDNA), also called transgene, superimposed on a defined genetic background. A tissue-specific promoter/enhancer drives the expression of a gene or cDNA in a defined spatial-temporal pattern. The transgene remains under the control of the engineered regulatory elements of the gene, however, the expression pattern of the transgene also depends on host genetic elements at the site of integration. The engineered expression of certain genes or hybrid genes can be lethal during early development. On the other hand, a transgene would be expressed in all cells that utilize the transgene promoter/enhancer.

2.3. Germline Gene Disruption (Knock-Out Mice)

In this model system, mice are generated carrying a mutation at a particular genetic locus. The gene of interest is disrupted by homologous recombination in embryonic stem cells, these are transferred into blastocysts to generate chimeric mice. Once the offspring are bred true they will carry the genotype of the embryonic stem cells with the designed altered alleles. This strategy yielded several mouse strains carrying targeted mutations of genes with particular interest to neuro-oncology such as *PTEN, TP53, p16^{INK4A}-p19^{ARF}*, and retinoblastoma *(RB)*. Some of these genes are required for development; thus homozygous adult animals cannot be obtained. For example, homozygous disruption of

PTEN causes embryonic lethality *(222,268)*. In the heterozygous state, *PTEN* leads to the development of tumors in other organs, such as lymphomas or sarcomas *(222)*, thus limiting the lifespan of the animals before they develop gliomas. Many genes in mammalian organisms are members of multigene families providing functional redundancy.

The expression of genes through transgenic mice or disruption of genes in the germline of mice makes it difficult to identify genes that are sufficient for tumorigenesis. First, a certain gene might be essential for development, and loss of this gene product might lead to embryonic lethality. Second, all cells of mice with engineered germline mutations carry the mutant allele or transgene. Because the allele is ubiquitous in all cells this might alter cell physiology in a multitude of different cells, cell types, and their tissue interactions, thus making interpretation difficult. Third, while mutations in certain genes, e.g., *TP53, PTEN*, make the individual susceptible to tumorigenesis, all cells in mice generated by "knock-out" or transgenic approach carry the same altered allele. During multistep carcinogenesis, additional mutations may be acquired in different cells or cell typesthat might be cumbersome to identify. These problems can be prevented with tissue specific expression of *cre* recombinases in combination with germline "knock-in" of *lox* sites flanking the tumor suppressor gene in question *(174,319)*. This allows the "knock-out" of defined genes in a particular cell lineage of an intact animal, as shown recently for *PTEN* in central nervous system (CNS) progenitor cells *(109)*.

2.4. Somatic Cell Gene Transfer Using Retroviral Vectors

A complementary strategy to germline mutation has been developed using somatic cell gene transfer utilizing retroviral vectors. For example, replication-competent Moloney murine leukemia virus *(287)* has been used as an expression vector in mice. This was accomplished by virus infection of brains of neonatal mice. Because the virus is replication-competent, it spreads throughout the tissue, infecting many cells and different cell types even during the course of tumor progression. Thus, replication competent vectors themselves may act as insertional mutagens either activating or inactivating unidentified genes cooperating in gliomagenesis. In fact, insertion mutagenesis through replication competent virus might aid to identify novel genes contributing to gliomagenesis *(1)*. Because Moloney-based vectors have a broad host range, the tumors of different cells of origin might be obtained within the same animal. Replication-deficient avian leukemia virus (ALV) offers additional high selectivity. The ALV utilizes for infection a specific receptor, named *tv-a* (Fig. 1). The receptor is encoded by tumor virus susceptibility locus A producing a transmembrane and a myristoylated form with extracellular receptor domain *(12,13)*. The cDNA of such of the myristoylated receptor form has been cloned and introduced into the germline of mice under the control of tissue specific promoters *(89,127,131)* (Fig. 1A). Thus, the receptor will be expressed in specific cell types depending on the promoter employed; for example either in the embryonic neural progenitor cells (*nestin* promoter in *Ntv-a* mice), astrocytes (*GFAP* promoter in *Gtv-a* mice), or in all tissues (β-*actin* promoter) (Fig. 1B). The *Ntv-a* transgene utilizes a modified *nestin* promoter that have been shown to direct expression to the CNS progenitor cells; polyadenylation is provided by SV40 sequences *(127)*. The *Gtv-a* transgene contains a 2.2–kb fragment of the *GFAP* promoter driving expression of the quail *tv-a* cDNA and a fragment from the mouse protamine gene (MP-1) supplying an intron and signal for polyadenylation *(127)*. Only the cells that express the receptor are susceptible to infection; cells not expressing the receptor are immune to infection (Fig. 1C). The retroviral genome integrates into the host genome, allowing expression of the viral oncogene (line in Fig. 1B). Integration of the proviral DNA requires at least one round of DNA replication of the *tv-a* expressing cell. Infection can be carried out by injection of the virus suspension (RCAS) or by injection of a chicken cell line, DF-1, *(132)* producing the virus (Fig.1B). The viruses are injected into a particular site of a tissue at a certain time of development. The experiments employing the RCAS/*tv-a* system summarized in Subheading 5 of this chapter all have been carried out by injection of virus producing cells into brains

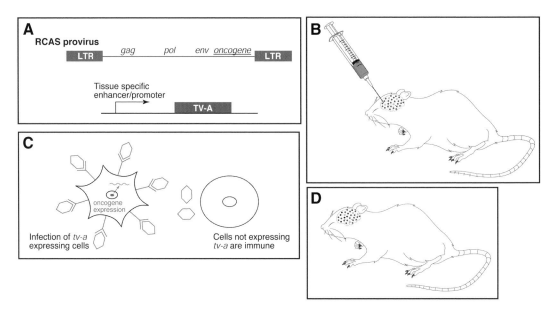

Fig. 1. Generation of somatic mutations through the RCAS/TVA system. Panel A shows the construction of a replication competent avian leukemia virus (green) carrying a particular oncogene. The long terminal repeats (LTR), and the viral genes *gag, pol, env* are required for virus production. Mice are generated carrying the virus receptor TV-A (red) under the control of a tissue specific enhancer/promoter. In this review TV-A is under the control of two enhancers/promoters driving the expression in the central nervous system, GFAP (astrocytes, in *Gtv-a* mice) and nestin (progenitor cells, in *Ntv-a* mice) respectively. Panel B shows the injection of RCAS (green) into the target tissue, where a certain target population expresses the TV-A (red). Panel C shows that cells expressing the RCAS receptor, TV-A (red) are infected by RCAS (green) and express the oncogene (waved green line), cells not expressing the TV-A are immune. Expression of the oncogene requires integration of the provirus in the host genome. Integration of proviral DNA requires at least one round of replication of the host DNA. Therefore, only replicating cells also expressing TVA are infected and express the oncogene in their progeny. Panel D demonstrates the expression of the oncogene in RCAS infected target population of the brain.

of newborn mice. These injected virus-producing cells are very sparse 2 d after injection and not detectable 7 d after injection *(132)*. Such approaches establish somatic mutations with a clear defined cell type of origin. The main limitation of the RCAS vector is the restricted size of the insert (approx 2.5 kb) that can be efficiently retained in repeated replications and subsequent infections. Furthermore, only a small number of cells are infected. Thus, the probability of acquiring secondary mutations is very low and cells giving rise to tumors are likely to have acquired genetic alterations sufficient for tumor formation through RCAS vector mediated gene transfer. Mice expressing *tv-a* under cell-type specific promoters may be bred to other strains carrying other mutations, for example, deletions of *TP53* or *INK4A-ARF (128)*. This allows the investigation of the biological consequences of a gene transferred via RCAS into a cell type of a particular tissue in mice with a clearly defined genetic background.

RCAS vectors carrying various oncogenes, marker genes, and recombinases have been generated and rigorously employed for analysis *(91)*. A detailed discussion of the system and a complete listing of RCAS vectors, are available at http://rex.nci.nih.gov/RESEARCH/basic/varmus/tva/web/tva2. html.

The specificity mediated by the retrovirus/host cell interaction can be experimentally coupled by precise stereotactic injection. Thus, RCAS vectors infect only cells in a defined anatomical region that are dividing and express the viral receptor, *tv-a.* An elegant combination of these three factors in addition to other experiments contributed to the identification of neural stem cells in the adult mouse brain *(78)*. In this case, a specific population of astrocytes in the subventricular zone of the brain of adult *Gtv-a* mice was targeted stereotactically and then infected with RCAS carrying a marker gene (alkaline phosphatase). This allowed lineage tracing of this population that has the capacity to differentiate into neurons. Thus, RCAS vectors might be utilized to express genes in the neural lineage. Currently available mutant mouse strains are listed in the Mouse Tumor Biology (MTB) Database (Jackson laboratory, Bar Harbor, ME) accessible through http://www.informatics.jax.org, or the Mouse Repository of the Mouse Models of Human Cancers Consortium (MMHCC) established by the National Cancer Institute (Frederick, MD) via http://www.web.ncifcrf.gov/researchresources/ mmhcc. Summaries of the workshops of the MMHCC can be obtained through http://emice.nci. nhi.gov/.

3. SIGNALING PATHWAYS CONTRIBUTING TO THE FORMATION OF GLIOMAS

A wealth of information about signaling molecules relevant to gliomagenesis has been gathered through screening for mutations, and from basic research in cell and developmental biology of the nervous system. Mutations have been found in receptor tyrosine kinases (RTK), their signal transducers, and in components of the cell-cycle. For example, amplification and mutations of *EGFR* are found in 30 to 50 % of human glioblastomas *(309,310)*. Other mutations include RTK and their growth factors such as *PDGF/PDGFR (93)*, *IGFR (246)*, molecules involved in signal transduction such as *C-MYC (283)*, *PTEN/MMAC1 (71,81,178,231,295)* and cell-cycle regulatory components such as *CDK4 (242)*, *CDK6 (62)*, *cyclin D1 (39)*, *MDM2 (23,233–235)*, *INK4A-ARF* locus *(209,210, 249,298)*, *TP53 (22,29,296,297)*, and *RB (137,286)*.

3.1. Receptor Tyrosine Kinases and Signal Transduction

At least three different pathways are activated through RTK: the RAS/MAP kinase, the AKT pathway, and protein kinase C (PKC) summarized in Fig. 2. The cellular signaling pathways required for normal cell physiology are abnormally regulated in transformed glioma cells. Some of the studies summarized below were carried out in fibroblasts or other nonglial systems and remain to be validated in glial cells. EGFR-mediated mitogenesis requires ligand-driven dimerization of receptor monomers that stimulates the intrinsic tyrosine kinase activity of the transmembrane receptor. Tyrosine phosphorylation of the receptor, and signaling through coupling of adapter molecules such as SOS, Grb2, Shc activate PLCγ (phospholipase C), Ras/MAPK, and PI3-kinase/AKT pathways (for review, *see* ref. 247). Receptor-ligand internalization and lysosomal breakdown attenuates this pathway.

3.1.1. Ras/Raf/MAPK Pathway

Ras belongs to a superfamily of GTPases existing in an inactive (GDP-bound) and an active (GTP-bound) conformation. The guanine nucleotide exchange factors (GEFs) catalyze the release of GDP, allowing GTP to bind. GTP has a higher intracellular concentration than GDP. Ras is inactivated by GTPase activating proteins, called GAPs. GAPs through their GTPase activity hydrolyze GTP to GDP and thus inactivate Ras. Activated mutant Ras has been found in different human cancers, e.g., colon and lung cancers, but not in astrocytomas *(105,181,199)*. However, increased activity of Ras-GTP has been reported in high-grade astrocytomas *(112)*. Activation of Ras-GTP in astrocytomas is mediated through constitutively active RTKs upstream of Ras *(90)*. Neurofibromin, the gene product of *NF1*, inactivates Ras-GTP through hydrolysis of GTP (for review, *see* ref. 57). Neurofibromin belongs to the evolutionary highly conserved family of GAP proteins (GTPase activating proteins). The inactivation of *NF1* leads to activation of Ras. Ras regulates the Ras/Raf1/Erk pathway, and the Rac/cdc42/Rho cascade that have been shown to activate transcription factors *(10,70)*, translation initiation factors *(97)*, components of cell-cycle control *(110,241)*, apoptosis, and affect cycotskeletal

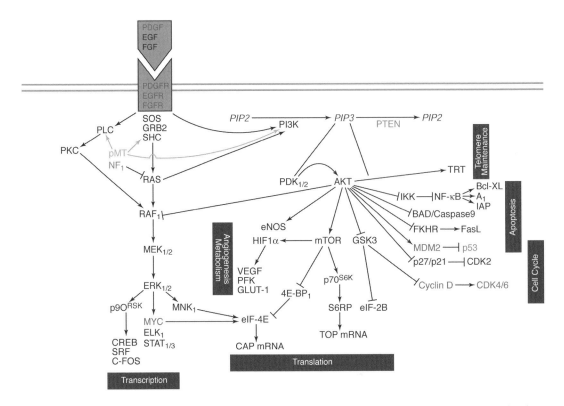

Fig. 2. Oncogenic signal transduction pathway mediated by receptor tyrosine kinases. The ligand stimulates the intrinsic transmembrane receptor tyrosine kinase (RTK) activity that leads to the activtion of PLC/PKC (left), Ras/Raf/Erk pathway after recruitment of adapter molecules such as Sos, Grb2, and Shc (middle) and the PI3K/AKT pathway (right). The phospholipids PtdIns(3,4)P$_2$ and PtdIns(3,4,5)P$_3$ (*PIP2* and *PIP3* in italic) are substrates of PI3-kinase and PTEN phosphatase. PtdIns(3,4,5)P$_3$ binds the pleckstrin homology (PH) domains of PDK1/2 and AKT resulting in their activation. Activated Ras also regulates the Rac/CDC42/Rho pathway. GTP-RAS is inactivated by NF-1-like GTP-ase activating proteins (GAPs). The different signaling pathways affect different functions of cellular physiology indicated in blue boxes. Mutations occurring in human gliomas are denoted in red (gain-of-function mutations) and green (loss-of-function mutations). *PDGF, EGFR, PDGFR, FGFR* amplifications and activating mutations are reported in sporadic gliomas. Deletions and inactivating mutations of *NF1* (neurofibromin) are reported in patients with neufibromatosis type I who are predisposed to gliomas. *PTEN* is deleted or mutated some families with multiple cancer types, inherited hamartoma syndromes, such as Cowden's disease, Bannayan-Riley-Ruvalcaba-syndrome and L'hermitte-Duclos disease as well as in the majority of high-grade gliomas. Polyoma middle T (pMT in orange) activates PLC, the Ras pathway via SHC and PI3K. Some substrates downstream of the Ras/Raf/Erk and PI3K/AKT pathways, such as *MYC, MDM2, Cyclin D, CDK4/6* are also found to by amplified in sporadic gliomas.

rearrangement *(70)*. For example, the Ras/Raf1/Erk pathway has been shown to effect cell-cycle control by various mechanisms. In fibroblasts, for example, PDGF-mediated Ras/Erk activation leads to the induction of cyclin D1 and a decrease of the G$_1$ cyclin inhibitor, p27^{KIP1} *(300)*. Furthermore, the Ras induces p19^{ARF} and growth arrest even in the absence of p21$^{WAF1/CIP1}$ and p27^{KIP1} *(110)*. Ras also induces the transcription of *MDM2,* and in the absence of p19^{ARF}, inactivates p53 *(241)* (*see* Subheading 3.2 for discussion). Thus, the Ras/Raf1/Erk pathway controls the G$_1$ transition point of the cell-cycle.

3.1.2. PI3K/AKT Pathway

AKT is a serine/threonine kinase which itself is activated through second messengers generated by activation of PI3-kinase (phosphoinositide-3-kinase) *(19,44,49,66,95)*. RTK activation of PI3-kinase leads to the generation of PtdIns(3,4)P$_2$ and PtdIns(3,4,5)P$_3$. These lipids are membrane bound and activate PDK1/2 and AKT (also called PKB). AKT requires for its activation PtdIns(3,4,5)P$_3$ and is inhibited by PTEN, a 3'phosphoinositol phosphatase *(172,184,205,313)*, mediating the hydrolysis of PtdIns(3,4,5)P$_3$ to PtdIns(3,4)P$_2$. Thus, via its phospholipid second messengers (italic symbols in Fig. 2) PI3-kinase activates and PTEN inactivates AKT *(177)*. The gene encoding *PTEN*, maps to chromosome 10q23, and is deleted in a large percentage of high-grade astrocytomas as well as in a wide variety of other malignant tumors *(175,177,229)*. Mutant *PTEN* is also found in familiar cancer and hamartoma syndromes *(71,186–188)*. There are three isoforms of AKT in the human genome with equivalent transforming potential *(196)*. In gastric and ovarian cancers AKT isoforms were found to be amplified *(53,263)*; however, amplification or activating mutations of AKT have yet not been described in human astrocytomas. In contrast to primary astrocytes, glioblastoma cells display high AKT activity and high levels of the PI3-kinase products PtdIns(3,4,5)P$_3$ and PtdIns(3,4)P$_2$ *(175,229,313)*. Transfer of *PTEN* into human glioma cells inhibits AKT activation and induces anoikis *(69)*. AKT regulates many biological processes, such as survival and apoptosis, transcription, translation, invasion and migration, cell-cycle control, and angiogenesis *(279)*. PTEN modulates cell migration and invasion through dephosphorylation of focal adhesion kinase (FAK) *(274,275)* and hydrolysis of PtdIns(3,4,5)P$_3$. AKT modulates by phosphorylation several of its downstream targets, including the mammalian target of rapamycin (mTOR) *(4,223,232,248)*, proapoptotic genes such as caspase 9 *(43)* and BAD *(67,68)*, forkhead transcription factor (FKHR) *(24,33,34,162,272)*, IKK, an inhibitor of the transcription factor NF-κB *(155,216,221,243)*, and glycogensynthasekinase-3β (GSK-3β) *(64,72)*. Through these signal transducers AKT indirectly regulates transcription, translation and the cell-cycle, stimulates cell survival, inhibits apoptosis, and influences angiogenesis, metabolism, and telomere maintenance *(279)*. *PTEN* expression in glioblastoma cells regulates angiogenesis in orthotopic brain tumor models *(307)*. This might be mediated via the transcription factor HIF1α, which is stabilized by AKT activity in glioblastoma cells *(325)*. In nonglial systems a remarkable cross-talk between Ras/Raf1/Erk and the PI3K/AKT has been demonstrated. For example, Ras has been shown to activate PI3-kinase *(217)*, whereas AKT inhibits Raf1 *(244,323)*. Some of these pathways are specific for certain stages of differentiation and remain to be validated in astrocytes. There is a remarkable degree of convergence between the Ras/Raf1/Erk and the PI3K/AKT pathways. Both pathways, for example, converge on the level of translational control *(31,32,103)*. The PI3K/AKT pathway via GSK-3β and mTOR and the Ras/Raf/Erk pathway via myc induce or activate translation initiation factors. However, these pathways remain to be validated in astrocytes and glioma cells. The cell-cycle is also regulated by AKT through several mechanisms *(85)*. For example, AKT stabilizes cyclin D *(74,204)*, and induces cytoplasmic localization of p21^{WAF1} and p27^{KIP1} *(60,102,107,266,279, 308,321)*. Thus, progression through G$_1$ phase of the cell-cycle is under the control of AKT. PTEN in contrast inhibits S phase entry by the recruitment of p27^{KIP1} into cyclin E/CDK2 complexes, and thus arrests glioblastoma cells in G$_1$ *(52,106,175)*. PI3K/AKT also promotes translocation of MDM2 to the nucleus where it complexes and inactivates p53 *(193)*. In the presence of PTEN, MDM2 fails to translocate into the nucleus and is retained in the cytoplasm where it is degraded *(193)*. Thus, PTEN allows p53 to stay in the nucleus and execute its functions in cell-cycle control and apoptosis. The sensitization of glioblastoma cells to chemotherapy after introduction of *PTEN* might be due to inactivation of *MDM2* and thereby activation of *TP53*, as well as the activation of other proapoptotic genes such as *BAD (120,218)*. TP53 provides an feedback loop through mediating the transcription of *PTEN (264)*. Thus, *TP53 via PTEN* influences indirectly the activity of PI3K/AKT.

3.1.3. Protein Kinase C Pathway

There exists yet another pathway through which RTKs act. Activation of EGF, PDGF, or FGF receptors leads to enhanced activity of PLC-γ *(211,212,247)*. This is accomplished by direct interaction of the cytoplasmic domain of RTKs with the SH2 domain of PLC-γ. PLC is also activated through polyoma middle T antigen (pMT) via a direct interaction *(135)*. Thus, pMT and RTKs activate Ras/ Raf/Erk, PI3K/AKT, and PLC pathways. This is particularly noteworthy because pMT and activated EGFR induce gliomas in mice with the appropriate genetic background *(129,130)*. PLC-γ hydrolyzes PtdIns(4,5)P$_2$ generating two second messengers, diacylglycerol and Ins(1,4,5)P$_3$. Diacylglycerol is an activator of the protein kinase C (PKC) and Ins(1,4,5)P$_3$ leads to the mobilization of Ca^{++} pools required for the activation of conventional isoforms of PKC. The calcium and phospholipid-dependent serine/threonine kinase, PKC, is the downstream target of PLC and has been implicated in growth control of astrocytes and glioblastoma cells *(15–17,20,252)*. Which of the multiple isoforms of PKC *(9,211)* contributes to glioma formation is not known.

3.2. Cell-cycle Regulation

Multiplication of cells requires duplication of DNA during S-phase and cell division during M-phase. During G$_1$-phase, extracellular cues determine whether the cell replicates DNA and divides or enters a quiescent state (G$_0$). The time point at which the decision is made to enter S-phase is called the "restriction point" and is usually late in G$_1$-phase *(220)*. There is a second restriction point at the G$_2$/M transition. A group of serine/threonine kinases, called cyclin-dependent kinases (CDK), mediate the ordered transition from G$_1$ to S-phase and from G$_2$ to M-phase *(256)*. The regulatory subunits of CDK are called cyclins and activate CDKs. These holoenzymes contain a regulatory subunit (cyclin), a catalytic subunit (CDK) plus other proteins forming a complex. The transition through G$_1$ requires activation of CDK4 and CDK6 by cyclin D, through the G$_1$/S requires CDK2 activation by cyclin E, through S-phase requires CDK2 activation by cyclin A, and through G$_2$/M requires CDK1 (CDC2) activation by cyclin B (see Fig. 3).

3.2.1. p16^{INK4A}/Cyclin D/CDK4/RB/E2F Pathway

The activity of CDK complexes is inhibited by various cyclin dependent kinase inhibitors (CDKI). These inhibitory proteins include the INK4 proteins (Inhibitor of cdk4), inhibiting the cyclin D dependent kinases CDK4 and CDK6, and p21$^{WAF1/CIP1}$, p27^{KIP1} and p57^{KIP2}, which inhibit cyclin E-CDK2 and cyclin A-CDK2. There are four INK4 proteins: p16^{INK4A}, p15^{INK4B}, p18^{INK4C}, and p19^{INK4D} (for review, *see* refs. *254,255*). The genes encoding p16 and p15 are both located on human chromosome 9 *(226)*, p18 is on chromosome 1, and p19 is on chromosome 19. The *p16^{INK4A}* locus also encodes the *p14^{ARF}* locus which is generated by an alternate reading frame *(154,227,228)*, and will be discussed in Subheading 3.2.2. The RB protein, the gene product of the RB locus, is the substrate of cyclin D-CDK4/6 and cyclin E-CDK2. In the hypophosphorylated state, RB is inactive and forms a complex with E2F. After phosphorylation of RB, E2F is released from the complex and mediates the transcription of S-phase specific genes *(51,139,149,150,208)*. E2F isoforms 1–3 are required for proliferation *(310)*. In fact, ectopic expression of E2F1 can trigger quiescent cells to

---

Fig. 3. *(opposite page)* **(A)** Cell-cycle arrest pathway. The cell-cycle is driven by a successive activation of cyclin dependent kinases (CDK) denoted inside the wheel. The activation is mediated through catalytic subunits called cyclins. At the G$_1$/S restriction point the p16^{INK4A}/Cyclin D/CDK4/RB and the p14^{ARF}/MDM2/p53 pathways converge. P16^{INK4A} inhibits cyclin D/CDK4 kinase. CyclinD/CDK4 kinase phosphorylates the RB/ E2F complex *(156)*. Phosphorylation of RB releases E2F acting as a transcription factor *(94)*. E2F-1 stimulates the transcription of genes required for DNA-replication *(150)* and of p14^{ARF} *(14)*. p14^{ARF} sequesters MDM2 *(305)* and thus indirectly stabilizes p53. MDM2 is a ubiquitin ligase leading to the proteolytic degradation of p53 *(119)*. p53 activates transcription of MDM2 thus providing a feedback loop *(312)* and p21, which inhibits the

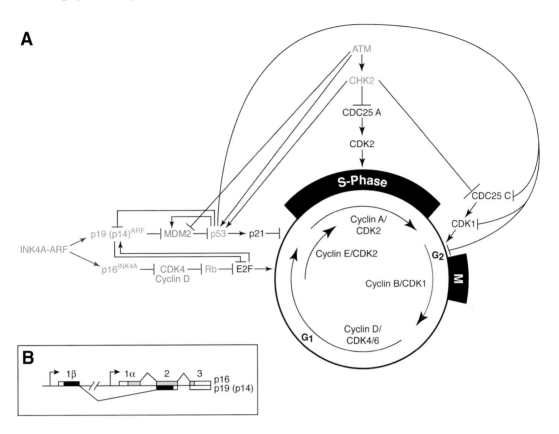

cyclin E/CDK2 kinase required for G_1/S transit. p19^{ARF} (the mouse homolog of p14^{ARF}) also sequester E2F species *(189)*. Therefore, p14(19)^{ARF} can act independently of p53 function. Thus p14^{ARF} coordinates the p16^{INK4A}/cyclin D/CDK4/RB and the MDM2/TP53 pathways.

P53 acts at two different checkpoints: G_1/S transition via induction of p21$^{CIP1/WAF1}$ and G_2/M transition. The transcription of p21$^{CIP1/WAF1}$ is induced by p53 *(86)*. p21$^{CIP1/WAF1}$ inhibits cyclin E/CDK2 required for G_1/S transition and also plays a role on sustained G_2 arrest after DNA damage *(35)*. The p53 mediated G_2/M arrest is mediated by inhibition of transcription of CDC25C *(165)* and induction of 14-3-3σ, which sequesters CDK1 (CDC2) *(48)*. CHK2 and ATM phosphorylate p53 *(45,124)*. ATM also phosphorylates MDM2 *(157)*. The phosphorylation of either p53 or MDM2 stabilizes p53 by inhibiting its interaction with MDM2 and subsequent proteolytic degradation. ATM is serine/threonine kinase activated after DNA damage induced by irradiation *(47)*. ATM activates CHK2, a serine/threonine kinase *(50,282)*. CHK2 phosphorylates and thus inhibits the phosphatases CDC25A *(88)* and CDC25C *(190)*. P53 also activates transcription of *PTEN (264)*, thus indirectly inhibiting the PI3K/AKT pathway denoted in Fig. 2. Consistent with its central role in signal transduction p53 has been shown to mediate cell-cycle control, apoptosis, senescence, and angiogenesis.

Mutations occurring in human gliomas are denoted (red) such as amplifications, or loss-of-function mutations (green), e.g., deletions or inactivating mutations. For example, deletions or inactivating mutations of *TP53* and *INK4A-ARF* have been reported in familiar cancer syndromes and in sporadic glioma. Germline mutations in *CHK2*, like *TP53*, have been reported in Li-Fraumeni syndrome, which includes gliomas. Primary brain tumors, including high-grade astrocytomas, among other tumor types where described in Ataxia-Telangiectasia. Gene amplifications of *CDK4/6, cyclin D*, and *MDM2* and deletions of *RB* were described in sporadic gliomas.

(**B**) *INK4A-ARF* locus. Both p19^{ARF} and 16^{INK4A} are encoded by the same gene but transcribed from different promoters. Exon 1β is transcribed in p19^{ARF} and exon 1α in p16^{INK4A}. Exons 1α and 1β are both spliced to exon 2 that is translated in different reading frames. The transcript of *p16^{INK4A}* contains exons 1α, 2 and 3, whereas the transcript of *p19^{ARF}* contains exon 1β and 2. Mutant mice deficient in *p16^{INK4A}/p19^{ARF}* described in Subheading 5 and Table 2, carry alleles disrupted in exons 2 and 3 *(251)*. (Adapted from ref. *254.*)

enter S-Phase *(144)*. Ectopic expression of E2F in gliomas has also been shown to induce the expression of Bcl-2 and p21$^{WAF1/CIP1}$ *(104)*. This is consistent with the reported increased levels of p21$^{WAF1/}$^{CIP1} in gliomas *(148)* and the high levels of Bcl-2 in gliomas carrying wild type *TP53 (2,215)*. p21$^{WAF1/}$^{CIP1} inhibits CDK1 (CDC2) and CDK2, but activates the cyclin D/CDK4 kinase complex *(54,170)*.

3.2.2. The p19 ^{ARF}/MDM2/p53 Pathway

P53 acts at the G$_1$/S transition point as an inducer of p21$^{WAF1/CIP1}$, as well as during the G$_2$/M transition. In addition, p53 mediates the induction of apoptosis after DNA damage *(173,225,245,273,293)*. p53 is inhibited by MDM2, which itself is inhibited by p19^{ARF} (alternate reading frame, in human p14^{ARF}) *(254)*. MDM2 (originally isolated from mouse double minute chromosomes) binds to the transactivation domain of p53, activating a ubiquitin ligase and initiates proteosomal destruction *(167)*. P53 itself activates the transcription of *MDM2,* thus providing a feedback loop *(312)*. P19^{ARF} binds to MDM2 and sequesters the complex in nucleolar structures *(276)*. MDM2 is activated by Ras/Raf/MEK/MAP kinase *(241)* on one hand, and by the PI3-kinase/AKT pathway on the other *(192–194,322)*. P53 provides feedback loop by activating the transcription of *PTEN* (264), and thus the activity of the PI3K/AKT pathway. p14^{ARF} (the human homolog of murine p19^{ARF}) is induced by E2F, myc, and Ras *(219,323)*. Thus, the Ras/Raf/MEK/MAP kinase pathway can act indirectly through CDK4/cyclin D, and the phosphorylation of pRB and release of E2F-1 can lead to the accumulation of p14^{ARF} and inhibition of MDM2 *(241,254)*. On the other hand, p19^{ARF} targets E2F-1, 2, 3 species for degradation *(189)*. Thus, p14^{ARF} links the *RB* and *TP53* pathways *(14)*. p53-independent functions of p19^{ARF} were shown in mice nullizygous for *ARF, TP53,* and *MDM2* *(301)*. These *p19^{ARF}/MDM2/p53* "triple knock-out mice" and *p19^{ARF}/p53* "double knock-out mice" develop a broad range of tumor types and multiple tumors compared to *p19^{ARF} (151)* and *p53* "single knock-out mice" *(141)*. However, gliomas were not reported in the *p19^{ARF}/MDM2/p53* or *p19^{ARF}/p53* nullizygous mice *(301)* in contrast to *p19^{ARF}* deficient mice *(151)*. Absence of *MDM2* leads to embryonic lethality, but can be rescued by absence of *TP53 (146,201)*. Mice deficient of both *PTEN* and *p16^{INK4A}/p19^{ARF}* develop a large variety of tumors, and earlier then either parent strain; however, gliomas were not reported in *PTEN/ p16^{INK4A}/p19^{ARF}* compound mutant mice either *(318)*. These studies showed also a gene dosage effect for either disrupted gene on the survival of the compound mutant strain. In summary, p19^{ARF}/MDM2/p53 have a physical and functional interaction in tumor surveillance.

3.2.3. Mutations and Alteration of Gene Expression Affecting the Cell Cycle in Human Astrocytomas

Mutations in various components of the cell-cycle are often found in gliomas. For example, familial gliomas have been ascribed to germline mutations of *TP53* and the *p16^{INK4A}/p14^{ARF}* locus *(169,206,270,271)*. Mutations in *TP53* have been described in Li-Fraumeni syndrome with a wide variety of cancers *(176,185)*. The autosomal-dominant inherited melanoma and nervous system tumor syndrome manifesting with astrocytomas, neurofibromas, schwannomas, and meningiomas in the absence of *NF1* mutations has been associated with deletions or mutations in *p16^{INK4A}* and *p14^{ARF} (8)*, and with deletions of *p14^{ARF}* in a setting of intact *p16^{INK4A}* and *p15^{INK4B} (230)*. The p16/cyclin D/CDK4/RB pathway is affected by mutations or deletions of *p16^{INK4A}* or *RB*, amplification or high expression of cyclin D or CDK4 which have been described in astrocytomas *(137)*. The human p19^{ARF} (murine p14^{ARF})/MDM2/p53 pathway is also affected in gliomas through mutations of *TP53* and amplifications of *MDM2* or mutations and deletions of *p14^{ARF} (136)*. Mutations affecting the p14^{ARF}/MDM2/TP53 pathway are particularly common in high-grade gliomas *(136)*. These mutations appear to form complementation groups, for example, some glioblastomas show amplification of *CDK4* without mutations of *CDKN2* (p16^{INK2A} and p15^{INK2B}), whereas others show deletion of *CDKN2* without amplification of *CDK4 (249)*. Either mutation can lead to activation of CDK4, phosphorylation of RB and release of E2F from the RB/E2F complex. Another example of complementary mutations is the amplification of *MDM2* in glioblastomas, which leads to the inactivation *TP53* even in the absence of mutant *TP53 (234)*. The complementation of *TP53* and *MDM2* in human gliomagenesis reflects the physical and genetic interactions of *MDM2* and *TP53* shown on the subcellular level and in mouse models *(99,119,145–147,157,167,201,202,301–303)*. *MDM2* and *CDK4* are located in the same chromosomal region, 12q13 to 12 q14, and amplifications in malignant gliomas often affect both genes *(235)*, thus inactivating both the p16^{INK4A}/cyclinD/CDK4/RB/E2F pathway and the p14^{ARF}/MDM2/p53 pathway. The amplicons have been carefully mapped in human gliomas. These studies show two centers of amplification, one at the *CDK4* locus and the other at the *MDM2* locus *(235)*, with discontinuous amplification of the genes in between suggesting independent selection.

The expression of p16^{INK4A} is also affected by epigenetic events. For example, DNA methylation of the *p16^{INK4A}* locus is seen in 24% of gliomas silencing the expression of p16 in the absence of mutations or deletions *(61,100)*. Therefore, genetic and epigenetic events affect the G$_1$-S transition point and its common alteration in gliomas suggests that this is a prerequisite for gliomagenesis. There are several mouse models with targeted deletions in *p16^{INK4A}*, *p19^{ARF}* or both *(151–153,166, 251,253,255)*. Sarcomas and lymphomas were the most common tumor types in mice carrying inactivated alleles for *p16^{INK4A}/p19^{ARF}* or *p19^{ARF}* alone *(151)*. Only the *p19^{ARF}* deficient mice have been reported to develop occasional gliomas *(151)*. There are two independently generated strains deficient solely *p16^{INK4A} (166,253)*. Either strain carries the capacity to develop melanomas under appropriate genetic cross and treatment with chemical carcinogens *(166,253)*; tumors affecting the CNS have not yet been described in this system. One of the strains has a low incidence of sarcomas and melanomas *(253)*, and no other phenotype was described suggesting that absence of *p16^{INK4A}* alone is insufficient to yield gliomas. The role of the G$_1$-S transition point has been investigated in astrocytes obtained from *p16^{INK4A}-19^{ARF}* deficient mice *(251)* and by infection of *Gtv-a* astrocytes with RCAS/CDK4 *(130)*.

The expression of these signaling molecules was also studied in human gliomas using DNA microarray technology. Consistent with the genetic studies described earlier, these investigations showed overexpression of *EGFR, CDK4*, and human telomerase reverse transcriptase (hTRT) almost exclusively in glioblastomas *(46)*. By contrast, as demonstrated on these DNA microarrays the expression of *TP53, RB, PTEN, p14^{ARF}* and *p16^{ARF}*, is lost or severely reduced in most gliomas *(46)*.

As mentioned previously, *TP53* is often mutated in Li-Fraumeni syndrome *(185)*. Another gene, encoding the checkpoint kinase 2 (CHK2), has recently been identified to be mutated in families with Li-Fraumeni syndrome, including patients with gliomas *(18,288)*. CHK2 is part of the ATM/CHK2/CDC25A/CDK2 pathway *(11,88,257,258,320)*. ATM (Ataxia-telangiectasia mutated) is a serine/threonine protein kinase activated by DNA double strand brakes caused by ionizing radiation. Through a cascade of phosphatases and kinases, *ATM* and *CHK2* regulates cell-cycle progression *(50,88,190,191,320)*. ATM, CHK2, and *TP53* through direct and indirect mechanisms interact with each other *(11,88,320)*. Germline mutations in any of these genes predispose to gliomas and other tumors. ATM is related to a similar kinase, ataxia-telangiectais related (ATR) that phosphorylates and thus activates the checkpoint kinase 1 (CHK1) *(320)*. The abrogation of the CHK 1/2 and ATM/ATR mediated pathways might potentiate effect of irradiation or chemotherapy on glioblastoma cells *(113,125)*. However, the precise role of CHK2, ATM, and CDC25, as well as their partners ATR and CHK1 in normal astrocytes and their role in gliomagenesis is poorly understood.

4. CELLS OF ORIGIN FOR GLIOMAS

The identification of cells of origin is important for any kind of tumor. Several experimental approaches suggest possible cells of origin for gliomas.

4.1. Mutation Analysis of Mixed Oligoastrocytomas and Gliosarcomas

A detailed analysis of mutations in morphologically different compartments of the same tumor allows a lineage analysis of these compartments, and possibly conclusions about the cell of origin. The presence of the same genetic profile in two morphologically distinct cell types would suggest the same cell of origin. Mixed oligoastrocytomas containing areas astrocytic and oligodendroglial differentiation have been shown to carry the same loss of heterozygosity for 1p and 19q *(164)*. Thus, the astrocytic and the oligodendroglial component most likely share a common cell of origin in these tumors. Also, gliosarcomas, carrying areas of glial as well as sarcomatous differentiation have been studied. Dissection of the glial and the sarcomatous elements and comparison of the *TP53* sequence revealed identical mutations in both components *(22,203)*. Similar observations were made with comparative genomic hybridization (CGH) and fluorescent *in situ* hybridization (FISH) of microdissected glial and sarcomatous components of several gliosarcomas *(28)*. These data suggest that a common precursor has the capacity to differentiate into the glial and the mesenchymal components of gliosarcomas carrying the same mutation. However, a detailed study exploring the amplification of *cyclin D* and *CDK4* in microdissected glial and sarcomatous areas of a gliosarcoma showed amplification of *CCND3* (cyclin D3) and *CDK4* only in the sarcomatous, but not the glial tumor cells *(39)*. Comparative genomic hybridization (CGH) of each compartment revealed gains of 7q in both compartments but 6p21 amplification only in the sarcomatous areas *(39)*. These results suggest that the sarcomatous and glial compartments may have derived from the same cell of origin, and that the sarcomatous component acquired new mutations and subsequently lost glial differentiation characteristics.

4.2. Developmental Biology Studies

Rodent cortical cultures showed a broad potential of progenitor cells in the brain *(284)*. Using heterotopic and heterochronic grafts the differentiation potential of brain-derived cells was studied *(277,278)*. These investigations show that brain-derived cells have the capacity to differentiate into myeloid cells after transplantation into irradiated mice *(27)*, into skeletal muscle after transplantation into regenerating muscle *(101)*, and into derivatives of all three germ layers after microinjection into blastocysts *(59)*. However, the exact identity of the grafted cells has not yet been determined. There are further clues from the study of growth and survival factors in developmental and neurobiology. For example, while EGF is vital to neural stem cell proliferation and survival *(239,291)*, PDGF is crucial during normal glial development *(195,213)*.

There are at least three isoforms of PDGFs A,B,C and they act in various combinations of homo- and heterodimers *(121)*. During embryogenesis, PDGF is expressed by neurons and astrocytes *(316)*, whereas the PDGFα receptor is expressed by glial progenitors and neurons *(317)*. Mice lacking the PDGF homodimer have a reduced number of glial progenitors and oligodendrocytes compared with control mice *(98)*. Mice carrying *PDGF-AA* under the control of neuron-specific enolase promoter show an increase in the number of glial precursors that generate abnormally localized oligodendrocytes *(40)*. PDGF ligand and receptor expression was shown in low-grade astrocytomas, in addition to *TP53* mutations *(111,122)*. Expression of the PDGFα receptor *(73)* and amplifications of the *PDGF a* gene *(260)* have been found in oligodendrogliomas. This is in contrast to mutations of *TP53* that are found rarely in oligodendrogliomas *(26,214, 299)*.

EGF is required by the stem cells in the ventricular zone for survival and proliferation *(36,37,180)*. There are several mutant forms of the receptor: the hypomorph *EGFR* allele, *waved 2 (183)*, and the mice carrying a disruption of the *EGFR (197,198, 259,281)*. The *EGFR* hypomorph, *waved 2*, show a decreased number of astrocytes and a smaller subventricular zone compared to normal mice *(183)*. Mice carrying a targeted deletion of *EGFR* result in embryonic lethality with cortical dysgenesis, neuronal ectopias and reduced numbers of astrocytes *(197,198,259,281)*. Thus, the *EGFR* plays an essential role in early development of the CNS. On the other hand, overexpression of *EGFR* via retroviral transfer results in proliferation of stem cells as well as premature astrocytic differentiation *(37)*. EGF-responsive stem cells in the ventricular and subventricular zone retain the capacity to generate all three major cell types in vitro *(238)*. Neural stem cells transplanted into the lateral ventricle remain undifferentiated with simultaneous infusion of EGF, but differentiate into astrocytes without simultaneous infusion of EGF *(96)*. There is evidence that EGFR-mediated signaling pathways play a role in gliomas. The *EGFR* is the often mutated or amplified in high-grade astrocytomas. Approximately 40% of glioblastomas with *EGFR* amplification express active forms of EGFR (also called EGFRvIII, ΔEGFR, or del2-7EGFR), lacking a portion of the extracellular ligand binding domain *(134,309)*, and are thus constitutively autophosphorylated and activated *(82–84)*. This was also studied by retroviral-mediated transfer of an active form of EGFR (EGFR*) into astrocytes and CNS/progenitors. The *EGFR** fragment used for this study contained a human *EGFR* cDNA that lacked the sequences corresponding to exons 2 to 7 *(129)*. RCAS-mediated transfer or *EGFR** into *Gtv-a* or *Ntv-a* mice carrying an inactivated *INK4A-ARF* locus lead to glioma formation (described in Subheading 5.5.).

Recently, studies were begun to study the function of gene in CNS progenitors using conditional mutants. This is particularly useful for genes that lead to embryonic lethality when all somatic cells are in the homozygous deficient state. Using the *cre/loxP* recombinase system, mice were generated lacking *PTEN* in *nestin*-expressing cells *(109)*. These mice die shortly after birth, and their brains show a proportional increase in overall brain structures with altered histology in cortex, hippocampus, and cerebellum. Cells in the ventricular zone show an increase in BRDU staining, consistent with a decrease in cell-cycle time, and a decreased apoptosis *(109)*. Cell fate commitment of progenitor cells was not affected in these mice. Thus, *PTEN* regulates the proliferation of the neural stem/progenitor cells in vivo. Similar studies were also carried out expressing the *cre* recombinase under the control of *GFAP* promoter and enhancer *(7,168)*. Unexpectedly, *PTEN* deletions were noted in neural cells, whereas in astrocytes the *cre* recombinase was expressed at a very low level. The neuronal soma-size was increased and cerebellar pathology similar to L'hermitte-Duclos disease. These results are consistent with the essential role of *PTEN* in the control of CNS progenitor cell proliferation.

4.3. Gene Transfer Into Somatic Cells

Gene transfer into a specific cell type or specific stages of differentiation allows one to study the effect of a particular gene on its descendents *(89,127,129)*. For example, the combined transfer of activated AKT and Ras yields glioblastomas only after transfer into nestin-expressing CNS-progenitor cells (*Ntv-a*), but not after transfer into GFAP-expressing astrocytes (*Gtv-a*) *(128)*. The activated form of the *EGFR* yields lesions resembling gliomas in both *Gtv-a* and *Ntv-a* mice *(129)*. However, these gliomas are more common in *Ntv-a* mice, suggesting that these tumors arise from a more primitive precursor. Glial cells represent a heterogeneous population, and it is unclear at this point which glial cell is the cell-of-origin of tumors in either *Gtv-a* and *Ntv-a* mice.

5. MOUSE GLIOMA MODELS WITH DEFINED GENETIC ALTERATIONS

Several mouse models were generated in mice with defined genetic alterations. The histology of these tumors is similar to that of human gliomas. The generation of these gliomas employed several strategies including transgenic mice, mice with targeted genetic disruption, somatic gene transfer into multiple or defined cell types, and their combinations. The models carry features similar to diffuse astrocytomas, low-grade and anaplastic oligodendrogliomas, and mixed gliomas. A synopsis of the different mouse models, including defined genetic alterations, cell-of-origin, and glioma histology is provided in Table 2.

5.1. Diffuse Astrocytomas

Low-grade diffuse astrocytomas (World Health Organization [WHO] grade II) have been generated in transgenic mouse lines employing several different transgenes.

Table 2
Glioma Models Using Genetically Engineered Mice

Germline mutations Gene disruption	Transgene	Somatic gene transfer	Cell of origin/affected cells	Tumor	Reference
	GFAP/v-src		All GFAP-expressing cells (astrocytes)	Low-grade (early) and high grade (late) astrocytomas	301
	GFAP/^{V12}H-Ras		All GFAP-expressing cells (astrocytes)	Heterozygous: predominantly single low-grade (WHO II) astrocytomas. Homozygous: predominantly multifocal high-grade (WHO III) astrocytomas.	76
	GFAP/EGFRvIII or GFAP/EGFR(wt)		All astrocytes	No tumor but increased number of astrocytes	77
	GFAP/V12H-Ras plus GFAP/EGFRvIII		All astrocytes	Oligodendrogliomas and mixed oligoastrocytomas	77
Ink4a/arf$^{-/+}$ or 53$^{-/+}$	S100β/v-erbB		Astrocytes	Low-grade oligodendrogliomas	304
	S100β/v-erbB		Astrocytes	High-grade Oligodendrogliomas	304
	GFAP/SV40-lgT$_{121}$		Astrocytes (SV lgT)	High-grade astrocytoma (WHOIII)	314
Pten$^{+/-}$	GFAP/SV40-lgT$_{121}$		All cells (Pten)	Accelerated high-grade astrocytoma (WHOIII)	314
NF1$^{-/+}$; p53$^{-/+}$ in cis			All cells in animal	Astrocytomas, grades II to IV (predominantly GBM). Strain specific penetrance of astrocytoma phenotype.	234
		Murine retrovirus/ PDGF B-chain	Mixed cell population in brain	GBM (astrocytoma, WHO grade IV), PNET	285

P53 or $(p16^{ink4a}/p19^{arf})^{+/-}$	Murine retrovirus/ PDGF B-chain	Mixed population in brain; all cells (gene disruption)	High-grade gliomas (accelerated growth and increased frequency)	123
$(p16^{INK4A}/p19^{ARF})^{-/-}$	K-Ras plus Akt	Infected nestin-producing CNS progenitor cell (Nt-va)	GBM (astrocytoma, WHO grade IV)	126
$(p16^{INK4A}/p19^{ARF})^{-/-}$	K-Ras plus Akt	Infected astrocytes (Gt-va)	No tumors	126
$(p16^{INK4A}/p19^{ARF})^{-/-}$	K-Ras	Astrocytes	CNS Sarcoma	288
$(p16^{INK4A}/p19^{ARF})^{+/+}$	K-Ras plus Akt	CNS progenitor cells (Nt-va)	Gliosarcoma (WHO IV)	288
$(p16^{INK4A}/p19^{ARF})^{-/-}$	K-Ras plus Akt	Astrocyte (Gt-va)	Gliosarcoma, spindle cell glioblastoma, giant cell glioblastoma (WHO IV)	288
$(p16^{INK4A}/p19^{ARF})^{+/+}$	PDGF-B	Infected nestin-producing CNS progenitor cells(Nt-va)	Low-grade oligo (WHO II)	65
$(p16^{INK4A}/p19^{ARF})^{-/-}$	PDGF-B	Infected nestin-producing CNS progenitor cells (Nt-va)	High-grade oligo (WHO III)	65
$(p16^{INK4A}/p19^{ARF})^{+/+}$	PDGF-B	Infected astrocytes (Gt-va)	Mixed oligoastrocytomas	65
	PDGF-B	Infected astrocytes (Gt-va)	Mixed oligoastrocytomas	129
$p19^{ARF-/-}$	Polyoma middle T	Infected astrocytes (Gt-va)	Mixed oligoastrocytomas	129
		All cells in animal	Oligodendrogliomas	149

Gliomas can be generated by various combinations of germline mutations and somatic gene transfers (see Table 1). Germline modifications include gene disruptions and inherited transgenes. Somatic gene transfer employs replication deficient or replication competent viruses. The listed mutations can affect all or only a subset of cells or a particular cell lineage of the entire animal (see Subheading 5 for discussion).

In one example, a transgene containing the *GFAP* promoter/enhancer and ^{V12}*H-Ras* which was introduced into the murine germline *(76)*. One of several lines developed solitary tumors similar to low-grade astrocytomas (WHO grade II) in 80% in the animals and multiple tumors resembling anaplastic astrocytomas (WHO grade III) in 20% of the animals when the transgene was in the heterozygous state. In the homozygous state, these animals developed multifocal tumors resembling anaplastic astrocytomas (WHO grade III). The median survival time was with 4 wk, significantly shorter in the homozygous mice compared to 3 mo in the heterozygous mice *(76)*.

In another system, the transgene contains the *v-src* kinase under the control of *GFAP* regulatory elements *(305)*. After a follow-up for 65 wk, 14.4% of these mice developed small proliferative foci and astrocytomas developed in the brain and spinal cord. The lesions were similar to low-grade astrocytomas at early stage and displayed histological characteristics of anaplastic astrocytoma (WHO grade III) and glioblastoma multiforme (WHO grade IV) *(305)*.

Mice carrying a heterozygous copy of *NFI* and *TP53* also developed low-grade astrocytoma *(236)*. NFI is an inhibitor of Ras (Fig. 2), indicating the central role of Ras in gliomagenesis.

5.2. Glioblastoma Multiforme

High-grade gliomas (WHO grade IV) have been generated in transgenic mice and by somatic gene transfer employing retroviral vectors.

5.2.1. Mice Carrying Germline Mutations

Transgenic mice carrying *GFAP/*^{V12}*H-Ras (76)* developed glioblastomas. Cell lines from *GFAP/* ^{V12}*H-Ras* induced astrocytomas showed abnormal karyotypes, as well as overexpression of *MDM2*, *EGFR*, and *CDK4*, and absent expression of *p16^{INK4A}*, *p19^{ARF}* and *PTEN (76)*. From these experiments it is unclear which gene(s) in addition to ^{V12}*H-Ras* is/are sufficient to generate gliomas. Transgenic mice carrying *GFAP/v-src* developed anaplastic astrocytomas, and some tumors had histological characteristics of glioblastoma multiforme *(305)*. A detailed genetic or karyotypic study of *GFAP/v-src* induced glioblastomas has not yet been reported. Glioblastomas were also observed in mice carrying inactivated alleles of *NF1* and *TP53 (236)*. The mice were generated with inactivated alleles of *TP53* and *NF1* on the same chromosome (mouse chromosome 11). These animals developed astrocytomas, WHO grade II to IV. The astrocytomas also showed loss of the wild-type alleles of *NFI* and *TP53*. There was a notable strain-specific effect on brain tumor formation in these *NFI-TP53* deficient compound mice. Mice carrying an inactivated alleles of either *NF1* or *TP53* are also predisposed to tumors *(79,118,141,142)*. However, glioblastomas were not reported from mice carrying single disrupted alleles of either *TP53* or *NF1*. Therefore, an interaction between Ras and p53 plays a central role in the formation of glioblastoma multiforme.

Retroviral gene transfer was used to generate mice expressing various oncogenes in CNS progenitor cells (nestin positive; *Ntv-a*) or astrocytes (GFAP positive; *Gtv-a*). In this study, two RCAS viruses were injected simultaneously: The G12D mutant (activated) form of *K-ras* and an activated form *AKT* (designated AKT-Myr Δ11-60, carrying an HA- tag on its carboxy terminus) *(3)*. The combination of both oncogenes induced glioblastoma multiforme in mice within 9 wk *(128)*. A typical example is shown in Fig. 4. Tumors were not observed with either oncogene alone, or with the combination in *Gtv-a* mice. Therefore, either oncogene requires the other oncogene in the appropriate cell-of-origin to generate glioblastoma multiforme in mice *(128)*. Mating of mice carrying an inactivated allele *p16^{INK4A}-p19^{ARF}* into mice of *Ntv-a* or *Gtv-a* background allows one to study the effect of either oncogene in the absence of *p16^{INK4A}* and *p19^{ARF}*. In such a situation the combination of K-ras and AKT accelerates the development of glioblastomas in the *Ntv-a* background and permits the development of glioblastomas in the *Gtv-a* background. Interestingly, transfer of K-Ras into *Ntv-a* mice carrying the *p16^{INK4A}-p19^{ARF}* deletion yields gliosarcoms in 30% of offspring (unpublished data). This is not seen with the transfer of either ^{G12D}K-Ras or AKT alone into *Gtv-a* mice. However, the combined transfer of ^{G12D}K-Ras or AKT into *Gtv-a* mice carrying an inactivated allele of *INK4A-ARF* produces spindle-cell gliomas and gemistocytic astrocytomas (unpublished data). Thus, the production of gliomas with the combination of ^{G12D}Kras and AKT in the *Gtv-a* background requires the

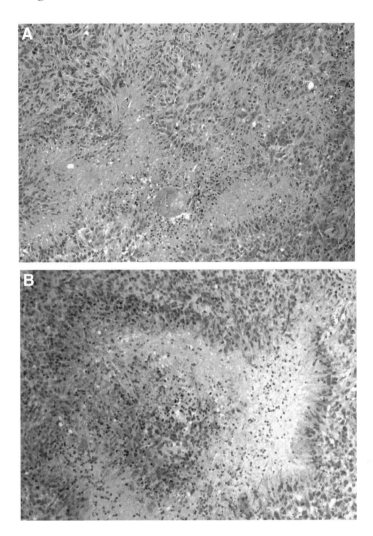

Fig. 4. Glioblastoma multiforme. High-grade astrocytoma with morphologic features identical to those of human glioblastomas (WHO grade IV) generated after combined introduction of ^{G12D}K-RAS together with AKT into *Ntv-a* transgenic mice. A. Malignant astrocytes are characterized by pleomorphic nuclei and prominent eosinophilic cytoplasm. An area of central necrosis is in the middle of the field. B. Expression of glial fibrillary acidic protein (GFAP) in tumor cells palisading around serpiginous zones of necrosis. (A, x100, H&E; B, x40, GFAP.)

inactivation of *p16^{INK4A}-p19^{ARF}*. An acceleration of tumor development in *PTEN*-deficient mice was also seen when these mice were bred with *p16^{INK4A}-p19^{ARF}*–deficient mice to generate *PTEN/ p16^{INK4a}/p19^{ARF}* compound mutant mice *(318)*. These animals developed a wide variety of tumors, however, gliomas were not reported.

5.3. Oligodendrogliomas

High-grade oligodendrogliomas (WHO grade III) are generated after the transfer of the gene encoding PDGF-B into *Ntv-a* mice carrying an inactivated allele of *INK4A-ARF* background *(65)*. A typical

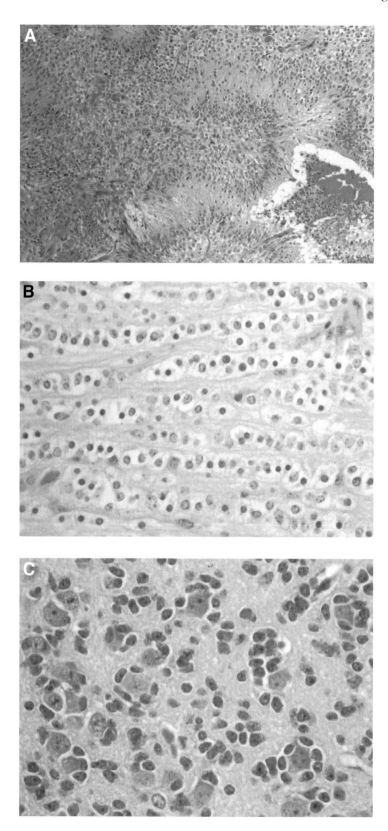

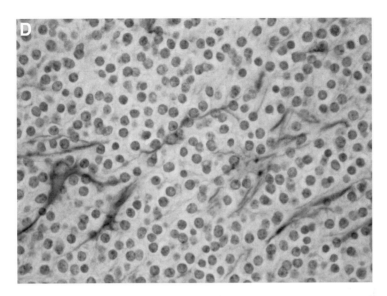

Fig. 5. Oligodendroglioma. High-grade (anaplastic) oligodendrogliomas generated by transfer of PDGF-B into *Ntv-a* mice, whose background includes an inactivated allele of INK4A-ARF. **(A)** foci of necrosis with surrounding pseudopalisading of tumor cells are seen. Detailed fields **(B,C,D)** show morphologic features of individual tumor cells with oligodendroglial differentiation, with uniform, rounded nuclei, surrounded by prominent cleared cytoplasm (perinuclear halos). Panel B, shows diffuse infiltration of cerebral white matter by oligodendroglioma cells, which line up in queues between bundles of myelinated axons. Panel C shows perineuronal satellitosis (clustering of tumor cells around neuronal cell bodies) by oligodendroglioma cells infiltrating the gray matter of the cerebral cortex. The same secondary structures of Scherer (perineuronal satellitosis, perivascular satellitosis, subpial infiltration, intrafascicular queuing) that are seen in human oligodendrogliomas are also typical of the mouse tumors. As in panel D, GFP immunostaining labels only entrapped reactive astrocytes; neoplastic oligodendrocytes are negative. Mouse oligodendrogliomas are also negative for neuronal differentiation markers such as synaptophysin and NeuN (not illustrated). (A, ×40 H&E; B, ×100, H&E; C, ×100, H&E; D, ×100, GFAP.)

example is shown in Fig. 5. This is consistent with the observation of oligodendrogliomas in mice after transfer of *PDGF-B* chain through Mo-MULV into newborn mice *(287)*. A second series of experiments using transgenic mice carrying the viral *erbB*, an active homologue of EGFR, from the S-100β promoter (which is active in astrocytes and glial precursors) also leads to oligodendrogliomas *(304)*. Thus, the ectopic expression of RTK growth factors may lead to oligodendroglioma formation. Mice carrying disrupted alleles of *p19^{ARF}* develop oligodendrogliomas (151), in contrast to *p16^{INK4A}/p19^{ARF}* –deficient mice that do not develop gliomas *(251)*. The reason for this discrepancy is unclear, but may involve differences in the genetic background. Finally, a variety of primary brain tumors were seen after infection of newborn mouse brains with replication-competent virus expressing the *PDGF-B* chain *(251)*. The tumors included high-grade gliomas including glioblastoma and oligodendrogliomas, in addition to tumors resembling primitive neuroectodermal tumors (PNETs). Because approximately half of human oligodendrogliomas demonstrate deletions of chromosomes 1p and 19q, and malignant gliomas often show loss of chromosome 10q, the syntenic chromosomal regions were in *PDGF*-induced mouse gliomas *(65)*. This was studied by FISH for regions syntenic to these human loci (murine 3, 84.9 cM and murine 4, 46.6 and 81.5 cM for human 1p; murine 7, 4-5.5 and 23.0 cM for human 19q). There was no evidence for loss of any of these regions. Therefore, those common mutations implicated in human oligodendrogliomas appear not to be required in PDGF- induced gliomas in mice.

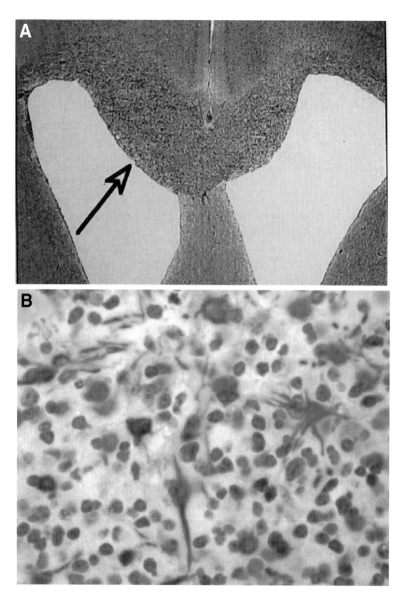

Fig. 6. Mixed oligoastrocytoma. Transfer of polyoma middle T antigen into *Gtv-a* mice. A butterfly growth pattern with invasive spread of tumor cells along the corpus callosum can be seen (**A**). Cells exhibiting astrocytic features have abundant eosinophilic cytoplasms and fibrillary processes and are strongly immunoreactive for GFAP, while those cells that exhibit oligodendroglial morphologic features have regular, round nuclei and perinuclear halos and are not immunoreactive for GFAP (**B**). (A, ×20, H&E; B, ×100, GFAP.)

5.4. Mixed Oligoastrocytoma

Polyoma middle T antigen stimulates several signal transduction pathways and activates SHC (leading to Ras activation), PI3-kinase (leading to AKT activation), PLC and SRC *(6,41,44,75,135,265)* (*see also* arrows in Fig. 2). The transfer of polyoma middle T antigen into *Gtv-a* mice via RCAS leads to mixed oligoastrocytomas (Fig. 6) *(131)*. These tumors were seen at 9 wk in 9 of 33 mice. The histologic features of these tumors were similar to anaplastic astrocytomas, anaplastic oligodendrogliomas, and anaplastic mixed oligoastrocytomas. Polyoma middle T does not require additional genetic modification in contrast to the induction of gliomas by *EGFR (129),* or glioblastomas by ^{G12D}K-Ras/AKT in the *Gtv-a* background. Mixed gliomas were also seen after the transfer of *PDGF* into *Gtv-a* mice *(65).* The histology of these tumors is very similar to those induced after transfer of polyoma middle T antigen.

5.5. Unclassified Gliomas

As described in Subheading 3, mutations and amplifications of *EGFR* are the most frequent in human astrocytomas. In the mouse model a constitutively active form for the EGFR (EGFR*) was used. Gliomas are produced after transfer of a constitutively active allele of *EGFR** into either *Ntv-a* or *Gtv-a* mice carrying a deletion at the *INK4A-ARF* locus; the induction of tumors is accelerated in mice carrying the *Ntv-a* transgene compared to *Gtv-a*. Transfer of the activated *EGFR** in either strains carrying an intact *INK4A-ARF* locus do not form tumors *(129).* Thus, the activated EGFR* receptor requires the inactivation of the *INK4A-ARF* locus in order to yield gliomas. As mentioned earlier, the *INK4A-ARF* locus encodes two different transcripts and proteins in alternate reading frames: $p16^{INK4A}$ and $p19^{ARF}$ (the mouse homologue of human $p14^{ARF}$). It is not known which of these two proteins is required to be inactive to yield gliomas in combination with a truncated version of EGFR.

5.6. Cell Migration and Proliferation

Cell Migration and proliferation without the induction of tumors was seen after transfer of *bFGF* (basic fibroblast growth factor) into *Gtv-a* mice *(132).* Which additional oncogene and/or mutation are required to induce gliomas in combination with *bFGF* remains unknown.

6. CONCLUDING REMARKS

The mouse models show a remarkable similarity to human gliomas. However, there are some important differences. When humans become symptomatic the tumor volume is usually much larger than observed in glioma models of mice. On the other hand, this might allow us to model the earliest stages of tumor induction in vivo and progression, which are not possible in humans. Furthermore, human gliomas usually show a larger number of genetic changes and aneuploid karyotypes *(25,26,42).* The diversity of genetic changes in human high-grade astrocytomas, therefore, is certainly more complex than in experimental mouse systems. Mice have the advantage of modeling tumors with defined genetic elements. The induction of glioblastomas by the combination of AKT and ^{G12D}K-Ras is a typical example *(128).* Differences between human and mice in their requirement for tumor development in different species were reported, e.g., the retinoblastoma oncogene. Mutations of the retinoblastoma oncogene lead to retinoblastoma in humans but not in mice carrying disrupted alleles of the same gene *(58,140,171).* Thus, different species may have different requirements for tumor development *(117,133).* The nature of these species differences requires further investigation. Another important difference between human and mice is the additional requirement of ectopically expressed *hTRT* (human telomerase reverse transcriptase) for malignant transformation of human cells, including astrocytes, along with other oncogenes such as Ras, and SV40 large T antigen, known to disrupt the *RB* and *TP53* pathway, respectively *(114,240,262).* Ectopic expression of *hTRT* to generate gliomas is not required in mice. This might be a result of high telomerase activity and longer telomeres in murine somatic cells compared to their human counterpart *(158).* However, consistent with the murine model system Ras and AKT cooperate in human astrocytes to generate glioblastoma multiforme (WHO grade IV) *(261,262).*

In this context, another interesting question that emerges is which mutation or ectopically expressed gene becomes necessary for maintenance vs induction of tumors. This has been addressed in mice using transgenes under the control of inducible enhancers/promoters. For example, using a tetracycline inducible system it was shown that expression of Ras is required for the maintenance of melanoma *(55,56)* and lung cancer *(92)* in mice. Similar studies have not been carried out for gliomas. This is of particular interest for murine glioblastoma multiforme induced by AKT and ^{G12D}K-Ras. For example, it is unclear in which order their activity is required for glioma induction, or whether their continued expression is required.

In addition to cell autonomous functions required for induction and maintenance of the tumorigenic phenotype, other tumor-associated requirements can be studied such as angiogenesis and the host immune response to the tumor. Early stages of astrocytomas arising in *GFAP/v-src* transgenic mice have been shown to express VEGF even at early stages *(280)*. Furthermore, the endothelial cells in these mice showed the induction of *flt-1, flk-1 (VEGFR2), tie-1,* and *tie-2 (280)*.

The age distribution in human gliomagenesis requires special attention. Gliomas can occur at any time in humans, but peak during adulthood. Mouse glioma models based on somatic transfer presented here (*see* Subheading 5 and Table 2) all utilized the introduction of expression vectors during the newborn period *(65,127–132,287)*. Malignant astrocytomas occur also in childhood but may utilize different genetic pathways than in adults *(224,267)*. Because humans glioblastoma occurs most commonly in the fifth decade of life, the question arises which cell types give rise to high-grade astrocytomas in later part of life. In adult mice, astrocytes of the subventricular zone *(77,78)*, and the hippocampus *(250)* can give rise to neurons. These are areas particularly susceptible to malignant transformation after exposure to chemical carcinogens *(160)*. Whether these populations of astrocytes in adult animals can give rise to gliomas after somatic gene transfer warrants further investigation.

Finally, murine glioma models provide an excellent system to search for surrogate markers and to test therapeutic agents for specific molecular targets. In fact, *PTEN*-deficient glioblastoma cells and embryonic stem (ES) cells are particularly susceptible to the FRAP/mTOR inhibitor CCI-779 *(207,219)*. Mouse models in combination with imaging technology, such as MRI *(92,305)*, or whole body fluorescent markers *(315)*, might allow the monitoring of the response of these tumors to these agents in the entire animal. Thus, with mouse models it might be possible to test specific therapeutic modalities on tumors induced with defined genetic elements.

7. GLOSSARY

AKT Protein serine-threonine kinase, acting as an oncogene, originally identified as an oncogene of murine retrovirus AKT8, which was isolated from spontaneous thymoma of a mouse strain designated AKR. There are three human AKT isoforms. AKT is activated by PI3-kinase and inhibited by the phosphatase PTEN.

ALV Avian leukosis virus.

ATM Ataxia-telangiectasia mutated. ATM is a serine protein kinase activated after DNA damage caused by ionizing irradiation. ATM phosphorylates CHK2, p53, and MDM2. Ataxia-teleangiectasia is an autosomal-recessive recessive disorder which consists of cerebellar degeneration, mild dementia, telangiectasias, increased susceptibility to infections secondary to deficient B-cell function and tumors, particularly lymphomas and primary brain tumors.

CDK2 Cyclin dependent kinase 2, a serine/threonine kinase, sequentially activated by the E-type cyclins during G_1/S transition and the A-type cyclins during S-phase.

CDK4/CDK6 Cyclin dependent kinases 4 and 6 are involved in early G_1 -phase of the cell-cycle, are activated by D-type cyclins and inhibited by p16^{INK4A}.

CDKI Cyclin dependent kinase inhibitors. Proteins that inhibit cell-cycleprogression by binding to and inhibiting CDKs. These include, on one hand, INK4s (p15^{INK4B}, p16^{INK4A}, p 18^{INK4C}, p19^{INK4D}) inhibiting CDK4 and 6, which are activated by cyclin D; on the other hand p21$^{WAF1/CIP1}$, p27^{KIP1}, and p57 ^{KIP2} inhibiting CDK2.

CHK2 The checkpoint kinase CHK2 is serine/threonine kinase activated by ATM after DNA-damage resulting in G_2-M arrest. CHK2 phosphorylates, and thus inactivates the phosphatases CDC25A and CDC25C.

DAG Diacylglycerol. Is produced upon hydrolysis of PtdIns(4,5)P$_2$ by PLC; activator of conventional isoforms of PKC.

E2F Transcription factor known to activate transcription of S-phase specific genes, e.g., subunits of DNA polymerases and topisomerase. E2F is inactive when complexed with the hypophosphorylated RB and is released after phosphorylation of RB.

eNOS Endothelial nitric oxide synthase regulates of tumor blood flow and vascular permeability. eNOS is activated by phosphorylation through the PI3K/AKT pathway.

ERK Extracellular regulated kinase, activated by Ras/Raf. Erk phosphorylates and activates transcription factors, such as Elk1, STAT 1/2, myc.

EGF Epithelial derived growth factor (*see* Subheading 4.2). In human astrocytomas the receptor for EGF, *EGFR*, carries activating mutations is commonly amplified. The oncogene *erbB2* of the avian erythroblastosis virus has high homology the EGFR family.

FGF Fibroblast growth factor (*see* Subheading 4.2)

HIF1a Hypoxia-inducible factor 1 is a transcription factor mediating the expressing of VEGF, phosphofructokinase, and the glucose transporter 1 (GLUT1). HIF1a is activated via PI3K/AKT/mTOR. Under nonhypoxic conditions HIF1a forms a complex with von-Hippel-Lindau (VHL) protein, is ubiquinated, and undergoes proteolytic degradation.

INK4A Inhibitor of cdk4 inhibits cyclin D-dependent kinases CDK4, and thus G_1-S transition. Synonyms of INK4A are MTS-1 (multiple tumor suppressor-1) and CDKN2. INK4A is on human chromosome 9.

TP53 Tetrameric transcription factor acting as tumor-suppressor (encodes human p53). P53 is involved in cell-cycle arrest, apoptosis, angiogenesis. Other family members include p63 and p73. P53 is located on human chromosome 17. Germline mutations of p53 are found in Li-Fraumeni syndrome. The p53 tumor suppressor was first described in 1979 as an interacting protein with the transforming large T-antigen of simian virus 40.

MDM2 Murine double minute 2 protein that inactivates p53 by ubiquination. MDM2 is inactivated by AKT phosphorylation.

MEK MAP kinase is activated by Raf1 and phosphorylates and activates ERK.

MRI Magnetic resonance imaging.

mTOR Mammalian target of rapamycin is a serine/threonine kinase and is activated by AKT. The mTOR is also called FKBP-rapamycin-associated protein (FRAP) or rapamycin and FKBP12 target (RAFT). It plays a crucial role in translational control through activation of $p70^{S6K}$ and inhibition of 4EBP1, and transcription through activating HIF1a.

NFI Neurofibromin, a GTPase-activating protein (GAP) inhibiting RAS. Mutations of NFI are found in neurofibromatosis type I.

P16^{INK4A}/p14^{ARF} locus generates two transcripts in alternate reading frame: $p16^{INK4A}$ inhibiting CDK4 (thus regulating cyclin D/RB/E2F) and $p14^{ARF}$ (mouse homolog $p19^{ARF}$) inhibiting MDM2 (thus limiting the MDM2 mediated ubiquination of p53) (*see also* Fig. 3). The *INK4A-ARF* locus is located on human chromosome 9.

$p70^{S6K}$ A cytoplasmic protein kinase that is activated by mTOR and regulates protein translation through its phosphorylation of the 40S ribosomal protein subunit S6. S6 mediates translation of 5'-terminal oligopyrimidine-rich tract (5'-TOP) mRNAs. These mRNAs encode primarily ribosomal proteins.

PDGF Platelet derived growth factor is highly related to *v-sis*, the transforming protein of simian sarcoma virus (SSV) (*see* Subheading 4.2).

PFK 6-Phosphofructo-2-kinase/fructose-2,6-bisphosphatase-3 is a key enzyme in glycolysis required also for the synthesis of the precursors of purines and pyrimidines, particularly in rapidly dividing tumor cells. PFK is activated via PI3K/AKT/mTOR.

PKC Protein kinase C (conventional isoforms are activated by calcium and diacylglycerol [DAG], produced by PLC)

PLC Phospholipase C, a polyphosphoinositide phosphodiesterase, activated by RTK. PLC hydrolyzes phoshatidylinositol-(4,5)-bisphosphate (PIP_2) to Inositol-(1,4,5)-trisphosphate (IP_3) and diacylglycerol (DAG). IP3 leads to release of Ca from intracellular stores, and DAG activates PKC.

PTEN Phosphatase and tensin homolog deleted from chromosome 10, also known as MMAC1 (mutated in multiple advanced cancers) or TEP1 (TGF-regulated and epithelial cell-enriched phosphatase). This lipid and protein phosphatase is involved in cell proliferation and survival, angiogenesis, and translational control. *PTEN* is located on human chromosome 10q23 and is deleted in a variety of human tumors. Germline mutations of *PTEN* are found in Cowden's disease, Bannayan-Riley-Ruvalcaba-syndrome, and L'hermitte-Duclos disease.

RAS A 21- kDa protein with GTPase acitivity, existing in different isoforms primarily, K-RAS, H-RAS, and N-RAS. K-RAS in contrast to H-RAS and N-RAS is essential for mouse development. Mutations for K-RAS are commonly found in human colon and pancreatic cancers, N-RAS in leukemias. RAS is inhibited by NF1. K-RAS and H-RAS are oncogenes originally identified in murine sarcoma viruses Ki-MSV (Kirsten) and Ha-MSV (Harvey). Ki-MSV and Ha-MSV are closely related, but independent isolates obtained from rat sarcomas that developed after inoculation with murine leukemia viruses. ^{G12D}K-RAS carries an activating mutation exchanging glycine (G) at position 12 to aspartic acid (D).

RB Retinoblastoma oncoprotein forms a complex with E2F. When RB is phosphorylated by CDK4 or CDK6, E2F is released and mediates the transcription of genes required for S –phase, RCAS Replication competent ALV splice acceptor is a retroviral expression vector based on ALV. This virus is specific for chicken and quail cells and replicates to high titer in these cells. It is unable to infect mammalian cells, because the receptor for this virus, a protein named tv-a, is not produced in mammals.

RTK Receptor tyrosine kinase. These include receptors such as EGF (EGF), IGF (IGFR), FGF (FGFR), and PDGF (PDGFR). Activation of RTK through adapter molecules such as Sos, Grb2, Shc activates Ras/Raf/ Erk, and the AKT pathway via PI3-kinase, and PKC through PLC.

SH2 Src homology-2 domain functions in protein-protein interaction. It is found in proteins interacting with the cytoplasmic domain of RTK.

TOP 5'terminal oligopyrimidine-rich tract. TOP are found in ribosomal proteins. The translation of these ribosomal proteins is controlled by PI3K/AKT via p70^{S6K}.

TV-A The tumor virus susceptibility locus A codes for the receptor, TV-A, for ALV. The receptor exists in two forms: transmembrane and myristoylated.

ACKNOWLEDGMENTS

We are grateful to David Thaler, The Rockefeller University, New York for his critical comments on this manuscript. This work was supported in part by the Searle Scholars foundation and NIH grant U01CA894314-1.

REFERENCES

1. Afanasieva T.A., Pekarik V., Grazia D'Angelo M., Klein M.A., Voigtlander T., Stocking C., Aguzzi A. 2001. Insertional mutagenesis of preneoplastic astrocytes by Moloney murine leukemia virus. *J. Neurovirol.* **7:**169–181.
2. Alderson L.M., Castleberg R.L., Harsh G.R.T., Louis D.N., Henson J.W. 1995. Human gliomas with wild-type p53 express bcl-2. *Cancer Res.* **55:**999–1001.
3. Aoki M., Batista O., Bellacosa A., Tsichlis P., Vogt P.K. 1998. The akt kinase: molecular determinants of oncogenicity. *Proc. Natl. Acad. Sci. USA* **95:**14,950–14,955.
4. Aoki M., Blazek E., Vogt P.K. 2001. A role of the kinase mTOR in cellular transformation induced by the oncoproteins P3k and Akt. *Proc. Natl. Acad. Sci. USA* **98:**136–141.
5. Arch E. M., Goodman B.K., Van Wesep R.A., Liaw D., Clarke K., Parsons R, et al. 1997. Deletion of PTEN in a patient with Bannayan-Riley-Ruvalcaba syndrome suggests allelism with Cowden disease. *Am. J. Med. Genet.* **71:**489–493.
6. Auger K.R., Carpenter C.L., Shoelson S.E., Piwnica-Worms H., Cantley L.C. 1992. Polyoma virus middle T antigen-pp60c-src complex associates with purified phosphatidylinositol 3-kinase in vitro. *J. Biol. Chem.* **267:**5408–5415.
7. Backman S.A., Stambolic V., Suzuki A., Haight J., Elia A., Pretorius J., et al. 2001. Deletion of Pten in mouse brain causes seizures, ataxia and defects in soma size resembling Lhermitte-Duclos disease. *Nat. Genet.* **29:**396–403.
8. Bahuau M., Vidaud D., Jenkins R.B., Bieche I., Kimmel D.W., Assouline B., et al. 1998. Germ-line deletion involving the INK4 locus in familial proneness to melanoma and nervous system tumors. *Cancer Res.* **58:**2298–2303.
9. Barry O.P., Kazanietz M.G. 2001. Protein kinase C isozymes, novel phorbol ester receptors and cancer chemotherapy. *Curr. Pharm. Des.* **7:**1725–1744.
10. Bar-Sagi D., Hall A. 2000. Ras and Rho GTPases: a family reunion. *Cell* **103:**227–238.
11. Bartek J., Falck J., Lukas J. 2001. CHK2 kinase—a busy messenger. *Nat. Rev. Mol. Cell Biol.* **2:**877–886.
12. Bates P., Rong L., Varmus H.E., Young J.A., Crittenden L.B. 1998. Genetic mapping of the cloned subgroup A avian sarcoma and leukosis virus receptor gene to the TVA locus. *J. Virol.* **72:**2505–2508.
13. Bates P., Young J.A., Varmus H.E. 1993. A receptor for subgroup A Rous sarcoma virus is related to the low density lipoprotein receptor. *Cell* **74:**1043–1051.
14. Bates S., Phillips A.C., Clark P.A., Stott F., Peters G., Ludwig R.L., Vousden K.H. 1998. p14ARF links the tumour suppressors RB and p53. *Nature* **395:**124–125.
15. Begemann M., Kashimawo S.A., Choi Y.A., Kim S., Christiansen K.M., Duigou G., et al. 1996. Inhibition of the growth of glioblastomas by CGP 41251, an inhibitor of protein kinase C, and by a phorbol ester tumor promoter. *Clin. Cancer Res.* **2:**1017–1030.
16. Begemann M., Kashimawo S.A., Heitjan D.F., Schiff P.B., Bruce J.N., Weinstein I.B.. 1998. Treatment of human glioblastoma cells with the staurosporine derivative CGP 41251 inhibits CDC2 and CDK2 kinase activity and increases radiation sensitivity. *Anticancer Res.* **18:**2275–2282.
17. Begemann M., Kashimawo S.A., Lunn R.M., Delohery T., Choi Y.J., Kim S., et al. 1998. Growth inhibition induced by Ro 31-8220 and calphostin C in human glioblastoma cell lines is associated with apoptosis and inhibition of CDC2 kinase. *Anticancer Res.* **18:**3139–3152.

18. Bell D.W., Varley J.M., Szydlo T.E., Kang D.H., Wahrer D.C., Shannon K.E., et al. 1999. Heterozygous germ line hCHK2 mutations in Li-Fraumeni syndrome. *Science* **286:**2528–2531.

19. Bellacosa A., Testa J.R., Staal S.P., Tsichlis P.N. 1991. A retroviral oncogene, akt, encoding a serine-threonine kinase containing an SH2-like region. *Science* **254:**274–277.

20. Benzil D.L., Finkelstein S.D., Epstein M.H., Finch P.W. 1992. Expression pattern of alpha-protein kinase C in human astrocytomas indicates a role in malignant progression. *Cancer Res.* **52:**2951–2956.

21. Bhatia S., Sklar C. 2002. Second Cancers in survivors of childhood cancers. *Nature Reviews Cancer* **2:**124–132.

22. Biernat W., Aguzzi A., Sure U., Grant J.W., Kleihues P., Hegi M.E. 1995. Identical mutations of the p53 tumor suppressor gene in the gliomatous and the sarcomatous components of gliosarcomas suggest a common origin from glial cells. *J. Neuropathol. Exp. Neurol.* **54:**651–656.

23. Biernat W., Kleihues P., Yonekawa Y., Ohgaki H. 1997. Amplification and overexpression of MDM2 in primary (de novo) glioblastomas. *J. Neuropathol. Exp. Neurol.* **56:**180–185.

24. Biggs W.H. 3rd, Meisenhelder J., Hunter T., Cavenee W.K., Arden K.C. 1999. Protein kinase B/Akt-mediated phosphorylation promotes nuclear exclusion of the winged helix transcription factor FKHR1. *Proc. Natl. Acad. Sci. USA* **96:**7421–7426.

25. Bigner S.H., Bjerkvig R., Laerum O.D. 1985. DNA content and chromosomal composition of malignant human gliomas. *Neurol. Clin.* **3:**769–784.

26. Bigner S.H., Rasheed B.K., Wiltshire R., McLendon R.E. 1999. Morphologic and molecular genetic aspects of oligodendroglial neoplasms. *Neuro-oncol.* **1:**52–60.

27. Bjornson C.R., Rietze R.L., Reynolds B.A., Magli M.C., Vescovi A.L. 1999. Turning brain into blood: a hematopoietic fate adopted by adult neural stem cells in vivo. *Science* **283:**534–537.

28. Boerman R.H., Anderl K., Herath J., Borell T., Johnson N., Schaeffer-Klein J., et al. 1996. The glial and mesenchymal elements of gliosarcomas share similar genetic alterations. *J. Neuropathol. Exp. Neurol.* **55:**973–981.

29. Bogler O., Huang H.J., Kleihues P., Cavenee W.K. 1995. The p53 gene and its role in human brain tumors. *Glia* **15:**308–327.

30. Bredel M., Pollack I.F., Hamilton R.L., James C.D. 1999. Epidermal growth factor receptor expression and gene amplification in high-grade non-brainstem gliomas of childhood. *Clin. Cancer Res.* **5:**1786–1792.

31. Brown E.J., Beal P.A., Keith C.T., Chen J., Shin T.B., Schreiber S.L. 1995. Control of p70 s6 kinase by kinase activity of FRAP in vivo. *Nature* **377:**441–446.

32. Brown E.J., Schreiber S.L. 1996. A signaling pathway to translational control. *Cell* **86:**517–520.

33. Brownawell A.M., Kops G.J., Macara I.G., Burgering B.M. 2001. Inhibition of nuclear import by protein kinase B (Akt) regulates the subcellular distribution and activity of the forkhead transcription factor AFX. *Mol. Cell Biol.* **21:** 3534–3546.

34. Brunet A., Bonni A., Zigmond M.J., Lin M.Z., Juo P., Hu L.S., et al. 1999. Akt promotes cell survival by phosphorylating and inhibiting a Forkhead transcription factor. *Cell* **96:**857–88.

35. Bunz F., Dutriaux A., Lengauer C., Waldman T., Zhou S., Brown J.P., et al. 1998. Requirement for p53 and p21 to sustain G2 arrest after DNA damage. *Science* **282:**1497–1501.

36. Burrows R.C., Lillien L., Levitt P. 2000. Mechanisms of progenitor maturation are conserved in the striatum and cortex. *De. Neurosci.* **22:**7–15.

37. Burrows R.C., Wancio D., Levitt P., Lillien L. 1997. Response diversity and the timing of progenitor cell maturation are regulated by developmental changes in EGFR expression in the cortex. *Neuron* **19:**251–267.

38. Burton E.C., Lamborn K.R., Forsyth P., Scott J., O'Campo J., Uyehara-Lock J.,et al. 2002. Aberrant p53, mdm2, and Proliferation Differ in Glioblastomas from Long-Term Compared with Typical Survivors(1). *Clin. Cancer. Res.* **8:**180–187.

39. Buschges R., Weber R.G., Actor B., Lichter P., Collins V.P., Reifenberger G. 1999. Amplification and expression of cyclin D genes (CCND1, CCND2 and CCND3) in human malignant gliomas. *Brain Pathol.* **9:**435–42; discussion 432–433.

40. Calver A.R., Hall A.C., Yu W.P., Walsh F.S., Heath J.K., Betsholtz C., Richardson W.D. 1998. Oligodendrocyte population dynamics and the role of PDGF in vivo. *Neuron* **20:**869–882.

41. Campbell K.S., Ogris E., Burke B., Su W., Auger K.R., Druker B.J., et al. 1994. Polyoma middle tumor antigen interacts with SHC protein via the NPTY (Asn-Pro-Thr-Tyr) motif in middle tumor antigen. *Proc. Natl. Acad. Sci. USA* **91:** 6344–6348.

42. Campomenosi P., Ottaggio L., Moro F., Urbini S., Bogliolo M., Zunino A., et al. 1996. Study on aneuploidy and p53 mutations in astrocytomas. *Cancer Genet. Cytogenet.* **88:**95–102.

43. Cardone M.H., Roy N., Stennicke H.R., Salvesen G.S., Franke T.F., Stanbridge E., et al. 1998. Regulation of cell death protease caspase-9 by phosphorylation. *Science* **282:**1318–1321.

44. Carpenter C.L., Auger K.R., Chanudhuri M., Yoakim M., Schaffhausen B., Shoelson S., Cantley L.C.. 1993. Phosphoinositide 3-kinase is activated by phosphopeptides that bind to the SH2 domains of the 85-kDa subunit. *J. Biol. Chem.* **268:**9478–9483.

45. Caspari T. 2000. How to activate p53. *Curr. Biol.* **10:**R315–R317.

46. Chakravarti A., Delaney M.A., Noll E., Black P.M., Loeffler J.S., Muzikansky A., Dyson N.J. 2001. Prognostic and pathologic significance of quantitative protein expression profiling in human gliomas. *Clin. Cancer Res.* **7:**2387–2395.

47. Chan D.W., Son S.C., Block W., Ye R., Khanna K.K., Wold M.S., et al. 2000. Purification and characterization of ATM from human placenta. A manganese-dependent, wortmannin-sensitive serine/threonine protein kinase. *J. Biol. Chem.* **275:**7803–7810.

48. Chan T.A., Hermeking H., Lengauer C., Kinzler K.W., Vogelstein B. 1999. 14–3-3Sigma is required to prevent mitotic catastrophe after DNA damage. *Nature* **401:**616–620.

49. Chan T.O., Rittenhouse S.E., Tsichlis P.N. 1999. AKT/PKB and other D3 phosphoinositide-regulated kinases: kinase activation by phosphoinositide-dependent phosphorylation. *Annu. Rev. Biochem.* **68:**965–1014.

50. Chaturvedi P., Eng W.K., Zhu Y., Mattern M.R., Mishra R., Hurle M.R., et al. 1999. Mammalian Chk2 is a downstream effector of the ATM-dependent DNA damage checkpoint pathway. *Oncogene* **18:**4047–4054.

51. Chellappan S.P., Hiebert S., Mudryj M., Horowitz J.M., Nevins J.R. 1991. The E2F transcription factor is a cellular target for the RB protein. *Cell* **65:**1053–1061.

52. Cheney I.W., Neuteboom S.T., Vaillancourt M.T., Ramachandra M., Bookstein R. 1999. Adenovirus-mediated gene transfer of MMAC1/PTEN to glioblastoma cells inhibits S phase entry by the recruitment of p27Kip1 into cyclin E/CDK2 complexes. *Cancer Res.* **59:**2318–2323.

53. Cheng J.Q., Godwin A.K., Bellacosa A., Taguchi T., Franke T.F., Hamilton T.C., et al. 1992. AKT2, a putative oncogene encoding a member of a subfamily of protein-serine/threonine kinases, is amplified in human ovarian carcinomas. *Proc. Natl. Acad. Sci. USA* **89:**9267–9271.

54. Cheng M., Olivier P., Diehl J.A., Fero M., Roussel M.F., Roberts J.M., Sherr C.J. 1999. The p21(Cip1) and p27(Kip1) CDK 'inhibitors' are essential activators of cyclin D-dependent kinases in murine fibroblasts. *Embo. J.* **18:**1571–1583.

55. Chin L., Merlino G., DePinho R.A. 1998. Malignant melanoma: modern black plague and genetic black box. *Genes Dev.* **12:**3467–3481.

56. Chin L., Tam A., Pomerantz J., Wong M., Holash J., Bardeesy N., et al. 1999. Essential role for oncogenic Ras in tumour maintenance. *Nature* **400:**468–472.

57. Cichowski K., Jacks T.. 2001. NF1 tumor suppressor gene function: narrowing the GAP. *Cell* **104:**593–604.

58. Clarke A.R., Maandag E.R., van Roon M., van der Lugt N.M., van der Valk M., Hooper M.L., et al. 1992. Requirement for a functional Rb-1 gene in murine development. *Nature* **359:**328–30.

59. Clarke D.L., Johansson C.B., Wilbertz J., Veress B., Nilsson E., Karlstrom H., Lendahl U., Frisen J. 2000. Generalized potential of adult neural stem cells. *Science* **288:**1660–1663.

60. Collado M., Medema R.H., Garcia-Cao I., Dubuisson M.L., Barradas M., J. Glassford, et al. 2000. Inhibition of the phosphoinositide 3-kinase pathway induces a senescence-like arrest mediated by p27Kip1. *J. Biol. Chem.* **275:**21,960–21,968.

61. Costello J.F., Berger M.S., Huang H.S., Cavenee W.K. 1996. Silencing of p16/CDKN2 expression in human gliomas by methylation and chromatin condensation. *Cancer Res.* **56:**2405–2410.

62. Costello J.F., Plass C., Arap W., Chapman V.M., Held W.A., Berger M.S., et al. 1997. Cyclin-dependent kinase 6 (CDK6) amplification in human gliomas identified using two-dimensional separation of genomic DNA. *Cancer Res* **57:**1250–1254.

63. Crafts D., Wilson C.B. 1977. Animal models of brain tumors. *Natl. Cancer Inst.* Monogr **46:**11–17.

64. Cross D.A., Alessi D.R., Cohen P., Andjelkovich M., Hemmings B.A. 1995. Inhibition of glycogen synthase kinase-3 by insulin mediated by protein kinase B. *Nature* **378:**785–789.

65. Dai C., Celestino J.C., Okada Y., Louis D.N., Fuller G.N., Holland E.C. 2001. PDGF autocrine stimulation dedifferentiates cultured astrocytes and induces oligodendrogliomas and oligoastrocytomas from neural progenitors and astrocytes in vivo. *Genes Dev.* **15:**1913–1925.

66. Datta K., Bellacosa A., Chan T.O., Tsichlis P.N. 1996. Akt is a direct target of the phosphatidylinositol 3-kinase. Activation by growth factors, v-src and v-Ha-ras, in Sf9 and mammalian cells. *J. Biol. Chem.* **271:**30,835–30,839.

67. Datta S.R., Brunet A., Greenberg M.E. 1999. Cellular survival: a play in three Akts. *Genes Dev.* **13:**2905–2927.

68. Datta S.R., Dudek H., Tao X., Masters S., Fu H., Gotoh Y., Greenberg M.E. 1997. Akt phosphorylation of BAD couples survival signals to the cell-intrinsic death machinery. *Cell* **91:**231–241.

69. Davies M.A., Lu Y., Sano T., Fang X., Tang P., LaPushin R., et al. 1998. Adenoviral transgene expression of MMAC/PTEN in human glioma cells inhibits Akt activation and induces anoikis. *Cancer Res.* **58:**5285–5290.

70. Davis R. J. 2000. Signal transduction by the JNK group of MAP kinases. *Cell* **103:**239–252.

71. De Vivo I., Gertig D.M., Nagase S., Hankinson S.E., O'Brien R., Speizer F.E., et al. 2000. Novel germline mutations in the PTEN tumour suppressor gene found in women with multiple cancers. *J. Med. Genet.* **37:**336–341.

72. Delcommenne M., Tan C., Gray V., Rue L., Woodgett J., Dedhar S. 1998. Phosphoinositide-3-OH kinase-dependent regulation of glycogen synthase kinase 3 and protein kinase B/AKT by the integrin-linked kinase. *Proc. Natl. Acad. Sci. USA* **95:**11,211–11,216.

73. Di Rocco F., Carroll R.S., Zhang J., Black P.M. 1998. Platelet-derived growth factor and its receptor expression in human oligodendrogliomas. *Neurosurgery* **42:**341–346.

74. Diehl J.A., Cheng M., Roussel M.F., Sherr C.J. 1998. Glycogen synthase kinase-3beta regulates cyclin D1 proteolysis and subcellular localization. *Genes Dev.* **12:**3499–3511.

75. Dilworth S.M., Brewster C.E., Jones M.D., Lanfrancone L., Pelicci G., Pelicci P.G. 1994. Transformation by polyoma virus middle T-antigen involves the binding and tyrosine phosphorylation of Shc. *Nature* **367**:87–90.

76. Ding H., Roncari L., Shannon P., Wu X., Lau N., Karaskova J., et al. 2001. Astrocyte-specific expression of activated p21-ras results in malignant astrocytoma formation in a transgenic mouse model of human gliomas. *Cancer Res.* **61**: 3826–3836.

77. Ding H., Shannon P., Lau N., Wu X., Roncari L., Baldwin R.L., et al. 2003. Oligodendrogliomas result from the expression of an activated mutant epidermal growth factor receptor in a RAS transgenic mouse astrocytoma model. *Cancer Res.* **63**:1106–1113.

78. Doetsch F., Caille I., Lim D.A., Garcia-Verdugo J.M., Alvarez-Buylla A. 1999. Subventricular zone astrocytes are neural stem cells in the adult mammalian brain. *Cell* **97**:703–716.

79. Doetsch F., Garcia-Verdugo J.M., Alvarez-Buylla A. 1999. Regeneration of a germinal layer in the adult mammalian brain. *Proc. Natl. Acad. Sci. USA* **96**:11,619–11,624.

80. Donehower L.A., Harvey M., Slagle B.L., McArthur M.J., Montgomery C.A. Jr., Butel J.S., Bradley A. 1992. Mice deficient for p53 are developmentally normal but susceptible to spontaneous tumours. *Nature* **356**:215–221.

81. Duerr E.M., Rollbrocker B., Hayashi Y., Peters N., Meyer-Puttlitz B., Louis D.N., et al. 1998. PTEN mutations in gliomas and glioneuronal tumors. *Oncogene* **16**:2259–2264.

82. Ekstrand A.J., James C.D., Cavenee W.K., Seliger B., Pettersson R.F., Collins V.P. 1991. Genes for epidermal growth factor receptor, transforming growth factor alpha, and epidermal growth factor and their expression in human gliomas in vivo. *Cancer Res.* **51**:2164–2172.

83. Ekstrand A.J., Longo N., Hamid M.L., Olson J.J., Liu L., Collins V.P., James C.D. 1994. Functional characterization of an EGF receptor with a truncated extracellular domain expressed in glioblastomas with EGFR gene amplification. *Oncogene* **9**:2313–2320.

84. Ekstrand A.J., Sugawa N., James C.D., Collins V.P. 1992. Amplified and rearranged epidermal growth factor receptor genes in human glioblastomas reveal deletions of sequences encoding portions of the N- and/or C-terminal tails. *Proc. Natl. Acad. Sci. USA* **89**:4309–4313.

85. El-Deiry W.S. 2001. Akt takes centre stage in cell-cycle deregulation. *Nat. Cell Biol.* **3**:E71—E73.

86. El-Deiry W.S., Tokino T., Velculescu V.E., Levy D.B., Parsons R., Trent J.M., et al. 1993. WAF1, a potential mediator of p53 tumor suppression. *Cell* **75**:817–825.

87. Elexpuru-Camiruaga J., Buxton N., Kandula V., Dias P.S., Campbell D., McIntosh J., et al. 1995. Susceptibility to astrocytoma and meningioma: influence of allelism at glutathione S-transferase (GSTT1 and GSTM1) and cytochrome P-450 (CYP2D6) loci. *Cancer Res.* **55**:4237–4239.

88. Falck J., Mailand N., Syljuasen R.G., Bartek J., Lukas J. 2001. The ATM-Chk2-Cdc25A checkpoint pathway guards against radioresistant DNA synthesis. *Nature* **410**:842–847.

89. Federspiel M.J., Bates P., Young J.A., Varmus H.E., Hughes S.H. 1994. A system for tissue-specific gene targeting: transgenic mice susceptible to subgroup A avian leukosis virus-based retroviral vectors. *Proc. Natl. Acad. Sci. USA* **91**:11,241–11,245.

90. Feldkamp M.M., Lala P., Lau N., Roncari L., Guha A. 1999. Expression of activated epidermal growth factor receptors, Ras-guanosine triphosphate, and mitogen-activated protein kinase in human glioblastoma multiforme specimens. *Neurosurgery* **45**:1442–1453.

91. Fisher G.H., Orsulic S., Holland E., Hively W.P., Li Y., Lewis B.C., et al. 1999. Development of a flexible and specific gene delivery system for production of murine tumor models. *Oncogene* **18**:5253–5260.

92. Fisher G.H., Wellen S.L., Klimstra D., Lenczowski J.M., Tichelaar J.W., Lizak M.J., et al. 2001. Induction and apoptotic regression of lung adenocarcinomas by regulation of a K-Ras transgene in the presence and absence of tumor suppressor genes. *Genes Dev.* **15**:3249–3262.

93. Fleming T.P., Saxena A., Clark W.C., Robertson J.T., Oldfield E.H., Aaronson S.A., Ali I.U. 1992. Amplification and/or overexpression of platelet-derived growth factor receptors and epidermal growth factor receptor in human glial tumors. *Cancer Res.* **52**:4550–4553.

94. Flemington E.K., Speck S.H., Kaelin W.G. Jr. 1993. E2F-1-mediated transactivation is inhibited by complex formation with the retinoblastoma susceptibility gene product. *Proc. Natl. Acad. Sci. USA* **90**:6914–6918.

95. Franke T.F., Yang S.I., Chan T.O., Datta K., Kazlauskas A., Morrison D.K., et al. 1995. The protein kinase encoded by the Akt proto-oncogene is a target of the PDGF-activated phosphatidylinositol 3-kinase. *Cell* **81**:727–736.

96. Fricker-Gates R.A., Winkler C., Kirik D., Rosenblad C., Carpenter M.K., Bjorklund A. 2000. EGF infusion stimulates the proliferation and migration of embryonic progenitor cells transplanted in the adult rat striatum. *Exp. Neurol.* **165**:237–247.

97. Frodin M., Gammeltoft S. 1999. Role and regulation of 90 kDa ribosomal S6 kinase (RSK) in signal transduction. *Mol. Cell Endocrinol.* **151**:65–77.

98. Fruttiger M., Karlsson L., Hall A.C., Abramsson A., Calver A.R., Bostrom H., et al. 1999. Defective oligodendrocyte development and severe hypomyelination in PDGF-A knockout mice. *Development* **126**:457–467.

99. Fuchs S.Y., Adler V., Buschmann T., Wu X., Ronai Z. 1998. Mdm2 association with p53 targets its ubiquitination. *Oncogene* **17**:2543–2547.

100. Fueyo J., Gomez-Manzano C., Bruner J.M., Saito Y., Zhang B., Zhang W., et al. 1996. Hypermethylation of the CpG island of p16/CDKN2 correlates with gene inactivation in gliomas. *Oncogene* **13**:1615–1619.

101. Galli R., Borello U., Gritti A., Minasi M.G., Bjornson C., Coletta M., et al. 2000. Skeletal myogenic potential of human and mouse neural stem cells. *Nat. Neurosci.* **3**:986–991.

102. Gesbert F., Sellers W.R., Signoretti S., Loda M., Griffin J.D. 2000. BCR/ABL regulates expression of the cyclin-dependent kinase inhibitor p27Kip1 through the phosphatidylinositol 3-Kinase/AKT pathway. *J. Biol. Chem.* **275**: 39,223–39,230.

103. Gingras A.C., Gygi S.P., Raught B., Polakiewicz R.D., Abraham R.T., Hoekstra M.F., et al. 1999. Regulation of 4E-BP1 phosphorylation: a novel two-step mechanism. *Genes Dev.* **13**:1422–1437.

104. Gomez-Manzano C., Mitlianga P., Fueyo J., Lee H.Y., Hu M., Spurgers K.B., et al. 2001. Transfer of E2F-1 to human glioma cells results in transcriptional up-regulation of Bcl-2. *Cancer Res.* **61**:6693–6697.

105. Gomori E., Doczi T., Pajor L., Matolcsy A. 1999. Sporadic p53 mutations and absence of ras mutations in glioblastomas. *Acta. Neurochir.* (Wien) **141**:593–599.

106. Gottschalk A.R., Basila D., Wong M., Dean N.M., Brandts C.H., Stokoe D., Haas-Kogan D.A. 2001. p27Kip1 is required for PTEN-induced G1 growth arrest. *Cancer Res.* **61**:2105–2111.

107. Graff J.R., Konicek B.W., McNulty A.M., Wang Z., Houck K., Allen S., et al. 2000. Increased AKT activity contributes to prostate cancer progression by dramatically accelerating prostate tumor growth and diminishing p27Kip1 expression. *J. Biol. Chem.* **275**:24,500–24,505.

108. Grossman S.A., Osman M., Hruban R., Piantadosi S. 1999. Central nervous system cancers in first-degree relatives and spouses. *Cancer Invest.* **17**:299–308.

109. Groszer M., Erickson R., Scripture-Adams D.D., Lesche R., Trumpp A., Zack J.A, et al. 2001. Negative regulation of neural stem/progenitor cell proliferation by the Pten tumor suppressor gene in vivo. *Science* **294**:2186–2189.

110. Groth A., Weber J.D., Willumsen B.M., Sherr C.J., Roussel M.F. 2000. Oncogenic Ras induces p19ARF and growth arrest in mouse embryo fibroblasts lacking p21Cip1 and p27Kip1 without activating cyclin D-dependent kinases. *J. Biol. Chem.* **275**:27,473–27,480.

111. Guha A., Dashner K., Black P.M., Wagner J.A., Stiles C.D. 1995. Expression of PDGF and PDGF receptors in human astrocytoma operation specimens supports the existence of an autocrine loop. *Int. J. Cancer* **60**:168–173.

112. Guha A., Feldkamp M.M., Lau N., Boss G., Pawson A. 1997. Proliferation of human malignant astrocytomas is dependent on Ras activation. *Oncogene* **15**:2755–2765.

113. Guha C., Guha U., Tribius S., Alfieri A., Casper D., Chakravarty P., et al. 2000. Antisense ATM gene therapy: a strategy to increase the radiosensitivity of human tumors. Gene Ther. **7**:852–858.

114. Hahn W.C., Counter C.M., Lundberg A.S., Beijersbergen R.L., Brooks M.W., Weinberg R.A.. 1999. Creation of human tumour cells with defined genetic elements. *Nature* **400**:464–468.

115. Hamilton S.R., Liu B., Parsons R.E., Papadopoulos N., Jen J., Powell S.M., et al. 1995. The molecular basis of Turcot's syndrome. *N. Engl. J. Med.* **332**:839–847.

116. Hann B., Balmain A. 2001. Building 'validated' mouse models of human cancer. *Curr. Opin. Cell Biol.* **13**:778–784.

117. Harlow E. 1992. Retinoblastoma. For our eyes only. *Nature* **359**:270–271.

118. Harvey M., McArthur M.J., Montgomery C.A. Jr., Bradley A., Donehower L.A. 1993. Genetic background alters the spectrum of tumors that develop in p53-deficient mice. *Faseb J.* **7**:938–943.

119. Haupt Y., Maya R., Kazaz A., Oren M. 1997. Mdm2 promotes the rapid degradation of p53. *Nature* **387**:296–299.

120. Hayakawa J., Ohmichi M., Kurachi H., Kanda Y., Hisamoto K., Nishio Y., et al. 2000. Inhibition of BAD phosphorylation either at serine 112 via extracellular signal-regulated protein kinase cascade or at serine 136 via Akt cascade sensitizes human ovarian cancer cells to cisplatin. *Cancer Res.* **60**:5988–5994.

121. Heldin C.H., Westermark B. 1999. Mechanism of action and in vivo role of platelet-derived growth factor. *Physiol. Rev.* **79**:1283–1316.

122. Hermanson M., Funa K., Hartman M., Claesson-Welsh L., Heldin C.H., Westermark B., Nister M. 1992. Platelet-derived growth factor and its receptors in human glioma tissue: expression of messenger RNA and protein suggests the presence of autocrine and paracrine loops. *Cancer Res.* **52**:3213–3219.

123. Hesselager G., Uhrbom L., Westermark B., Nister M. 2003. Complementary effects of platelet-derived growth factor autocrine stimulation and p53 or Ink4a-Arf deletion in a mouse glioma model.*Cancer Res.* **63**:4305–4309.

124. Hirao A., Kong Y.Y., Matsuoka S., Wakeham A., Ruland J., Yoshida H., et al. 2000. DNA damage-induced activation of p53 by the checkpoint kinase Chk2. *Science* **287**:1824–1827.

125. Hirose Y., Berger M.S., Pieper R.O. 2001. Abrogation of the Chk1-mediated G(2) checkpoint pathway potentiates temozolomide-induced toxicity in a p53-independent manner in human glioblastoma cells. *Cancer Res.* **61**:5843–5849.

126. Hogan B., Costantini F., Lacy E. 1986. *Manipulating the Mouse Embryo*, CSH Press, Cold Spring Harbor, New York.

127. Holland E.C. 2000. A mouse model for glioma: biology, pathology, and therapeutic opportunities. *Toxicol. Pathol.* **28**:171–177.

128. Holland E.C., Celestino J., Dai C., Schaefer L., Sawaya R.E., Fuller G.N. 2000. Combined activation of Ras and Akt in neural progenitors induces glioblastoma formation in mice. *Nat. Genet.* **25**:55–57.

129. Holland E.C., Hively W.P., DePinho R.A., Varmus H.E. 1998. A constitutively active epidermal growth factor receptor cooperates with disruption of G1 cell-cycle arrest pathways to induce glioma-like lesions in mice. *Genes Dev.* **12**:3675–3685.

130. Holland E.C., Hively W.P., Gallo V., Varmus H.E. 1998. Modeling mutations in the G1 arrest pathway in human gliomas: overexpression of CDK4 but not loss of INK4a-ARF induces hyperploidy in cultured mouse astrocytes. *Genes Dev.* **12**:3644–3649.

131. Holland E.C., Li Y., Celestino J., Dai C., Schaefer L., Sawaya R.A., Fuller G.N. 2000. Astrocytes give rise to oligodendrogliomas and astrocytomas after gene transfer of polyoma virus middle T antigen in vivo. *Am. J. Pathol.* **157**:1031–1037.

132. Holland E.C., Varmus H.E. 1998. Basic fibroblast growth factor induces cell migration and proliferation after glia-specific gene transfer in mice. *Proc. Natl. Acad. Sci. USA* **95**:1218–1223.

133. Holliday R. 1992. Of mice and men. *Nature* **360**:270–271.

134. Humphrey P.A., Wong A.J., Vogelstein B., Friedman H.S., Werner M.H., Bigner D.D., Bigner S.H. 1988. Amplification and expression of the epidermal growth factor receptor gene in human glioma xenografts. *Cancer Res.* **48**:2231–2238.

135. Ichaso N., Dilworth S.M. 2001. Cell transformation by the middle T-antigen of polyoma virus. *Oncogene* **20**:7908–7916.

136. Ichimura K., Bolin M.B., Goike H.M., Schmidt E.E., Moshref A., Collins V.P. 2000. Deregulation of the p14ARF/ MDM2/p53 pathway is a prerequisite for human astrocytic gliomas with G1-S transition control gene abnormalities. *Cancer Res.* **60**:417–424.

137. Ichimura K., Schmidt E.E., Goike H.M., Collins V.P. 1996. Human glioblastomas with no alterations of the CDKN2A (p16INK4A, MTS1) and CDK4 genes have frequent mutations of the retinoblastoma gene. *Oncogene* **13**:1065–1672.

138. Ilgren E.B., Kinnier-Wilson L.M., Stiller C.A. 1985. Gliomas in neurofibromatosis: a series of 89 cases with evidence for enhanced malignancy in associated cerebellar astrocytomas. *Pathol. Annu.* **20(Pt 1)**:331–358.

139. Ishida S., Huang E., Zuzan H., Spang R., Leone G., West M., Nevins J.R. 2001. Role for E2F in control of both DNA replication and mitotic functions as revealed from DNA microarray analysis. *Mol. Cell Biol.* **21**:4684–4699.

140. Jacks T., Fazeli A., Schmitt E.M., Bronson R.T., Goodell M.A., Weinberg R.A. 1992. Effects of an Rb mutation in the mouse. *Nature* **359**:295–300.

141. Jacks T., Remington L., Williams B.O., Schmitt E.M., Halachmi S., Bronson R.T., Weinberg R.A. 1994. Tumor spectrum analysis in p53-mutant mice. *Curr. Biol.* **4**:1–7.

142. Jacks T., Shih T.S., Schmitt E.M., Bronson R.T., Bernards A., Weinberg R.A. 1994. Tumour predisposition in mice heterozygous for a targeted mutation in Nf1. *Nat. Genet.* **7**:353–361.

143. Jay V., Edwards V., Varela-Stavrinou M., Rutka J. 1997. Unique intracerebral tumor with divergent differentiation in a patient presenting as NF2: report of a case with features of astrocytoma, ependymoma, and PNET. *Ultrastruct. Pathol.* **21**:57–71.

144. Johnson D.G., Schwarz J.K., Cress W.D., Nevins J.R. 1993. Expression of transcription factor E2F1 induces quiescent cells to enter S phase. *Nature* **365**:349–352.

145. Jones S.N., Hancock A.R., Vogel H., Donehower L.A., Bradley A. 1998. Overexpression of Mdm2 in mice reveals a p53-independent role for Mdm2 in tumorigenesis. *Proc. Natl. Acad. Sci. USA* **95**:15,608–15,612.

146. Jones S.N., Roe A.E., Donehower L.A., Bradley A. 1995. Rescue of embryonic lethality in Mdm2-deficient mice by absence of p53. *Nature* **378**:206–208.

147. Jones S.N., Sands A.T., Hancock A.R., Vogel H., Donehower L.A., Linke S.P., Wahl G.M., Bradley A. 1996. The tumorigenic potential and cell growth characteristics of p53-deficient cells are equivalent in the presence or absence of Mdm2. *Proc. Natl. Acad. Sci. USA* **93**:14,106–14,111.

148. Jung J.M., Bruner J.M., Ruan S., Langford L.A., Kyritsis A.P., Kobayashi T., et al. 1995. Increased levels of p21WAF1/ Cip1 in human brain tumors. *Oncogene* **11**:2021–2028.

149. Kaelin W.G. Jr., Krek W., Sellers W.R., DeCaprio J.A., Ajchenbaum F., Fuchs C.S., et al. 1992. Expression cloning of a cDNA encoding a retinoblastoma-binding protein with E2F-like properties. *Cell* **70**:351–364.

150. Kalma Y., Marash L., Lamed Y., Ginsberg D. 2001. Expression analysis using DNA microarrays demonstrates that E2F-1 up-regulates expression of DNA replication genes including replication protein A2. *Oncogene* **20**:1379–1387.

151. Kamijo T., Bodner S., van de Kamp E., Randle D.H., Sherr C.J. 1999. Tumor spectrum in ARF-deficient mice. *Cancer Res.* **59**:2217–2222.

152. Kamijo T., van de Kamp E., Chong M.J., Zindy F., Diehl J.A., Sherr C.J., McKinnon P.J. 1999. Loss of the ARF tumor suppressor reverses premature replicative arrest but not radiation hypersensitivity arising from disabled atm function. *Cancer Res.* **59**:2464–2469.

153. Kamijo T., Weber J.D., Zambetti G., Zindy F., Roussel M.F., Sherr C.J. 1998. Functional and physical interactions of the ARF tumor suppressor with p53 and Mdm2. *Proc. Natl. Acad. Sci. USA* **95**:8292–8297.

154. Kamijo T., Zindy F., Roussel M.F., Quelle D.E., Downing J.R., Ashmun R.A., et al. 1997. Tumor suppression at the mouse INK4a locus mediated by the alternative reading frame product p19ARF. *Cell* **91**:649–659.

155. Kane L.P., Shapiro V.S., Stokoe D., Weiss A. 1999. Induction of NF-kappaB by the Akt/PKB kinase. *Curr. Biol.* **9**: 601–604.

156. Kato J., Matsushime H., Hiebert S.W., Ewen M.E., Sherr C.J. 1993. Direct binding of cyclin D to the retinoblastoma gene product (pRb) and pRb phosphorylation by the cyclin D-dependent kinase CDK4. *Genes Dev.* **7:**331–342.

157. Khosravi R., Maya R., Gottlieb T., Oren M., Shiloh Y., Shkedy D. 1999. Rapid ATM-dependent phosphorylation of MDM2 precedes p53 accumulation in response to DNA damage. *Proc. Natl. Acad. Sci. USA* **96:**14,973–14,977.

158. Kipling D. 1997. Telomere structure and telomerase expression during mouse development and tumorigenesis. *Eur. J. Cancer* **33:**792–800.

159. Kleihues P., Cavenee W.K. 2000. *Pathology and Genetics of Tumours of the Nervous System*. IARC Press, Lyon, France.

160. Kleihues P., Lantos P.L., Magee P.N. 1976. Chemical carcinogenesis in the nervous system. *Int. Rev. Exp. Pathol.* **15:** 153–232.

161. Kleihues P., Schauble B., zur Hausen A., Esteve J., Ohgaki H. 1997. Tumors associated with p53 germline mutations: a synopsis of 91 families. *Am. J. Pathol.* **150:**1–13.

162. Kops G.J., de Ruiter N.D., De Vries-Smits A.M., Powell D.R., Bos J.L., Burgering B.M. 1999. Direct control of the Forkhead transcription factor AFX by protein kinase B. *Nature* **398:**630–634.

163. Korf B.R. 2000. Malignancy in neurofibromatosis type 1. *Oncologist* **5:**477–485.

164. Kraus, J. A., J. Koopmann, P. Kaskel, D. Maintz, S. Brandner, J. Schramm, et al. 1995. Shared allelic losses on chromosomes 1p and 19q suggest a common origin of oligodendroglioma and oligoastrocytoma. *J. Neuropathol. Exp. Neurol.* **54:**91–95.

165. Krause K., Haugwitz U., Wasner M., Wiedmann M., Mossner J., Engeland K. 2001. Expression of the cell cycle phosphatase cdc25C is down-regulated by the tumor suppressor protein p53 but not by p73. *Biochem. Biophys. Res. Commun.* **284:**743–770.

166. Krimpenfort P., Quon K.C., Mooi W.J., Loonstra A., Berns A. 2001. Loss of p16Ink4a confers susceptibility to metastatic melanoma in mice. *Nature* **413:**83–86.

167. Kubbutat M.H., Jones S.N., Vousden K.H. 1997. Regulation of p53 stability by Mdm2. *Nature* **387:**299–303.

168. Kwon C.H., Zhu X., Zhang J., Knoop L.L., Tharp R., Smeyne R.J., et al. 2001. Pten regulates neuronal soma size: a mouse model of Lhermitte-Duclos disease. *Nat. Genet.* **29:**404–411.

169. Kyritsis A.P., Bondy M.L., Xiao M., Berman E.L., Cunningham J.E., Lee P.S., et al. 1994. Germline p53 gene mutations in subsets of glioma patients. *J. Natl. Cancer Inst.* **86:**344–349.

170. LaBaer J., Garrett M.D., Stevenson L.F., Slingerland J.M., Sandhu C., Chou H.S., et al. 1997. New functional activities for the p21 family of CDK inhibitors. *Genes Dev.* **11:**847–862.

171. Lee E.Y., Chang C.Y., Hu N., Wang Y.C., Lai C.C., Herrup K., et al. 1992. Mice deficient for Rb are nonviable and show defects in neurogenesis and haematopoiesis. *Nature* **359:**288–294.

172. Lee J.O., Yang H., Georgescu M.M., Di Cristofano A., Maehama T., Shi Y., et al. 1999. Crystal structure of the PTEN tumor suppressor: implications for its phosphoinositide phosphatase activity and membrane association. *Cell* **99:**323–334.

173. Levine A.J., Momand J., Finlay C.A. 1991. The p53 tumour suppressor gene. *Nature* **351:**453–456.

174. Lewandoski M. 2001. Conditional control of gene expression in the mouse. *Nat. Rev. Genet.* **2:**743–755.

175. Li D. M., Sun H. 1998. PTEN/MMAC1/TEP1 suppresses the tumorigenicity and induces G1 cell cycle arrest in human glioblastoma cells. *Proc.Natl. Acad. Sci. USA* **95:**15,406–15,411.

176. Li F.P., Fraumeni J.F. Jr. 1969. Soft-tissue sarcomas, breast cancer, and other neoplasms. A familial syndrome? *Ann. Intern. Med.* **71:**747–752.

177. Li J., Simpson L., Takahashi M., Miliaresis C., Myers M.P., Tonks N., Parsons R. 1998. The PTEN/MMAC1 tumor suppressor induces cell death that is rescued by the AKT/protein kinase B oncogene. *Cancer Res.* **58:**5667–5672.

178. Li J., Yen C., Liaw D., Podsypanina K., Bose S., Wang S.I., et al. 1997. PTEN, a putative protein tyrosine phosphatase gene mutated in human brain, breast, and prostate cancer. *Science* **275:**1943–1947.

179. Liaw D., Marsh D.J., Li J., Dahia P.L., Wang S.I., Zheng Z., et al. 1997. Germline mutations of the PTEN gene in Cowden disease, an inherited breast and thyroid cancer syndrome. *Nat. Genet.* **16:**64–67.

180. Lillien L., Raphael H. 2000. BMP and FGF regulate the development of EGF-responsive neural progenitor cells. *Development* **127:**4993–5005.

181. Lohr M., Maisonneuve P., Lowenfels A.B. 2000. K-Ras mutations and benign pancreatic disease. *Int. J. Pancreatol.* **27:**93–103.

182. Lossignol D., Grossman S.A., Sheidler V.R., Griffin C.A., Piantadosi S. 1990. Familial clustering of malignant astrocytomas. *J. Neurooncol.* **9:**139–145.

183. Luetteke N.C., Phillips H.K., Qiu T.H., Copeland N.G., Earp H.S., Jenkins N.A., Lee D.C. 1994. The mouse waved-2 phenotype results from a point mutation in the EGF receptor tyrosine kinase. *Genes Dev.* **8:**399–413.

184. Maehama T., Dixon J.E. 1998. The tumor suppressor, PTEN/MMAC1, dephosphorylates the lipid second messenger, phosphatidylinositol 3,4,5-trisphosphate. *J Biol. Chem.* **273:**13,375–13,378.

185. Malkin D., Li F.P., Strong L.C., Fraumeni J.F. Jr., Nelson C.E., Kim D.H., et al. 1990. Germ line p53 mutations in a familial syndrome of breast cancer, sarcomas, and other neoplasms. *Science* **250:**1233–1238.

186. Marsh D.J., Coulon V., Lunetta K.L., Rocca-Serra P., Dahia P.L., Zheng Z., et al. 1998. Mutation spectrum and geno-

type-phenotype analyses in Cowden disease and Bannayan-Zonana syndrome, two hamartoma syndromes with germline PTEN mutation. *Hum. Mol. Genet.* **7:**507–515.

187. Marsh D.J., Dahia P.L., Zheng Z., Liaw D., Parsons R., Gorlin R.J., Eng C. 1997. Germline mutations in PTEN are present in Bannayan-Zonana syndrome. *Nat. Genet.* **16:**333–334.

188. Marsh D.J., Kum J.B., Lunetta K.L., Bennett M.J., Gorlin R.J., Ahmed S.F.,. et al. 1999. PTEN mutation spectrum and genotype-phenotype correlations in Bannayan-Riley-Ruvalcaba syndrome suggest a single entity with Cowden syndrome. *Hum. Mol. Genet.* **8:**1461–1472.

189. Martelli F., Hamilton T., Silver D.P., Sharpless N.E., Bardeesy N., Rokas M., et al. 2001. p19ARF targets certain E2F species for degradation. *Proc. Natl. Acad. Sci. USA* **98:**4455–4460.

190. Matsuoka S., Huang M., Elledge S.J. 1998. Linkage of ATM to cell cycle regulation by the Chk2 protein kinase. *Science* **282:**1893–1897.

191. Matsuoka S., Rotman G., Ogawa A., Shiloh Y., Tamai K., Elledge S.J. 2000. Ataxia telangiectasia-mutated phosphorylates Chk2 in vivo and in vitro. *Proc. Natl. Acad. Sci. USA* **97:**10,389–10,394.

192. Mayo L.D., Dixon J.E., Durden D.L., Tonks N.K., Donner D.B. 2001. PTEN protects p53 from Mdm2 and sensitizes cancer cells to chemotherapy. *J. Biol. Chem.* **277:**5484–5489.

193. Mayo L.D., Donner D.B. 2001. A phosphatidylinositol 3-kinase/Akt pathway promotes translocation of Mdm2 from the cytoplasm to the nucleus. *Proc. Natl. Acad. Sci. USA* **98:**11,598–11,603.

194. Mayo M.W., Madrid L.V., Westerheide S.D., Jones D.R., Yuan X.J., Baldwin A.S. Jr., Whang Y.E. 2002. PTEN blocks TNF-induced NF-kappa B-dependent transcription by inhibiting the transactivation potential of the p65 subunit. *J. Biol. Chem.* **277:**11,116–11,125.

195. McKinnon R.D., Matsui T., Dubois-Dalcq M., Aaronson S.A. 1990. FGF modulates the PDGF-driven pathway of oligodendrocyte development. *Neuron* **5:**603–614.

196. Mende I., Malstrom S., Tsichlis P.N., Vogt P.K., Aoki M. 2001. Oncogenic transformation induced by membrane-targeted Akt2 and Akt3. *Oncogene* **20:**4419–4423.

197. Miettinen P.J., Berger J.E., Meneses J., Phung Y., Pedersen R.A., Werb Z., Derynck R. 1995. Epithelial immaturity and multiorgan failure in mice lacking epidermal growth factor receptor. *Nature* **376:**337–341.

198. Miettinen P.J., Chin J.R., Shum L., Slavkin H.C., Shuler C.F., Derynck R., Werb Z. 1999. Epidermal growth factor receptor function is necessary for normal craniofacial development and palate closure. *Nat. Genet.* **22:**69–73.

199. Minamoto T., Mai M., Ronai Z. 2000. K-ras mutation: early detection in molecular diagnosis and risk assessment of colorectal, pancreas, and lung cancers—a review. *Cancer Detect. Prev.* **24:**1–12.

200. Miyagi K., Mukawa J., Kinjo N., Horikawa K., Mekaru S., Nakasone S., et al. 1995. Astrocytoma linked to familial ataxia-telangiectasia. *Acta. Neurochir. (Wien)* **135:**87–92.

201. Momand J., Zambetti G.P., Olson D.C., George D., Levine A.J. 1992. The mdm-2 oncogene product forms a complex with the p53 protein and inhibits p53-mediated transactivation. *Cell* **69:**1237–1245.

202. Montes de Oca Luna R., Wagner D.S., Lozano G. 1995. Rescue of early embryonic lethality in mdm2-deficient mice by deletion of p53. *Nature* **378:**203–206.

203. Mueller W., Lass U., Herms J., Kuchelmeister K., Bergmann M., von Deimling A. 2001. Clonal analysis in glioblastoma with epithelial differentiation. *Brain Pathol.* **11:**39–43.

204. Muise-Helmericks R.C., Grimes H.L., Bellacosa A., Malstrom S.E., Tsichlis P.N., Rosen N. 1998. Cyclin D expression is controlled post-transcriptionally via a phosphatidylinositol 3-kinase/Akt-dependent pathway. *J. Biol. Chem.* **273:**29,864–29,872.

205. Myers M.P., Pass I., Batty I.H., Van der Kaay J., Stolarov J.P., Hemmings B.A., et al. 1998. The lipid phosphatase activity of PTEN is critical for its tumor supressor function. *Proc. Natl. Acad. Sci. USA* **95:**13,513–13,518.

206. Nakamura M., Watanabe T., Klangby U., Asker C., Wiman K., Yonekawa Y., Kleihues P., Ohgaki H. 2001. p14ARF deletion and methylation in genetic pathways to glioblastomas. *Brain Pathol.* **11:**159–168.

207. Neshat M.S., Mellinghoff I.K., Tran C., Stiles B., Thomas G., Petersen R., et al. 2001. Enhanced sensitivity of PTEN-deficient tumors to inhibition of FRAP/mTOR. *Proc. Natl. Acad. Sci. USA* **98:**10,314–10,319.

208. Nevins J.R. 1992. E2F: a link between the Rb tumor suppressor protein and viral oncoproteins. *Science* **258:**424–429.

209. Newcomb E.W., Alonso M., Sung T., Miller D.C. 2000. Incidence of p14ARF gene deletion in high-grade adult and pediatric astrocytomas. *Hum. Pathol.* **31:**115–119.

210. Nishikawa R., Furnari F.B., Lin H., Arap W., Berger M.S., Cavenee W.K., Su Huang H.J. 1995. Loss of P16INK4 expression is frequent in high grade gliomas. *Cancer Res.* **55:**1941–1945.

211. Nishizuka Y. 1992. Intracellular signaling by hydrolysis of phospholipids and activation of protein kinase C. *Science* **258:**607–614.

212. Nishizuka Y. 1995. Protein kinase C and lipid signaling for sustained cellular responses. *Faseb J.* **9:**484–496.

213. Noble M., Murray K., Stroobant P., Waterfield M.D., Riddle P. 1988. Platelet-derived growth factor promotes division and motility and inhibits premature differentiation of the oligodendrocyte/type-2 astrocyte progenitor cell. *Nature* **333:**560–562.

214. Ohgaki H., Eibl R.H., Wiestler O.D., Yasargil M.G., Newcomb E.W., Kleihues P. 1991. p53 mutations in nonastrocytic human brain tumors. *Cancer Res.* **51:**6202–6205.

215. Ono Y., Tamiya T., Ichikawa T., Matsumoto K., Furuta T., Ohmoto T., et al. 1997. Accumulation of wild-type p53 in astrocytomas is associated with increased p21 expression. *Acta. Neuropathol. (Berl)* **94:**21–27.

216. Ozes O.N., Mayo L.D., Gustin J.A., Pfeffer S.R., Pfeffer L.M., Donner D.B. 1999. NF-kappaB activation by tumour necrosis factor requires the Akt serine-threonine kinase. *Nature* **401:**82–85.

217. Pacold M.E., Suire S., Perisic O., Lara-Gonzalez S., Davis C.T., Walker E.H., et al. 2000. Crystal structure and functional analysis of Ras binding to its effector phosphoinositide 3-kinase gamma. *Cell* **103:**931–943.

218. Page C., Lin H.J., Jin Y., Castle V.P., Nunez G., Huang M., Lin J. 2000. Overexpression of Akt/AKT can modulate chemotherapy-induced apoptosis. *Anticancer Res.* **20:**407–416.

219. Palmero I., Pantoja C., Serrano M. 1998. p19ARF links the tumour suppressor p53 to Ras. *Nature* **395:**125–126.

220. Pardee A.B. 1989. G1 events and regulation of cell proliferation. *Science* **246:**603–608.

221. Pianetti S., Arsura M., Romieu-Mourez R., Coffey R.J., Sonenshein G.E. 2001. Her-2/neu overexpression induces NF-kappaB via a PI3-kinase/Akt pathway involving calpain-mediated degradation of IkappaB-alpha that can be inhibited by the tumor suppressor PTEN. *Oncogene* **20:**1287–1299.

222. Podsypanina K., Ellenson L.H., Nemes A., Gu J., Tamura M., Yamada K.M., et al. 1999. Mutation of Pten/Mmac1 in mice causes neoplasia in multiple organ systems. *Proc. Natl. Acad. Sci. USA* **96:**1563–1568.

223. Podsypanina K., Lee R.T., Politis C., Hennessy I., Crane A., Puc J., et al. 2001. An inhibitor of mTOR reduces neoplasia and normalizes p70/S6 kinase activity in Pten+/- mice. *Proc. Natl. Acad. Sci. USA* **98:**10,320–10,325.

224. Pollack I.F., Finkelstein S.D., Woods J., Burnham J., Holmes E.M., Hamilton R.L., et al. 2002. Expression of p53 and prognosis in children with malignant gliomas. *N. Engl. J. Med.* **346:**420–427.

225. Prives C., Manley J.L. 2001. Why is p53 acetylated? *Cell* **107:**815–818.

226. Quelle D.E., Ashmun R.A., Hannon G.J., Rehberger P.A., Trono D., Richter K.H., et al. 1995. Cloning and characterization of murine p16INK4a and p15INK4b genes. *Oncogene* **11:**635–645.

227. Quelle D.E., Cheng M., Ashmun R.A., Sherr C.J. 1997. Cancer-associated mutations at the INK4a locus cancel cell cycle arrest by p16INK4a but not by the alternative reading frame protein p19ARF. *Proc. Natl. Acad. Sci. USA* **94:** 669–673.

228. Quelle D.E., Zindy F., Ashmun R.A., Sherr C.J. 1995. Alternative reading frames of the INK4a tumor suppressor gene encode two unrelated proteins capable of inducing cell cycle arrest. *Cell* **83:**993–1000.

229. Ramaswamy S., Nakamura N., Vazquez F., Batt D.B., Perera S., Roberts T.M., Sellers W.R. 1999. Regulation of G1 progression by the PTEN tumor suppressor protein is linked to inhibition of the phosphatidylinositol 3-kinase/Akt pathway. *Proc. Natl. Acad. Sci. USA* **96:**2110–2115.

230. Randerson-Moor J.A., Harland M., Williams S., Cuthbert-Heavens D., Sheridan E., Aveyard J., et al. 2001. A germline deletion of p14(ARF) but not CDKN2A in a melanoma-neural system tumour syndrome family. *Hum. Mol. Genet.* **10:** 55–62.

231. Rasheed B.K., Stenzel T.T., McLendon R.E., Parsons R., Friedman A.H., Friedman H.S., et al. 1997. PTEN gene mutations are seen in high-grade but not in low-grade gliomas. *Cancer Res.* **57:**4187–4190.

232. Raught B., Gingras A.C., Sonenberg N. 2001. The target of rapamycin (TOR) proteins. *Proc. Natl. Acad. Sci. USA* **98:** 7037–7044.

233. Reifenberger G., Ichimura K., Reifenberger J., Elkahloun A.G., Meltzer P.S., Collins V.P. 1996. Refined mapping of 12q13-q15 amplicons in human malignant gliomas suggests CDK4/SAS and MDM2 as independent amplification targets. *Cancer* Res **56:**5141–5145.

234. Reifenberger G., Liu L., Ichimura K., Schmidt E.E., Collins V.P. 1993. Amplification and overexpression of the MDM2 gene in a subset of human malignant gliomas without p53 mutations. *Cancer Res.* **53:**2736–2739.

235. Reifenberger G., Reifenberger J., Ichimura K., Meltzer P.S., Collins V.P. 1994. Amplification of multiple genes from chromosomal region 12q13-14 in human malignant gliomas: preliminary mapping of the amplicons shows preferential involvement of CDK4, SAS, and MDM2. *Cancer Res.* **54:**4299–4303.

236. Reilly K.M., Loisel D.A., Bronson R.T., McLaughlin M.E., Jacks T. 2000. Nf1;Trp53 mutant mice develop glioblastoma with evidence of strain-specific effects. *Nat. Genet.* **26:**109–113.

237. Relling M.V., Rubnitz J.E., Rivera G.K., Boyett J.M., Hancock M.L., Felix C.A., et al. 1999. High incidence of secondary brain tumours after radiotherapy and antimetabolites. *Lancet* **354:**34–39.

238. Reynolds B.A., Weiss S. 1996. Clonal and population analyses demonstrate that an EGF-responsive mammalian embryonic CNS precursor is a stem cell. *Dev. Biol.* **175:**1–13.

239. Reynolds B.A., Weiss S. 1992. Generation of neurons and astrocytes from isolated cells of the adult mammalian central nervous system. *Science* **255:**1707–1710.

240. Rich J.N., Guo C., McLendon R.E., Bigner D.D., Wang X.F., Counter C.M. 2001. A genetically tractable model of human glioma formation. *Cancer Res.* **61:**3556–3560.

241. Ries S., Biederer C., Woods D., Shifman O., Shirasawa S., Sasazuki T.et al. 2000. Opposing effects of Ras on p53: transcriptional activation of mdm2 and induction of p19ARF. *Cell* **103:**321–330.

242. Rollbrocker B., Waha A., Louis D.N., Wiestler O.D., von Deimling A. 1996. Amplification of the cyclin-dependent

kinase 4 (CDK4) gene is associated with high cdk4 protein levels in glioblastoma multiforme. *Acta. Neuropathol.* (Berl) **92:**70–74.

243. Romashkova J.A., Makarov S.S. 1999. NF-kappaB is a target of AKT in anti-apoptotic PDGF signalling. *Nature* **401:** 86–90.

244. Rommel C., Clarke B.A., Zimmermann S., Nunez L., Rossman R., Reid K., et al. 1999. Differentiation stage-specific inhibition of the Raf-MEK-ERK pathway by Akt. *Science* **286:**1738–1741.

245. Ryan K.M., Phillips A.C., Vousden K.H. 2001. Regulation and function of the p53 tumor suppressor protein. *Curr. Opin. Cell Biol.* **13:**332–337.

246. Sara V.R., Prisell P., Sjogren B., Persson L., Boethius J., Enberg G. 1986. Enhancement of insulin-like growth factor 2 receptors in glioblastoma. *Cancer Lett.* **32:**229–234.

247. Schlessinger J. 2000. Cell signaling by receptor tyrosine kinases. *Cell* **103:**211–225.

248. Schmelzle T., Hall M.N. 2000. TOR, a central controller of cell growth. *Cell* **103:**253–262.

249. Schmidt E.E., Ichimura K., Reifenberger G., Collins V.P. 1994. CDKN2 (p16/MTS1) gene deletion or CDK4 amplification occurs in the majority of glioblastomas. *Cancer Res.* **54:**6321–6324.

250. Seri B., Garcia-Verdugo J.M., McEwen B.S., Alvarez-Buylla A. 2001. Astrocytes give rise to new neurons in the adult mammalian hippocampus. *J. Neurosci.* **21:**7153–7160.

251. Serrano M., Lee H., Chin L., Cordon-Cardo C., Beach D., DePinho R.A. 1996. Role of the INK4a locus in tumor suppression and cell mortality. *Cell* **85:**27–37.

252. Sharif T.R., Sasakawa N., Sharif M. 2001. Regulated expression of a dominant negative protein kinase C epsilon mutant inhibits the proliferation of U-373MG human astrocytoma cells. *Int. J. Mol. Med.* **7:**373–380.

253. Sharpless N.E., Bardeesy N., Lee K.H., Carrasco D., Castrillon D.H., Aguirre A.J., et al. 2001. Loss of p16Ink4a with retention of p19Arf predisposes mice to tumorigenesis. *Nature* **413:**86–91.

254. Sherr C. J. 2001. The INK4a/ARF network in tumour suppression. *Nat. Rev. Mol. Cell Biol.* **2:**731–737.

255. Sherr C. J. 2001. Parsing Ink4a/Arf: "pure" p16-null mice. *Cell* **106:**531–534.

256. Sherr C. J. 2000. The Pezcoller lecture: cancer cell cycles revisited. *Cancer Res.* **60:**3689–3695.

257. Shiloh Y. 2001. ATM and ATR: networking cellular responses to DNA damage. *Curr. Opin. Genet. Dev.* **11:**71–77.

258. Shiloh Y., Kastan M.B. 2001. ATM: genome stability, neuronal development, and cancer cross paths. *Adv. Cancer Res.* **83:**209–254.

259. Sibilia M., Steinbach J.P., Stingl L., Aguzzi A., Wagner E.F. 1998. A strain-independent postnatal neurodegeneration in mice lacking the EGF receptor. *Embo. J.* **17:**719–731.

260. Smith J.S., Wang X.Y., Qian J., Hosek S.M., Scheithauer B.W., Jenkins R.B., James C.D. 2000. Amplification of the platelet-derived growth factor receptor-A (PDGFRA) gene occurs in oligodendrogliomas with grade IV anaplastic features. *J. Neuropathol. Exp. Neurol.* **59:**495–503.

261. Sonoda Y., Ozawa T., Aldape K.D., Deen D.F., Berger M.S., Pieper R.O. 2001. Akt pathway activation converts anaplastic astrocytoma to glioblastoma multiforme in a human astrocyte model of glioma. *Cancer Res.* **61:**6674–6678.

262. Sonoda Y., Ozawa T., Hirose Y., Aldape K.D., McMahon M., Berger M.S., Pieper R.O. 2001. Formation of intracranial tumors by genetically modified human astrocytes defines four pathways critical in the development of human anaplastic astrocytoma. *Cancer Res.* **61:**4956–4960.

263. Staal S. P. 1987. Molecular cloning of the akt oncogene and its human homologues AKT1 and AKT2: amplification of AKT1 in a primary human gastric adenocarcinoma. *Proc. Natl. Acad. Sci. USA* **84:**5034–5037.

264. Stambolic V., MacPherson D., Sas D., Lin Y., Snow B., Jang Y., Benchimol S., Mak T.W. 2001. Regulation of PTEN transcription by p53. *Mol. Cell* **8:**317–325.

265. Summers S.A., Lipfert L., Birnbaum M.J. 1998. Polyoma middle T antigen activates the Ser/Thr kinase Akt in a PI3-kinase-dependent manner. *Biochem. Biophys. Res. Commun* **246:**76–81.

266. Sun H., Lesche R., Li D.M., Liliental J., Zhang H., Gao J., et al. 1999. PTEN modulates cell cycle progression and cell survival by regulating phosphatidylinositol 3,4,5,-trisphosphate and Akt/protein kinase B signaling pathway. *Proc. Natl. Acad. Sci. USA* **96:**6199–6204.

267. Sung T., Miller D.C., Hayes R.L., Alonso M., Yee H., Newcomb E.W. 2000. Preferential inactivation of the p53 tumor suppressor pathway and lack of EGFR amplification distinguish de novo high grade pediatric astrocytomas from de novo adult astrocytomas. *Brain Pathol.* **10:**249–259.

268. Suzuki A., de la Pompa J.L., Stambolic V., Elia A.J., Sasaki T., del Barco Barrantes I., et al. 1998. High cancer susceptibility and embryonic lethality associated with mutation of the PTEN tumor suppressor gene in mice. *Curr. Biol.* **8:** 1169–1178.

269. Swenberg J.A. 1977. Chemical- and virus-induced brain tumors. *Natl. Cancer Inst. Monogr.* **46:**3–10.

270. Tachibana I., Smith J.S., Sato K., Hosek S.M., Kimmel D.W., Jenkins R.B. 2000. Investigation of germline PTEN, p53, p16(INK4A)/p14(ARF), and CDK4 alterations in familial glioma. *Am. J. Med. Genet.* **92:**136–141.

271. Tada K., Shiraishi S., Kamiryo T., Nakamura H., Hirano H., Kuratsu J., et al. 2001. Analysis of loss of heterozygosity on chromosome 10 in patients with malignant astrocytic tumors: correlation with patient age and survival. *J. Neurosurg.* **95:**651–659.

272. Takaishi H., Konishi H., Matsuzaki H., Ono Y., Shirai Y., Saito N., et al. 1999. Regulation of nuclear translocation of forkhead transcription factor AFX by protein kinase B. *Proc. Natl. Acad. Sci. USA* **96**:11836–11841.

273. Takimoto R., El-Deiry W.S. 2001. DNA replication blockade impairs p53-transactivation. *Proc. Natl. Acad. Sci. USA* **98**:781–783.

274. Tamura M., Gu J., Danen E.H., Takino T., Miyamoto S., Yamada K.M. 1999. PTEN interactions with focal adhesion kinase and suppression of the extracellular matrix-dependent phosphatidylinositol 3-kinase/Akt cell survival pathway. *J. Biol. Chem.* **274**:20,693–20,703.

275. Tamura M., Gu J., Matsumoto K., Aota S., Parsons R., Yamada K.M. 1998. Inhibition of cell migration, spreading, and focal adhesions by tumor suppressor PTEN. *Science* **280**:1614–1617.

276. Tao W., Levine A.J. 1999. P19(ARF) stabilizes p53 by blocking nucleo-cytoplasmic shuttling of Mdm2. *Proc. Natl. Acad. Sci. USA* **96**:6937–6941.

277. Temple S. 2001. The development of neural stem cells. Nature **414**:112–117.

278. TempleS. 2001. Stem cell plasticity—building the brain of our dreams. *Nat. Rev. Neurosci.* **2**:513–520.

279. Testa J. R., Bellacosa A. 2001. AKT plays a central role in tumorigenesis. *Proc. Natl. Acad. Sci. USA* **98**:10,983–10,985.

280. Theurillat J.P., Hainfellner J., Maddalena A., Weissenberger J., Aguzzi A. 1999. Early induction of angiogenetic signals in gliomas of GFAP-v-src transgenic mice. *Proc. Natl. Acad. Sci. USA* **154**:581–590.

281. Threadgill D.W., Dlugosz A.A., Hansen L.A., Tennenbaum T., Lichti U., Yee D., et al. 1995. Targeted disruption of mouse EGF receptor: effect of genetic background on mutant phenotype. *Science* **269**:230–234.

282. Tominaga K., Morisaki H., Kaneko Y., Fujimoto A., Tanaka T., Ohtsubo M., et al. 1999. Role of human Cds1 (Chk2) kinase in DNA damage checkpoint and its regulation by p53. *J. Biol. Chem.* **274**:31,463–31,467.

283. Trent J., Meltzer P., Rosenblum M., Harsh G., Kinzler K., Mashal R., et al. 1986. Evidence for rearrangement, amplification, and expression of c-myc in a human glioblastoma. *Proc. Natl. Acad. Sci. USA* **83**:470–473.

284. Tsai R. Y., McKay R.D. 2000. Cell contact regulates fate choice by cortical stem cells. *J. Neurosci.* **20**:3725–3735.

285. Ueki K., Nishikawa R., Nakazato Y., Hirose T., Hirato J., Funada N., et al. 2002. Correlation of Histology and Molecular Genetic Analysis of 1p, 19q, 10q, TP53, EGFR, CDK4, and CDKN2A in 91 Astrocytic and Oligodendroglial Tumors. *Clin. Cancer Res.* **8**:196–201.

286. Ueki K., Ono Y., Henson J.W., Efird J.T., von Deimling A., Louis D.N. 1996. CDKN2/p16 or RB alterations occur in the majority of glioblastomas and are inversely correlated. *Cancer Res.* **56**:150–153.

287. Uhrbom L., Hesselager G., Nister M., Westermark B. 1998. Induction of brain tumors in mice using a recombinant platelet-derived growth factor B-chain retrovirus. *Cancer Res* **58**:5275–5279.

288. Uhrbom L., Dai C., Celestino J.C., Rosenblum M.K., Fuller G.N., Holland E.C. 2003. Ink4a-Arf loss cooperates with Kras activation in astrocytes and neural progenitors to generate glioblastomas of various morphologies depending on acivated Akt. *Cancer Res.* **62**:5551–5558.

289. Vahteristo P., Tamminen A., Karvinen P., Eerola H., Eklund C., Aaltonen L.A., et al. 2001. p53, CHK2, and CHK1 genes in Finnish families with Li-Fraumeni syndrome: further evidence of CHK2 in inherited cancer predisposition. *Cancer Res.* **61**:5718–5722.

290. van Dyke R., Jacks T. 2002. Cancer modeling in the modern era: progress and challenges. *Cell* **108**:135–144.

291. Vescovi A.L.,Reynolds B.A., Fraser D.D., Weiss S. 1993. bFGF regulates the proliferative fate of unipotent (neuronal) and bipotent (neuronal/astroglial) EGF-generated CNS progenitor cells. *Neuron* **11**:951–966.

292. von Deimling A., Eibl R.H., Ohgaki H., Louis D.N., von Ammon K., Petersen I., et al. 1992. p53 mutations are associated with 17p allelic loss in grade II and grade III astrocytoma. *Cancer Res.* **52**:2987–2990.

293. Vousden K.H. 2000. p53: death star. *Cell* **103**:691–694.

294. Walter A.W., Hancock M.L., Pui C.H., Hudson M.M., Ochs J.S., Rivera G.K., et al. 1998. Secondary brain tumors in children treated for acute lymphoblastic leukemia at St Jude Children's Research Hospital. *J. Clin. Oncol.* **16**:3761–3767.

295. Wang S.I., Puc J., Li J., Bruce J.N., Cairns P., Sidransky D., Parsons R. 1997. Somatic mutations of PTEN in glioblastoma multiforme. *Cancer Res.* **57**:4183–4186.

296. Watanabe K., Sato K., Biernat W., Tachibana O., von Ammon K., Ogata N., et al. 1997. Incidence and timing of p53 mutations during astrocytoma progression in patients with multiple biopsies. *Clin. Cancer Res.* **3**:523–530.

297. Watanabe K., Tachibana O., Sata K., Yonekawa Y., Kleihues P., Ohgaki H. 1996. Overexpression of the EGF receptor and p53 mutations are mutually exclusive in the evolution of primary and secondary glioblastomas. *Brain Pathol.* **6**:217–223; discussion 23–24.

298. Watanabe T., Nakamura M., Yonekawa Y., Kleihues P., Ohgaki H. 2001. Promoter hypermethylation and homozygous deletion of the p14ARF and p16INK4a genes in oligodendrogliomas. *Acta. Neuropathol. (Berl)* **101**:185–189.

299. Watanabe T., Yokoo H., Yokoo M., Yonekawa Y., Kleihues P., Ohgaki H. 2001. Concurrent inactivation of RB1 and TP53 pathways in anaplastic oligodendrogliomas. *J. Neuropathol. Exp. Neurol.* **60**:1181–1189.

300. Weber J.D., Hu W., Jefcoat S.C. Jr., Raben D.M., Baldassare J.J. 1997. Ras-stimulated extracellular signal-related kinase 1 and RhoA activities coordinate platelet-derived growth factor-induced G1 progression through the independent regulation of cyclin D1 and p27. *J. Biol. Chem.* **272**:32,966–32,971.

301. Weber J.D., Jeffers J.R., Rehg J.E., Randle D.H., Lozano G., Roussel M.F., et al. 2000. p53-independent functions of the p19(ARF) tumor suppressor. *Genes Dev.* **14**:2358–2365.

302. Weber J.D., Kuo M.L., Bothner B., DiGiammarino E.L., Kriwacki R.W., Roussel M.F., Sherr C.J. 2000. Cooperative signals governing ARF-mdm2 interaction and nucleolar localization of the complex. *Mol. Cell Biol.* **20**:2517–2528.

303. Weber J.D., Taylor L.J., Roussel M.F., Sherr C.J., Bar-Sagi D. 1999. Nucleolar Arf sequesters Mdm2 and activates p53. *Nat. Cell Biol.* **1**:20–26.

304. Weiss W.A., Burns M.J., Hackett C., Aldape K., Hill J.R., Kuriyama H., et al. 2003. Genetic determinants of malignancy in a mouse model for oligodendrogliomas. *Cancer* Cell **63**:1589–1595.

305. Weissenberger J., Steinbach J.P., Malin G., Spada S., Rulicke T., Aguzzi A. 1997. Development and malignant progression of astrocytomas in GFAP-v-src transgenic mice. *Oncogene* **14**:2005–2013.

306. Weissleder R. 2002. Scaling down imaging: molecular mapping of cancer in mice. *Nature Reviews Cancer* **2**:11–18.

307. Wen S., Stolarov J., Myers M.P., Su J.D., Wigler M.H., Tonks N.K., Durden D.L. 2001. PTEN controls tumor-induced angiogenesis. *Proc. Natl. Acad. Sci. USA* **98**:4622–4627.

308. Weng L.P., Brown J.L., Eng C. 2001. PTEN coordinates G(1) arrest by down-regulating cyclin D1 via its protein phosphatase activity and up-regulating p27 via its lipid phosphatase activity in a breast cancer model. *Hum. Mol. Genet.* **10**:599–604.

309. Wong A.J., Bigner S.H., Bigner D.D., Kinzler K.W., Hamilton S.R., Vogelstein B. 1987. Increased expression of the epidermal growth factor receptor gene in malignant gliomas is invariably associated with gene amplification. *Proc. Natl. Acad. Sci. USA* **84**:6899–6903.

310. Wong A.J., Ruppert J.M., Bigner S.H., Grzeschik C.H., Humphrey P.A., Bigner D.S., Vogelstein B. 1992. Structural alterations of the epidermal growth factor receptor gene in human gliomas. *Proc. Natl. Acad. Sci. USA* **89**:2965–2969.

311. Wu L., Timmers C., Maiti B., Saavedra H.I., Sang L., Chong G.T., et al. 2001. The E2F1-3 transcription factors are essential for cellular proliferation. *Nature* **414**:457–462.

312. Wu X., Bayle J.H., Olson D., Levine A.J. 1993. The p53-mdm-2 autoregulatory feedback loop. *Genes Dev.* **7**:1126–1132.

313. Wu X., Senechal K., Neshat M.S., Whang Y.E., Sawyers C.L. 1998. The PTEN/MMAC1 tumor suppressor phosphatase functions as a negative regulator of the phosphoinositide 3-kinase/Akt pathway. *Proc. Natl. Acad. Sci. USA* **95**:15,587–15,591.

314. Xiao A., Wu H., Pandolfi P.P., Louis D.N., VanDyke T. 2002. Astrocyte inactivation of the pRb pathwy predisposes mice to malignant astrocytoma development that is accelerated by PTEN mutation. *Cancer Cell* **1**:157–168.

315. Yang M., Baranov E., Moossa A.R., Penman S., Hoffman R.M. 2000. Visualizing gene expression by whole-body fluorescence imaging. *Proc. Natl. Acad. Sci. USA* **97**:12,278–12,282.

316. Yeh H.J., Ruit K.G., Wang Y.X., Parks W.C., Snider W.D., Deuel T.F. 1991. PDGF A-chain gene is expressed by mammalian neurons during development and in maturity. *Cell* **64**:209–216.

317. Yeh H.J., Silos-Santiago I., Wang Y.X., George R.J., Snider W.D., Deuel T.F. 1993. Developmental expression of the platelet-derived growth factor alpha-receptor gene in mammalian central nervous system. *Proc. Natl. Acad. Sci. USA* **90**:1952–1956.

318. You M.J., Castrillon D.H., Bastian B.C., O'Hagan R.C., Bosenberg M.W., Parsons R., et al. 2002. Genetic analysis of Pten and Ink4a/Arf interactions in the suppression of tumorigenesis in mice. *Proc. Natl. Acad. Sci. USA* **99**:1455–1460.

319. Yu Y., Bradley A. 2001. Engineering chromosomal rearrangements in mice. *Nat. Rev. Genet.* **2**:780–790.

320. Zhou B.B., Elledge S.J. 2000. The DNA damage response: putting checkpoints in perspective. *Nature* **408**:433–439.

321. Zhou B.P., Liao Y., Xia W., Spohn B., Lee M.H., Hung M.C. 2001. Cytoplasmic localization of p21Cip1/WAF1 by Akt-induced phosphorylation in HER-2/neu-overexpressing cells. *Nat. Cell Biol.* **3**:245–252.

322. Zhou B.P., Liao Y., Xia W., Zou Y., Spohn B., Hung M.C. 2001. HER-2/neu induces p53 ubiquitination via Akt-mediated MDM2 phosphorylation. *Nat. Cell Biol.* **3**:973–982.

323. Zimmermann S., Moelling K. 1999. Phosphorylation and regulation of Raf by Akt (protein kinase B). *Science* **286**:1741–1744.

324. Zindy F., Eischen C.M., Randle D.H., Kamijo T., Cleveland J.L., Sherr C.J., Roussel M.F. 1998. Myc signaling via the ARF tumor suppressor regulates p53-dependent apoptosis and immortalization. *Genes Dev.* **12**:2424–2433.

325. Zundel W., Schindler C., Haas-Kogan D., Koong A., Kaper F., Chen E., et al. 2000. Loss of PTEN facilitates HIF-1-mediated gene expression. *Genes Dev.* **14**:391–396.

5

Biology of Brain Metastasis

Minsoo Kang, Takamitsu Fujimaki,
Seiji Yano, and Isaiah J. Fidler

Brain metastases, which develop in up to 35% of all cancer patients, are a major cause of death from cancer. Development of improved therapies requires the understanding of the biology of brain metastasis. A relevant in vivo model for brain metastasis is essential. The intracarotid injection of murine or human cancer cells into syngeneic or immune-incompetent mice produces metastasis in different regions of the brain. This site-specific metastasis is not due to patterns of initial cell arrest, motility, or invasiveness, but rather to the ability of tumor cells to proliferate in the brain parenchyma or the meninges. The blood–brain barrier is intact in metastases that are smaller than 0.25 mm in diameter. Although in larger metastases the blood–brain barrier is leaky, the lesions are resistant to many chemotherapeutic drugs. These data demonstrate that the development of brain metastasis represents the end result of multiple interactions between tumor cells and the unique microenvironment of the brain.

1. INTRODUCTION

Because most deaths from cancer are caused by metastases that are resistant to conventional therapy (39), there is an urgent need to develop effective regimens against disseminated cancer. Brain metastases develop in up to 35% of all cancer patients, usually representing the final stage of the disease (120). In the United States, between 80,000 (3) and 170,000 (121) patients develop brain metastases each year. Because of this frequent occurrence and the fact that cancers in other organs can be more effectively controlled, brain metastases are becoming a major cause of death from cancer. A better understanding of molecular mechanisms that regulate the process of metastasis and of the multiple interactions between metastatic cells and host factors can provide a biological foundation for the design of more effective therapies.

2. IN VIVO ORTHOTOPIC MODEL OF BRAIN METASTASIS

To examine the biology of brain metastasis, Schackert and Fidler (133) developed a procedure of injecting neoplastic cells into the internal or external carotid arteries, hence producing a model to study experimental brain cancer metastasis. To develop this model, murine K-1735 melanoma cells that have a high metastatic potential (45,124), were injected into the carotid arteries of syngeneic mice. In a parallel experiment, the melanoma cells were injected directly into the cerebrum by direct implantation to verify that these cells, once in the brain, could proliferate into grossly visible lesions.

From: *Contemporary Cancer Research: Brain Tumors*
Edited by: F. Ali-Osman © Humana Press Inc., Totowa, NJ

Unlike that of rats *(95),* the common carotid artery of mice is too short to allow proper injection of cells without leakage into surrounding tissues; therefore in mice, the cells are introduced into the internal or external carotid artery *(121,122).* Mice are anesthetized by intraperitoneal injection of pentobarbital sodium, restrained on a corkboard on the back, and placed under a dissecting microscope. After a midline incision over the thyroid glands and exposure of the trachea, the carotid artery is prepared for an injection distal to the point of bifurcation into internal and external carotid arteries. A ligature of 5–0 silk suture is placed in the distal part of the common carotid artery. A second ligature is then placed and tied loosely proximal to the injection site. A sterile cotton tip applicator is inserted under the artery just distal to the injection site to elevate the carotid artery. This procedure controls bleeding from the carotid artery by regurgitation from distal vessels. The artery is then nicked with a pair of microscissors, and a less than 30-gauge glass cannula is inserted into the blood vessel lumen. To assure proper delivery, the cells are injected slowly and the cannula is removed. The second ligature is tightened and the skin is closed with sutures (Fig. 1).

Because the injection of cells into the carotid artery of mice simulates the hematogenous spread of tumor emboli to the brain, the technique can be used to examine the last steps of the metastatic process: release of tumor cells into the circulation, arrest in capillaries, penetration and extravasation into the brain through the blood–brain barrier, and continuous growth of cells in the brain tissue *(39,122).*

The internal carotid artery supplies the brain parenchyma, whereas the external carotid artery supplies the musculature and glands in the head and neck region as well as the meninges. For this reason, Schackert and Fidler *(133)* first examined whether the injection into the internal and external carotid arteries would influence the growth of tumor cells in the brain.

For the highly metastatic K-1735 cells, both routes of injection resulted in the development of highly melanotic lesions in the brain parenchyma. Distant metastases developed in the lungs and heart, but the mice died from the brain lesions *(134).* In some syngeneic C3H/HeN mice, tumor cells injected into the external carotid artery produced tumors in the neck and cheek. The injection of nonmetastatic K-1735 cells *(45)* into the internal, but not external, carotid artery produced melanotic lesions in the brain parenchyma *(134).* The difference in tumorigenicity may reside in the fact that the nonmetastatic cells injected into the internal carotid artery reach the brain tissue in high numbers and can then proliferate, whereas the number of tumor cells introduced into the external carotid artery may be insufficient to produce metastatic lesions in the brain *(53,133).* The nonmetastatic K-1735 cells die rapidly in the circulation *(39,40,124,135),* which may explain the absence of extracranial lesions.

3. SITE-SPECIFIC BRAIN METASTASIS

The search for the mechanisms that regulate the pattern of metastasis began more than a century ago. In 1889, Paget *(115)* questioned whether the distribution of metastases was a result of chance. He analyzed hundreds of autopsy records of women with breast cancer and discovered a nonrandom pattern of visceral metastases. This finding suggested that the process of metastasis was not owing to chance but, rather, that certain tumors (the "seed") have a specific affinity for the milieu of certain organs (the "soil"). Metastases resulted only when the seed and soil were compatible *(115).*

In 1929, Ewing *(29)* challenged Paget's seed and soil theory and hypothesized that metastatic dissemination occurs by purely mechanical factors such as the anatomical structure of the vascular system. These explanations have been evoked separately or together to explain the secondary site preference of certain types of neoplasms. Sugarbaker *(148),* in a review of clinical studies on secondary site preferences of malignant neoplasms, concluded that common *regional* metastatic involvement could be attributed to anatomical or mechanical considerations, such as different venous circulation or lymphatic drainage to regional lymph nodes, but that *distant* organ colonization by metastatic cells from numerous types of cancers established their own patterns of site specificity *(148).*

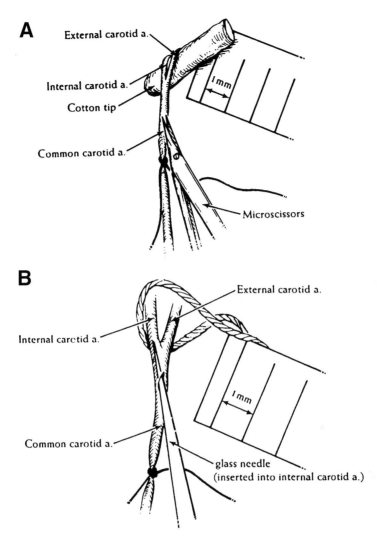

Fig. 1. Methodology for injecting tumor cells into the carotid artery of mice. The right side carotid artery is exposed. The carotid artery is elevated by insertion of a cotton-tip applicator distal to the injection site to collapse the artery (**A**). This procedure allows the insertion of a glass cannula without bleeding (**B**). (From ref. *5*.)

Clinical observations of cancer patients and studies with experimental rodent tumors have revealed that certain tumors produce site-specific metastasis independent of vascular anatomy, rate of blood flow, and number of tumor cells delivered *(38,39,41,89)*. For example, malignant melanoma will produce brain metastasis in most patients *(149)*. Of these brain metastases, 49% are intraparenchymal, 22% are leptomeningeal, and 32% are dural *(82,93,149)*.

To determine whether mouse melanomas also produce site-specific brain metastasis, cells from the K-1735 melanoma syngeneic to C3H/HeN mice *(45)* and the B16 melanoma syngeneic to C57BL/6 *(42)* were injected into the internal carotid arteries of syngeneic or nude mice. Regardless of the route of injection, the K-1735 cells produced melanotic lesions only in the brain parenchyma of 151 of 167 mice, whereas B16 cells produced lesions only in the meninges and ventricles of 49 of 49 mice *(134)*. The unique patterns of experimental brain metastases were therefore not a result of the circulatory system of the brain *(33,141)*.

Studies on the distribution and fate of hematogenously disseminated radiolabeled tumor cells have concluded that tumor cells can reach the microvasculature of many organs, but the growth of the arrested cells into clinically relevant metastases occurs in only some organ sites *(40)*. Subsequent to the injection of radiolabeled murine melanoma cells into the internal carotid artery, most cells were trapped in the vasculature of the brain. For both K-1735 and B16 melanoma, only a few cells reached the meninges. The K-1735 cells failed to proliferate in the meninges, but the B16 cells grew rapidly *(95)*. These data confirm that initial tumor cell arrest in the microvasculature does not predict the development of progressively growing metastases *(40,69)*.

To further determine the factors responsible for the organ-site metastases, somatic cell hybrids between the B16 and K-1735 cells were created by fusion *(53)*. K-1735/K-1735 hybrid cells produced lesions only in the brain parenchyma of C57BL/6 x C3H/HeNF1 or nude mice, whereas B16/K-1735 hybrid cells produced lesions only in the meninges and ventricles, as did hybrid cells of B16/B16. In only 2 of 21 mice injected in the internal carotid artery, few cells grew into the brain parenchyma from ventricular lesions (Table 1).

Subsequent to intracarotid injection, tumor cells must reach the microvasculature of the brain, arrest, extravasate into the organ parenchyma, and then proliferate into measurable lesions. Theoretically, the difference in site-specific brain metastasis observed between the different melanomas could have been a result of the differences in behavior at different steps of the metastatic process. Using the melanoma cell lines and somatic hybrids, differences in cell arrest, extravasation, and growth that could account for the presence or absence of brain parenchymal metastases were determined *(53)*.

The arrest of cells in the capillary bed is regulated by multiple factors, including adhesion molecules and the size of circulating emboli *(43,107)*. The expression of cell surface CD44 has been shown to play a role in organ-specific homing of lymphocytes *(70)* and brain metastases *(84,102,127,155)*. This molecule binds to components of the extracellular matrix such as fibronectin, hyaluronate, and collagen types I and IV *(11,68,70)*. Although the expression of CD44 on mouse or human melanomas has been correlated with metastatic potential *(11,68)*, neither expression of cell surface CD44 nor formation of homotypic aggregates correlated with initial cell arrest as measured by using [^{125}I]IdUrd-labeled cells. As shown previously *(69,135)*, initial cell arrest in brain parenchyma or meninges did not predict the development of metastases.

Once cells arrest in a capillary bed, they can extravasate into the organ parenchyma. Increased cell motility *(90)* and production of degradative enzymes facilitate this process *(87,104,106)*. Motility did not suffer among the melanoma cells, but the production of collagenase IV did. Specifically, B16 cells did not produce measurable gelatinase A activity (72-kDa), whereas K-1735 cells did. However, both B16/K-1735 hybrid cells (that produced lesions in the meninges) and the K-1735/K-1735 hybrid cells (that produced lesions in the brain parenchyma) expressed similar levels of gelatinase A activity. Therefore, the expression of gelatinase A did not explain why the B16 melanoma cells or K-1735/B16 hybrid cells failed to grow in the brain parenchyma *(53)*.

Because the growth of cells at a metastatic site is essential to the development of measurable lesions, the tumorigenic properties of the melanoma cells and hybrids were determined subsequent to direct intracerebral injection. Both B16 cells and B16/K-1735 hybrid cells grew in the brain parenchyma. The B16 cells produced well-defined lesions, whereas the B16/K-1735 hybrid cells were invasive, probably because they produce gelatinases. Subsequent to inoculation of the cells into the cisterna magna (subarachnoid space), the B16 cells, K-1735 cells, B16/K-1735 hybrid cells, and K-1735/K-1735 hybrid cells grew rapidly on the leptomeninges. B16 cells did not infiltrate the brain parenchyma, whereas the K-1735 cells and hybrid cells did. Because the B16 and B16/K-1735 hybrid cells did not proliferate in the brain parenchyma (except after direct intracerebral injection), the failure to grow after intracarotid injection could be the result of the absence of stimulatory growth factors or the presence of inhibitory growth factors in the microenvironment *(109)*.

The different melanoma cell and hybrids were cultured in the presence of several growth factors previously shown to influence growth *(78)*. Epidermal growth factor (EGF), basic fibroblast growth

Table 1
Site-Specific Experimental Brain Metastasis Produced by Murine B16
Melanoma Cells, K-1735r Melanoma Cells, and Somatic Cell Hybrids

Cells [a]	Tumori-genicity [b]	Tumor growth in the brain			Mean survival (d)
		Parenchyma	Meninges	Ventricle	
K-1735 C-4	7/7	7/7	0/7	0/7	26
K-1735 C-4N	7/7	7/7	0/7	0/7	24
K-1735 C-4H	8/8	8/8	0/8	0/8	30
B16BL-6	9/9	0/9	9/9	3/9	18
B16BL-6-6N	9/9	0/9	9/9	3/9	19
C-4N/C-4H	15/15	15/15	0/15	0/15	28
B16BL-6N/ C-4H Clone 2	5/5	1/5 [c]	5/5	4/5	29
B16BL-6N/ C-4H Clone 8	5/5	1/5 [c]	5/5	2/5	28
B16BL-6N/ C-4H Clone 9	6/6	0/6	6/6	2/6	28
B16BL-6/ C-4H Clone 12	5/5	0/5	5/5	5/5	28
B16 BL-6/ C-4H Clone 21	5/5	1/5 [c]	5/5	3/5	27

[a] Mice were injected in the internal carotid artery with 1×10^5 viable tumor cells. Moribund mice were killed and necropsied. The presence of brain metastasis was confirmed by histological examination.
[b] Number of positive mice/number of mice injected.
[c] Small intraparenchymal lesions adjacent to meningeal or ventricular tumors.

factor (bFGF), or platelet-derived growth factor (PDGF) did not influence the growth of any of the cell lines tested. Significant differences were found when the cells were cultured with transforming growth factor-β (TGF-β). In addition to its effect on cell proliferation *(32)* and differentiation *(16)*, TGF-β also regulates many biological processes, such as glycolysis *(12)*, angiogenesis *(129)*, extracellular matrix metabolism *(74)*, and protein phosphorylation *(85)*. TGF-β can interact with hormones *(79)* and growth factors such as EGF *(151)*, PDGF *(2)*, and bFGF *(5)*. Both TGF-β_1 and TGF-β_2 stimulated the growth of K-1735 and K-1735/K-1735 hybrid cells, but TGF-β_1 and TGF-β_2 inhibited the growth of B16 and B16/K-1735 hybrid cells. Previous reports have shown that the level of TGF-β binding to its receptors on tumor cells correlates with growth inhibition *(32,56)*. Indeed, TGF-β bound to B16 and B16/K-1735 cells at a higher level than to K-1735 cells alone. Because the concentration of TGF-β_2 is high in the brain *(47,100,130,153)*, the failure of B16 or B16/K-1735 hybrid cells to produce intraparenchymal brain metastases could be a result of their sensitivity to growth inhibition by TGF-β.

All but one human melanoma produced experimental brain metastases following intracarotid artery injection. The melanoma metastases were located in the meninges, ventricle, and parenchyma. Each melanoma line produced a slightly different pattern of growth. However, one striking feature was that two cell lines derived from two different brain parenchyma metastases from two different patients had a preference for growth in the brain parenchyma. The cell lines derived from lymph node or subcutaneous metastases of patients grew more frequently in the meninges or ventricles than in the brain parenchyma of the nude mice (Table 2).

Table 2
**Experimental Brain Metastasis After the Injection of Human
Melanoma Cells Into the Internal Carotid Artery of Nude Mice**

Cells	Tumori-genicity [a]	Tumor growth in the brain [b]			Necropsy (d) [c]	Lung metastasis [a]
		Parenchyma	Meninges	Ventricle		
A375-SM	8/10	2/8	2/8	5/8	22–30	2/10
DX-3	8/10	4/8	8/8	0/8	30–44	2/10
DM-4	7/9	2/5	4/7	1/7	90	2/9
TXM-13	8/8	7/8	4/8	2/8	50–75	1/8
TXM-31-3	0/10	0	0	0	180	0/10
TXM-31-4	3/10	2/3	2/3	0/3	45–110	2/10
TXM-40	9/10	9/9	4/9	0/9	65–165	0/10

[a] Number of mice with tumors/number of mice injected with 1×10^5 viable tumor cells in the internal carotid artery.

[b] Number of mice with one or more lesions in the specific site/number of tumor-positive mice.

[c] Time of necropsy is recorded for mice with brain tumors (except for TXM-31-3). Asymptomatic animals from groups injected with TXM-13-3 and TXM-31-4 cells were killed 140 or 180 d after injection, and no tumor lesions were found in histologic sections of the brain.

The biological behavior of different human melanoma cell lines and cells isolated from fresh surgical specimens of cutaneous melanoma, lymph node metastases, and brain metastases was determined subsequent to intracisternal implantation in nude mice *(54,135)*. The ability of human melanoma cells to grow in the brain parenchyma was inversely correlated with their sensitivity to the antiproliferative effects of TGF-β_2. One interpretation is that the brain-metastases-derived cell lines were already selected in the patient for the ability to proliferate in the presence of TGF-β_2 *(54)*.

4. ANGIOGENESIS AND BRAIN METASTASIS

Tumors are biologically heterogeneous and contain subpopulations of cells with different angiogenic, invasive, and metastatic properties *(46)*. As stated previously, to produce metastasis, tumor cells must complete a series of sequential and selective steps *(46,124)*. Failure to complete even one step eliminates the cells from the process *(4)*. Recent studies indicate that to produce brain metastasis, tumor cells must reach the vasculature of the brain, attach to the microvessel endothelial cells, extravasate into the parenchyma, proliferate (by responding to growth factors), and induce angiogenesis *(28,53,110,134*; Fig. 2).

The growth and spread of neoplasm is dependent on the establishment of adequate blood supply, i.e., angiogenesis *(13,48,66,67,88)*. The process of angiogenesis consists of multiple, sequential, and interdependent steps *(38)*. It begins with local degradation of the basement membrane surrounding capillaries, followed by invasion of the surrounding stroma by the underlying endothelial cells in the direction of the angiogenic stimulus. Endothelial cell migration is accompanied by the proliferation of endothelial cells at the leading edge of the migrating column. Endothelial cells then organize into three-dimensional structures to form new capillary tubes *(38)*. The onset of angiogenesis involves a change in the local equilibrium between positive and negative regulatory molecules *(13,26,38,66,67)*. Some of the major angiogenic factors include bFGF, interleukin-8 (IL-8), platelet-derived endothelial cell growth factor (PD-ECGF), PDGF, hepatocyte growth factor (HGF), and vascular endothelial growth factor (VEGF) *(26,30,44,49,66)*.

Angiogenesis can occur by either sprouting or nonsprouting processes *(128)*. Sprouting angiogenesis occurs by branching (true sprouting) of new capillaries from pre-existing vessels. Nonsprouting

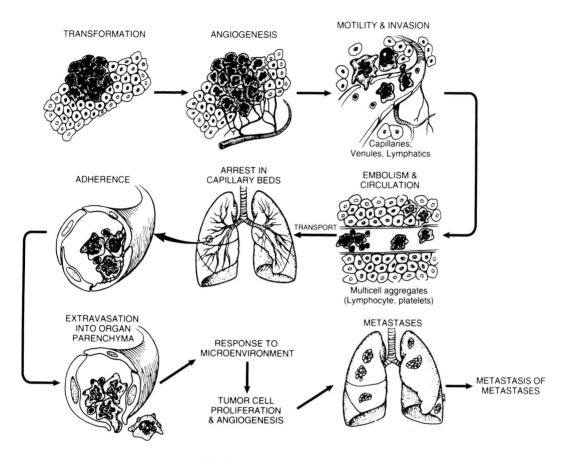

Fig. 2. The metastatic process.

angiogenesis results from the enlargement, splitting, and fusion of pre-existing vessels produced by proliferation of endothelial ells within the wall of a vessel. Transcapillary pillars (or transluminal bridges) are sometimes observed in enlarged vessels produced by nonsprouting angiogenesis *(128)*. This type of angiogenesis can concurrently occur with sprouting angiogenesis in the vascularization of organs or tissues such as the lung, heart, and yolk sac during development *(128)*. The mechanism of nonsprouting angiogenesis in metastasis is not yet known, but VEGF, also calledvascular permeability factor, which plays a pivotal role in developmental, physiological, and pathological neovascularization *(15,35,36,140)*, is a candidate molecule.

VEGF is a 34- to 45-kDa dimeric glycosylated protein with structural homology to PDGF *(77)*. VEGF stimulates the proliferation and migration of endothelial cells and induces the expression of metalloproteinases and plasminogen activity by these cells *(37,83,118,152)*. VEGF functions as a survival factor for endothelial cells, because it has been shown that VEGF is required for maintenance of newly formed vessels in a natural developmental setting of retina vascularization and in a model of tumor angiogenesis *(1,8)*. VEGF and its receptors are expressed in a wide spectrum of brain tumors and brain metastases *(9,97,112,119,147)*. Moreover, expression of VEGF in tumor cells enhances tumor growth and metastasis in several animal models by stimulating vascularization (increased microvessel density) *(18,20,113)*. Although its mechanism still remains speculative, VEGF increases vascular permeability and generates peritumoral edema in brain tumors *(91)*.

The molecular mechanism of angiogenesis in experimental brain metastasis was investigated subsequent to intracarotid injection of cells from six different human cancer cell lines (proven to produce visceral metastasis). Colon carcinoma (KM12SM) and lung adenocarcinoma (PC14PE6 and PC14Br) cells produced large, fast-growing parenchymal brain metastases, whereas lung squamous cell carcinoma (H226), renal cell carcinoma (SN12PM6), and melanoma (TXM13) cells produced only a few slow-growing brain metastases. Rapidly progressing brain metastases contained many enlarged blood vessels. The expression of VEGF mRNA and protein by the tumor cells directly correlated with angiogenesis and growth of brain metastasis. Causal evidence for the essential role of VEGF in this process was provided by transfecting PC14PE6 and KM12SM cells with antisense-*VEGF165* gene, which significantly reduced the diameter/number of enlarged vessels and decreased the incidence of brain metastasis. In contrast, transfection of H226 human lung squamous carcinoma cells with sense-*VEGF121* or sense-*VEGF165* neither enhanced nor inhibited formation of brain metastases. Collectively, the results indicate that VEGF expression is essential but not sufficient for production of progressively growing brain metastasis.

Several lines of evidence suggest that VEGF levels must reach a threshold before it functions in physiological and pathological conditions *(18,91)*. For example, a decrease in VEGF secretion to 20–30% of parental glioma cells inhibits in vivo growth *(17)*. Because angiogenesis consists of several distinct steps *(10,83)* that can be regulated by VEGF *(35,83)*, a decrease in VEGF could inhibit angiogenesis in the brain. Indeed, our data show that decreasing VEGF production (by antisense transfection) to 20–50% of parental cell level, which is accompanied by reduced biological activity (measured by human dermal microvascular endothelial cell proliferation), was associated with inhibition of both angiogenesis and brain metastasis formation. Therefore, results of this experimental work provides strong evidence that reduction of VEGF production could be a therapeutic target. Newer and more efficient vector system for optimizing gene delivery and gene expression will be necessary to deliver the antisense-VEGF gene therapies. Among these are various inhibitors of VEGF and its receptors (Flt-1 and Flk-1/KDR), such as humanized neutralizing antibody for VEGF *(123)*, dominant-negative VEGF *(143)*, VEGF receptor tyrosine kinase inhibitors *(50)*, soluble VEGF receptors *(81,86,146)*, antisense-VEGF *(131)*, and dominant-negative Flk-1 *(59,92,98,99)*. These data suggest that anti-angiogenesis therapy targeting VEGF/VEGF receptor signal transduction pathway may be useful for controlling brain metastasis.

5. EFFECT OF BRAIN MICROENVIRONMENT ON TUMOR CELL PHENOTYPE

Metastatic K-1735 murine melanoma cells are amelanotic in culture or in the subcutis of syngeneic C3H/HeN mice. However, when injected into the internal carotid artery, these cells produce melanotic brain metastases. The melanocortins are a complex family of peptides with a variety of biological activities that include the control of melanocyte growth, pigment production, and morphological changes associated with increased differentiation *(27)*. Many reports indicate that α-melanocyte-stimulating hormone 3 (α-MSH3) increases darkening of the skin and hair by stimulating melanogenesis *(14,21)*. This process involves α-MSH binding to the melanocyte-stimulating hormone receptor (MSH-R) and activation of the heterotrimeric guanine nucleotide-binding protein Gs, which in turn activates adenylyl cyclase and elevates cyclic adenosine monophosphate (cAMP) to activate tyrosinase, the rate-limiting enzyme in melanin synthesis *(64,117)*. Many, but not all, cultured melanoma cells *(55)* or normal melanocytes *(51,65,139)* respond to α-MSH by increased pigmentation. Similarly, not all normal melanocytes respond to α-MSH in vivo *(14)*. Various mechanisms to explain this phenomenon have been proposed. The differences in response of normal and transformed melanocytes to α-MSH can be from a lack of MSH-R expression and/or to downstream defects in the cAMP signal transduction pathway *(71,132)*. The recent cloning and sequencing of the cDNA encoding the human and mouse MSH-R genes should allow for the determination of why different melanocytes respond differently to α-MSH *(19,101)*.

Recent reports from our laboratory have shown that the organ microenvironment profoundly influences the biological behavior of tumor cells, including production of degradative enzymes *(31,41,58,105)*, angiogenesis *(63,144)*, resistance to chemotherapy *(25)*, and induction of terminal differentiation *(126)*. We therefore examined whether the brain microenvironment could also influence the expression of the MSH-R as a potential mechanism for the site-specific regulation of melanogenesis in K-1735 melanoma cells. The steady-state expression of MSH-R mRNA transcripts in K-1735 and B16 cells as well as their somatic cell hybrids were analyzed as was the function of MSH-R in induction of cell proliferation, melanin production, and intracellular cAMP accumulation in response to α-MSH *(125)*. The production of melanin in tumor cells growing in the brain directly correlates with induction of MSH-R steady-state mRNA transcripts. K-1735 cells isolated from brain metastases and implanted into the subcutis or grown in culture lost MSH-R transcripts and became amelanotic. In contrast to K-1735 cells, B16-BL6 melanoma cells that constitutively produce melanin, constitutively express a high level of MSH-R mRNA. Somatic cell hybrids between K-1735 and B16 cells also produce melanin and express high level of MSH-R mRNA regardless of the site of growth, suggesting the dominance of the B16 phenotype *(125)*. Treatment with α-MSH failed to upregulate MSH-R expression in cultures K-1735 cells or to maintain MSH-R expression in K-1735 cells isolated from brain metastases to be grown in culture. Responsiveness to α-MSH as determined by cell proliferation, melanin production, and intracellular accumulation of cAMP directly correlated with MSH-R expression. These data demonstrate that a specific organ environment influences the phenotype of metastatic cells by regulation of specific genes that encode for cell surface receptors *(125)*.

6. BLOOD–BRAIN BARRIER IN BRAIN METASTASIS

The microvasculature of the brain parenchyma is lined by a continuous, nonfenestrated endothelium with tight junctions and little pinocytic vesicle activity *(60,75,116,150)*. This structure, designated as the blood–brain barrier, limits the entrance of circulating macromolecules into the brain parenchyma. The blood–brain barrier and the lack of a lymphatic system are responsible for maintaining the brain as an immunologically privileged site *(33,96,137)*, and protecting the brain against the entry of most drugs and invasion of microorganisms *(142)*. The blood–brain barrier does not prevent the invasion of the brain parenchyma by circulating metastatic cells. In fact, the integrity of the blood–brain barrier is altered in some brain tumors and in metastases *(22,23,52,73,80,111,145, 154,156)*. Indeed, some but not all neoplastic cells can affect the integrity of this structure *(108,138, 145,156)*.

In general, primary brain neoplasms and brain metastases are resistant to treatment by most chemotherapeutic drugs *(137,142,158)*, and this resistance has been attributed to the inability of drugs to cross the blood–brain barrier *(57,61,62)*. However, because this structure is morphologically, biochemically, and functionally heterogeneous in different regions of the brain *(7,34, 114,116,150)*, its relationship to the failure to eradicate brain metastases with anticancer drugs was unclear.

We investigated the functional viability of the blood–brain barrier in an experimental animal model to study the establishment, progression, and therapy of brain metastases *(53,121,136,157)*. Eight different human tumor cell lines were injected into the internal carotid artery of nude mice *(157)*. The tumors produced lesions in different regions of the brain and the pattern of lesions varied from diffuse to solitary with well-defined margins. Of several molecular tracers used to study the permeability of the blood–brain barrier, we chose sodium fluorescein. Despite its low molecular weight (MW 376), this hydrosoluble molecule is excluded from the barrier by an intact blood–brain barrier *(76,103)*. Sodium fluorescein is not sensitive to minor or transient changes in blood–brain barrier permeability, and unlike horseradish peroxidase, it is not transported into brain tissue by nonspecific endocytosis *(94)*. This molecule is therefore most suitable for studies of blood–brain barrier functions in brain metastases.

Table 3
Size of Experimental Brain Metastasis and Permeability of the Blood–Brain
Barrier to Sodium Fluorescein

Tumor cells [a]	Size of brain metastases (mm^2) [b]		Status of the blood–brain barrier [c]
	Median	Range	
A375 SM melanoma	0.0004	0.003–0.006	Intact
	3.7	1.6–9.1	Permeable
TXM-34 melanoma	0.2	0.08–0.2	Intact
	1.7	0.3–10.1	Permeable
KM12L4 colon carcinoma	0.06	0.003–0.2	Intact
	1.2	0.3–16.7	Permeable
SN12 renal carcinoma	0.2	0.02–0.2	Intact
	0.8	0.3–3.9	Permeable
MDA-435 breast carcinoma	0.1	0.02–0.2	Intact
	0.5	0.3–0.9	Permeable
MDA-468 breast carcinoma	0.01	0.007–0.1	Intact
	4.3	0.3–6.5	Permeable

[a] 1×10^5 viable tumor cells were injected into the internal carotid artery of nude mice. The mice were killed at different intervals thereafter ($n = 3$).

[b] The data are median size in mm^2 of at least 20 brain lesions.

[c] Permeability of the blood–brain barrier was determined by vascular retention of sodium fluorescein.

Before studying the function of the blood–brain barrier in such brain lesions, we ruled out that the procedure of intracarotid injection, which is followed by ligation of the artery, or the entry of a bolus of tumor cells into the brain damages the endothelial cells of the cerebromicrovessels and, thus, change the permeability of the blood–brain barrier *(157)*.

Leakage through the blood–brain barrier may be a result of endothelial alterations brought about by tumor cells in the perivascular space *(6)*. Several ultrastructural studies concluded that brain tumors disrupt adjacent endothelium *(72,145)*. In our study with eight different human tumor cell lines, the lesions in the brain parenchyma were either well demarcated with well-defined margins or diffuse lesions throughout a region of the parenchyma. We found that the solitary well-defined lesions had a lower density of blood vessels than normal brain tissue. The blood–brain barrier is known to become permeable in ischemic regions of the brain where increased endothelial pinocytosis, opening of the interendothelial tight junctions, and damage to endothelial cells have all been observed *(24)*. We found that degeneration and central necrosis often occurred in large (> 0.5 mm in diameter, 0.2 mm^2) brain metastases. Therefore, in these lesions, damage to endothelial cells may compromise the integrity of the blood–brain barrier (Table 3).

We have previously reported that the blood–brain barrier was intact in established mouse UV-2237 fibrosarcoma brain metastases *(136)*. Two human melanoma cell lines (TXM-13, TXM-18) growing in the brain parenchyma of nude mice produced the same phenomenon. The common characteristic to the brain metastases produced by mouse and human tumors was their diffuse pattern of growth. The permeability of the blood–brain barrier in this lesion was not increased as compared with normal brain tissue unless the tumor cell clusters coalesced to form large tumor masses. Transplantation of quail avascularized embryonic mesodermal tissue into the brain of chick embryos and an in vivo study of endothelial cell-astrocyte interaction *(60)* demonstrated that signals arising within the brain, rather than a programmed commitment of the endothelial cells, are responsible for the function of the blood–brain barrier. The integrity of the barrier around small lesions (metastases) shows that the barrier can repair after passage of metastatic cells into the brain parenchyma. Moreover, the interaction of astrocytes with endothelial cells and elongated cytoplasmic processes of oligodendrocytes are likely to be important in maintaining a functional blood–brain barrier *(150)*. A growing tumor mass may disturb this interaction, especially if it depends on contact between astrocytes and endothelial cells. In any event, the normal brain tissue interspread among the small tumor clusters or surrounding small tumor lesions might be responsible for the normal function of the blood–brain barrier.

The experimental data show that the permeability of the blood–brain barrier in experimental brain metastases produced by different human tumor cells after injection into the carotid artery of nude mice was determined by the size and pattern of growth of the lesions. Because the blood–brain barrier is not intact in experimental brain metastases that exceed 0.2 mm^2, the resistance to chemotherapy may be a result of other mechanisms

7. CONCLUSIONS

The development of a relevant in vivo mouse model of brain metastasis has been invaluable for studies of the biology of this fatal consequence of systemic cancer. The intracarotid injection of different tumor cells produces metastases in different regions of the brain. This site-specific metastasis correlates with the ability of tumor cells to proliferate in the brain and induce angiogenesis. Hence, the development of brain metastasis represents the end result of multiple interactions between tumor cells and the unique microenvironment of the brain.

REFERENCES

1. Alon T., Hemo I., Itin A., Pe'er J., Stone J., Keshet E.1995. Vascular endothelial growth factor acts as a survival factor for newly formed retinal vessels and has implications for retinopathy of prematurity. *Nat. Med.* **10**:1024–1028.
2. Anzano M.A., Roberts A.B., Sporn M.B. 1986. Anchorage-independent growth of primary rat embryo cells is induced by platelet-derived growth factor and inhibited by type-beta transforming growth factor. *J.Cell. Physiol.* **126**:312–318.
3. Arbit E,, Wronski M. 1995.. The treatment of brain metastases. *Neurosurg. Quart.***5**:1–17.
4. Aukerman S.L., Price J.E., Fidler I.J. 1986. Different deficiencies in the prevention of tumorigenic-low-metastatic murine K-1735 melanoma cell from producing metastasis. *J. Natl. Cancer Inst.* **77**:915–924.
5. Baird A., Drukin T. 1986. Inhibition of endothelial cell proliferation by type-beta transforming growth factor: interaction with acid and basic fibroblast growth factors. *Biochem. Biophys. Res. Commun.* **138**:476–482.
6. Ballinger, W.E., Jr., Schimpff, R.D. 1979 An experimental model for cerebral metastasis: preliminary light and ultrastructural studies. *J. Neuropath. Exp. Neurol.* **38**:19–34.
7. Baur H.C., Tonsch U., Amberger A., Bauer H. 1990. Gamma-glutamyl-transpeptidase (GGPT) and Na$^+$- K$^+$-ATPase activities in different subpopulations of cloned cerebral endothelial cells: response to glial stimulation. *Biochem. Biophys. Res. Commun.* **168**:358–363.
8. Benjamin L.E., Keshet E. 1997 Conditional switching of vascular endothelial growth factor (VEGF) expression in tumors: induction of endothelial cell shedding and repression of hemangioblastoma-like vessels by VEGF withdrawal. *Proc. Natl. Acad. Sci. USA* **94**:8761–8766.
9. Berkman R.A., Merrill M.J., Reinhold W.C., Monacci W.T., Saxena A., Clark W.C., et al. 1993. Expression of the vascular permeability factor/vascular endothelial growth factor gene in central nervous system neoplasms. *J. Clin. Invest.* **91**:513–159
10. Bicknell R. 1997. Mechanistic insights into tumor angiogenesis, in *Tumor Angiogenesis* (Bicknell, R., Lewis, C.E., Ferrara, N., eds.), Oxford University Press, New York, pp.19–28.
11. Birch M., Mitchell S., Hart I.R. 1991. Isolation and characterization of human melanoma cell variants expressing high and low levels of CD44. *Cancer Res.* **51**:6660–6667.
12. Boener P., Resnick R.J., Racker E. 1985. Stimulation of glycolysis and amino uptake in NRK-49F cells by transforming growth factor-β and epidermal growth factor. *Proc. Natl. Acad. Sci. USA* **82**:1350–1353.
13. Bouck N., Stellmach V., Hsu S.C. 1996. How tumors become angiogenic. *Adv. Cancer Res.*.**69**:135–174.
14. Burchill S.A., Virden R., Thody A.J. 1989. Regulation of tyrosinase and its processing in the hair follicular melanocytes of the mouse during melanogenesis and pharmacomelanogenesis. *J. Invest. Dermatol.* **93**:236–240.
15. Carmeliet P., Ferreira V., Breier G., Pollefeyt S., Kieckens L., Gertsenstein M., et al. 1996. Abnormal blood vessel development and lethality in embryos lacking a single *VEGF* allele. *Nature* **380**:435–439.
16. Chakrabarty C., Fan D., Varani J. 1990. Modulation of differentiation and proliferation in human colon carcinoma cells by transforming growth factor-β$_1$ and -β$_2$. *Int. J. Cancer* **46**:493–499.

17. Cheng S.Y., Huang H.J., Nagane M., Ji X.D., Wang D., Shih C.C., et al. 1996. Suppression of glioblastoma angiogenicity and tumorigenicity by inhibition of endogenous expression of vascular endothelial growth factor. *Proc. Natl. Acad. Sci. USA* **93**:8502–8507.

18. Cheng S.Y., Nagane M., Huang H.S., Cavenee W.K. Intracerebral tumor-associated hemorrhage caused by overexpression of the vascular endothelial growth factor isoforms VEGF121 and VEGF165 but not VEGF 189. *Proc. Natl. Acad. Sci. USA* **94**:12,081–12,087.

19. Chhajlani V., Wiberg J.E.S. 1992. Molecular cloning and expression of the human melanocyte-stimulating hormone receptor cDNA. *FEBS Lett.* **3**:417–420.

20. Claffey, K.P., Brown L.F., del Aguila L.F., Tognazzi K., Yeo K.T., Manseau E.J., Dvorak H.F. 1996. Expression of vascular permeability factor/vascular endothelial growth factor by melanoma cells increases tumor growth, angiogenesis, and experimental metastasis. *Cancer Res.* **56**:172–181.

21. Clive D., Snell D.S. 1972. Effect of MSH on mammalian hair color. *J. Invest. Dermatol.* **49**:314–321.

22. Coomber B.L., Stewart P.A., Hayakawa K. Farrell C.L., Del Maestro R.F. 1987. Quantitative morphology of human glioblastoma multiforme microvessels: structural basis of blood-brain barrier defect. *J. Neurooncol.* **5**:299–307.

23. Debbage P.L., Gabius H.J. Bise K., Marguth F. 1988. Cellular glyco-conjugates and their potential endogenous receptors in the cerebral microvasculature of man: a glycohistochemical study. *Eur. J. Cell Biol.* **46**:425–434.

24. Dietrich W.D., Busto R., Hailey M., Valdes I. 1990. The importance of brain temperature in alterations of the blood-brain barrier following cerebral ischemia. *J. Neuropathol. Exp. Neurol.* **49**:486–497.

25. Dong Z., Radinsky R., Fan D., Tsan R., Bucana C.D., Wilmanns C., Fidler I.J. 1994. Organ-specific modulation of steady-state mdr gene expression and drug resistance in murine colon cancer cells. *J. Natl. Cancer Inst.* **86**:913–920.

26. Dvorak H.F. 1988. Tumors: wounds that do not heal. *N. Engl. J. Med.* **315**:1650–1659.

27. Eberle A.N. 1988. *The Melanotropins: Chemistry, Physiology, and Mechanisms of Action*, Karger, Basel, Switzerland.

28. Ellis L.M., Fidler I.J. 1996. Angiogenesis and metastasis. *Eur. J. Cancer* **32A**:2451–2460.

29. Ewing J. 1928. Neoplastic *Diseases*, 6th edition, Saunders, Philadelphia, PA.

30. Ezekowitz R.A.B., Mulliken J.B., Folkman J. 1992. Interferon alpha-2a therapy for life-threatening hemangiomas of infancy. *N. Engl. J. Med.* **326**:1456–1463.

31. Fabra A., Nakajima M., Bucana C.D., Fidler I.J. 1992. Modulation of the invasive phenotype of human colon carcinoma cells by fibroblasts from orthotopic or ectopic organs of nude mice. *Differentiation* **52**:101–110.

32. Fan D., Chakrabarty C., Seid C., Bell C.W., Schackert H., Morikawa K., Fidler I.J. 1989. Clonal stimulation or inhibition of human colon carcinomas and human renal carcinomas mediated by transforming growth factor-β_1. *Cancer Commun.* **1**:117–125.

33. Felgenhauser K. 1986. The blood-brain barrier redefined. *J. Neurol.* **233**:193–194.

34. Fenstermacher J., Gross P., Sposito N., Acuff V., Petterson S., Gruber K. 1988. Structural and functional variations in capillary system within the brain. *Ann. NY Acad. Sci.* **529**:21–30.

35. Ferrara N. 1997. The role of vascular endothelial growth factor in the regulation of blood vessel growth, in *Tumor Angiogenesis* (Bicknell R., Lewis C.E., Ferrara N.,eds), Oxford University Press, New York, pp.185–199.

36. Ferrara N., Carver-Moore K., Chen H., Dowd M., Lu L., O'Shea K.S., et al. 1996.. Heterozygous embryonic lethality induced by targeted inactivation of the *VEGF* gene. *Nature (Lond)* **380**:439–442.

37. Ferrara N., Henzel W.J. 1989. Pituitary follicular cells secrete a novel heparin-binding growth factor specific for vascular endothelial cells. *Biochem. Biophys. Res. Commun.* **161**:851–859.

38. Fidler I.J. 1999. Critical determinants of cancer metastasis: rationale for therapy. *Cancer Chemother. Pharmacol.* **43**:S3 – S10.

39. Fidler I.J. 1990. Critical factors in the biology of human cancer metastasis: twenty-eighth GHA Clowes Memorial Award Lecture. *Cancer Res.* **50**:6130–6138.

40. Fidler I.J. 1970. Metastasis: quantitative analysis of distribution and fate of tumor emboli labeled with ^{125}I-5-iodo-2'-deoxyuridine. *J. Natl. Cancer Inst.* **45**:773–782.

41. Fidler I.J. 1995. Modulation of the organ microenvironment for the treatment of cancer metastasis. *J. Natl. Cancer Inst.* **84**:1588–1592.

42. Fidler I.J. 1973. Selection of successive tumor lines for metastasis. *Nature (New Biol)* **242**:148–149.

43. Fidler I.J. 1973. The relationship of embolic homogeneity, number, size and viability to the incidence of experimental metastasis. *Eur. J. Cancer* **9**:223–227.

44. Fidler I.J., Ellis L.M. 1994. The implications of angiogenesis for the biology and therapy of cancer metastasis. *Cell* **79**:185–188.

45. Fidler I.J., Gruys E., Cifone M.A., Barnes Z., Bucana C.D. Demonstration of multiple phenotypic diversity in murine melanoma of recent origin. *J. Natl. Cancer Inst.* **67**:947–956.

46. Fidler I.J, Kripke M. 1977. Metastasis results from preexisting variant cells within a malignant tumor. *Science (Washington, DC)* **197**:893–895.

47. Flanders K.C., Ludecke G., Engles S., Cissel D.S., Roberts A.B., Kondaiah P., et al. 1991.. Localization and actions of transforming growth factor-β in the embryonic nervous system. *Develop.* **113**:183–191.

48. Folkman J. 1995. Clinical application of research on angiogenesis. *N. Engl. J. Med.* **333**:1757–1763.

49. Folkman J., Klagsbrun M. 1987. Angiogenic factors. *Science* **235**:442–447.
50. Fong T.A., Shawver L.K., Sun L., Tang C., App H., Powell T.J., et al. 1999.. SU5416 is a potent and selective inhibitor of the vascular endothelial growth factor receptor (Flk-1/KDR) that inhibits tyrosine kinase catalysis, tumor vascularization, and growth of multiple tumor types. *Cancer Res.* **59**:99–106.
51. Friedman P.S., Wren F., Buffey J., MacNeil S. 1990. α-MSH causes a small rise in cAMP but has no effect on basal or ultraviolet-stimulated melanogenesis in human melanocytes. *Br. J. Dermatol.* **123**:145–151.
52. Front D., Israel O., Kohn S., Nir I. 1984. The blood-brain barrier of human brain tumors: correlation of scintigraphic and ultrastructural findings (concise communication). *J. Nucl. Med.* **25**:461–465.
53. Fujimaki T., Fan D., Staroselsky A.H., Gohji K., Bucana C.D., Fidler I.J. 1993. Critical factors regulating site-specific brain metastasis of murine melanomas. *Int. J. Oncol.* **3**:789–799.
54. Fujimaki T., Price J.E., Fan D., Bucana C.D., Itoh K., Kirino T., Fidler I.J. 1996. Selective growth of human melanoma cells in the brain parenchyma of nude mice. *Melanoma Res.***6**:363–371.
55. Fuller B.B., Meyskins F.L. 1981. Endocrine responsiveness in human melanocytes and melanoma cells in culture. *J. Natl. Cancer Inst.* **66**:799–802.
56. Geiser A.G., Burnester J.K., Wevvink R., Roberts A.B., Sporn M.B. 1992. Inhibition of growth by transforming growth factors following fusion of two nonresponsive human carcinoma cell lines. *J. Bio. Chem.* **267**:2588–2593.
57. Genka S., Deutsch J., Stahle P.L., Shetty U.H., John V., Robinson C., et al. 1990. Brain and plasma pharmacokinetics and anticancer activities of cyclophosphamide and phosphamide mustard in the rat. *Cancer Chemother. Phamacol.* **27**:1–7.
58. Gohji K., Fidler I.J., Fabra A., Bucana C.D., von Eschenbach A.C., Nakajima M.1994. Regulation of gelatinase production in metastatic renal cell carcinoma by organ-specific fibroblasts. *Japan J. Cancer Res.* **85**:152–160.
59. Goldman C.K., Kendall R.L., Cabrera G., Soroceanu L., Heike Y., Gillespie G.Y., et al. 1998. Paracrine expression of a native soluble vascular endothelial growth factor receptor inhibits tumor growth, metastasis, and mortality rate. *Proc. Natl.Acad. Sci. USA* **95**:8795–8800.
60. Goldstein G.W. 1988. Endothelial cell-astrocyte interaction: a cellular model of the blood-brain barrier. *Ann. NY. Acad. Sci.* **529**:31–39.
61. Gregoire N. 1989. The blood-brain barrier. *J. Neuroradiol.* **16**:238–250.
62. Greig N.H. 1987. Optimizing drug delivery to brain tumors. *Cancer Treat. Rev.* **13**:1–28.
63. Greig N.H., Soncrant T..T, Shetty H.U., Momma S., Smith Q.R., Rapoport S.I. 1990. Brain uptake and anticancer activities of vincristine and vinblastine are restricted by their low cerebrovascular permeability and binding to plasma constituents in rat. *Cancer Chemother. Phamacol.***26**:263–268.
64. Gutman M., Singh R.K., Xie K., Bucana C.D., Fidler I.J. 1995. Regulation of IL-8 expression in human melanoma cells by the organ environment. *Cancer Res.* **55**:2470–2475.
65. Halaban R., Pomerantz S.H., Marshall S., Lambert D.T., Lerner A.B. 1983. Regulation of tyrosinase in human melanocytes grown in culture. *J. Cell Biol.* **97**:480–488.
66. Halaban R., Pomerantz S.H., Marshall S., Lerner A.B. 1984. Tyrosinase activity ant its abundance in Cloudman melanoma cells. *Arch. Biochem. Biophys.* **230**:383–387.
67. Hanahan D., Folkman J. 1996. Patterns and emerging mechanisms of the angiogenic switch during tumorigenesis. *Cell* **86**:353–364.
68. Harris A.L. 1998. Antiangiogenesis therapy and strategies for integrating it with adjuvant therapy: recent results. *Cancer Res.* **152**:342–352.
69. Hart I.R., Birch M., Marshall J.F. 1991. Cell adhesion receptor expression during melanoma progression and metastasis. *Cancer Metastasis Rev.* **10**:115–128.
70. Hart I.R., Fidler I.J. 1980. Role of organ selectivity in the determination of metastatic patterns of B16 melanoma. *Cancer Res.* **40**:2281–2287.
71. Haynes B.F., Telen M.J., Hale L.P., Denning S.M. 1989. CD44 – a molecule involved in leukocyte adherence and T-cell activation. *Immunol. Today* **10**:423–428.
72. Hill S., Buffey J., Thody A.J., Oliver I., Bleehen S.S., MacNeil S. 1989. Investigation of the regulation of pigmentation in melanocyte-stimulating hormone responsive and unresponsive cultured B16 murine melanoma cells. *Pigm. Cell Res.* **2**:161–166
73. Hirano A., Zimmerman H.M. 1972. Fenestrated blood vessels in metastatic renal carcinoma in the brain. *Lab. Invest.* **26**:465–468.
74. Iannotti F., Fleschi C., Alfano B., Picozzi P., Mansi L., Pozzili C., et al. 1987. Simplified, noninvasive PET measurement of blood brain barrier permeability. *J. Comput. Assist Tomogr.* **11**:390–397.
75. Ignotz R.A., Massague J. 1986. Transforming growth factor-β stimulates the expression of fibronectin and collagen and their incorporation into the extracellular matrix. *J. Biol. Chem.* **261**:4337–4347.
76. Johansson B.B. 1990. The physiology of the blood-brain barrier. *Adv. Exp. Med. Biol.* **274**:25–39.
77. Kawamura S., Schuere L., Goetz A., Kempski O. Schumucker B., Baethmann A. 1990. An improved closed cranial window technique for investigation of blood-brain barrier function and cerebral vasomotor control in the rat. *Int. J. Microcir. Clin. Exp.* **9**: 369–383.

78. Keck P.J., Hauser S.D., Krivi G., Sanzo K., Warren T., Feder J., Connolly D.T. 1989. Vascular endothelial growth factor, an endothelial cell mitogen related to PDGF. *Science* **246:**1309–1312.

79. Kerbel R.S. Expression of multi-cytokine resistant and multi-growth factor independence in advanced stage metastatic cancer: malignant melanoma as a paradigm. *Am. J. Pathol.* **141:**519–524.

80. Knabbe C., Lippman M.E., Wakefield L.M., Flanders A.K., Derynck R., Dickson R.B. 1987. Evidence that transforming growth factor is a hormonally regulated negative growth factor in human breast cancer cells. *Cell 1987;***48:**417–428.

81. Kohn S., Front D., Nir I. 1989. Blood-brain barrier permeability of human gliomas as determined by quantitation of cytoplasmic vessels of the capillary endothelium and scintigraphic findings. *Cancer Invest.* **7:**313–321.

82. Kong H.L., Hecht D., Song W., Kovesdi I., Hackett N.R., Yayon A., Crystal R.G. 1998. Regional suppression of tumor growth by *in vivo* transfer of a cDNA encoding a secreted form of the extracellular domain of flt-1 vascular endothelial growth factor receptor. *Hum. Gene Ther.* **9:**823–833.

83. Kornblith P.L., Walker M.D., Cassady J.R. 1985. Neoplasm of the central nervous system, in *Cancer: Principles and Practice of Oncology*, 2nd ed. (DeVita, Jr V.T., Hellman S., Rosenberg S.A., eds.), Lippincott, Philadelphia, PA, pp.1437–1566.

84. Kumar R., Yoneda J., Bucana C.D., Fidler I.J. 1998. Regulation of distinct steps of angiogenesis by different angiogenic molecules. *Int. J. Oncol.* **12:**749–757

85. Kuppner M.C., van Meir E., Gauthier T., Hamou M.F., de Tribolet N. 1992. Differential expression of the CD44 molecule in human brain tumors. *Int. J. Cancer* **50:**572–577.

86. Laiho M., deCaprio J.A., Ludlow J.W., Livingston D.M., Massague J. 1990. Growth inhibition by TGF-β linked to suppression of retinoblastoma protein phosphorylation. *Cell* **62:**175–185.

87. Lin P., Sankar S., Shan S., Dewhirst M.W., Polverini P.J., Quinn T.Q., Peters K.G. 1998. Inhibition of tumor growth by targeting tumor endothelium using a soluble vascular endothelial growth factor receptor. *Cell Growth Differ.* **9:**49–58.

88. Liotta L.A., Rao C.N., Barsky S.H. 1983. Tumor invasion and the extracellular matrix. *Lab. Invest.* **49:**636–649.

89. Liotta L.A., Steeg P.S., Stetler-Stevenson W.G. 1991. Cancer metastasis and angiogenesis: an imbalance of positive and negative regulation. *Cell* **64:**327–332.

90. Liotta L.A., Stetler-Stevenson W.G. 1991. Tumor invasion and metastasis: an imbalance of positive and negative regulation. *Cancer Res.* **51:**5054S–5059S.

91. Lotan R., Amos B., Watanabe H., Raz A. 1992. Suppression of motility factor receptor expression by retinoic acid. *Cancer Res.* **52:**4878–4884.

92. Machein M.R., Plate K.H. 2000 VEGF in brain tumors. *J. Neurooncol.* **50:**109–120.

93. Machein M.R. Risau W., Plate K.H. 1999. Antiangiogenic gene therapy in rat glioma model using a dominant-negative vascular growth factor receptor 2. *Hum. Gene Ther.* **10:**1117–1128.

94. Madjewicz S.T., Karakousis C., West C.R., Caracanadas J., Avellanosa A.M. 1984. Malignant melanoma brain metastases: a review of Roswell Park Memorial Institute experience. *Cancer* **53:**2550–2562.

95. Malmgren L.T., Olsson Y. 1980. Differences between the peripheral and the central nervous system in permeability to sodium fluorescein. *J. Comp. Neurol.* **191:**103–117.

96. Mandybur T.I. 1981. Metastatic brain tumors induced by injection of syngeneic tumor cells into cerebral artery circulation in rats. *Acta. Neuropathol.* **53:**57–64.

97. Medawar P.B. 1948. Immunity to homologous grafted skin: III. The fate of skin homografts transplanted to the brain, to subcutaneous tissue, and to the anterior chamber of the eye. *Br. J. Exp. Pathol.* **29:**58–69.

98. Meister B., Grunebach F., Bautz F. Brugger W., Fink F.M., Kanz L., Mohle R. 1999. Expression of vascular endothelial growth factor (VEGF) and its receptors in human neuroblastoma. *Eur. J. Cancer* **35:**445–449.

99. Millauer B., Longhi M.P., Plate K.H., Shawver L.K., Risau W., Ullrich A., Strawn L.M. 1996. Dominant-negative inhibition of flk-1 suppresses the growth of many tumors in vivo. *Cancer Res.* **56:**1615–1620.

100. Millauer B., Shawver L.K., Plate K.H., Risau W., Ullrich A. 1994. Glioblastoma growth inhibited in vivo by a dominant-negative Flk-1 mutant. *Nature* **367:**576–579.

101. Miller D.A., Lee A. Pelton R.W., Chen E.Y., Moses H.L., Derynck R. 1989. Murine transforming growth factor-β$_2$ cDNA sequence and expression in adult tissues and embryos. *Mol. Endocrinol.* **3:**1108–1114.

102. Mountjoy K.G., Robbins L.S., Mortrud M.T., Cone R.D. 1992. The cloning of a family of genes that encode the melanocortin receptors. *Science* (*Washington, DC*) **257:**1248–1251.

103. Nagasaka S., Tanabe K.K., Bruner J.M., Saya H., Sawaya R.E., Morrison R. 1995. Alternative splicing of the hyaluronic acid receptor CD44 in the normal human brain and in brain tumors. *J. Neurosurg.* **82:**858–863.

104. Nakagawa Y., Fujimoto N., Matsumoto K., Cervos Navarro J. 1990. Morphological changes in acute cerebral ischemia after occlusion and reperfusion in the rat. *Adv. Neurol.* **52:**21–27.

105. Nakajima M., Irimura T., Di Ferrante N., Nicolson G. 1983. Heparin sulfate degradation: relation to tumor invasive and metastatic properties of mouse B16 melanoma sublines. *Science* **220:**611–613.

106. Nakajima M., Morikawa K., Fabra A., Bucana C.D., Fidler I.J. 1990. Influence of organ environment on extracellular matrix degradative activity and metastasis of human colon carcinoma cells. *J. Natl. Cancer Inst.* **82:**1890–1898.

107. Nakajima M., Welch D.R., Belloni P.N., Nicolson G.L. 1987. Degradation of basement membrane type IV collagen and lung subendothelial matrix by rat mammary adenocarcinoma cell clones of differing metastatic potential. *Cancer Res.* **47:**4869–4876.

108. Nicolson G.L. 1989. Metastatic tumor cell interaction with endothelium, basement membrane and tissue. *Curr. Opin. Cell Biol.* **1:**1009–1019.

109. Nicolson G.L. 1990. Organ specificity of cancer metastasis is determined, in part, by tumor cell properties and cytokines expressed at particular organ sites. *Am. Assoc. Cancer Res.* **31:**506–507.

110. Nicolson G.L., Cavanaugh P.G., Inoue T. 1992. Differential stimulation of the growth of lung-metastasizing tumor cells by lung (paracrine) growth factors: identification of transferrin-like mitogens in lung tissue-conditioned medium (monograph). *J. Natl. Cancer Inst.* **13:**153–161.

111. Nicolson G.L., Menter D.G., Herrmann J.L., Yun A., Cavanaugh P., Marchetti D. 1996. Brain metastasis: role of trophic, autocrine, and paracrine factors in tumor invasion and colonization of the central nervous system. *Curr. Topics Microbiol. Immunol.* **213:**89–115.

112. Nir I., Levanon D., Iosilevsky G. 1989. Permeability of blood vessels in experimental gliomas: uptake of ^{99}Tc-glucoheptonate and alteration in blood-brain barrier as determined by cytochemistry and electron microscopy. *Neurosurgery* **25:**523–532.

113. Nishikawa R., Cheng S.Y., Nagashima R., Huanh H.J., Cavenee W.K., Matsutani M. 1998. Expression of vascular endothelial growth factor in human brain tumors. *Acta. Neuropathol.* **96:**453–462.

114. Oku T., Tjuvajev J.G., Miyagawa T., Sasajima T., Joshi A., Joshi R., et al. 1998. Tumor growth modulation by sense and antisense vascular endothelial growth factor gene expression: effects on angiogenesis, vascular permeability, blood volume, blood flow, fluorododeoxyglucose uptake, and proliferation of human melanoma intracerebral xenografts. *Cancer Res.* **58:**4185–4192.

115. Owman C., Hardebo J.E. 1988. Functional heterogeneity of the cerebrovascular endothelium. *Brain Behav. Evol.* **32:**65–75.

116. Paget S. 1889. The distribution of secondary growths in cancer of the breast. *Lancet* **1:**571–573.

117. Pardridge W.M., Oldendorf W.H., Cancilla P., Frank H.J. 1986. Blood-brain barrier: interface between internal medicine and the brain clinical conference. *Ann. Intern. Med.* **105:**82–95.

118. Pawelek J., Wong G., Sansone J., Morowitz J. 1973. Molecular controls in mammalian pigmentation. *Yale J. Biol. Med.* **46:**430–443.

119. Pepper M.S., Ferrara N., Orci L., Montesana R. 1991. Vascular endothelial growth factor (VEGF) induces plasminogen activators and plasminogen activator inhibitor type 1 in microvascular endothelial cells. *Biochem. Biophys. Res. Commun.* **181:**902–908.

120. Pietsch T., Valter M.M., Wolf H.K., von Deimling A., Huang H.J., Cavenee W.K., Wiestler O.D. 1997. Expression and distribution of vascular endothelial growth factor protein in human brain tumors. *Acta. Neuropathol.* **93:**109–117

121. Posner J.B. 1996. Brain metastases: 1995. A brief review. *J. Neurooncol.* **27:**287–293.

122. Posner J.B. 1992. Management of brain metastases. *Rev. Neurol. (Paris)* **148:**477–487.

123. Poste G., Fidler I.J. 1980. The pathogenesis of cancer metastasis. *Nature (Lond)* **283:**139–146.

124. Presta L.G., Chen H., O'Connor S.J., Chisholm V., Meng Y.G., Krummen L., et al. 1997. Humanization of antivascular endothelial growth factor monoclonal antibody for the therapy of solid tumors and other disorders. *Cancer Res.* **57:**4593–4599.

125. Price J.E., Aukerman S.L., Fidler I.J. 1986. Evidence that the process of murine melanoma metastasis is sequential and selective and contains stochastic elements. *Cancer Metastasis Rev.* **46:**5172–5178.

126. Radinsky R., Beltran P.J., Tsan R., Zhang R., Cone R.D., Fidler I.J. 1995. Transcriptional induction of the melanocyte stimulating hormone receptor in brain metastases of murine K-1735 melanoma. *Cancer Res.* **55:**141–148.

127. Radinsky R., Fidler I.J., Price J.E., Esumi N., Tsan R., Petty C.M., et al. 1994. Terminal differentiation and apoptosis in experimental lung metastases of human osteogenic sarcoma cells by wild type p53. *Oncogene* **9:**1877–1883.

128. Radotra B., McCormick D., Crockard A. 1994. CD44 plays a role in adhesive interactions between glioma cells and extracellular matrix components. *Neuropathol. Appl. Neurobiol.* **20:**399–405.

129. Risau W. 1997. Mechanisms of angiogenesis. *Nature (Lond)* **386:**671–674.

130. Roberts A.B., Sporn M.B., Assoian R.K., Smith J.M., Roche N.S., Wakefield L.M., et al. 1986. Transforming growth factor type β: rapid induction of fibrosis and angiogenesis in vivo and stimulation of collagen formation in vitro. *Proc. Natl. Acad. Sci. USA* **83:**4167–4717.

131. Saad B., Constam D.B., Ortmann R., Moos M., Fontana A., Achachner M. 1991. Astrocyte-derived TGF-β$_1$ and NGF differently regulate neural recognition molecule expression by cultured astrocytes. *J. Cell Biol.* **115:**471–484.

132. Saleh M., Stacker S.A., Wilks A.F. 1996. Inhibition of growth of C6 glioma cells in vivo by expression of antisense vascular endothelial growth factor sequence. *Cancer Res.* **393:**393–401.

133. Salomon Y., Zohar M., DeJordy J.O., Eshel Y., Shafir I., Lieba H., et al. 1993. Signaling mechanisms controlled by melanocortins in melanoma, lacrimal, and brain astroglia cells. *Ann. NY Acad. Sci.* **680:**364–380.

134. Schackert G., Fidler I.J. 1988. Development of in vivo models for studies of brain metastasis. *Int. J. Cancer* **41:**589–594.

135. Schackert G., Fidler I.J. 1988. Site-specific metastasis of mouse melanomas and a fibrosarcoma in the brain or the meninges of syngeneic animals. *Cancer Res.* **48:**3478–3484.

136. Schackert G. Price J.E., Zhang R.D., Bucana C.D., Itoh K., Fidler I.J. 1990. Regional growth of different human melanomas as metastases in the brain of nude mice. *Am. J. Pathol.* **136:**95–101.

137. Schackert G., Simmons R.D., Buzbee T.M., Hume D.A., Fidler I.J. 1988. Macrophage infiltration into experimental brain metastases: occurrence through an intact blood-brain barrier. *J. Natl. Cancer Inst.* **80:**1027–1034.

138. Scheinberg L.C., Edelman F.L., Levy W.A. 1964. Is the brain "an immunologically privileged site"? *Arch. Neurol.* **11:**248–264.

139. Schlingemann R.O. Rivetveld F.J., De Wall R.M., Ferrone S. 1990. Expression of the high molecular weight melanoma-associated antigen by pericytes during angiogenesis in tumor and in healing wounds. *Am. J. Pathol.* **136:**1393–1405.

140. Seechrun P., Thody A.J. 1990. The effect of UV-irradiation and MSH on tyrosinase activity in epidermal melanocyte of the mouse. *J. Dermatol. Sci.* **1:**283–288.

141. Senger D.R., Galli S.J., Devorak A.M., Perruzzi C.A., Harvey V.S., Devorak H.F. 1982. Tumor cells secrete a vascular permeability factor that promotes accumulation of ascites fluid. *Science (Washington, DC)* **219:**983–985.

142. Shapiro W.R. Hiesiger E.M., Cooney G.A., Gasler G.A., Lipschutz L.E., Posner J.B. 1990. Temporal effects of dexamethasone on blood-to-brain and blood-to-tumor transport of ^{14}C-alpha-aminoisobutyric acid in rat C6 glioma. *J. Neurooncol.* **8:**997–1041.

143. Shapiro W.R., Shapiro J.R. 1986. Principles of brain tumor chemotherapy. *Semin. Oncol.* **13:**56–69.

144. Siemeister G., Schirner M., Reusch P., Barleon B., Marme D., Martiny-Baron G. 1998. An antagonistic vascular endothelial growth factor (VEGF) variant inhibits VEGF-stimulated receptor autophosphorylation and proliferation of human endothelial cells. *Proc. Natl. Acad. Sci. USA* **95:**4625–4629.

145. Singh R.K., Gutman M., Radinsky R., Bucana C.D. Fidler I.J. 1994. Expression of interleukin-8 correlates with the metastatic potential of human melanoma cells in nude mice. *Cancer Res.***54:**3242–3247.

146. Steward P.A., Hayakawa K., Farrell C.L., Del Maestro R.F. 1987. Quantitative study of microvessel ultrastructure in human peritumoral brain tissue: evidence for a blood-brain barrier defect. *J. Neurosurg.* **67:**697–705.

147. Strawn L.M., McMahon G. App H., Schreck R., Kuchler W.R., Longhi M.P., et al. 1996. Flk-1 as a target for tumor growth inhibition. *Cancer Res.* **56:**3540–3545.

148. Strugar J., Rothbart D., Harrington W., Criscuolo G.R. 1994. Vascular permeability factor in brain metastases: correlation with vasogenic brain edema and tumor angiogenesis. *J. Neurosurg.* **81:**560–566.

149. Sugarbaker E.V. 1979. Cancer metastasis: a product of tumor-host interactions. *Curr. Prob. Cancer* **3:**1–59.

150. Takakura K., Sano K., Hojo S., Hirano A. 1982. Metastatic Tumors of the Central Nervous System. Tokyo, Japan: Igaku-Shoin, Ltd.

151. Tomlinson E. Theory and practice of site-specific drug delivery. *Adv. Drug Del. Rev.* **1:**187–198.

152. Tucker R.F., Shipley G.D., Moses H.L., Holley R.W. Growth inhibitor from BSC-1 cells closely related platelet type beta transforming growth factor. *Science* **226:**705–707.

153. Unemori E., Ferrara N., Bauer E.A., Amento E.P. Vascular endothelial growth factor induces interstitial collagenase expression in human endothelial cells. *J. Cell Physiol.* **153:**557–562.

154. Unsicker K., Flanders K.C., Cissel D.S., Lafyatis R., Sporn M.B. 1991. Transforming growth factor-beta isoforms in the adult rat central and peripheral nervous system. *Neuroscience* **44:**513–525.

155. Vriesendorp F.J., Peagram C., Bigner D.D., Groothuis D.R. 1987. Concurrent measurement of blood flow and transcapillary transport in xenotransplanted human gliomas in immunosuppressed rats. *J. Natl. Cancer Inst.* **79:**123–130.

156. Weber G.F., Ashkar S. 2000. Molecular mechanisms of tumor dissemination in primary and metastatic brain cancers. *Brain Res. Bull.* **53:**421–424.

157. Zagzag D., Goldenberg M., Brem S. 1989. Angiogenesis and blood-brain barrier breakdown modulate CT contrast enhancement: an experimental study in a rabbit brain-tumor model. *AJR* **153:**141–146.

158. Zhang R., Price J.E., Fujimaki T., Bucana C.D., Fidler I.J. 1992. Differential permeability of the blood-brain barrier in experimental brain metastases produced by human neoplasms implanted into nude mice. *Am. J. Pathol.* **141:**1115–1124.

6

Analysis of Neural Precursor Cells in the Context of Origin of Brain Tumors, Their Treatment, and Repair of Treatment-Associated Damage

Mark Noble and Joerg Dietrich

1. INTRODUCTION

The treatment of any disease always begins with a correct diagnosis. It is here, before any treatment has been initiated, that enormous problems are faced by those involved in investigating brain tumors. Despite longstanding attempts to generate unambiguous diagnostic criteria for tumors of the central nervous system (CNS), the extent of disagreement between neuropathologists diagnosing the same tumor is often considerable (17,47,53,91). The importance of this disagreement cannot be understated. If pathologists are going to place identical tumors in different categories, then further analyses of outcomes as they pertain to diagnosis are severely compromised.

Perhaps somewhat paradoxically, one of the best arguments supporting the need for improving upon current classification systems comes from the limited successes that have occurred with existing approaches. For example, one tumor group that often appears to be morphologically distinct is the oligodendroglioma. Using existing criteria, it has become clear that approx 70% of patients with oligodendrogliomas respond positively to chemotherapy. By contrast, as few as 5% of individuals with astrocytomas of a comparable degree of malignancy receive similar benefit from such treatment (26,57,110). More specifically, individuals who present with malignant oligodendroglioma and loss of heterozygosity (LOH) on chromosome 1 and 19 exhibit longer recurrence-free survival after chemotherapy than patients with other genetic changes (18). These data provide a clear example of the importance of classification; by focusing attention on individuals with oligodendrogliomas, it is clear that chemotherapy does indeed work for some types of brain tumors.

The recognition that a high proportion of patients with oligodendrogliomas are responsive to chemotherapy raises the question of whether there are other patient groups for whom chemotherapy might be exceptionally useful, if we only had a means of prospectively recognizing such individuals. Thus, what is of crucial concern is whether the small subsets of treatment-responsive patients currently diagnosed with astrocytomas or glioblastomas might themselves be members of specific biological classes that perhaps reflect the origin of the tumor. How might these individuals be recognized? How canthe existing classification systems be improved so that patients with the same tumor type are recognized?

From: *Contemporary Cancer Research: Brain Tumors*
Edited by: F. Ali-Osman © Humana Press Inc., Totowa, NJ

2. MULTIPLE CELL TYPES OF THE DEVELOPING AND MATURE CENTRAL NERVOUS SYSTEM

One approach to glioma diagnosis that has potential merit is to apply information that has been obtained through the study of the normal cellular populations that contribute to the development and function of the CNS. Indeed, the hope that such an approach is a useful one is strongly rooted even in the names used to describe different types of neural tumors, in which there is a longstanding tradition of attempting to correlate tumor cytology with the characteristics of particular neural cell types. Moreover, the proposal that a lineage-based approach to tumor diagnosis would be of value would be consistent with experiences in the treatment of tumors of the hematopoietic system, for which the normal cellular lineage to which a tumor is related seems to be closely correlated with the likelihood of that tumor responding to particular kinds of treatment *(3,63,92)*.

If one believes that there is value in categorizing brain tumors in respect to their relationship with normal neural lineages and cell types, then it is critical to have a firm understanding of the complexity of the CNS itself. This is a rapidly evolving area of research that has advanced far beyond the classifications found in the field of neuropathology.

At present, the following precursor cell populations have been identified in the developing and/or mature CNS:

Multipotent neuroepithelial stem cells (NSCs) generate the neural cell types of the CNS *(60,104,117)*. There are at least two different groups of NSCs, one of which can be grown in monolayer cultures and requires basic fibroblast growth factor (FGF-2) as a mitogen. The second NSC population is generally grown in neurosphere cultures, and requires epidermal growth factor (EGF) as a mitogen *(86–88,111)*. Both of these populations express the same differentiation potential. It also has been suggested that a population of glial fibrillary acidic protein (GFAP, an intermediate filament protein found in abundance in astrocytes) expressing cells that resides in the subventricular zone may also have the ability to generate all of the different cell types of the CNS *(25)*.

NSCs appear to give rise to differentiated progeny through the intermediate generation of lineage-restricted precursor cells able to generate neurons or glia, but not both *(58,84,85)*. Neuron-restricted precursor (NRP) cells can generate a range of different neuronal phenotypes, including motor neurons and dopaminergic neurons, but do not generate glial cells *(43,58)*. Glial-restricted precursor (GRP) cells, in contrast, can give rise to at least three of the major known CNS glial cell types (i.e., oligodendrocytes, type-1 astrocytes, type-2 astrocytes) *(75,85)*. Both GRP cells and NRP cells can be generated from NSCs in vitro, and also can be directly isolated from the CNS of developing rats.

GRP cells appear to give rise to oligodendrocytes, the myelin-forming cells of the CNS, through the intermediate generation of bipotential cells limited to the generation, at least in vitro, of oligodendrocytes and type-2 astrocytes *(36,73,75)*. These intermediate cells are known as oligodendrocyte-type-2 astrocyte (O2A) progenitor cells, also named oligodendrocyte precursor cells (OPCs) *(83)*. GRP cells and O2A/OPCs differ in multiple properties, including response to a multitude of mitogens, survival factors and differentiation-inducing factors *(36,75)*. Moreover, GRP cells readily generate astrocytes when transplanted in vivo *(39)*, a cell type not generated from primary O2A/OPCs following transplantation *(29)*.

Other neural precursor cells that have been reported are the A2B5[+] astrocyte precursor cells present in embryonic (E17) spinal cord described by Miller and colleagues *(31,32)*, the putative astrocyte precursor cells from the embryonic mouse cerebellum described by Seidman et al. *(96)*, the astrocyte precursor cells described by Mi and Barres *(61)*, and the pre-O2A progenitor cell described by Grinspan and colleagues *(38)*.

Finally, in this particular context, it is critical to note that the adult CNS also contains NSCs, and at least some glial precursor cells (as discussed later). However, we are still far from understanding the richness of the precursor cells of the adult CNS.

3. COMPLEXITY WITHIN SINGLE LINEAGES

As if the above collection of precursor cells were not already complex enough, it also is becoming clear that even within individual precursor cell populations great complexity can exist. This has been studied in some detail in the O2A/OPC lineage, for which recent studies indicate the existence of marked differences in self-renewal and differentiation characteristics of O2A/OPCs isolated from cortex, optic nerve, and optic chiasm *(80)*. For example, in conditions in which optic nerve-derived O2A/OPCs generate oligodendrocytes within 2 d, oligodendrocytes arise from chiasm-derived cells after 5 d and from cortical O2A/OPCs after only 7–10 d. Such differences, which appear to be cell-intrinsic (and may be related to intracellular redox state), are manifested both in reduced percentages of clones producing oligodendrocytes and in a lesser representation of oligodendrocytes in individual clones. In addition, responsiveness of optic nerve-, chiasm- and cortex-derived O2A/OPCs to thyroid hormone (TH) and ciliary neurotrophic factor (CNTF), well-characterized inducers of oligodendrocyte generation, was inversely related to the extent of self-renewal observed in basal division conditions. Thus, these different populations have intrinsically different probabilities of undergoing extensive division. Whether they also differ in their migratory or survival characteristics remains to be determined.

Another example of heterogeneity in the O2A/OPC lineage is seen with cells isolated from adult animals. The O2A/OPCs of the perinatal optic nerve generate a second precursor cell population that is specific to adult tissue. This bipotential glial precursor cell, the O2A/OPC$^{(adult)}$, exhibits a much slower cell-cycle time and also a much slower migration rate than its perinatal counterpart *(120,122)*. Whereas the O2A/OPCs$^{(adult)}$ can transiently express a rapidly dividing phenotype *(121)*, it currently appears that this cell is intrinsically unable to rapidly generate the large numbers of oligodendrocytes that can be generated from its perinatal counterpart.

It is unlikely that phenotypic heterogeneity will be a unique feature of O2A/OPCs. Indeed, we already have seen evidence of GRP cell heterogeneity in the embryonic rat spinal cord, with cells from the ventral and dorsal half of the cord showing differences in response to inducers of differentiation *(36)*. As most of the discoveries thus far made through the studies of O2A/OPCs have turned out to be indicative of general biological principles, it seems likely that a good deal of biological heterogeneity remains to be discovered in precursor cell populations of the CNS.

We have proposed that the heterogeneity that exists within the O2A/OPC lineage reflects the physiological requirements of the tissue from which each population is isolated. For example, myelination has long been known to progress in a caudal-rostral direction, beginning in the spinal cord significantly earlier than in the brain *(33,46,55)*. Even within a single CNS region, myelination is not synchronous. In the rat optic nerve, for example, myelinogenesis occurs along a retinal-to-chiasmal gradient, with regions of the nerve nearest the retina becoming myelinated first *(33,100)*. The cortex itself shows the widest range of timing for myelination, both initiating later than many other CNS regions *(33,46,55)* and exhibiting an ongoing myelinogenesis that can extend over long periods of time. This latter characteristic is seen perhaps most dramatically in the human brain, for which it has been suggested that myelination may not be complete until after several decades of life *(11,124)*.

The characteristics of the various O2A/OPC populations we have isolated from the developing CNS are consistent with the hypothesis that differences in the timing of myelinogenesis may be a result of, at least in part, local utilization of oligodendrocyte precursor cell populations with fundamentally different properties. In the optic nerve, where myelination starts early and is completed relatively rapidly, the O2A/OPCs isolated from young postnatal rats undergo limited self-renewal before generating oligodendrocytes. In contrast, O2A/OPCs isolated from the cortex—where the process of myelination starts later and occurs over a longer period of time—tend to undergo much more self-renewal and to generate oligodendrocytes over a much more prolonged time course.

The properties of O2A/OPCs^{adult} are also consistent with being associated with the physiological requirements of adult tissue. These slowly dividing cellsthat have a tendency to undergo asymmetric self-renewing divisions even under conditions in which their perinatal counterparts all differentiate *(123)*, seem much more appropriate in their phenotype to adult tissues.

The above studies on CNS development suggest that even if oligodendrogliomas are related to the oligodendrocyte lineage, there is still a wide range of cell types from which these tumors could originate. There is no similar body of knowledge on the complexity of astrocyte lineages, but it seems likely that this will be at least as complex as that of oligodendrocyte lineages. Thus, it is ever more apparent that the developmental complexity of the normal cells that are the likely cells of origin of tumors far exceeds the current complexity of tumor classification systems, whether cytologically or molecularly based. It is also of potential interest that the genetic characteristics of oligodendrogliomas and oligoastrocytomas may differ depending on site of tumor location *(65,126)*. Could these differences be reflective of the different properties of glial precursor cells isolated from different regions of the CNS *(80)*?

If the biological properties of the cell of origin of a tumor are important in the behavior of the tumor itself, then it will be of considerable importance to develop better means of relating the tumors of the CNS to the normal cells that contribute to the development and function of this complex tissue. Is it possible, for example, that apparently similar tumors of childhood and adulthood express different properties because they are derived from cells with fundamentally different biological properties? Is it further possible that part of the differing behavior of tumors that appear to be of a single-cellular lineage actually represent origination from a biologically diverse population of potential founder cells?

4. EXPERIMENTAL MODELING OF GLIOMAS SUGGESTS ADDITIONAL LEVELS OF COMPLEXITY

An increasingly used approach to analyzing the underlying principles of tumor development, and the relationship between tumor origin and tumor cytology, is to express defined oncogenes in specific cell types. Three approaches have been used to examine the effects of inducing neoplastic changes in targeted populations. One approach uses specific promoter elements to express in particular populations either oncogenes or receptors for viruses that can be used to introduce oncogenes into cells. A second uses transgenic animals expressing particular oncogenes, or with compromised expression of tumor suppressor genes, as a source of purified cells that can be studied for their properties. A third approach begins with cell purification, followed by genetic modification of cells in vitro to express particular oncogenes. These approaches can also be combined with each other. This important area of research can only be touched upon briefly in this chapter, and the reader is referred to a variety of publications (*see* refs. *7,8,22–24,40,50,75,107,118*).

One of the striking outcomes of studies in which tumors are generated using the above described targeting mechanisms, is the diversity of approaches that result in the formation of high-grade (i.e., malignant) gliomas. For example, such tumors result from expression of constitutively active mutant ras in astrocytes *(23)*, in astrocytes and neural progenitors cells that have lost expression of Ink4a-Arf *(107)* owing to expression of constitutively active epidermal growth factor receptors (EGFR) in neural precursor cells or astrocytes lacking the p16(INK4a) and p19(ARF) tumor suppressor genes *(7)*, and from O-2A/OPCs engineered to express mutated ras and myc genes *(8)*. Such results are consistent with the hypothesis that there are multiple pathways that can lead to the generation of high-grade gliomas.

Some results obtained by using the approaches described above suggest, quite surprisingly, that particular tumor phenotypes may be associated more with the oncogenes that are expressed than with the putative cell type of tumor origin. For example, overexpression of the EGFR under the control of the putatively astrocyte specific promoter for the S100β protein is associated with the generation of tumors that resemble low-grade oligodendrogliomas *(118)*. Similarly, mating of animals that express a truncated EGFR (an oncogenic mutation found in many gliomas) *(66)* under control of the putatively astrocyte-specific promoter for GFAP with animals that express a constitutively active v(12)Ha-ras oncogene under control of the same promoter leads to tumors that histologically appear to be oligodendrogliomas and mixed oligoastrocytomas *(24)*. In contrast, animals expressing only the GFAP-v(12)Ha-ras construct developed astrocytomas of varying grades of malignancy *(23,24)*.

Still, other studies in which the receptor for avian leukosis virus (ALV) is expressed in transgenic mice under control of the GFAP promoter (thus allowing specific introduction of oncogenes into expressing cells by infection with ALV) have yielded related conclusions *(22)*. In these studies, an ALV encoding platelet-derived growth factor (PDGF) was used to infect cells in vitro. Resultant cells expressed a glial progenitor-like phenotype, but were able to generate cells that looked like astrocytes when PDGF-mediated signaling was pharmacologically inhibited. Moreover, intracranial infection with PDGF-encoding ALV of mice in which ALV receptor expression was controlled by the nestin or the GFAP promoter, was associated with the generation of tumors with cytological features of oligodendrogliomas or, in the latter case, oligoastrocytomas.

One suggested explanation for the generation of oligodendrogliomas by expressing oncogenes in astrocytes, is that it is the oncogenes that dictate tumor type. Another possibility, however, is that the GFAP promoter is expressed in precursor cells as well as in astrocytes (an outcome consistent with observations on stem cells of the adult subventricular zone *(4)*, and with our own ongoing analyses of gene expression in glial development; M. Noble and C. Pröschel, work in progress); thus, the results obtained may reflect targeting of both precursor cells and astrocytes with this promoter. Similarly, the association of PDGF overexpression with the development of oligodendrogliomas may reflect the known importance of this mitogen for O-2A/OPCs *(74)*. If these interpretations are correct, then the surprising generation of oligodendrogliomas in the above studies would be consistent with the hypothesis that oligodendrogliomas are tumors of glial precursor cells—although with possible origins in a variety of different glial precursor cells. The validity of such a hypothesis—and the extent the ability of different origins to lead to high-grade gliomas is mirrored by analogous outcomes for oligodendrogliomas— remains to be determined, but it is clear that these important in vivo studies are further enriching our appreciation of the complexity of tumor development.

5. TUMOR CELL HETEROGENEITY

To make matters still more complex, it is clear that tumors can not be treated as a homogeneous mass of identical cells *(72)*. Remarkable heterogeneity can be found within a tumor of a single patient. Indeed, extensive karyotypic heterogeneity within one tumor may exist even in low-grade gliomas *(21)*. For example, analysis of 38 distinct regions of a low-grade oligoastrocytoma with relatively homogeneous histology revealed an enormous diversity of cellular populations, ranging from diploid to tetraploid in karyotype. Multiple spatially discrete tumor areas were often, but not invariably, associated with particular karyotypes. It was also possible to identify tumor regions that appeared to be genetically unstable as indicated by an abundance of nonclonal karyotypes. Malignant gliomas also show considerable heterogeneity, indicating that progression is not associated with the emergence of a single dominant cellular phenotype or genotype *(97,98)*. More recent studies have confirmed and extended earlier findings of intratumor genetic heterogeneity *(52,62,99)*.

Tumor cells from the same patient may also exhibit substantial functional heterogeneity in growth potential. For example, it was suggested almost 20 yr ago that brain tumors contain distinct "stem cell" populations *(97)*. Hyperdiploid variants of tumor cells isolated from malignant gliomas exhibited a greater sensitivity to chemotherapeutic agents such as carmustine than did near-diploid cells isolated from the same tumor. The explicit suggestion was made that these near-diploid cells are the stem cells that repopulate the tumor mass. More recent studies have confirmed that it is indeed possible to isolate, from both brain tumors and breast cancers, cells with stem cell-like characteristics *(2,42)*. In the case of breast cancer, it appears that these cells are a minority tumor subpopulation in which resides the ability to form new tumors in immunocompromised mice *(2)*.

In addition to the above contributions to heterogeneity, cells from gliomas can undergo a poorly understood redifferentiation—apparently both in vitro and in vivo—to yield mesenchymal-like cells *(13,45,119)*. These mesenchymal derivatives of gliomas have been studied very little, but it is clear that they are transformed cells that can form tumors when transplanted into host animals. It is also clear that the mesenchymal derivatives of glial-like glioma cells share the molecular abnormalities of their parental tumor cells. At this stage, nothing is known about the extent to which such diversity contributes to the challenges of treating gliomas.

6. CELLULAR FUSION AND TUMOR HETEROGENEITY

Another possible contributor to tumor heterogeneity is the fusion of different cell types. For example, analysis of the mechanism by which hematopoietic stem cells (HSCs) repair the damaged liver in mice with a liver-specific metabolic disorder (which originally was thought to be from the generation of liver cells by HSCs) has shown that repair results from fusion of HSC-derived progeny with liver cells *(105,115,125)*. Subsequently, the resultant hybrid cells adopt a phenotype different from their "parental" cells by expressing genes of the HSC derivatives as well as of the liver cells themselves. Similarly, early studies interpreted in favor of blood cell generation of brain may also be the result of cell fusion *(116)*.

Cell fusion has long been suggested to play a role in tumor evolution and progression to a more malignant phenotype *(27,49,81)*. It now seems important to consider the possibility that if HSC-derived progeny can fuse with normal cells, and tumor cells themselves seem to have a higher probability of undergoing fusion events than normal cells, that fusion of nontumor cells with tumor cells may represent still another contributor to tumor heterogeneity.

7. BRAIN TUMOR CLASSIFICATION AND THE FUTURE

The disparity between neuropathological classification and our understanding of development and differentiation in the CNS creates a significant opportunity for productive interactions between developmental neurobiologists and the oncology and neuropathology communities. The question of whether accurate biological lineage assignment is correlated with treatment outcome—as appears to be the case for other tumors—cannot be answered without the tools to make such assignments. Moreover, without unambiguous diagnosis of different classes of brain tumors, it is inherently more difficult to identify therapies that might only be effective on tumor groups that so far are not recognized as being biologically distinct. Thus, there is a strong rationale for developmental neurobiologists to be working together with clinicians to develop diagnostic systems that reflect the potential complexity of this diverse group of tumors.

One approach to the creation of improved means of tumor diagnosis is to analyze patterns of gene expression in these tumors. Such an approach has the advantage that one can examine expression of thousands of genes at one time. Microarray analysis of some tumors suggests that, in at least some cases, patterns of gene expression are associated with responsiveness to different therapeutic approaches and thus may be of prognostic utility *(79,108)*.

However, microarray analysis is not without its limitations. For example, microarray analysis provides no information on levels of protein expression (which may show little correlation with levels of gene expression), on the activation state of individual proteins, or on the metabolic state of the tumor. In addition, it is not clear to what extent patterns of gene and protein expression seen within a tumor mass are indicative of the biology of those tumor cells that have migrated away from their primary site of origin. If these migratory cells of a malignant glioma represent the critical source of recurrence following surgical removal *(12)*, it may be that their biology is the most critical of all to understand.

It also is important to point out the implications of intratumor heterogeneity for attempts to develop molecular classifications of tumors. Within the gliomas, one wonders about the extent to which such information will be representative of the tumor as contrasted with an average over multiple populations within the tumor. To this end, it will be of importance to conduct such microarray analyses on multiple biopsies taken from different regions of the tumor, so as to begin to understand the extent of diversity of gene expression that might exist within a single tumor mass.

One of the major disadvantages to microarray analysis is that it is difficult to see how this approach will become as readily integrated into the majority of neuropathology practices as, for example, immunohistochemical analysis of antigen expression in tumor bioposies. Thus, once genes of potential diagnostic value are identified it will be critical to move as quickly as possible to generation of antibodies and complementary deoxyribonucleic acid (cDNA) probes that can be used to analyze biopsy specimens.

One of the most important sources of diagnostic antibodies may come from attempts to identify markers useful in distinguishing among the multiple neural precursor cells discussed earlier. This is in fact a commonly accepted practice, and one that likely deserves continued attention. For example, current attempts to develop more robust diagnostics for oligodendrogliomas freely rely on the hypothesis that these tumors are related in some manner to oligodendrocytes or the precursor cells for oligodendrocytes. Thus, antibodies against the alpha isoform of the receptor for PDGF and the NG2 proteoglycan—both of which have been suggested to label oligodendrocyte precursor cells—have been proposed as useful markers of oligodendrogliomas *(69)*. Similarly, expression of the olig2 transcription factor—which also has been proposed as a marker of cells of the oligodendrocyte lineage—has been mooted as a useful marker for oligodendrogliomas *(54,56)*. However, such expression may also be seen in astroctyomas and glioblastomas *(14,54)*.

8. COGNITIVE IMPAIRMENT AND THE VULNERABILITY OF CENTRAL NERVOUS SYSTEM PRECURSOR CELLS AND OLIGODENDROCYTES TO RADIATION AND CHEMOTHERAPY

A different manner in which the precursor cells of the CNS are important in cancer research comes from the analysis of the potential role of damage to these populations by standard treatment regimens. It is becoming increasingly apparent that traditional approaches to cancer therapy are often associated with adverse neurological events. These neurological sequelae are seen in treatment regimes ranging from chemotherapy of primary breast carcinoma to radiation therapy of brain tumors. Even based on the figures available from recent publications (which represent only a beginning appreciation of this general problem), it seems likely that there are significant numbers of individuals for whom such neurotoxicity is a serious concern.

Even though there are still many cancer treatments for which cognitive changes and other neurological sequelae have not been noted in the literature, it nonetheless appears that these adverse effects may be frequent. In 1997, the Cancer Statistics Branch of NCI estimated the prevalence of cancer in the United States at nearly nine million. If cognitive impairment associated with treatment were to only effect 2.5% of this population, the total number of patients for whom this issue would be a concern is of similar size to the population of individuals with chronic spinal cord injury. As discussed in more detail later, recent studies raise the spectre that such complications may occur in significantly more than 2.5% of individuals treated for cancer. Lowered IQ scores and other evidence of cognitive impairment are relatively frequent in children treated for brain tumors or leukemias, thus presenting survivors and their families with considerable challenges in respect to the ability of these children to achieve normal lives. Data for patients treated for non-CNS tumors are only beginning to emerge, and give grounds for further concern. For example, some studies suggest that as many as 30% of women treated with standard chemotherapy regimes for primary breast carcinoma show significant cognitive impairment 6 mo after treatment *(94,109)*. As some of the compounds used in the treatment for breast cancer (cyclophosphamide, methotrexate, and 5-fluorouracil) are used fairly widely in different other cancer types, it would not be surprising to find problems emerging in other patient populations as more testing is conducted. Thus, current trends support the view that the numbers of individuals for whom cognitive impairment associated with cancer treatment is a problem may be as great as for many of the more widely recognized neurological syndromes.

Neurological complications have been most extensively studied in respect to radiation therapy to the brain, and these studies indicate the presence of a wide range of potential adverse effects. Radiation-induced neurological complications include radionecrosis, myelopathy, cranial nerve damage, leukoencephalopathy, and dopa-resistant Parkinson syndromes *(44)*. Imaging studies have documented extensive white matter damage in patients receiving radiation to the CNS *(112)*. Cognitive impairment associated with radiotherapy has also been reported in many of these patients. For example, in examination of 31 children aged 5–15 yr, who had received radiotherapy for posterior fossa tumorsand been off therapy for at least 1 yr, long-term cognitive impairment occurred in most cases *(37)*. Neurotoxicity also affects older patients, presenting as cognitive dysfunction, ataxia, or dementia as a consequence of leukoencephalopathy and brain atrophy *(95)*. In adults, subcortical dementia occurs 3–12 mo after cerebral radiotherapy *(112)*.

Although chemotherapy has been less well studied than radiation in terms of its adverse effects on the CNS, it is becoming increasingly clear that many chemotherapeutic regimens are associated with neurotoxicity. Multiple reports have confirmed cognitive impairment in children and adults after cancer treatment. In particular, improvements in survival for children with leukemias or brain tumors treated with radiotherapy and chemotherapy have led to increasing concerns on qualityoflife issues for long-term survivors, in which neuropsychological testing has revealed a high frequency of cognitive deficits *(5,34,37,89,113)*. Cetingul et al. *(19)* recently reported performance and total IQ scores were significantly reduced in children treated for acute lymphoblastic leukemia who had completed therapy at least 1 yr before and survived more than 5 yr after diagnosis. Indeed, it is felt that neurotoxicity of chemotherapy is frequent, and may be particularly hazardous when combined with radiotherapy *(19,95)*. For example, in computed tomography (CT) studies of patients receiving both brain radiation and chemotherapy, all patients surviving a malignant glioma for more than 4 yr developed leukencephalopathy and brain atrophy *(102)*.

Cognitive impairment is not only a problem for children with leukemia and for adult brain tumor patients *(6,35,93)*, but may also represent a significant problem for adults treated for non-CNS cancers. For example, recent studies indicate that there is a substantial risk for breast cancer patients who received adjuvant chemotherapy to develop cognitive impairment *(15,94)*, especially in case of high-dose chemotherapy *(109)*.

In general, an increasing number of reports underline the importance of rigorous neuropsychological and neurocognitive assessment of cancer patients during follow-up *(20,89,106,113)*. It also seems likely that the current evaluations of the extent of cognitive impairment associated with cancer therapy represent an underestimate of the extent of neurological damage that actually is occurring in these patients. It is difficult to find studies in which patients are cognitively evaluated before and after tumor treatment. Thus, those patients whose cognitive abilities are above average at the beginning of treatment may find that a 10% decrement in function is not associated with their being judged as cognitively impaired by standard diagnostic techniques—despite any differences in ability these individuals (or those close to them) may notice. Moreover, there is no consensus that exists as to what tests are most appropriate in studying cognitive impairment that may be associated with cancer therapy. If it emerges that the actual functions that are impaired are not adequately measured by the tests employed, this would add another source of underestimation of the extent to which cognitive damage is associated with the application of radiation or chemotherapy to the brain.

9. RADIATION AND THE CENTRAL NERVOUS SYSTEM: A WIDE VARIETY OF ADVERSE EFFECTS

It is clear that we are still far from being able to abandon radiation and chemotherapy as major means of treating cancer, thus raising the challenge of how to mitigate the adverse consequences of these treatments. It is broadly appreciated that prolongation of life must be also connected to the quality of that life, thus such conditions play an increasingly important role in evaluation of medical interventions. Only by understanding the underlying biology of adverse neurological consequences of chemotherapy and radiotherapy will we be able to develop means of protecting against this damage without sacrificing the value of these treatments in prolonging lifespan in many individuals.

Potential clues to the biological basis for cognitive impairment have come from studies on the effects of radiation on the brain, for which dose-limiting neurotoxicity has long been recognized *(82, 90)*. On a cellular basis, radiation appears to cause damage to both dividing and nondividing CNS cells. Recent studies have shown that irradiation causes apoptosis in precursor cells of the dentate gyrus subgranular zone of the hippocampus *(78,103)* and in the subependymal zone *(9)*, both of which are sites of continuing precursor cell proliferation in the adult CNS. Such damage is also associated with long-term impairment of subependymal repopulation. In addition, it seems clear that nondividing cells, such as oligodendrocytes, are killed by irradiation *(51)*. Damage to oligodendrocytes is consistent with clinical evidence, where radiation-induced neurotoxicity has been associated with diffuse myelin and axonal loss in the white matter, with tissue necrosis and diffuse spongiosis of the white matter characterized by the presence of vacuoles that displaced the normally-stained myelin sheets and axons *(112)*.

There is considerable discussion as to whether the damage caused by radiation represents a direct or indirect effect of radiation on the brain. Although some damage in vivo may well be secondary consequences of vascular damage, evidence also has been provided that radiation is directly damaging to important CNS populations, such as oligodendrocyte precursor cells *(41)*.

10. CHEMOTHERAPY AND THE CENTRAL NERVOUS SYSTEM: A FIELD IN NEED OF DEVELOPMENT

Despite the clear evidence for neurotoxicity of at least some forms of chemotherapy, studies on the effects of chemotherapeutic compounds on cells of the brain are surprisingly rare. It has been found, in vivo, that a single-dose application of methotrexate into the ventricles is associated with ventricular dilatation, oedema, and visible destruction of the ependymal cell layer lining the ventricles and the surrounding brain tissue *(64)*. Numerous glial cells with pyknotic nuclei were observed in the gray and white matter, with increased numbers of microglial cells. There was also a rapid reduction in the number of nuclei per unit area in the rostral extension of the subependymal plate, with a 30% reduction seen 1–2 d after methotrexate administration. A similar reduction in mitotic figures was seen. This morphological study did not provide detailed information on effects on individual cell types.

Our own studies on chemotherapy-associated damage to the CNS were initiated to determine whether there might exist a lineage-related basis for the differential response of oligodendrogliomas and astrocytomas to treatment revealed vulnerability of normal CNS cells to chemotherapy. In these studies *(76)* we found that carmustine (BCNU; an alkylating agent widely used in the treatment of brain tumors, myeloma, and both Hodgkin's and non-Hodgkin's lymphoma) was toxic for oligodendrocytes at doses that would be routinely achieved during treatment. In contrast, astrocytes were relatively resistant to this drug, and O2As/OPCs showed intermediate levels of sensitivity.

The sensitivity of oligodendrocytes to BCNU raises the disturbing issue of whether the normal cells of the brain are damaged by exposure to chemotherapeutic agents. This work is currently in progress, but early results have raised the possibility that multiple neural precursor cells (including, so far, glia-restricted precursor cells, neuron-restricted precursor cells, and O2A progenitor cells), as well as oligodendrocytes, are at least as sensitive to death induced by chemotherapeutic agents as are cancer cells themselves (J. Dietrich and M. Noble, unpublished observations).

Our observations on the vulnerability of oligodendrocytes to chemotherapeutic agents seem to be consistent with clinical reports. For example, two longitudinal studies using magnetic resonance imaging (MRI) and proton spectroscopy have shown that white matter changes in the CNS induced by high-dose chemotherapy with BCNU, cisplatin, and cyclophosphamide for breast cancer could occur in up to 70% of individuals, usually with a delayed onset of several months after treatment *(16,101)*. As mentioned earlier, white matter damage is even more likely to occur when both brain radiation and chemotherapy are applied, as has been reported in CT studies demonstrating that all individuals who survive a malignant glioma for more than 4 yr developed diffuse damage to the white matter (i.e., leukoencephalopathy) and brain atrophy *(102)*. To add still another level of complexity to attempts to better understand CNS damage associated with cancer treatment, older adults are less able to tolerate the adverse effects of chemotherapy than younger adults, which reveals a second period of particular vulnerability. The physiological basis for the increased vulnerability of older adults is not known, but it will be particularly important to determine whether identical treatment protocols cause different levels of CNS damage in young vs older adults.

11. SELECTIVE KILLING OF TUMOR CELLS VS REPAIR OF COLLATERAL DAMAGE TO NORMAL TISSUE

The observation that normal cells of the brain can be damaged by radiation and chemotherapeutic agents makes it of paramount importance to discover means of selectively killing cancer cells or of repairing the damage, or both, caused to the normal brain by cancer treatment. Tumor cells do sometimes differ from normal cells in ways that might be exploited for therapeutic benefit. For example, many gliomas express a truncated form of the EGFR that is constitutively active in the absence of ligand binding *(30,67)*. Exposure to pharmacological agents that selectively inhibit this mutant receptor appear to enhance the sensitivity of glioma cell lines to cisplatin, and might therefore be useful when applied in combination with conventional chemotherapy *(68)*. Whether the combined application of such sensitizing agents with traditional therapies will sufficiently enhance killing so as to allow use of doses of chemotherapeutic agents or radiation that do not cause damage to the brain is wholly unknown.

If dose-limiting neurotoxicity of multiple chemotherapeutic agents and of radiation is as problematic as we currently believe, then it is important to ask how the damage induced by these compounds can be repaired. Cell transplantation techniques offer one possibility. However, owing to the diffuse nature of the damage that is likely to be associated with chemotherapy, repair of such damage represents a potentially different category of problem than the repair of focal injury or degeneration. It is also unclear whether repair of the CNS without repair of vasculature damaged by radiation will be of long-term value. Nonetheless, it seems crucial to define more clearly the cellular compartments damaged by radiation or chemotherapy, or both, as a prelude to the analysis of cell protection and/or cell replacement strategies in affected brains. It is important to re-emphasize, in this regard, that concern with this problem is not unique to the issue of brain tumors, but could represent a problem relevant to treatment of multiple types of cancers.

In addition to potential utility in repair, transplantation of neural stem cells might itself offer therapeutic opportunities related to the outright killing of tumor cells, as indicated by two recent innovative studies. Benedetti and colleagues *(10)* have reported that neural stem cells genetically modified to produce interleukin-4 (to promote immune attack against the tumor cells) can promote tumor regression and prolong survival in mice injected intracranially with the GL261 mouse glioma cell line. Aboody et al. *(1)* have explored independently and in a different manner the potential utility of neural stem cells as therapeutic delivery systems. Neural stem cells were engineered to produce cytosine deaminase (which converts 5-fluorocytosine to the oncolytic drug 5-flourouracil), and transplantation of these genetically modified stem cells into the CNS of mice harboring a glioma cell line was able to cause objective reduction in tumor mass in vivo when animals were treated with 5-fluorocytosine.

One of the particularly encouraging results to emerge from the studies of Aboody et al. *(1)*, was that the extensive migratory capacity of neural stem cells enables transplanted cells to home to the primary tumor mass when injected at a distance from the tumor. Moreover, neural stem cells were seen to migrate away from the site of injection to become juxtaposed with tumor cells that had themselves migrated out into the CNS parenchyma. The reason this result is exceptionally exciting is that one of the most difficult treatment problems associated with gliomas arises from the fact that these tumor cells migrate great distances in the normal brain. These distant cells cannot be removed surgically, and unacceptable levels of CNS damage are associated with radiation applied over a large enough volume to kill these cells.

There are still many questions that must be answered before it is clear whether neural stem cells can be of use in the treatment of brain tumors. Among the questions that need to be assessed in preclinical studies, some of the most important are those related to determining in more detail whether stem cells can really preferentially migrate toward tumor cells present in small numbers, and perhaps even distributed as individual cells. The information provided by Aboody et al. *(1)* is insufficient to distinguish unambiguously between the hypothesis that stem cells are able to "track down" individual tumor cells and the possibility that the instances in which these cells are co-localized instead represent utilization of identical migratory substrates by tumor cells and stem cells. Both of these influences may be relevant, as stem cells might be expected to migrate toward a source of growth factor production (as occurs in a tumor mass), but it also is possible that tumor cells migrate along identical substrate pathways to those used by normal migratory CNS cells.

If migration along identical substrate pathways is the predominant reason that transplanted stem cells and tumor cells are juxtaposed, this would introduce a strong element of chance in the occurrence of this event. If so, the great majority of disseminated tumor cells might be expected to escape killing. As tumor cells that have migrated away from the central tumor mass play a major role in brain tumor recurrences, it is essential to determine with greater accuracy the extent to which neural stem cells might be guided to small numbers of tumor cells. Precise quantitative experiments in which small tumors are established and then labeled neural stem cells are transplanted into and/or around the tumor bed, followed by determination of the frequency with which migratory tumor cells and migratory neural stem cells are in contact with each other are required to address these questions.

Closely correlated with the question of whether transplanted stem cells can successfully home to the location of dispersed tumor cells, are the issues of division and differentiation of the stem cells and the number of tumor cells that can be killed by a single stem cell. These are finely graded balances that are closely interrelated. If the stem cells continue to divide after transplantation, then it is possible that they will themselves create an inappropriate cell mass. If, in contrast, they do not divide (as appears to be the case in the present studies), then as tumor cells continue their own division they eventually will become too numerous for the therapeutically modified stem cells to kill directly. Thus, if the mode of tumor cell killing requires close proximity to the transplanted stem cells, as might be expected in the studies of Aboody et al. *(1)*, then action of the stem cells would be expected to only be temporarily effective. Moreover, if the transplanted stem cells differentiate into neurons or oligodendrocytes, then their migratory capacity will be compromised. It is possible, for these reasons, that killing of tumor cells and repair of CNS damage might require transplantation of two different stem cell populations, only one of which has been modified to kill the tumor cells. Still further considerations of importance are whether the therapeutic agent produced by the transplanted stem cells causes injury to normal brain cells, how to engineer the stem cells to cease producing the therapeutic agent when it is no longer necessary to do so, and whether the use of nonautologous stem cells eventually will trigger an immune reaction against the cells they produce, as discussed previously *(70,71)*.

For the patient with a malignant glioma, concern over a number of the above questions is an unrealistic luxury. In these very needy patients, it is likely that trials will go ahead before all relevant information is obtained in experimental animals, and it is critical that such clinical trials are designed so that knowledge is gained even in failure. Thus, if one does not see prolonged regression of tumor mass or enhancement of neurological function in clinical trials, how will it be possible to determine the reasons for this apparent failure? How can one identify variables that might be manipulated to obtain more successful outcomes? Such questions can only be answered by transplanting cells that are permanently labeled, and making certain that a thorough analysis will be conducted on the brains of patients who die at various time points after receiving stem cell transplants. Such a label could be intrinsic to the cell, as would be the case if neural stem cells from a male were transplanted into the CNS of a female patient (thus, enabling recognition of transplanted cells with Y chromosome-specific probes), or could be expressed because of genetic modification of the transplanted cells. It also will be important to determine whether the transplanted stem cells continue to partake in DNA synthesis.

BrdU (5-bromodeoxyuridine) administration to glioma patients has been used to label tumor cells before biopsy or surgery and also has been used as a radiosensitizing agent (as described, for example, in refs. *48,59,77,114*). BrdU is also incorporated by normal human brainstem cells or precursor cells that are engaged in DNA synthesis in situ in the CNS of patients with brain tumors *(28)*. Thus, it is well established that BrdU can be used to label dividing stem cells in the human CNS. In case division of transplanted stem cells continues for long periods after transplantation into the human CNS, the BrdU injection will need to be as close in time to the point of death as is possible in some patients to prevent dilution of label to undetectable levels. To allow for the possibility that cell-cycle times are long, it would be advantageous if BrdU delivery could be continuous over a period of 8–24 h. Appropriate informed consent would need to be obtained for all such experiments, but their importance warrants examination of this possibility. By combining the use of labeled stem cells with BrdU administration, it will be possible to obtain a great deal of information that will not be observable through standard neurological and radiological examination. The ability to unambiguously recognize transplanted cells will allow determination of whether they form aberrant growths, whether they become incorporated into the subventricular zone or other germinal zones, whether a population of dividing cells is retained for long periods, and whether the transplanted cells generate new neurons, oligodendrocytes, and astrocytes.

It also would be advantageous to determine whether the tumors of patients treated with this approach have any molecular characteristics (e.g., expression of a truncated or amplified receptor for EGF) that would allow tumor cells to be identified with immunohistochemical markers. Although it will not be possible in the human to quantify the apposition between stem cells and tumor cells with the accuracy that is possible in preclinical models, it is nonetheless important to use any means available to at least estimate the extent to which this hopedfor association actually occurs.

As discussed, the problems that remain to be resolved in obtaining benefit from this novel therapeutic approach are formidable ones. A particularly critical issue derives from the fact that neural stem (or precursor) cell transplantation is a treatment that might confer two wholly different kinds of benefits, one on survival and one on repair of CNS damage. Structuring clinical trials to gain useful insights into these distinct possibilities is particularly challenging, especially if obvious therapeutic success is not achieved in the first attempts.

As can be seen from the earlier considerations, the question of how we are going to kill brain tumor cells—and cancer cells in other parts of the body—without destroying the normal cells of the brain represents still one more point of intersecting interest between neurobiologists and the cancer community. It is unlikely that the answer to this question will come from any singular path of investigation, be it gene expression analysis or cell biology. Instead, it seems much more likely that the answer will come from the development of convergent therapies that target multiple components of the physiological differences between cancer cells and normal cells. The requirement to prevent death of normal tissue while at the same time killing tumor cells stresses the importance of returning to the long,unfinished business of understanding the metabolic—and not just the genetic—differences between cancer cells and normal cells.

REFERENCES

1. Aboody K.S., Brown A., Rainov N.G., Bower K.A., Liu S., Yang W., et al. 2000. Neural stem cells display extensive tropism for pathology in adult brain: evidence from intracranial gliomas. *Proc. Natl. Acad. Sci. USA* **97:**12,846–12,851.

2. Al-Hajj M., Wicha M.S., Benito-Hernandez A., Morrison S.J., Clarke M.F.. 2003. Prospective identification of tumorigenic breast cancer cells. *Proc. Natl. Acad. Sci. USA* **100:**3983–3988.

3. Alizadeh A.A., Staudt L.M. 2000. Genomic-scale gene expression profiling of normal and malignant immune cells. *Curr. Opin. Immunol.* **12:**219–225.

4. Alvarez-Buylla A., Garcia-Verdugo J.M. 2002. Neurogenesis in adult subventricular zone. *J. Neurosci.* **22:**629–634.

5. Appleton R.E., Farrell K., Zaide J., Rogers P. 1990. Decline in head growth and cognitive impairment in survivors of acute lymphoblastic leukaemia. *Arch. Dis. Child* **65:**530–534.

6. Archibald Y.M., Lunn D, Ruttan L.A., Macdonald D.R., Del Maestro R.F., Barr H.W., et al. 1994. Cognitive functioning in long-term survivors of high-grade glioma. *J. Neurosurg.* **80:**247–253.

7. Bachoo R.M., Maher E.A., Ligon K.L., Sharpless N.E., Chan S.S., You M.J., et al. 2002. Epidermal growth factor receptor and Ink4a/Arf: convergent mechanisms governing terminal differentiation and transformation along the neural stem cell to astrocyte axis. *Cancer Cell* **1:**269–277.

8. Barnett S.C., Robertson L., Graham D., Allan D., Rampling R. 1998. Oligodendrocyte-type-2 astrocyte (O-2A) progenitor cells transformed with c-myc and H-ras form high-grade glioma after stereotactic injection into the rat brain. *Carcinogenesis* **19:**1529–1537.

9. Bellinzona M., Gobbel G.T., Shinohara C., Fike J.R. 1996. Apoptosis is induced in the subependyma of young adult rats by ionizing irradiation. *Neurosci. Lett.* **208:**163–166.

10. Benedetti S., Pirola B., Pollo B., Magrassi L., Bruzzone M.G., Rigamonti D., et al. 2000. Gene therapy of experimental brain tumors using neural progenitor cells. *Nat. Med.* **6:**447–450.

11. Benes F.M., Turtle M., Khan Y., Farol P. 1994. Myelination of a key relay zone in the hippocampal formation occurs in the human brain during childhood, adolescence and adulthood. *Arch. Gen. Psychiat.* **51:**477–484.

12. Berens M.E., Giese A. 1999. "...those left behind." Biology and oncology of invasive glioma cells. *Neoplasia* **1:** 208–219.

13. Bigner S.H., Bullard D.E., Pegram C.N., Wikstrand C.J., Bigner D.D.. 1981. Relationship of in vitro morphologic and growth characteristics of established human glioma-derived cell lines to their tumorigenicity in athymic nude mice. *J. Neuropathol. Exp. Neurol.* **40:**390–409.

14. Bouvier C., Bartoli C., Aguirre-Cruz L., Virard I., Colin C., Fernandez C., et al. 2003. Shared oligodendrocyte lineage gene expression in gliomas and oligodendrocyte progenitor cells. *J. Neurosurg.* **99:**344–350.

15. Brezden C.B., Phillips K.A., Abdolell M., Bunston T., Tannock I.F. 2000. Cognitive function in breast cancer patients receiving adjuvant chemotherapy. *J. Clin. Oncol.* **18:**2695–2701.

16. Brown M.S., Stemmer S.M., Simon J.H., Stears J.C., Jones R.B., Cagnoni P.J., Sheeder J.L. 1998. White matter disease induced by high-dose chemotherapy: longitudinal study with MR imaging and proton spectroscopy. *AJNR Am. J. Neuroradiol.* **19:**217–221.

17. Bruner J.M., Inouye L., Fuller G.N., Langford L.A. 1997. Diagnostic discrepancies and their clinical impact in a neuropathology referral practice. *Cancer* **79:**796–803.

18. Cairncross J.G., Ueki K., Zlatescu M.C., Lisle D.K., Finkelstein D.M., Hammond R.R., et al. 1998. Specific genetic predictors of chemotherapeutic response and survival in patients with anaplastic oligodendrogliomas. *J. Natl. Cancer Inst.* **90:**1473–1479.

19. Cetingul N., Aydinok Y., Kantar M., Oniz H., Kavakli K., Yalman O., et al. 1999. Neuropsychologic sequelae in the long-term survivors of childhood acute lymphoblastic leukemia. *Pediatr. Hematol. Oncol.* **16:**213–220.

20. Cleeland C.S., Mendoza T.R., Wang X.S., Chou C., Harle M.T., Morrissey M., Engstrom M.C.. 2000. Assessing symptom distress in cancer patients: the M.D. Anderson Symptom Inventory. *Cancer* **89:**1634–1646.

21. Coons S.W., Johnson P.C., Shapiro J.R.. 1995. Cytogenetic and flow cytometry DNA analysis of regional heterogeneity in a low grade human glioma. *Cancer Res.* **55:**1569–1577.

22. Dai C., Celestino J.C., Okada Y., Louis D.N., Fuller G.N., Holland E.C.. 2001. PDGF autocrine stimulation dedifferentiates cultured astrocytes and induces oligodendrogliomas and oligoastrocytomas from neural progenitors and astrocytes in vivo. *Genes Dev.* **15:**1913–1925.

23. Ding H., Roncari L., Shannon P., Wu X., Lau N., Karaskova J., et al. 2001. Astrocyte-specific expression of activated p21-ras results in malignant astrocytoma formation in a transgenic mouse model of human gliomas. *Cancer Res.* **61:**3826–3836.

24. Ding H., Shannon P., Lau N., Wu X., Roncari L., Baldwin R.L., et al. 2003. Oligodendrogliomas result from the expression of an activated mutant epidermal growth factor receptor in a RAS transgenic mouse astrocytoma model. *Cancer Res.* **63:**1106–1113.

25. Doetsch F., Caille I., Lim D.A., Garcia-Verdugo J.M., Alvarez-Buylla A. 1999. Subventricular zone astrocytes are neural stem cells in the adult mammalian brain. *Cell* **97:**703–716.

26. Donahue B., Scott C.B., Nelson J.S., Rotman M., Murray K.J., Nelson D.F., et al. 1997. Influence of an oligodendroglial component on the survival of patients with anaplastic astrocytomas: a report of Radiation Therapy Oncology Group 83-02. *Int. J. Radiat. Oncol. Biol. Phys.* **38:**911–914.

27. Duelli D., Lazebnik Y. 2003. Cell fusion: A hidden enemy? *Cancer Cell* **3:**445–448.

28. Eriksson P.S., Perfilieva E., Bjork-Eriksson T., Alborn A.M., Nordborg C., Peterson D.A., Gage F.H. 1998. Neurogenesis in the adult human hippocampus. *Nat. Med.* **4:**1313–1317.

29. Espinosa de los Monteros A., Zhang M., De Vellis J. 1993. O2A progenitor cells transplanted into the neonatal rat brain develop into oligodendrocytes but not astrocytes. *Proc. Natl. Acad. Sci. USA* **90:**50–54.

30. Feldkamp M.M., Lala P., Lau N., Roncari L., Guha A. 1999. Expression of activated epidermal growth factor receptors, Ras-guanosine triphosphate, and mitogen-activated protein kinase in human glioblastoma multiforme specimens. *Neurosurgery* **45:**1442–1453.

31. Fok-Seang J., Miller H.R. 1992. Astrocyte precursors in neonatal rat spinal cord cultures. *J. Neurosci.* **12:**2751–2764.

32. Fok-Seang J., Miller R.H. 1994. Distribution and differentiation of A2B5+ glial precursors in the developing rat spinal cord. *J. Neurosci. Res.* **37:**219–235.

33. Foran D.R., Peterson A.C. 1992. Myelin acquisition in the central nervous system of the mouse revealed by an MBP-LacZ transgene. *J. Neurosci.* **12:**4890–4897.

34. Glauser T.A., Packer R.J. 1991. Cognitive deficits in long-term survivors of childhood brain tumors. *Childs Nerv. Syst.* **7:**2–12.

35. Gregor A., Cull A., Traynor E., Stewart M., Lander F., Love S. 1996. Neuropsychometric evaluation of long-term survivors of adult brain tumours: relationship with tumour and treatment parameters. *Radiother. Oncol.* **41:**55–59.

36. Gregori N., Pröschel C., Noble M., Mayer-Pröschel M. 2002. The tripotential glial-restricted precursor (GRP) cell and glial development in the spinal cord: Generation of bipotential oligodendrocyte-type-2 astrocyte progenitor cells and dorsal-ventral differences in GRP cell function. *J. Neurosci.* **22:**248–256.

37. Grill J., Renaux V.K., Bulteau C., Viguier D., Levy-Piebois C., Sainte-Rose C., et al. 1999. Long-term intellectual outcome in children with posterior fossa tumors according to radiation doses and volumes. *Int. J. Radiat. Oncol. Biol. Phys.* **45:**137–145.

38. Grinspan J.B., Stern J.L., Pustilnik S.M., Pleasure D. 1990. Cerebral white matter contains PDGF-responsive precursors to O2A cells. *J. Neurosci.* **10:**1866–1873.

39. Herrera J., Yang H., Zhang S.C., Proschel C., Tresco P., Duncan I.D., et al. 2001. Embryonic-derived glial-restricted precursor cells (GRP cells) can differentiate into astrocytes and oligodendrocytes in vivo. *Exp. Neurol.* **171:**11–21.

40. Hesselager G., Holland E.C.. 2003. Using mice to decipher the molecular genetics of brain tumors. *Neurosurgery* **53:** 685–694.

41. Hopewell J.W., van der Kogel A.J. 1999. Pathophysiological mechanisms leading to the development of late radiation-induced damage to the central nervous system. *Front Radiat. Ther. Oncol.* **33:**265–275.

42. Ignatova T.N., Kukekov V.G., Laywell E.D., Suslov O.N., Vrionis F.D., Steindler D.A. 2002. Human cortical glial tumors contain neural stem-like cells expressing astroglial and neuronal markers in vitro. *Glia* **39:**193–206.

43. Kalyani A., Piper D., Mujitaba T., Lucero M., Rao M. 1998. E-NCAM immunoreactive neuronal precursor cells differentiate into multiple neurotransmitter phenotypes. *J. Neurosci.* **18:**7856–7868.

44. Keime-Guibert F., Napolitano M., Delattre J.Y. 1998. Neurological complications of radiotherapy and chemotherapy. *J. Neurol.* **245:**695–708.

45. Kennedy P.G., Watkins B.A., Thomas D.G., Noble M.D. 1987. Antigenic expression by cells derived from human gliomas does not correlate with morphological classification. *Neuropathol. Appl. Neurobiol.* **13:**327–347.

46. Kinney H.C., Brody B.A., Kloman A.S., Gilles F.H. 1988. Sequence of central nervous sytem myelination in human infancy. II. Patterns of myelination in autopsied infants. *J. Neuropath. Exp. Neurol.* **47:**217–234.

47. Kraus J.A., Wenghoefer M., Schmidt M.C., von Deimling A., Berweiler U., Roggendorf W., et al. 2000. Long-term survival of glioblastoma multiforme: importance of histopathological reevaluation. *J. Neurol.* **247:**455–460.

48. Lamborn K.R., Prados M.D., Kaplan S.B., Davis R.L. 1999. Final report on the University of California-San Francisco experience with bromodeoxyuridine labeling index as a prognostic factor for the survival of glioma patients. *Cancer* **85:**925–935.

49. Larizza L., Schirrmacher V., Pfluger E. 1984. Acquisition of high metastatic capacity after in vitro fusion of a nonmetastatic tumor line with a bone marrow-derived macrophage. *J. Exp. Med.* **160:**1579–1584.

50. Lee J.C., Mayer-Proschel M, Rao M.S. 2000. Gliogenesis in the central nervous system. *Glia* **30:**105–121.

51. Li Y.Q., Wong C.S. 1998. Apoptosis and its relationship with cell proliferation in the irradiated rat spinal cord. *Int. J. Radiat. Biol.* **74:**405–417.

52. Loeper S., Romeike B.F., Heckmann N., Jung V., Henn W., Feiden W., et al. 2001. Frequent mitotic errors in tumor cells of genetically micro-heterogeneous glioblastomas. *Cytogenet. Cell Genet.* **94:**1–8.

53. Louis D.N., Gusella J.F.. 1995. A tiger behind many doors: multiple genetic pathways to malignant glioma. *Trends Genet.* **11:**412–415.

54. Lu Q.R., Park J.K., Noll E., Chan J.A., Alberta J., Yuk D., et al. 2001. Oligodendrocyte lineage genes (OLIG) as molecular markers for human glial brain tumors. *Proc. Natl. Acad. Sci. USA* **98:**10,851–10,856.

55. Macklin W.B., Weill C.L. 1985. Appearance of myelin proteins during development in the chick central nervous system. *Dev. Neurosci.* **7**:170–178.

56. Marie Y., Sanson M., Mokhtari K., Leuraud P., Kujas M., Delattre J.Y., et al. 2001. OLIG2 as a specific marker of oligodendroglial tumour cells. *Lancet* **358**:298–300.

57. Mason W., Louis D.N., Cairncross J.G. 1997. Chemosensitive gliomas in adults: which ones and why? *J. Clin. Oncol.* **15**:3423–3426.

58. Mayer-Pröschel M., Kalyani A., Mujtaba T., Rao M.S. 1997. Isolation of lineage-restricted neuronal precursors from multipotent neuroepithelial stem cells. *Neuron.* **19**:773–785.

59. McDermott M.W., Krouwer H.G., Asai A., Ito S., Hoshino T., Prados M.D. 1992. A comparison of CT contrast enhancement and BUDR labeling indices in moderately and highly anaplastic astrocytomas of the cerebral hemispheres. *Can. J. Neurol. Sci.* **19**:34–39.

60. McKay R. 1997. Stem cells in the central nervous system. *Science* **276**:66–71.

61. Mi H., Barres B.A. 1999. Purification and characterization of astrocyte precursor cells in the developing rat optic nerve. *J. Neurosci.* **19**:1049–1061.

62. Misra A., Chattopadhyay P., Dinda A.K., Sarkar C., Mahapatra A.K., Hasnain S.E., Sinha S. 2000. Extensive intratumor heterogeneity in primary human glial tumors as a result of locus non-specific genomic alterations. *J. Neurooncol.* **48**:1–12.

63. Moe P.J., Holen A. 2000. High-dose methotrexate in childhood all. *Pediatr.Hematol. Oncol.* **17**:615–622.

64. Morris G.M., Hopewell J.W., Morris A.D. 1995. A comparison of the effects of methotrexate and misonidazole on the germinal cells of the subependymal plate of the rat. *Br. J. Radiol.* **68**:406–412.

65. Mueller W., Hartmann C., Hoffmann A., Lanksch W., Kiwit J., Tonn J., et al. 2002. Genetic signature of oligoastrocytomas correlates with tumor location and denotes distinct molecular subsets. *Am. J. Pathol.* **161**:313–319.

66. Nagane M., Coufal F., Lin H., Bogler O., Cavenee W., Huang H. 1996. A common mutant epidermal growth factor receptor confers enhanced tumorigenicity on human glioblastoma cells by increasing proliferation and reducing apoptosis. *Cancer Res.* **56**:5079–5086.

67. Nagane M., Coufal F., Lin H., Bogler O., Cavenee W.K., Huang H.J. 1996. A common mutant epidermal growth factor receptor confers enhanced tumorigenicity on human glioblastoma cells by increasing proliferation and reducing apoptosis. *Cancer Res.* **56**:5079–5086.

68. Nagane M., Levitzki A., Gazit A., Cavenee W.K., Huang H.J. 1998. Drug resistance of human glioblastoma cells conferred by a tumor-specific mutant epidermal growth factor receptor through modulation of Bcl-XL and caspase-3-like proteases. *Proc. Natl. Acad. Sci. USA* **95**:5724–5729.

69. Nishiyama A., Chang A., Trapp B.D. 1999. NG2+ glial cells: a novel glial cell population in the adult brain. *J. Neuropathol. Exp. Neurol.* **58**:1113–1124.

70. Noble M. 2000. Can neural stem cells be used as therapeutic vehicles in the treatment of brain tumors? *Nat. Med.* **6**:369–370.

71. Noble M. 2000. Can neural stem cells be used to track down and destroy migratory brain tumor cells while also providing a means of repairing tumor-associated damage? *Proc. Natl. Acad. Sci. USA* **97**:12,393–12,395.

72. Noble M., Dietrich J. 2004. The complex identity of brain tumors: emerging concerns regarding origin, diversity and plasticity. *Trends Neurosci.* **27**:148–154.

73. Noble M., Murray K. 1984. Purified astrocytes promote the in vitro division of a bipotential glial progenitor cell. *EMBO-J.* **3**:2243–2247.

74. Noble M., Murray K., Stroobant P., Waterfield M.D., Riddle P. 1988. Platelet-derived growth factor promotes division and motility and inhibits premature differentiation of the oligodendrocyte/type-2 astrocyte progenitor cell. *Nature* **333**:560–562.

75. Noble M., Pröschel C., Mayer-Proschel M. 2004. Getting a GR(i)P on oligodendrocyte development. *Dev. Biol.* **265**:33–52.

76. Nutt C.L., Noble M., Chambers A.F., Cairncross J.G. 2000. Differential expression of drug resistance genes and chemosensitivity in glial cell lineages correlate with differential response of oligodendrogliomas and astrocytomas to chemotherapy. *Cancer Res.* **60**:4812–4818.

77. Onda K., Davis R.L., Shibuya M., Wilson C.B., Hoshino T. 1994. Correlation between the bromodeoxyuridine labeling index and the MIB-1 and Ki-67 proliferating cell indices in cerebral gliomas. *Cancer* **74**:1921–1926.

78. Peissner W., Kocher M., Treuer H., Gillardon F. 1999. Ionizing radiation-induced apoptosis of proliferating stem cells in the dentate gyrus of the adult rat hippocampus. *Brain Res. Mol. Brain Res.* **71**:61–68.

79. Pomeroy S.L., Tamayo P., Gaasenbeek M., Sturla L.M., Angelo M., McLaughlin M.E., et al. 2002. Prediction of central nervous system embryonal tumour outcome based on gene expression. *Nature* **415**:436–442.

80. Power J., Mayer-Proschel M., Smith J., Noble M. 2002. Oligodendrocyte precursor cells from different brain regions express divergent properties consistent with the differing time courses of myelination in these regions. *Dev. Biol.* **245**:362–375.

81. Rachkovsky M., Sodi S., Chakraborty A., Avissar Y., Bolognia J., McNiff J.M., et al. 1998. Melanoma x macrophage hybrids with enhanced metastatic potential. *Clin. Exp. Metastasis.* **16**:299–312.

82. Radcliffe J., Bunin G.R., Sutton L.N., Goldwein J.W., Phillips P.C. 1994. Cognitive deficits in long-term survivors of childhood medulloblastoma and other noncortical tumors: age-dependent effects of whole brain radiation. *Int. J. Dev. Neurosci.* **12:**327–334.

83. Raff M.C., Miller R.H., Noble M. 1983. A glial progenitor cell that develops in vitro into an astrocyte or an oligodendrocyte depending on the culture medium. *Nature* **303:**390–396.

84. Rao M., Mayer-Pröschel M. 1997. Glial restricted precursors are derived from multipotent neuroepithelial stem cells. *Dev. Biology* **188:**48–63.

85. Rao M., Noble M., Mayer-Pröschel M. 1998. A tripotential glial precursor cell is present in the developing spinal cord. *Proc. Natl. Acad. Sci. USA* **95:**3996–4001.

86. Reynolds B.A., Tetzlaff W., Weiss S. 1992. A Mulitpotent EGF-Responsive Striatal Embryonic Progenitor Cell Produces Neurons and Astrocytes. *J. Neuroscience* **12:**4565–4574.

87. Reynolds B.A., Weiss S. 1992. Generation of neurons and astrocytes from isolated cells of the adult mammalian cental nervous system. *Science* **225:**1707–1710.

88. Reynolds B.A., Weiss S. 1996. Clonal and population analyses demonstrate that an EGF-responsive mammalian embryonic CNS precursor is a stem cell. *Dev. Biol.* **175:**1–13.

89. Riva D., Giorgi C. 2000. The neurodevelopmental price of survival in children with malignant brain tumours. *Childs Nerv. Syst.* **16:**751–754.

90. Roman D.D., Sperduto P.W. 1995. Neuropsychological effects of cranial radiation: current knowledge and future directions. *Int. J. Radiat. Oncol. Biol. Phys.* **31:**983–998.

91. Rorke L.B. 1997. Pathologic diagnosis as the gold standard. *Cancer* **79:**665–667.

92. Rubnitz J.E. 2000. Molecular diagnostics in the treatment of childhood acute lymphoblastic leukemia. *J. Biol. Regul. Homeost. Agents* **14:**182–186.

93. Salander P., Karlsson T., Bergenheim T., Henriksson R. 1995. Long-term memory deficits in patients with malignant gliomas. *J. Neurooncol.* **25:**227–238.

94. Schagen S.B., Muller M.J., Boogerd W., Lindeboom J.. 1999. Cognitive deficits after postoperative adjuvant chemotherapy for breast carcinoma. *Cancer* **85:**640–650.

95. Schlegel U., Pels H., Oehring R., Blumcke I. 1999. Neurologic sequelae of treatment of primary CNS lymphomas. *J. Neurooncol.* **43:**277–286.

96. Seidman K., Teng A., Rosenkopf R., Spilotro P.,Weyhenmeyer J. 1997. Isolation, cloning and characterization of a putative type-1 astrocyte cell line. *Brain Res.* **753:**18–26.

97. Shapiro J.R., Shapiro W.R.. 1984. Clonal tumor cell heterogeneity. *Prog. Exp. Tumor Res.* **27:**49–66.

98. Shapiro J.R., Shapiro W.R. 1985. The subpopulations and isolated cell types of freshly resected high grade human gliomas: their influence on the tumor's evolution in vivo and behavior and therapy in vitro. *Cancer Metastasis Rev.* **4:** 107–124.

99. Shuangshoti S., Navalitloha Y., Kasantikul V., Shuangshoti S., Mutirangura A. 2000. Genetic heterogeneity and progression in different areas within high-grade diffuse astrocytoma. *Oncol. Rep.* **7:**113–117.

100. Skoff R.P., Toland D., Nast E. 1980. Pattern of myelination and distribution of neuroglial cells along the developing optic system of the rat and rabbit. *J. Comp. Neurol.* **191:**237–253.

101. Stemmer S.M., Stears J.C., Burton B.S., Jones R.B., Simon J.H. 1994. White matter changes in patients with breast cancer treated with high-dose chemotherapy and autologous bone marrow support. *AJNR Am. J. Neuroradiol.* **15:** 1267–1273.

102. Stylopoulos L.A., George A.E., de Leon M.J., Miller J.D., Foo S.H., Hiesiger E., Wise A. 1988. Longitudinal CT study of parenchymal brain changes in glioma survivors. *AJNR Am. J. Neuroradiol.* **9:**517–522.

103. Tada E., Parent J.M., Lowenstein D.H., Fike J.R. 2000. X-irradiation causes a prolonged reduction in cell proliferation in the dentate gyrus of adult rats. *Neuroscience* **99:**33–41.

104. Temple S., Qian X. 1996. Vertebrate neural progenitor cells: subtypes and regulation. *Curr. Op. Neurobiol.* **6:**11–17.

105. Terada N., Hamazaki T., Oka M., Hoki M., Mastalerz D.M., Nakano Y., et al. 2002. Bone marrow cells adopt the phenotype of other cells by spontaneous cell fusion. *Nature* **416:**542–545.

106. Troy L., McFarland K., Littman-Power S., Kelly B.J., Walpole E.T., Wyld D., Thomson D. 2000. Cisplatin-based therapy: a neurological and neuropsychological review. *Psychooncology* **9:**29–39.

107. Uhrbom L., Dai C., Celestino J.C., Rosenblum M.K., Fuller G.N., Holland E.C. 2002. Ink4a-Arf loss cooperates with KRas activation in astrocytes and neural progenitors to generate glioblastomas of various morphologies depending on activated Akt. *Cancer Res.* **62:**5551–5518.

108. van 't Veer L.J., Dai H., van De Vijver M.J., He Y.D., Hart A.A., Mao M, et al. 2002. Gene expression profiling predicts clinical outcome of breast cancer. *Nature* **415:**530–536.

109. van Dam F.S., Schagen S.B., Muller M.J., Boogerd W., vd Wall E., Droogleever Fortuyn M.E., Rodenhuis S. 1998. Impairment of cognitive function in women receiving adjuvant treatment for high-risk breast cancer: high-dose versus standard-dose chemotherapy. *J. Natl. Cancer Inst.* **90:**210–218.

110. van den Bent M.J. 2000. Chemotherapy of oligodendroglial tumours: current developments. *Forum (Genova)* **10:**108–118.

111. Vescovi A., Gritti A., Galli R., Parati E. 1999. Isolation and intracerebral grafting of nontransformed multipotential embryonic human CNS stem cells. *J. Neurotrauma* **16**:689–693.

112. Vigliani M.C., Duyckaerts C., Hauw J.J., Poisson M., Magdelenat H. 1999. Dementia following treatment of brain tumors with radiotherapy administered alone or in combination with nitrosourea-based chemotherapy: a clinical and pathological study. *J. Neurooncol.* **41**:137–149.

113. Waber D.P., Tarbell N.J. 1997. Toxicity of CNS prophylaxis for childhood leukemia. *Oncology (Huntingt)* **11**:259–264; discussion 264–265.

114. Wacker M.R., Hoshino T., Ahn D.K., Davis R.L., Prados M.D. 1994. The prognostic implications of histologic classification and bromodeoxyuridine labeling index of mixed gliomas. *J. Neurooncol.* **19**:113–122.

115. Wang X., Willenbring H., Akkari Y., Torimaru, Foster M., Al-Dhalimy M., et al. 2003. Cell fusion is the principal source of bone-marrow-derived hepatocytes. *Nature* **422**:897–901.

116. Weimann J.M., Johansson C.B., Trejo A., Blau H.M. 2003. Stable reprogrammed heterokaryons form spontaneously in Purkinje neurons after bone marrow transplant. *Nat. Cell Biol.* **5**:959–966.

117. Weiss S., Dunne C., Hewson J., Wohl C., Wheatley M., Peterson A.C., Reynolds B.A. 1996. Multipotent CNS Stem Cells are Present in the Adult Mammalian Spinal Cord and Ventricular Neuroaxis. *J. Neurosci.* **16**:7599–7609.

118. Weiss W.A., Burns M.J., Hackett C., Aldape K., Hill J.R., Kuriyama H., et al. 2003. Genetic determinants of malignancy in a mouse model for oligodendroglioma. *Cancer Res.* **63**:1589–1595.

119. Westphal M., Nausch H., Herrmann H.D. 1990. Antigenic staining patterns of human glioma cultures: primary cultures, long-term cultures and cell lines. *J. Neurocytol.* **19**:466–477.

120. Wolswijk G., Noble M. 1989. Identification of an adult-specific glial progenitor cell. *Development* **105**:387–400.

121. Wolswijk G., Noble M. 1992. Cooperation between PDGF and FGF converts slowly dividing O-2Aadult progenitor cells to rapidly dividing cells with characteristics of O-2Aperinatal progenitor cells. *J. Cell. Biol.* **118**:889–900.

122. Wolswijk G., Riddle P.N., Noble M. 1991. Platelet-derived growth factor is mitogenic for O-2A^{adult} progenitor cells. *Glia* **4**:495–503.

123. Wren D., Wolswijk G., Noble M. 1992. In vitro analysis of the origin and maintenance of O-2A^{adult} progenitor cells. *J. Cell. Biol.* **116**:167–176.

124. Yakovlev P.L., Lecours A.R. 1967. The myelogenetic cycles of regional maturation of the brain, in *Regional development of the brain in early life* (Minkowski A., et. al., ed.), Blackwell, Oxford. p. 3–70.

125. Ying Q.L., Nichols J., Evans E.P., Smith A.G.. 2002. Changing potency by spontaneous fusion. *Nature* **416**:545–548.

126. Zlatescu M.C., TehraniYazdi A., Sasaki H., Megyesi J.F., Betensky R.A., Louis D.N., Cairncross J.G. 2001. Tumor location and growth pattern correlate with genetic signature in oligodendroglial neoplasms. *Cancer Res.* **61**:6713–6715.

7

Biology of Primitive Neuroectodermal Tumors

John R. Hill, Shoichiro Ohta, and Mark A. Israel

1. INTRODUCTION

As a group, brain tumors are the most common tumors to occur in children. Primitive neuroecto-dermal brain tumors is a designation widely used clinically to identify a family of undifferentiated embryonal tumors of neuroepithelial origin. This group of tumors is widely recognized as including medulloblastoma, supratentorial primitive neuroectodermal tumors, and atypical teratoid/rhabdoid tumors. A variety of classification efforts, some described in this chapter, have sought to classify these tumors. Initially, they were grouped together simply on the basis of their histologic appearance, which did not reflect specific cellular lineages. The cellular morphology of these tumors mimicked the appearance of cells found largely only during embryonic development. Subsequent classification attempted to include in their evaluation more precise estimates of their cellular origin, their pathology, and the genetic alterations that contributed to their development. The most recent World Health Organization (WHO) classification of tumors of the nervous system is based largely upon the histologic appearance of individual tumor entities, but describes molecular and genetic characteristics of the entities they name where such information exists (79). This classification includes not only embryonal tumors of neuroepithelial tissue, but also less commonly occurring tumors such as medulloepithe-lioma and ependymoblastoma.

The histologic appearance of these embryonal tumors is typically characterized as densely packed, small round cells, with prominent nuclei, and little cytoplasm (79). Consistent with their embryonal designation is the finding that although these tumors can occur in adults, they are most typically seen in early childhood. This is particularly true of medulloblastoma, which is the most common and most extensively studied of this tumor group. In addition to histological classification, a number of clinical features of these tumors can be important in determining the prognosis for patients with individual tumors, and together these guide therapy. An understanding of the pathogenesis of tumors, and especially the genetic alterations that underlie the development of these tumors, can be of considerable importance for prognostication and ultimately, it is thought, for treatment.

Because these tumors most commonly arise in young children, the need for improved strategies for pathological classification, prognostication, and treatment is particularly compelling. Currently, the most effective available modalities of treatment—surgery, irradiation, and chemotherapy—are each particularly toxic to the developing brain (115). This makes current therapy a significant challenge requiring integration of efforts from diverse pediatric specialists not only from the traditional fields of oncology, but also from less obvious disciplines such as rehabilitation medicine and psychology. Our emerging understanding of the pathogenesis of these tumors and the commitment to develop more effective, less toxic therapeutic agents provide both the focus and the emphasis needed to move forward efforts to build more effective interventions based upon an understanding of the molecular events underlying tumor development.

From: *Contemporary Cancer Research: Brain Tumors*
Edited by: F. Ali-Osman © Humana Press Inc., Totowa, NJ

2. PRIMITIVE NEUROECTODERMAL TUMORS OF THE CENTRAL NERVOUS SYSTEM

2.1. Medulloblastoma

2.1.1. General Description

Medulloblastomas are embryonal tumors of the neuroepithelium that occur in the posterior fossa of the brain and have a propensity to spread throughout the neuroaxis, especially to the spinal cord. Median survival for all children with this tumor is approx 10 yr *(93,100,120)*. It is among the most common brain tumor to arise in childhood, accounting for approx 7–8% of all intracranial tumors and approx 18% of pediatric brain tumors *(74)*. These tumors are approximately twice as common in males than in females *(100)*. Other posterior fossa tumors occurring in childhood include atypical teratoid tumors, cerebellar astrocytomas, ependymomas, and brain stem gliomas. The incidence of medulloblastoma in the United States is approximately five cases per million per year or approx 400 new cases each year, and the incidence may be rising *(100)*. Caucasians are more frequently affected than Afro-Americans *(100)*. There is no country in which significantly higher or lower rates of medulloblastoma have been claimed. Medulloblastoma most often occurs in the first decade of life with a median age of incidence of approx 6–7 yr *(74,79,100)*. Children presenting at a young age may have a family history of medulloblastoma *(106,142)*. Rarely medulloblastoma occurs in adults *(96,125)*, and it has been reported in elderly patients *(75)*. Among adults, the tumor is most common in the first four decades of life.

2.1.2. Clinical Presentation and Treatment Approaches

The clinical presentation of medulloblastoma, like other tumors of childhood, is age dependent. In young children subtle presentations such as behavior changes, lethargy, or increasing head circumference may be the only presenting symptoms. Irritability and listlessness are also seen. Vomiting can occur in infants, but is more common in older children. On physical examination, bulging anterior fontanelles can sometimes be detected and open cranial sutures palpated. In older children, lethargy can be associated with a head tilt, truncal ataxia, and gait disturbances. Head tilt suggests a trochlear nerve palsy or encroachment of the tumor on the foramen magnum. Cerebellar tonsil herniation into the foramen magnum as a result of tumor compression is a life threatening complication of tumor growth. Older children present with a wide variety of symptoms related to tumor location, size, and the rapidity of tumor growth. The history of symptoms is typically short, measured in weeks to a couple of months, presumably because of the rapid growth of this tumor. Beyond infancy, children may also have symptoms such as severe headaches and vomiting in the morning associated with intracranial hypertension caused by tumor-mediated cerebrospinal fluid (CSF) obstruction in the recumbent position. These symptoms usually increase in intensity over the course of the untreated disease. In children with increased intracranial pressure, papilledema is a very common finding on funduscopic examination. Patients may also present with palsies of the fourth or sixth cranial nerves and complain of diplopia because of tumor-mediated compression of these nerves. Visual disturbances in older children can occur as the result of papilledema, but severe visual loss at presentation is uncommon. The speech of patients with untreated medulloblastoma may also be impaired, but this too is rare at presentation. If the history of symptoms prior to presentation is long enough, school performance may have deteriorated.

Medulloblastoma most commonly occurs in the midline, frequently in the cerebellar vermis. When located there, nystagmus may be present. A midline location is also commonly associated with a wide-based gait or other evidence of gait and truncal ataxia, although unilateral dysmetria may also be present. Sometimes patients complain of clumsiness and problems with tasks like handwriting. In adults, medulloblastoma frequently arises in a cerebellar hemisphere, causing unilateral syndromes of cerebellar dysfunction such as dysmetria. Leptomeningeal dissemination of tumor throughout the neuroaxis occurs as tumor growth progresses. Such dissemination can involve the cranial nerves, spinal cord, and rarely the convexity of the brain. Whereas there is a clear propensity for medullo-blastoma to metastasize throughout the CNS, rarely do systemic metastases of this tumor occur. Bone tends to be the major site of extraneural metastases *(14)*. Patients complaining of a stiff neck, extrem-ity weakness, or a radiculopathy may have spinal cord involvement, although these symptoms are not often present at a patient's initial presentation. Other symptoms associated with spread of the tumor to the spinal cord include back pain, difficulty walking, and loss of bladder and bowel control.

At the time of presentation it is important to ascertain whether there are tumor cells that have seeded the cerebral spinal fluid, but lumbar puncture in untreated brain tumor patients with increased intracranial pressure can cause herniation of the cerebellar tonsil. Whereas some surgeons choose to obtain fluid by puncture of the cisterna magna at the time of surgery, others will obtain fluid at the time of placing a ventricular drain, which some patients require. There is no agreed-upon approach for obtaining fluid, and some practitioners perform a lumbar puncture after surgery, although this can produce a false-positive result.

2.1.2.1. IMAGING STUDIES

Imaging studies play a primary role in the diagnosis of medulloblastoma, as they do in other brain tumors. Other modalities have been largely replaced by computed tomography (CT) and mag-netic resonance imaging (MRI). The CT appearance of medulloblastoma is typically a hyperdense mass in the midline in the cerebellum, commonly filling the fourth ventricle. Contrast-enhanced CT examination usually reveals a solid, intensely and homogenously enhancing mass. Medulloblas-toma enhances strongly following the intravenous administration of an enhancing agent, although the surrounding area is sometimes hypodense, indicating the presence of vasogenic edema. MRI is the imaging strategy of choice for medulloblastoma, because it is not encumbered by artifacts from bone that compromise CT images. Medulloblastoma typically appears as a hypodense mass in T1-weighted MR images prior to the administration of gadoliniumdiethylenetriamine pentacetic acid, an enhancing agent. On MRI examination, compression and displacement of the brain stem ventrally is sometimes observed (Fig. 1). Following administration of gadolinium, T1-weighted images usually reveal a homogenously enhancing, hyperintense mass with a surrounding area of edema. Compression of the brain stem and extension of the tumor into the spinal canal is best observed in these views. MRI is also effective in imaging metastatic lesions, and patients should have an MRI of the spine at the time of their evaluation. Metastases can be seen as foci, nodular, or diffuse contrast enhancing lesions of the leptomeninges (Fig. 2). These lesions may not enhance to the same degree that the primary tumor does. In patients with evidence of metastatic disease a skeletal survey can define the extent of bony involvement.

2.1.2.2. TREATMENT

Surgery, radiation therapy, and chemotherapy are used to treat medulloblastoma. All patients receive surgical treatment. The goals of surgery are to obtain tissue for precise diagnosis and to remove as much tumor as possible. At surgery the spread of tumor to areas adjacent to the tumor can also be assessed. Subarachnoid spread is a serious complication associated with early relapse. Where seeding has not occurred, it is often possible to remove all known tumor, and these patients, patients with a gross total resection, are known to have a better prognosis than patients in which the tumor cannot be totally removed. Involvement of the floor of the fourth ventricle sometimes precludes removing the entire tumor. Surgery usually relieves the obstruction of CSF flow associated with medulloblastoma, although a ventricular drain for shunting of CSF is usually placed at the time of operation and removed later if CSF does not accumulate following occlusion of the drain. Some patients require permanent drainage.

Whereas the clinical staging of patients with medulloblastoma has been compressed to the desig-nation of average-risk or high-risk patients, such designations are an important aspect of patient management that should occur following surgery *(5)*. A patient's risk for relapse is determined by age, the extent of resection, radiographic evidence of residual tumor and tumor spread, and CSF

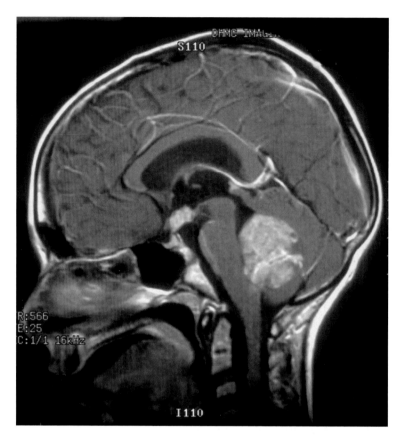

Fig. 1. MRI of a child with medulloblastoma. This is a T1 sagittal MR image following the injection of gadolinium, demonstrating an enhanced tumor in the posterior fossa compressing the brainstem.

cytology *(5,90)*. Patients older than 3 yr of age at diagnosis who do not have disseminated tumor and whose tumors that can be totally or almost totally resected, are considered average risk. Patients younger than 3 yr of age, with residual tumor following surgery or with evidence of tumor dissemination, are considered high risk. The presence of residual tumor following surgery should be assessed by a gadolinium-enhanced MRI. Patients for whom it is not possible to achieve a gross total resection, who have malignant cells in the CSF, residual tumor recognizable on MRI exam following surgery, or evidence of metastatic disease have a high risk of relapse and are treated more aggressively. Invasion of the brainstem is another feature of medulloblastoma widely regarded as a poor prognostic marker. Very recently, data have been presented suggesting that the pathological, cytological appearance of medulloblastoma *(44)* and molecular and genetic markers *(126)* are also of prognostic importance (see below).

   Radiotherapy is the most effective adjuvant to surgical intervention in the management of patients with medulloblastoma. Average risk children, those with no evidence of neuroaxis tumor spread beyond the primary site, should routinely receive postsurgical irradiation to the craniospinal axis 3000 cGy in 13 fractions with a boost to the primary tumor site totaling 5400 cGy, followed by adjuvant chemotherapy *(120)*. Patients receiving less than 3600 cGy to the neuroaxis without adjuvant chemotherapy have a significantly increased rate of neuroaxis recurrence *(146)*. High-risk patients should also be treated with 3600 cGy to the entire neuroaxis with boosts to primary and

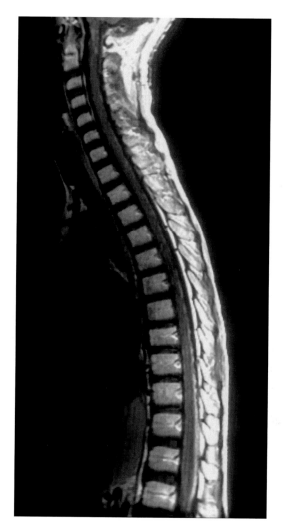

Fig. 2. Spinal MRI examination. This T1 image demonstrates evidence of drop metastases throughout the spinal canal.

gross metastatic disease sites, followed by adjuvant chemotherapy. Very young children (<3 yr) with medulloblastoma may be treated differently from older children in that chemotherapy can be used to delay the use of radiation therapy, which is associated with more severe long-term side effects in younger children *(42).* The severity of complications of radiotherapy is closely related to the age of the patient and include cognitive, psychological, and behavioral impairments, as well as neuroendocrine and growth disorders *(73,116,119,118).* Chemotherapy is now used in an effort to delay the use of radiation when this is possible. Life-threatening complications, including second malignancies and white matter necrosis, can occur years after the completion of therapy.

The role of chemotherapy in the management of patients with medulloblastoma is under study. Various regimens are widely used in conjunction with other modalities as initial therapy, and as noted earlier, in young children to delay the use of radiotherapy. Children with nondisseminated disease at the time of diagnosis have been reported to have as high as a 60% 5-yr disease-free survival rate after treatment with irradiation and chemotherapy given during and after radiation therapy *(120).*

Active regimens often include some of the following drugs: vincristine, cyclophosphamide, etoposide, cisplatin, lomustine, and prednisone. Chemotherapy is typically given to children with medulloblastoma after the completion of their radiotherapy. Children with disseminated disease are a highly problematic subgroup of patients to treat. Toxic side effects, which frequently occur following radiation therapy, are related to both the specific drug being used and the intensity with which a patient is treated. Whereas the role of chemotherapy for children with medulloblastoma that has disseminated throughout the neuroaxis is still under study, these children are at high risk for persistent or recurrent tumor and receive intensive therapy, both radiation therapy and chemotherapy (5,90,159). With the exception of the desmoplastic variant of medulloblastoma, the prognosis for all the histologic subgroups (see below) seems indistinguishable and has not been used as a means to guide therapy (52).

A significant proportion of children with medulloblastoma relapse. Most relapses occur within the first years after therapy, although late relapses are well documented (93). Because most children are treated with irradiation and radiation can cause extensive tissue damage, biopsy is sometimes necessary to distinguish tumor relapses from the symptoms of an expanding mass that are associated with radiation-induced brain necrosis. Most children today also receive either neo-adjuvant (for < 3 yr of age) or post-radiation adjuvant chemotherapy (for those > 3 yr of age). The choice of chemotherapy should be guided by the specific agents and the dose intensity of the treatment that the patient previously received. Few children can be cured following the recurrence of tumor (94), but myeloablative chemotherapy and autologous stem cell rescue at the time of relapse has provided some evidence that such approaches may be effective in a subgroup of such children (43,46).

2.1.3. Pathological Features

Primary brain tumors are classified by their site of origin and their histologic appearance. Bailey and Cushing were the first to use the term "medulloblastoma" to describe tumors found in the cerebellum of children. Medulloblastoma occurs in the posterior fossa, and although the precise cell of origin is not known, this tumor can be easily recognized. Most medulloblastomas in children arise in the vermis and project into the fourth ventricle. Larger tumors, typically found in older children, commonly involve the cerebellar hemispheres. At surgery, these tumors are typically pinkish-gray and soft, but firm to the touch (79). Cysts, areas of necrosis, or calcification are rare. Histologically, these tumors typically consist of sheets of small, round, blue (when stained with hematoxylin) cells, with little evidence of lineage-specific differentiation (Fig. 3). There is little or no stroma between the densely packed cells. Their undifferentiated appearance is characterized by scant cytoplasm and loosely packed chromatin. Most tumors have a high mitotic index and also, frequently, display cytologic evidence of ongoing apoptosis, which may be a prognostic indicator (63,84). Differentiation can sometimes be seen along astrocytic, neuronal, or even mesenchymal lines. In the case of neuronal differentiation, Homer-Wright rosettes may be seen and less commonly pseudorosettes formed by elongated cells surrounding acellular areas (Fig. 4).

There are several histologic variants of medulloblastoma, including desmoplastic, medullomyoblastoma, melanotic medulloblastoma, and large-cell medulloblastoma (81). Desmoplastic medulloblastoma is typically seen in adults and usually arises in the cerebellar hemisphere, a finding consistent with the clinical presentation that oftentimes has lateralizing features. Whereas histologically similar to medulloblastoma, the desmoplastic variant is characterized by nodules, islands of cells with round, regular nuclei surrounded by a dense reticulin network along which the tumor cells may be organized (Fig. 5). In these tumors, there are frequently contrasting areas of high and low cellularity. Cells within the nodules frequently exhibit cytologic evidence of neuronal differentiation, while the surrounding cells are more anaplastic and more mitotically active (Fig. 6). Mutations in the PTCH gene may occur specifically in this histologic variant of medulloblastoma (123). Medullomyoblastoma is characterized by the presence of striated or smooth muscle cells. Melanotic medulloblastoma is characterized by undifferentiated cells containing melanin. All variants of medulloblastoma can spread throughout the CNS, and systemic metastases, especially to bone, have been observed and documented

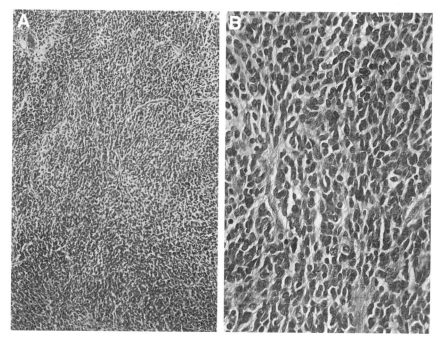

Fig. 3. Medulloblastoma. This hematoxylin and eosin stained histologic section demonstrates densely packed round to oval shaped cells with hyperchromatic nuclei and little cytoplasm. Low magnification (**A**), higher magnification (**B**).

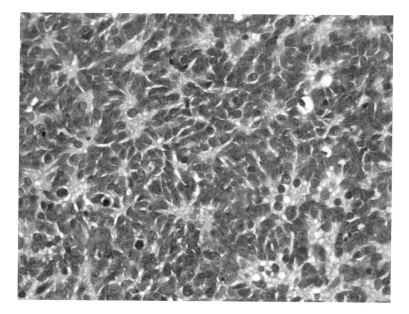

Fig. 4. Medulloblastoma with neuroblastic differentiation. This hematoxylin and eosin stained histologic section demonstrates the presence of Homer-Wright rosettes in which tumor cells surround pockets of neuropile.

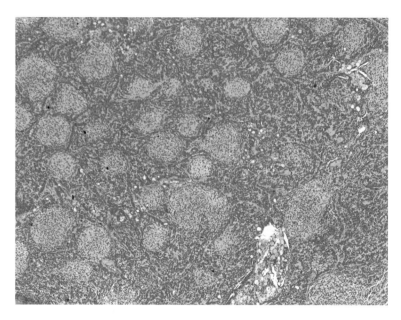

Fig. 5. Desmoplastic medulloblastoma. This hematoxylin and eosin stained histologic section demonstrates the nodular appearance of desmoplastic medulloblastoma. The pale nodular zones are surrounded by densely packed small round tumor cells that produce a dense reticulin network, which is not present within the nodules.

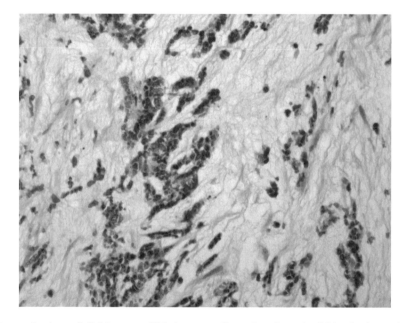

Fig. 6. Desmoplastic medulloblastoma. This hematoxylin and eosin stained histologic section reveals the streaming of anaplastic tumor cells on a fibrillary background of reticulin.

for varying histologies. Recently, a histologic grading system for medulloblastoma has been proposed *(44)*. This classification grew out of the observation that there may be a spectrum of tumors with varying degrees of anaplasia as evidenced by desmoplastic medulloblastoma with easily recognizable evidence of differentiation as compared to very undifferentiated large-cell medulloblastomas *(51,117)*. This grading system may be of clinical and prognostic value as the extent of anaplasia was associated with more aggressive clinical behavior *(44,117)*

2.1.4. Pathogenesis

Medulloblastoma is thought to arise from precursor cells of the external germinal layer of the cerebellum, although there remains some controversy regarding this point *(151,157)*. The cerebellar cortex includes a number of different types of neurons of which granule cells are the most abundant. In mice, the lack of granule cells is associated with gait disturbances, and it is thought that the major function of these cells is to modulate the activity of Purkinje cells, neurons that are key in the control of motor function. Other cells that have been proposed as a source of medulloblastoma are the undifferentiated cells of the medullary vellum that migrate to the external germinal layer, and neural stem cells present in the cerebellum. Whereas these cells probably persist physiologically in large numbers for only a short time after birth, residual precursor cells or stem cells could persist longer. All of these cell types appear cytologically similar to the undifferentiated cells of medulloblastoma. Granular cell precursors, found early in development in the external germinal layer, proliferate extensively, differentiate, and migrate to form the internal granular layer of the fully mature cerebellum. The failure of these cells to progress through the normal pathways of neuronal differentiation, may contribute to the development of medulloblastoma *(151)*. Compelling evidence supporting this hypothesis comes from the observation of Zic expression in medulloblastoma cells *(157)*. Zic, a novel zinc finger protein, is expressed primarily in the nuclei of the cerebellar granule cell lineage.

2.1.4.1. GENETIC FEATURES

The patterns of gene expression in tumors determine their biologic properties and pathologic behaviors. The expression of some genes in tumor cells may reflect the cell of origin, whereas others might result directly from events that underlie the pathogenesis of individual tumors. Medulloblastomas arise from cells of the nervous system as described earlier, and among the genes expressed in these tumors that reflect this origin and that may also contribute to the pathobiology of these tumors are neurotrophin receptors of the TRK family. TRK family members encode the high-affinity receptor tyrosine kinases that bind neurotrophins of the nerve growth factor family. During normal development TRK mediated signals are of major importance for nervous system morphogenesis and maturation. Whereas members of the TRK gene family have been found to be mutated in some tumor types and can contribute to the malignant transformation of normal cells in laboratory experiments, mutations of TRK genes have not been reported in medulloblastoma. However, the expression of TRKc in medulloblastoma has been widely recognized and its expression has been correlated with an improved prognosis *(60,136)*.

Another developmentally regulated gene that may be involved in the pathogenesis of medulloblastoma is PAX5, a member of the PAX family of homeobox genes *(85)*. PAX5 expression can be detected in medulloblastoma, but not in normal cerebellum. The potential role of homeobox-containing proteins such as PAX5, which have been found in medulloblastoma or other tumors, has not been well described. Similarly, genes known to play important roles in normal cerebellar development, such as molecules important for Notch-mediated signaling in external germinal layer cells *(138)*, may be important candidates for better understanding the pathology of tumors of the cerebellum but have not yet been explored in this context.

Mutations of genes whose expression is important for normal development, cellular proliferation, and cellular differentiation underlie the development of medulloblastoma as they underlie oncogenesis in many other tissues. Much of our knowledge of the specific genetic changes and the molecular pathways involved in the pathogenesis of medulloblastoma comes from the recognition of clinicians that, although most cases of medulloblastoma are sporadic and occur unexpectedly, rare cases do occur in association with other malignancies. Such associations occur in nevoid basal-cell carcinoma syndrome, Turcot's syndrome, and the Li Faumeni syndrome.

The nevoid basal cell carcinoma syndrome, or Gorlin's syndrome, is an autosomal dominantly inherited disorder characterized by multiple basal-cell carcinoma and, commonly, skeletal abnormalities. A variety of other tumors also occur in these patients, including brain tumors, especially medulloblastoma. Nonetheless, the incidence of medulloblastoma in patients with nevoid basal cell carcinoma syndrome is probably less than 5%, and when such tumors do occur, they occur early in life *(78,149)*. The gene altered in the nevoid basal cell carcinoma syndrome is the human homologue (PTCH) of the *Drosophilia melanogaster* gene, Patched. PTCH maps to human chromosome 9q22.3-9q31. Although loss of heterozygosity (LOH) at these loci is infrequent in sporadic medulloblastomas, it has been reported to be associated with a specific histologic variant of medulloblastoma called desmoplastic medulloblastoma *(134,150)*. Interestingly, desmoplastic medulloblastoma has been considered by others as a genetic entity that was distinguishable from medulloblastoma with a more classical histopathologic appearance based upon DNA content *(50)* and/or molecular cytogenetic analysis *(12,134)*. Patients with the nevoid basal cell carcinoma syndrome have germline alterations in one copy of the PTCH gene, and tumors that occur in these patients, including medulloblastoma, may have detectable evidence of the loss of the other allele, suggesting that inactivation of the cellular pathway in which PTCH is active may be necessary for tumor development *(155)*.

However, loss of the second PTCH allele in sporadic medulloblastomas that exhibit evidence for loss of one PTCH allele oftentimes cannot be documented, and recently haploinsufficiency of PTCH has been proposed as sufficient to predispose to the development of medulloblastoma *(165)*. This interpretation is based largely on the finding that Ptch +/– mice, which develop medulloblastoma *(57)*, also retain the wild type allele *(165)* and the tumors continue to express Ptch mRNA *(153)*. Nearly 15% of animals heterozygous for Ptch develop CNS tumors histologically indistinguishable from medulloblastoma in the posterior fossa by 10 mo of age, with a peak tumor incidence occurring between 16 and 24 wk of age. PTCH is thought to be a transmembrane receptor for the secreted ligand sonic hedgehog (SHH) and functions in collaboration with another transmembrane protein, smoothened (SMOH), to regulate organ development (Fig. 7) *(57)*. This pathway is particularly important in the developing CNS. The addition of SHH to cerebellar cells in culture leads to the proliferation of external germinal layer cells, and blocking SHH activity results in a decrease in the number of external germinal layer cells *(138)*. These findings are consistent with the model that the loss of PTCH or the enhanced activity of SHH results in increased downstream activity of the SHH/PTCH signaling pathway that might lead to increased cell proliferation and tumorigenesis.

Another gene whose role in the pathogenesis of medulloblastoma is less well understood, but which is likely to be important, is suppressor of fused (SUFU) *(145)*. Very recently, exciting work has shown that SUFU mutations occur in the germline of a subset of children with medulloblastoma, and there is a loss of the remaining wild-type allele in tumors that develop in these children. SUFU plays a role in the PTCH signaling pathway, and homozygous deletion of SUFU would be expected to result in activation of the SHH signaling pathway.

Although PTCH signaling remains under investigation, among the important downstream targets of PTCH activation are the GLI family of transcription factors. The activity of these transcription factors is regulated as a result of signaling through the PTCH/SHH pathway. Under physiologic circumstance, PTCH inhibits SMOH, which in turn modifies the function of GLI family members. When SHH binds and inactivates PTCH, SMOH relays the SHH signal into the cell, activating GLI1 and GLI2 activity, while repressing GLI3. Whereas GLI1 is expressed in medulloblastoma, GLI1 mutations have not been found in sporadic medulloblastoma. PTCH/SHH also regulates GLI, but whether this leads to inhibition or activation of downstream targets in medulloblastoma tissues is unknown.

Sonic Hedgehog Signaling Pathway

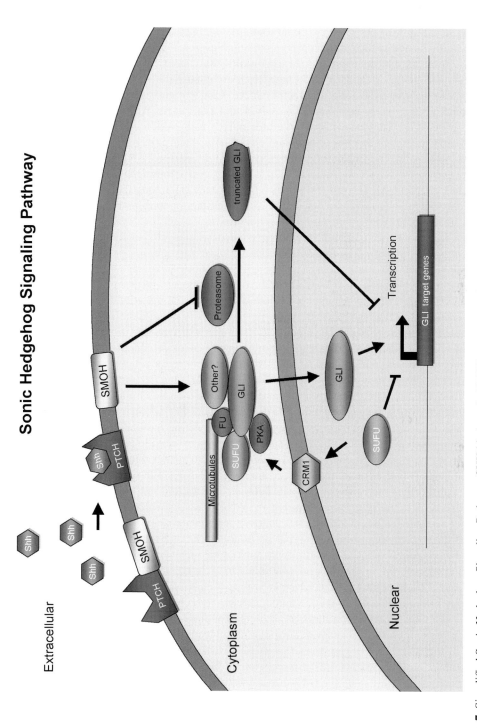

Fig. 7. Simplified Sonic Hedgehog Signaling Pathway. SHH binds to the PTCH receptor causing release of SMOH. SMOH blocks carboxyl-terminal cleavage of phosphorylated GLI (Zinc-finger transcription factors [GLI1, 2, and 3]) by the proteasome. FU and PKA are protein kinases that may phosphorylate GLIs to target them for proteasome-mediated modification. This prevents formation of c-terminal truncated GLIs that can act to repress transcription of GLI target genes. Either GLIs or truncated GLIs can translocate to the nucleus to transactivate or suppress transcription of various target genes. SUFU appears to block GLI transcriptional activity by binding to it in the nucleus and promoting its nuclear export via CRM1. SUFU also sequesters GLI in the cytoplasm and promotes its degradation.

Protein kinase A (PKA) appears to be a component of the protein complex downstream of PTCH/SHH signaling, which regulates GLI phosphorylation and proteasome-mediated modification, but to date PKA has not been implicated in the pathogenesis of medulloblastoma.

Turcot's syndrome is characterized by brain tumors that occur in patients with familial adenomatous polyposis (FAP) *(62)*. FAP is an autosomal dominant familial disorder that typically presents with osteoma, bone cysts, and colorectal cancer (CRC) in early adult life, secondary to extensive adenomatous polyps of the colon as a result of mutations in the APC gene. Typically, the colons of these patients are studded with innumerable polyps from which adenocarcinoma of the colon develops early in life. Both glial tumors and medulloblastoma have been described in such families. Glial tumors, typically glioblastoma multiforme, that develop in FAP patients are typically characterized by genomic evidence of microsatellite instability and somatic mutations in DNA mismatch repair genes including MLH1 and PMS2 *(62)*. These genes are among the DNA repair genes whose germ line mutation is known to be associated with hereditary nonpolyposis colorectal cancer, and it is possible that patients with colon cancer and glial tumors, though considered to have Turcot's syndrome, are pathophysiologically distinct from FAP patients who develop medulloblastoma *(147)*. Consistent with this idea is the finding that these patients typically have fewer polyps than are typically seen in FAP patients.

Medulloblastoma typically arises in a small subgroup of FAP patients with extensive polyposis and mutation of the APC gene *(62)*. In patients with extensive polyposis, mutations of the APC gene typically occur in the central region of the APC gene, the mutation cluster region (MCR), and result in expression of COOH-terminally truncated proteins. Loss of the wild type APC in colorectal tumors and medulloblastoma is consistent with the Knudson hypothesis that loss of function through inactivation of the second allele occurs during tumorigenesis when tumors arise in patients with familial predisposition syndromes. These tumors do not display evidence of DNA replication errors, suggesting that the mutation of APC is an initiating event in the development of these tumors *(67)*. Mutations in APC have been reported *(69)*, but most studies have been unable to find such mutations *(102)*. In contrast, mutations of β-catenin *((45,69,166)*, a cytoplasmic signaling molecule, and axin1 *(37)*, a scaffolding protein—both downstream of APC—have been found in medulloblastoma.

APC functions in the WNT signaling pathway, which plays important roles in development and cell proliferation in many tissues including the nervous system (Fig. 8). The activity of WNT signaling pathways is tightly regulated by the components of the pathway, and also by factors in the extracellular environment, particularly glycosaminoglycans. WNT genes, of which there are approx 20 in mammals, encode secreted ligands that bind to transmembrane receptors belonging to the FRIZZLED family *(39)*. FRIZZLED activation leads to signal transduction through the cytoplasmic disheveled (Dsh) protein which interacts with the constitutively active glycogen synthase kinase (GSK3). APC is complexed to GSK3 and the scaffolding protein, axin *(104)*. In the absence of a WNT signal this complex binds and phosphorylates the cytoplasmic protein β-catenin, a modification that targets it for degradation by a ubiquitin/proteasome-mediated pathway *(83)*. Activation of the WNT pathway leads to inhibition of GSK3 kinase, stabilization of β-catenin, and accumulation of β-catenin in the cell. This aberrant accumulation of β-catenin in the cytoplasm leads to nuclear transport of β-catenin where it binds to the HMG box of the transcription factors of the TCF/LEF family *(45)*. The β-catenin/TCF complex acts to modulate the transcription of such WNT target genes as CMYC and cyclin D. Importantly, activating mutations of β-catenin have been documented in sporadic medulloblastoma, as has the nuclear localization of β-catenin, an indication that the molecule is activated in these tumors *(60,157)*.

While functional aspects of the WNT signaling pathway have not been extensively studied in medulloblastoma, they have been studied in colonic tissue and tissue from colonic tumors. In colonic tissue, CMYC expression is repressed by wild type APC and activated by β-catenin, and these effects were mediated through TCF4 binding sites in the CMYC promoter, a finding consistent with the widely reported observation that CMYC expression is elevated in adenocarcinoma of the colon *(64)*.

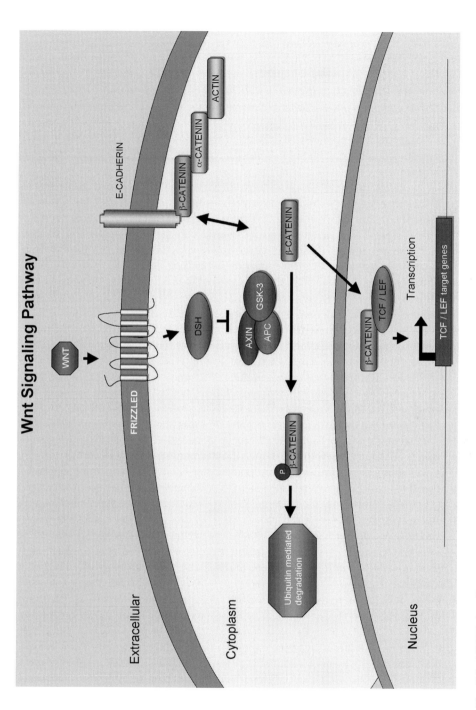

Fig 8. Simplified WNT signaling pathway. The WNT signaling pathway plays a significant role in organogenesis and embryonic fate determination. The WNT ligand binds the frizzled receptor that in turn activates disheveled (DSH). β-Catenin has multiple functions including bridging E-cadherin to the actin cytoskeleton. β-Catenin not associated with E-cadherin is phosphorylated by the GSK-3/APC/Axin complex. The phospho-β-catenin is degraded by the ubiquitination-mediated pathway. DSH blocks phosphorylation of β-catenin allowing it to accumulate in the cytoplasm and translocate to the nucleus, where it binds with TCF/LEF family of transcription factors and leads to expression of target genes including MYC, CYCLIN D1, and WISP.

These findings are consistent with a model in which the deletion of APC or the activation of β-catenin could result in overactivity of the WNT signaling pathway to give rise to colon cancer, and by extension to medulloblastoma *(103)*. Such a model is supported by the finding of increased expression of CMYC, and rarely, amplication of the CMYC gene in medulloblastoma tissues. β-Catenin may also contribute to the development of medulloblastoma as the result of disorder functioning in its role in cell–cell communication. Both mutations in β-catenin and cytoplasmic expression suggest this possibility. β-catenin binds to E-cadherin and N-cadherin transmembrane proteins that are important elements of adherens junctions required for cell-cell contacts. While there are data to indicate a role for these structures in the maintenance of epithelial layers and "contact inhibition" of cell growth, a role for this function in the pathogenesis of medulloblastoma has not been explored although cadherins are expressed in the brain *(129)*.

As discussed earlier, mutation of components of either the SHH or WNT signaling pathways can cause inappropriate, persistent activation of these pathways in medulloblastoma *(158,164)*. It is interesting to note that interactions occur between these two important pathways in the normal course of normal development. WNT signaling can act to positively or negatively regulate GLI2 transactivation activity and suppress GLI3 repressor activity during somite formation in the avian embryo *(29)*. Both GLI2 and GLI3 have been shown to have roles in modulating activation of GLI1 *(40)*. So WNT signaling might modulate GLI1 activity through regulating GLI2 and 3 activities. Conversely GLI proteins are capable of regulating WNT expression *(107)*. Therefore, dysregulation of one pathway could have an effect on the other and may contribute to the formation of medulloblastoma.

The Li Fraumeni syndrome is another inherited tumor predisposition in which affected individuals have developed medulloblastoma, although this is not one of the more common tumors these individuals develop *(80)*. The spectrum of tumors associated with this syndrome is wide. Li Fraumeni syndrome occurs as the result of inherited mutations in the TP53 tumor suppressor gene. The TP53 locus, located on chromosome 17p, has been examined in sporadic medulloblastomas, but mutations at this locus are uncommon *(2,8)*. MDM2 is a gene that encodes a protein important for the destruction of p53 and high levels of MDM2 can inactivate p53. Whereas the amplification of MDM2, which does occur in some tumors, has not been found to occur in medulloblastoma *(2)*, high levels of MDM2 expression have been detected in a subset of medulloblastoma and found to correlate with a poor prognosis *(56)*. p53 mediates a number of different biologies important for tumorigenesis, including genomic stability, cell-cycle arrest following DNA damage, and apoptosis, and alterations in genes in any of these pathways could be envisioned as an alternative means for inactivating one or another p53 function *(163)*.

Interestingly, a second locus on chromosome 17p23, telomeric to TP53, has been found to be frequently deleted in medulloblastoma, and suggests the presence of a tumor suppressor gene that is deleted in medulloblastomas *(34,99,124,139)*. Deletions at this locus have also been associated with an aggressive clinical course *(10,141)*.

CMYC and NMYC amplifications have been reported to occasionally occur in medulloblastoma tumors *(8,9,30,49,95)*. High-level MYC expression may be a marker of poor prognosis in medulloblastoma *(8,59,65)*.

In addition to the structural alterations in genes important for normal development and cellular proliferation that underlie the development of medulloblastoma, the inappropriate expression of genes may also contribute to tumorigenesis. Genes whose altered expression in medulloblastoma may be of clinical significance include TrkC *(108,136)*, ERBB, and RE1-silencing transcription factor (REST)/ neuron-restrictive silencer factor (NRSF) *(71,91)*. As discussed earlier, TrkC is a neurotrophin receptor that mediates transmembrane signal by the ligand NT-3 in neuronal progenitor cells. TrkC expression has been recognized to be a likely positive prognostic marker for children with medulloblastoma *(60,136)*. Importantly, expression of this tyrosine kinase receptor may mark a subgroup of patients whose tumor biology is different because of changes in biology mediated by TrkC. TrkC mediates NT-3 induced apoptosis of medulloblastoma in vitro, and TrkC expression is highly correlated with apoptosis in clinical specimens of medulloblastoma. The importance of these findings is supported by the observation that TrkC overexpression inhibits the growth of an intracerebral xenograft of medulloblastoma grown in immunosuppressed mice *(77)*. These findings speak to a potential role for TrkC in the pathologic behavior of medulloblastoma.

The epidermal growth factor receptor (EGFR) family of genes has also been implicated in the pathogenesis of medulloblastoma. Four EGFR family members EGFR, ERBB2, ERBB3, and ERBB4, have been examined in medulloblastoma. Whereas a mutant EGFR receptor, EGFRvIII, in which the extracellular domain has been deleted resulting in the formation of a new, tumor-specific antigen has been reported in medulloblastoma *(105)*, this finding has not been confirmed and evidence for the inappropriate expression of EGFR or ERBB3 has not been reported. High levels of other heregulin receptors have been reported in these tumors. Interestingly, while ERBB2 may be highly expressed in most medulloblastoma tumor tissues, it is not detectable during cerebellar development *(53)*. This finding and the observations that ERBB4 is both highly expressed in medulloblastoma and that the coexpression of ERBB2 and ERBB4 in medulloblastoma may be of prognostic significance for these patients *(54)*, suggest a role for these tyrosine kinase growth factor receptors in the pathogensis of medulloblastoma.

Another gene of potential biologic and therapeutic importance for patients with medulloblastoma is REST/NRSF. This transcription factor, which functions physiologically to inhibit the transcription of genes typically expressed in neuronal cells, is highly expressed in medulloblastoma. Suppression of this inhibition leads to the expression of these genes in medulloblastoma cells, and can induce apoptosis in these cells *(71,91)*. Inhibition of REST/NRSF function in xenografts of medulloblastoma by the injection of a recombinant adenovirus expressing a REST-VP16 chimeric protein inhibits medulloblastoma growth, suggesting a role for this gene in the pathogenesis of this tumor.

Both classical cytogenetics and more recently developed molecular strategies have been utilized to discover genes important in the pathogenesis of medulloblastoma. Genetic changes in addition to those mentioned earlier, especially isochromosome (17q), which is present in approx 30–50% of cases *(18)*, includes rearrangements of chromosomes 2p, 6q, 8p, 20q, 22p, 22q, and 26q *(17,26)*. Reciprocal translocations, common in childhood hematopoietic tumors, have rarely been detected in medulloblastoma *(7)*. More recently, comparative genomic hybridization has been used to examine medulloblastoma tumors for evidence of chromosomal amplification or deletion *(11,55,72,101,111,127,156)*. Comparative genomic hybridization analysis confirmed some of the allelic imbalances detected by conventional cytogenetic approaches, and has identified previously unrecognized chromosomal regions as being either amplified or deleted *(109,133)*. Among chromosomal regions found in multiple studies to be present in increased copy number in medulloblastoma are 2p, 7q, 13q, 17q, and 18q *(101,111,137)*. Similarly, loss of chromosomal DNA has been reported in multiple studies at 8p, 11q, 16q, and 17p *(101,111,137)*. Consistent with the loss of DNA from 17p has been the observation that 17p11.2 is commonly hypermethylated in medulloblastoma tumors *(48)*.

Other regions that have been reported to be presenting increased copy number include 1q, 2q, 3q, 4q, 6q, 7p, 8q, 9p, 11p, 14q, 17p, 18p, and 21q. Loss of chromosomal material has been reported at 1p, 5p, 10p, 11p, 13p, 18p, 20q, and 20p. Whether these chromosomal regions will harbor genes important for the pathogenesis of medulloblastoma or genes only indirectly involved is not known, but these sites do remain as focal points for pursuing future investigations.

2.1.4.2. POSSIBLE ENVIRONMENTAL FACTORS

There are no known environmental causes of medulloblastoma. Recent work in which the presence of viral sequences from the human polyoma virus, JC, were detected in some samples of medulloblastoma tissue was of particular interest because it was possible to demonstrate in a subset of these tumors the expression of JC T-antigen *(76,87)*. JC DNA was not detectable in brain tissue from healthy individuals. Although JC infection is ubiquitous in many populations, including the United States *(121)*, it is generally latent and undetectable in individuals who are immunocompetent.

Also, JC virus infection of hamsters can cause tumors that mimic medulloblastoma *(161)*, and transgenic mice in which JC virus T-antigen was expressed in the cerebellum developed medulloblastoma as well *(88)*. SV40 is another polyoma virus that is found, though less commonly, in the human population. SV40 sequences have also been detected in medulloblastoma tissues *(87,160)*, although these are not thought to be present in brain tissue from normal patients, and were not detectable from normal tissue present in the same histologic section from which tumor tissue containing SV40 sequences were detected *(70)*. These findings are significant in that both SV40 large T-antigen and JC virus large T-antigen inactivate both Rb and p53, important tumor suppressor genes in a wide range of human tumors, and JC virus T-antigen has been shown to interact directly with these tumor suppressors in tumor tissue from medulloblastoma arising in JC-expressing transgenic mice *(89)*. These findings suggest a role for disruption of the regulatory pathways in which p53 and Rb play important key roles *(61)*, a possibility strongly supported by the observation that Trp53-null mice in which Rb has been inactivated in cells of the external germinal layer develop medulloblastoma *(98)*.

2.2. Cerebral Primitive Neuroectodermal Tumor

2.2.1. General Description

Primitive neuroectodermal tumor (PNET) of the cerebrum or supratentorial PNET is an embryonal tumor distinguished from medulloblastoma primarily, but not exclusively, by its supratentorial location. Historically, these tumors have been known as cerebral neuroblastomas, although this name is rarely used now. Pineoblastomas, highly undifferentiated tumors of the pineal glands are probably distinct pathologic entities *(79)*. PNETs are thought to arise in cells of the primitive neuroepithelium. These tumors are histopathologically similar to medulloblastoma with varying proportions of features that suggest astrocytic or ependymal differentiation. Typically, they are poorly differentiated and appear histologically as sheets of small, round blue cells, although on occasion they may express evidence of differentiation along any of several lineages including neuronal, astrocytic, or melanocytic cell types. Because of this tumor's very anaplastic appearance and its aggressive pathological behavior, it is classified as grade IV by the WHO *(79)*. The incidence of this tumor type is unknown, but it is rare. Perhaps 2% of pediatric brain tumors are supratentorial PNETs, or approximately one-tenth as common as medulloblastoma. PNETs occur in children primarily, although they can rarely occur in adults.

2.2.2. Clinical Presentation and Treatment Approaches

The clinical presentation of PNET, like other brain tumors, reflects the site and the rapidity of tumor growth. Rapidly growing tumors can lead to symptoms associated with increased intracranial pressure including somnolence. Tumors arising in the cortex oftentimes are associated with headache. Seizures, though a more common symptom in low-grade astrocytic tumors involving the cortex, can also occur in patients with PNET. If these symptoms occur in the motor region, disturbances of gait or hemiplegia can be observed. Suprasellar tumors can compress the optic nerves, causing visual disturbances, or lead to endocrine disorders as a result of pituitary malfunctions. PNETs can disseminate throughout the neuroaxis, and patients should be evaluated by diagnostic imaging of the brain and spinal cord *(82)*.

As is the case for other tumors of the CNS, imaging is a key diagnostic and patient management tool. PNETs tend to be large tumors, with the exception of those arising at the base of the skull near the optic chiasm. These tumors rarely occur in the midline; most commonly, they are located in the frontal and temporal lobes causing them to become symptomatic earlier in their course. Whereas the CT appearance of PNET is similar to that of medulloblastoma and does not vary systematically among tumors arising at different locations in the CNS, the MRI appearance of PNETs may vary as a function of the site of origin. Tumors of the cortex may appear hypointense relative to adjacent grey

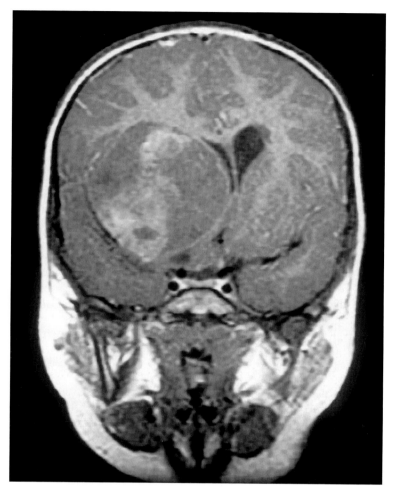

Fig. 9. MRI of a child with a primitive neuroectodermal tumor of the cerebrum. This is a T1 coronal MR image following the injection of gadolinium, demonstrating tumor enhancement and compression of the lateral ventricle.

matter, whereas in other regions a hypointense appearance on T1 images is more consistent with hemorrhage. T2 images are also hypointense, although cysts and regions of necrosis are hyperintense. Consistent with their high pathologic grade, PNETs enhance following the administration of gadolinium (Fig. 9). MRI of the entire neuroaxis, including the spine, should be performed with gadolinium to evaluate subarachnoid metastases on the surface of the brain and spinal cord, as well as within the spinal canal *(82)*.

There are no well established staging systems for cerebral PNET and no prognostic factors have been critically evaluated, although there is widespread agreement that patients with disseminated disease at presentation do poorly compared with patients with localized disease *(116)*. Based upon the experience of clinical investigators in the evaluation of patients with medulloblastoma and other primary brain tumors, more extensive surgical resections are likely to be associated with improved survival rates in patients who present without evidence of spread beyond the site of the primary tumor. Patients with disseminated tumor, unresectable tumor, or recurrent tumor are widely considered to be at highest risk *(128)*.

Surgery is the mainstay of therapy, and resecting the maximum amount of tumor that can be removed safely is important, though the extent of resection has not been as tightly linked to outcome in these patients as it has been in patients with medulloblastoma. Radiation therapy should then be used for virtually all children with this tumor type. The suggested tumor dose is 54 Gy using conventional fractionation. Craniospinal irradiation with 36 Gy is important because of the high rate of relapse at sites within the neuroaxis but distant from the primary tumor. Whereas randomized trials have indicated a role for adjuvant chemotherapy in improving the overall survival of children with medulloblastoma (35,114,128), there have not been sufficiently large groups of children with supratentorial PNET to pursue a systematic evaluation of such therapies in children with this tumor. There is not a defined role for chemotherapy, and there are no agents that are known to be efficacious in the treatment of this tumor. Nonetheless, because of the very poor prognosis for children with extensive disease or disease remaining after surgery, chemotherapy is widely used in the treatment of these patients. Multiagent therapy used for medulloblastoma is most commonly employed for this tumor as well, although the prognosis seems worse for children with supratentorial PNET than with medulloblastoma (35,114,128). Very young children with PNET may have a poorer prognosis than other children, but as described earlier, chemotherapy can be used to delay the initiation of radiation therapy in young children because of the known toxicities associated with high dose irradiation. While such children may respond to chemotherapy, currently available regimes are not sufficient to cure patients of these tumors (97). Importantly, chemotherapy and the underlying pathology associated with these tumors can also be associated with significant residual neurologic deficits.

2.2.3. Pathological Features

The pathologic classification of supratentorial PNET is an area of considerable research interest. It remains unclear, despite modern research strategies to address the question, whether embryonal, small round cell tumors of the CNS are most thoughtfully considered a single, although quite variable, pathologic entity reflecting the malignant transformation of primitive neuroectodermal cells or a disparate group of highly undifferentiated tumors. Whereas the histological features of embryonal, small round cell tumors occurring in different sites throughout the CNS, including medulloblastoma occurring in the posterior fossa, are similar, the prognosis for children with medulloblastoma and PNET is quite different (6,41,140). This difference may reflect fundamental biological differences between these two groups of tumors, and this could be the result of different cells of origin or differences in the malignant characteristics of these tumors. However, in both tumor types the extent of surgical resection is a key prognostic determinant (6,5,140), and one can easily imagine that obtaining complete or near complete resections is more easily achieved and more common in the posterior fossa than in supratentorial sites.

PNETs may grow to very large size, often with cystic areas, and typically appear as well circumscribed lesions, although microscopically they can be recognized as invariably invading adjacent tissue and frequently extending far beyond the anticipated margins. These tumors can have a variable desmoplastic component, which is typically collagenous in nature. Tumors with extensive desmoplasia tend to be firmer than those without a desmoplastic component. Hemorrhage is a common finding, and although these tumors frequently exhibit easily detectable apoptosis, necrosis is rare.

The histologic and cytologic appearance of these tumors mimics the appearance of medulloblastoma (Fig. 10). The cells are typically small with a low cytoplastic to nuclear ratio with a round, regular, basophilic nucleus (81). The mitotic index of these tumors is typically very high, and mitotic figures are readily detectable in many tumors. While the characteristic appearance of these tumors is very undifferentiated, there may be evidence of differentiation along divergent pathways including neuronal, astrocytic, and ependymol (Fig. 11). Immunohistochemical evidence of such differentiation is oftentimes necessary to demonstrate such differentiation. The finding of neuroendocrine differentiation as evidenced by the expression of synaptophysin and neuropeptides may be more common than generally appreciated, indicating that PNETs as well as medulloblastomas share phenotypic feature with neuroendocrine tumors.

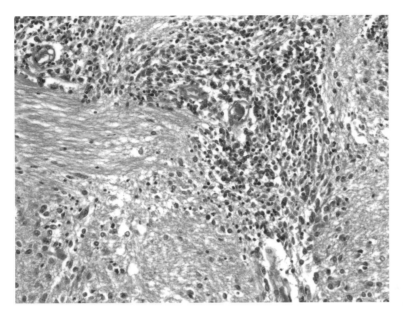

Fig. 10. Cerebral primitive neuroectodermal tumor. This hematoxylin and eosin stained histologic section reveals the highly cellular nature of these invasive tumors, which can also have well-demarcated regions delineating the adjacent brain tissue.

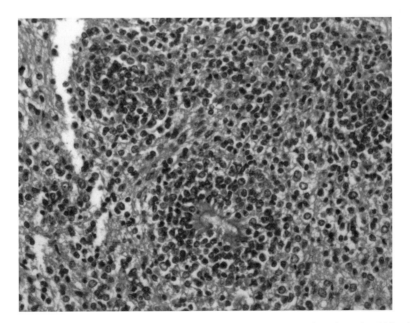

Fig. 11. PNET with pendymoblastic differentiation. This hematoxylin and eosin stained histologic section of a highly cellular PNET arising in the cerebrum shows cytologic ependymal features, but lacks the ependymal rosettes characteristic of pendymoma.

Nonetheless, there are several lines of investigation that suggest possible differences in medullo-blastoma and PNETs that could explain substantive differences in their pathophysiology. In addition to differences in the genetic alterations that are commonly observed in these tumors, there are cyto-logical and pathological differences have been reported. The detection of Zic expression in precursor cells of the external germinal layer of the cerebellum and in medulloblastoma is consistent with the origin of these tumors in this cell type *(157)*. Remarkably, this gene was not detected in PNETs, a finding interpreted as suggesting a distinctive origin for these, tumors *(157)*, a topic that has been extensively reviewed *(110,132)*. Like medulloblastomas synaptophysin, neuropeptides are oftentimes expressed in CNS PNETs, but a highly variable intermediate filament expression pattern suggests that these tumors are distinct from medulloblastomas *(58)*. These findings and their interpretation are consistent with the elegant, recently published studies in which genomic approaches to the evaluation of primitive embryonal tumors of the CNS provided strong evidence indicating that medulloblasto-mas and PNETS are molecularly distinctive entities *(126)*.

2.2.4. Pathogenesis

The histogenesis of PNETs as a group has been a controversial issue, and the cell of origin of these tumors is unknown. The i(17q) abnormality found in 30 to 50% of medulloblastomas does not occur in PNETs, and the aberrant hypermethylation of the major breakpoint cluster region at 17p11.2 in medulloblastomas also is not detectable in PNETs *(48)*. This finding is consistent with more global screens for genetic changes in these tumors. Studies utilizing comparative genomic hybridization strategies to examine chromosomal structure *(109,133)* or gene expression array technology to exam-ine patterns of gene expression *(126)* have detected evidence that distinguishes PNET from medullo-blastoma, which differ in location but not in histologic appearance. While no large or systematic studies of the molecular genetic abnormalities have been developed, there have been occasional reports of mutations in the TP53 gene and MYC gene expression, but these do not seem to be prominent features of these tumors.

2.3. Atypical Teratoid Tumors

2.3.1. General Description

While atypical teratoid/rhabdoid tumors (AT/RT) have not been as widely recognized as a distinc-tive pathological entity as other poorly differentiated tumors of childhood, recent studies have defined more clearly this entity, and it now is more widely appreciated *(113,130)*. AT/RTs typically contain extensive fields of undifferentiated malignant neuroectodermal cells that are indistinguish-able from medulloblastoma or PNET tissue until the presence of rhabdoid cells is recognized. While this tumor had been described earlier, a report from Rorke and colleagues *(132)* called attention to the distinguishing characteristics of this tumor's presentation and histologic appearance and focused attention on it as an important disease entity. Of particular importance in this regard was the recogni-tion of the rhabdoid appearance of some cells, while also noting the presence of mesenchymal and epithelial elements *(31)*. Rarely, these tumors occur in children who also have malignant rhabdoid tumors, most frequently occurring in the kidney *(1,28,47,68)*.

2.3.2. Clinical Presentation and Treatment Approaches

AT/RTs typically occur in infants and very young children. Kleihues and Cavanee *(79)* identified almost 200 cases that included only a few adults.. There was a slight preponderance in males, but this tumor occurs in individuals of both sexes with similar incidence. AT/RTs can occur throughout the CNS with almost an equal chance of occurring in the cerebrum and in the posterior fossa (Fig. 12). Importantly, it has been estimated that as many as a third of patients may have detectable metastases at the time of diagnosis *(4)*. Like other brain tumors, the clinical presentation is greatly influenced by the location of the tumor and the rapidity of its growth *(16)*. Typically, AT/RTs are clinically aggres-sive tumors. Rapid growth is often associated with a more dramatic and more rapidly developing

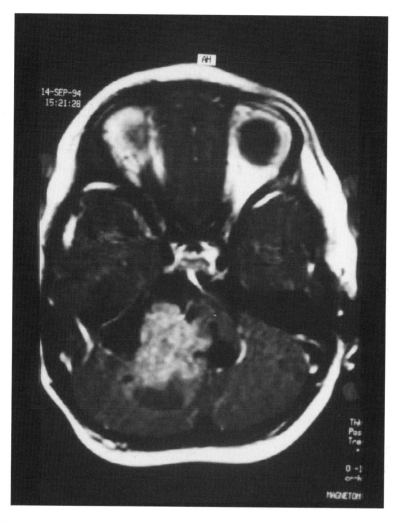

Fig. 12. MRI of child with an atypical teratoid/rhabdoid tumor of the cerebellum. This is a T1 axial MR image following the injection of gadolinium, demonstrating tumor enhancement.

clinical syndrome. In very young children, this can be predominantly nonspecific symptoms including failure to thrive and lethargy.

The appearance of AT/RTs by either CT or MRI is not different from that observed in other primitive neuroectodermal tumors of childhood *(32,162)*. These tumors do not appear as homogenous masses, though they enhance with gadolinium, emphasizing their infiltrative nature and the disruption of the blood barrier that typically characterizes them. Cysts and evidence of bleeding are sometimes present. Treatment includes surgery followed by radiotherapy and chemotherapy, although no prospective clinical trials have been conducted *(113)*. There is no standard or highly effective therapy known. Various chemotherapeutic regimens have been used *(27,66,152)* and cures have been reported *(112)*. Typically, this is a rapidly progressive neoplasm that responds poorly to available modalities of therapy *(112,113,130)*, although early experience with very intensive chemotherapeutic regimens seems hopeful *(66)*.

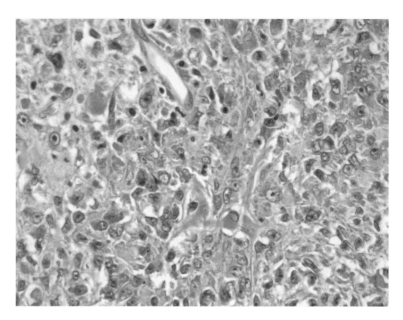

Fig. 13. AT/RT. This hematoxylin and eosin stained histologic section reveals typical rhabdoid cells that are round to oval in shape with eccentric nuclei and prominent nucleoli. The cytoplasm is finely granular with a tapering tail and contains dense pink regions that mimic the appearance of inclusion bodies.

2.3.3. Pathological Features

The macroscopic appearance of AT/RT is not characteristic, although obvious areas of necrosis and hemorrhage may be present. In contrast, the histologic appearance and immunohistochemical characteristics of these tumors are distinctive, which is consistent with the mesenchymal and epithelial elements that are always present, along with evidence of rapid growth, namely mitotic figures, cell death, and apoptosis. Cytologically, rhabdoid cells may be the prominent cell type easily visible or they may appear in nests or among monotonous fields of undifferentiated neuroepithelial cells (Fig. 13). Rhabdoid cells appear as medium-sized round cells with indented nuclei, conspicuous nucleoli, and prominent eosinophilic cytoplasmic inclusions *(13)*. Examination by electron microscopy

---

Fig. 14. *(opposite page)* The SWI/SNF complex has been implicated as a chromatin remodeling complex with ATPase activity that facilitates DNA access for various transcription factors, and can act as either a co-activator or a corepressor. The SNF5/INI1 protein appears to be a core protein of this complex of approx 10 proteins. Mutation of the SNF5/INI1 has been implicated in the development of rhabdoid tumors occurring at various locations. While specific regulation of SNF5/INI1 is poorly understood, the activity of the SWI/SNF complex appears to be cell-cycle dependent. SWI/SNF is phosphorylated and inactivated at the G2/M transition. SNF5/INI1 appears to be involved in a variety of pathways important for regulation of proliferation and apoptosis, though it is not clear whether it is involved independent of or as a component of the SWI/SNF complex. Dashed lines indicate regulatory pathways in which it is not yet understood whether SNF5/INI1 acts independently of other factors or as a component of the SWI/SNF complex. It appears to upregulate expression of ink4a, but it is unclear whether or not SNF5/INI1 is necessary for the SWI/SNF complexes that potentiate Rb mediated sequestering of E2F transcription factors to block cell-cycle progression. SNF5/INI1 may also bind directly with other transcription factors, such as p53 and c-myc to initiate SWI/SNF formation and transcription of various target genes of these transcription factors. In response to stress events, SNF5/INI1 may interact directly with GADD34 to induce growth arrest and apoptosis. SNF5/INI1 has also been shown to recruit HDAC1 to inhibit cyclin D1 expression, causing a G0/G1 arrest.

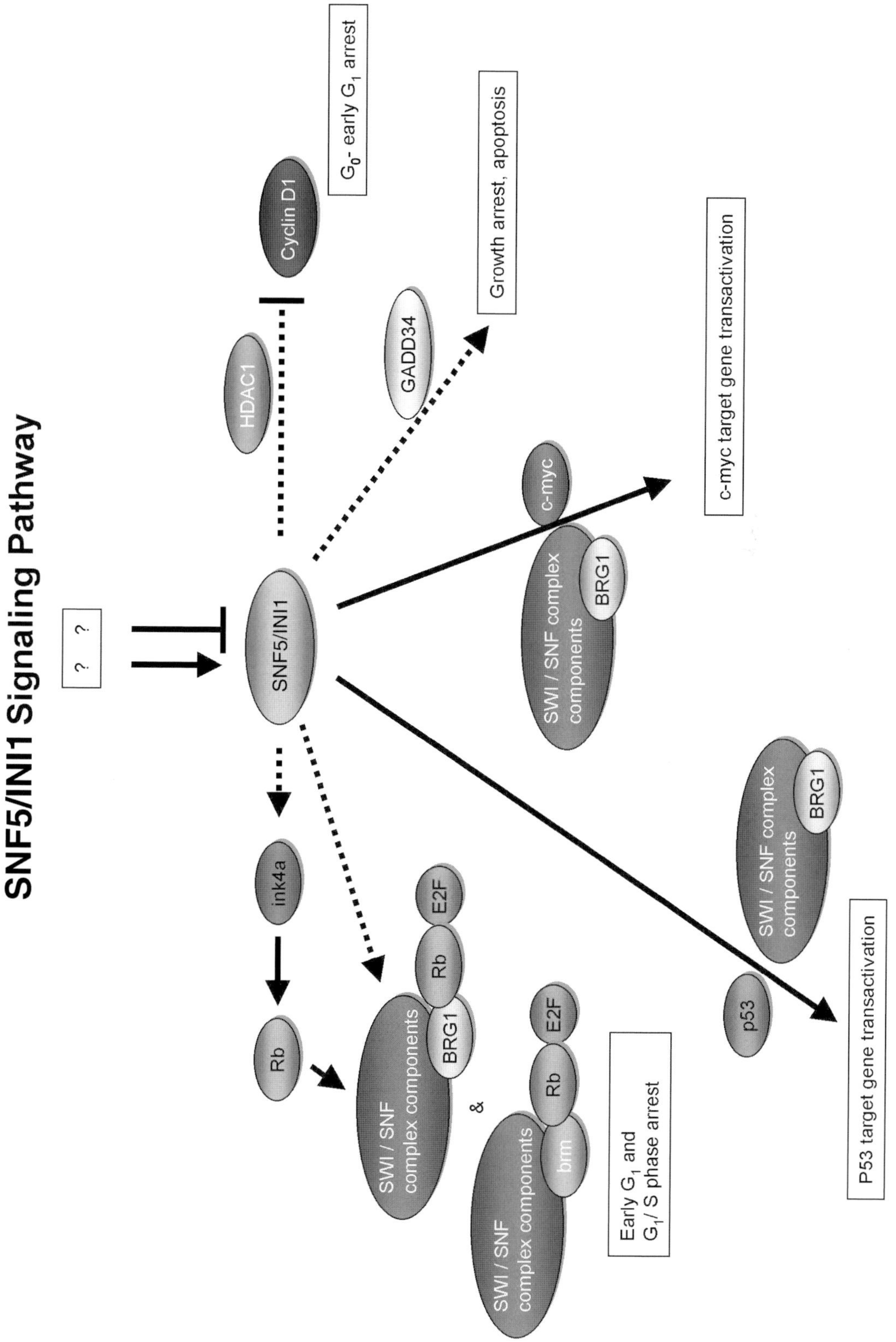
SNF5/INI1 Signaling Pathway
? ?
SNF5/INI1
HDAC1
Cyclin D1
G0- early G1 arrest
GADD34
Growth arrest, apoptosis
c-myc
SWI / SNF complex components
BRG1
c-myc target gene transactivation
SWI / SNF complex components
BRG1
p53
P53 target gene transactivation
ink4a
Rb
SWI / SNF complex components
BRG1
Rb
E2F
&
SWI / SNF complex components
brm
Rb
E2F
Early G1 and
G1 / S phase arrest

reveals prominent intermediate filaments *(15,25,36)*. Immunohistochemical analysis has been reported to show considerable intratumoral variation, but typically evidence of gene expression from both the epithelial and mesenchymal compartments is positive. Markers commonly used in this regard are epithelial membrane antigen, vimentin, smooth muscle actin, desmin, and cytokeratins. Germ cell markers are invariably negative. Neuroepithelial markers including glial fibrillary acidic protein and S-100 protein are generally detectable *(13,15,25)*.

2.3.4. Pathogenesis

The cell of origin of AT/RT is not known and the pathogenesis of these tumors is not understood. Deletion of chromosome 22 in these tumors has been recognized for some time *(21,22,19)*, and this led to the proposition that a tumor suppressor gene maps to 22q *(24,135)*. Shortly after the identification in a mutated gene, hSNF5/INI1, at this location in rhabdoid tumors of the kidney *(148)*, the same gene was found to be mutated in rhabdoid tumors of the CNS *(19)*. Subsequently, germline alterations in INI1 were reported in children who developed AT/RTs, and determination of the retention of only the mutated allele in tumor tissue lead to the formal description of INI1 as a classical tumor suppressor gene *(20,19,144)*. Alterations in this particular gene are important to screen for when no abnormality in chromosome 22 can be identified by cytogenetic approaches *(143)*. These findings and the designation of INI1 as a tumor suppressor gene are consistent with the observation that haploinsufficiency of Snf5/Ini1 in mice predisposes these genetically engineered animals to the development of rhabdoid tumors *(131)*.

The finding of deletions and mutations in INI1 is a reliable indicator that these are AT/RT, and can serve as a marker to distinguish these tumors from other primitive neuroectodermal brain tumors of childhood, especially medulloblastoma and PNET *(23)*. Mutations in this gene probably do not occur in medulloblastoma *(86)*. Distinguishing between AT/RT and PNET is important, because AT/RTs are aggressive tumors that respond poorly to available therapies, compared to other primitive embryonal tumors of the CNS.

The discovery of a central role for SNF5/INI1 in the pathogenesis of AT/RT has lead to considerable insight into how this tumor might develop (Fig. 14). SNF5/INI1 is a transcriptional regulator that is part of a multiprotein complex important for the positioning of nucleosomes along chromatin. SNF5/INI1 is one member of a group of proteins that includes hBRM and hBRG1. Interestingly, hBRG1 has been found to be mutated in cell lines derived from tumors of several different organ sites *(154)*. These proteins complex with SNF5/INI1 to form a critical part of the SWI/SNF complex, which is the critical mediator of nucleosome remodeling *(122)*. This important complex binds to transcription factors already bound to DNA, and exerts function in an ATP-dependent manner to facilitate nucleosome remodeling that enhances the expression of target genes. An important transcription factor with which SNF5/INI1 has been shown to interact is CMYC *(33)*. Other target genes of potential interest for tumor biologists include GAS41 *(38)*, TP53 *(92)*, and GADD34 *(3)*. GAS41 has been identified as binding to a translocation breakpoint protein site in leukemia *(38)*. p53 and GADD34 are important for apoptosis *(3,92)*. While it is not certain how deletions of SNF5/INI1 might lead to the altered expression of specific genes critical for the development of this tumor, it seems likely that a subset of SNF5/INI1 target genes will be found to play a critical role in biologic functions critical for the regulation of proliferation and differentiation of the cells in which AT/RTs arise.

REFERENCES

1. Adachi, Y., Takamatsu H., Noguchi H., Tahara H., Fukushige T., Takasaki T., et al. 2000. malignant rhabdoid tumor of the kidney occurring concurrently with a brain tumor: report of a case. *Surg. Today* **30**:298–301.
2. Adesina A.M., Nalbantoglu J., Cavenee W.K. 1994. p53 gene mutation and mdm2 gene amplification are uncommon in medulloblastoma. *Cancer Res.* **54**:5649–5651.
3. Adler H.T., Chinery R., Wu D.Y., Kussick S.J., Payne J.M., Fornace A.J. Jr., et al. 1999. Leukemic HRX fusion proteins inhibit GADD34-induced apoptosis and associate with the GADD34 and hSNF5/INI1 proteins. *Mol. Cell Biol.* **19**:7050–7060.

4. Agranovich A.L., Ang L.C., Griebel R.W., Kobrinsky N.L., Lowry N., Tchang S.P. 1992. Malignant rhabdoid tumor of the central nervous system with subarachnoid dissemination. *Surg. Neurol.* **37**:410–414.

5. Albright A.L., Wisoff J.H., Zeltzer P.M., Boyett J.M., Rorke L.B., Stanley P. 1996. Effects of medulloblastoma resections on outcome in children: a report from the Children's Cancer Group. *Neurosurgery* **38**:265–271.

6. Albright A.L., Wisoff J.H., Zeltzer P., Boyett J., Rorke L.B., Stanley P., et al. 1995. Prognostic factors in children with supratentorial (nonpineal) primitive neuroectodermal tumors. A neurosurgical perspective from the Children's Cancer Group. *Pediatr. Neurosurg.* **22**:1–7.

7. Aldosari N., Wiltshire R.N., Dutra A., Schrock E., McLendon R.E., Friedman H.S., et al. 2002. Comprehensive molecular cytogenetic investigation of chromosomal abnormalities in human medulloblastoma cell lines and xenograft. *Neuro-oncol.* **4**:75–85.

8. Aldosari N., Bigner S.H., Burger P.C., Becker L., Kepner J.L., Friedman H.S., McLendon R.E. 2002. MYCC and MYCN oncogene amplification in medulloblastoma. A fluorescence in situ hybridization study on paraffin sections from the Children's Oncology Group. *Arch. Pathol. Lab. Med.* **126**:540–44.

9. Badiali M., Pession A., Basso G., Andreini L., Rigobello L., Galassi E., Giangaspero 1991. N-myc and c-myc oncogenes amplification in medulloblastomas. Evidence of particularly aggressive behavior of a tumor with c-myc amplification. *Tumori* **77**:118–121.

10. Batra S.K., McLendon R.E., Koo J.S., Castelino-Prabhu S., Fuchs H.E., Krischer J.P., 1995. Prognostic implications of chromosome 17p deletions in human medulloblastomas. *J. Neurooncol.* **24**:39–45.

11. Bayani J., Thorner P., Zielenska M., Pandita A., Beatty B., Squire J.A. 1995. Application of a simplified comparative genomic hybridization technique to screen for gene amplification in pediatric solid tumors. *Pediatr. Pathol. Lab. Med.* **15**:831–844.

12. Bayani J., Zielenska M., Marrano P., Kwan Ng Y., Taylor M.D., Jay V., et al. 2000. Molecular cytogenetic analysis of medulloblastomas and supratentorial primitive neuroectodermal tumors by using conventional banding, comparative genomic hybridization, and spectral karyotyping. *J. Neurosurg.* **93**:437–448.

13. Behring B., Bruck W., Goebel H.H., Behnke J., Pekrun A., Christen H.J., Kretzschmar H.A. 1996. Immunohistochemistry of primary central nervous system malignant rhabdoid tumors: report of five cases and review of the literature. *Acta Neuropathol. (Berl)* **91**:578–586.

14. Berger M.S., Baumeister B., Geyer J.R., Milstein J., Kanev P.M., LeRoux P.D. 1991. The risks of metastases from shunting in children with primary central nervous system tumors. *J. Neurosurg.* **74**:872–877.

15. Bergmann M., Spaar H.J., Ebhard G., Masini T., Edel G., Gullotta F., Meyer H. 1997. Primary malignant rhabdoid tumours of the central nervous system: an immunohistochemical and ultrastructural study. *Acta Neurochir. (Wien)* **139**: 961–968; discussion 968–969.

16. Bhattacharjee M., Hicks J., Langford L., Dauser R., Strother D., Chintagumpala M., et al. 1997. Central nervous system atypical teratoid/rhabdoid tumors of infancy and childhood. *Ultrastruct. Pathol.* **21**:369–378.

17. Biegel J.A. 1999. Cytogenetics and molecular genetics of childhood brain tumors. *Neuro-oncol.* **1**:139–151.

18. Biegel J.A. 1997. Genetics of pediatric central nervous system tumors. *J. Pediatr. Hematol. Oncol.* **19**:492–501.

19. Biegel J.A., Zhou J.Y., Rorke L.B., Stenstrom C., Wainwright L.M., Fogelgren B. 1999. Germ-line and acquired mutations of INI1 in atypical teratoid and rhabdoid tumors. *Cancer Res.* **59**:74–79.

20. Biegel J.A., Fogelgren B., Wainwright L.M., Zhou J.Y., Bevan H., Rorke L.B. 2000. Germline INI1 mutation in a patient with a central nervous system atypical teratoid tumor and renal rhabdoid tumor. *Genes Chromosomes Cancer* **28**:31–37.

21. Biegel J.A., Burk C.D., Parmiter A.H., Emanuel B.S. 1992. Molecular analysis of a partial deletion of 22q in a central nervous system rhabdoid tumor. *Genes Chromosomes Cancer* **5**:104–108.

22. Biegel J.A., Rorke L.B., Emanuel B.S. 1989. Monosomy 22 in rhabdoid or atypical teratoid tumors of the brain. *N. Engl. J. Med.* **321**:906.

23. Biegel J.A., Fogelgren B., Zhou J.Y., James C.D., Janss A.J., Allen J.C., et al. 2000. Mutations of the INI1 rhabdoid tumor suppressor gene in medulloblastomas and primitive neuroectodermal tumors of the central nervous system. *Clin. Cancer Res.* **6**:2759–2763.

24. Biegel J.A., Allen C.S., Kawasaki K., Shimizu N., Budarf M.L., Bell C.J. 1996. Narrowing the critical region for a rhabdoid tumor locus in 22q11. *Genes Chromosomes Cancer* **16**:94–105.

25. Biggs P.J., Garen P.D., Powers J.M., Garvin A.J. 1987. Malignant rhabdoid tumor of the central nervous system. *Hum. Pathol.* **18**:332–337.

26. Bigner S.H., Vogelstein B. 1990. Cytogenetics and molecular genetics of malignant gliomas and medulloblastoma. *Brain Pathol.* **1**:12–18.

27. Blaney S., Berg S.L., Pratt C., Weitman S., Sullivan J., Luchtman-Jones L., Bernstein M. 2001. A phase I study of irinotecan in pediatric patients: a pediatric oncology group study. *Clin. Cancer Res.* **7**:32–37.

28. Bonnin J.M., Rubinstein L.J., Palmer N.F., Beckwith J.B. 1984. The association of embryonal tumors originating in the kidney and in the brain. A report of seven cases. *Cancer* **54**:2137–2146.

29. Borycki A., Brown A.M., Emerson, C.P. Jr. 2000. Shh and Wnt signaling pathways converge to control Gli gene activation in avian somites. *Development Supplement* **127**:2075–2087.

30. Bruggers C.S., Tai K.F., Murdock T., Sivak L., Le K., Perkins S.L., et al. 1998. Expression of the c-Myc protein in childhood medulloblastoma. *J. Pediatr. Hematol. Oncol.* **20:**18–25.

31. Burger P.C., Yu I.T., Tihan T., Friedman H.S., Strother D.R., Kepner J.L., et al. 1998. Atypical teratoid/rhabdoid tumor of the central nervous system: a highly malignant tumor of infancy and childhood frequently mistaken for medulloblastoma: a Pediatric Oncology Group study. *Am. J. Surg. Pathol.* **22:**1083–1092.

32. Caldemeyer K.S., Smith R.R., Azzarelli B., Boaz J.C. 1994. Primary central nervous system malignant rhabdoid tumor: CT and MR appearance simulates a primitive neuroectodermal tumor. *Pediatr. Neurosurg.* **21:**232–236.

33. Cheng S.W., Davies K.P., Yung E., Beltran R.J., Yu J., Kalpana G.V. 1999. c-MYC interacts with INI1/hSNF5 and requires the SWI/SNF complex for transactivation function. *Nat. Genet.* **22:**102–105.

34. Cogen P.H., Daneshvar L., Metzger A.K., Duyk G., Edwards M.S., Sheffield V.C. 1992. Involvement of multiple chromosome 17p loci in medulloblastoma tumorigenesis. *Am. J. Hum. Genet.* **50:**584–589.

35. Cohen B.H., Zeltzer P.M., Boyett J.M., Geyer J.R., Allen J.C., Finlay J.L, et al. 1995. Prognostic factors and treatment results for supratentorial primitive neuroectodermal tumors in children using radiation and chemotherapy: a Childrens Cancer Group randomized trial. *J. Clin. Oncol.* **13:**1687–1696.

36. Cossu A., Massarelli G., Manetto V., Viale G., Tanda F., Bosincu L., et al. 1993. Rhabdoid tumours of the central nervous system. Report of three cases with immunocytochemical and ultrastructural findings. *Virchows Arch. A. Pathol. Anat. Histopathol.* **422:**81–85.

37. Dahmen R.P., Koch A., Denkhaus D., Tonn J.C., Sorensen N., Berthold F., et al. 2001. Deletions of AXIN1, a component of the WNT/wingless pathway, in sporadic medulloblastomas. *Cancer Res.* **61:**7039–7043.

38. Debernardi S., Bassini A., Jones L.K., Chaplin T., Linder B., de Bruijn D.R., et al. 2002. The MLL fusion partner AF10 binds GAS41, a protein that interacts with the human SWI/SNF complex. *Blood* **99:**275–281.

39. Dierick H., Bejsovec A. 1999. Cellular mechanisms of wingless/Wnt signal transduction. *Curr. Top. Dev. Biol.* **43:**153–190.

40. Ding Q., Motoyama J., Gasca S., Mo R., Sasaki H., Rossant J., Hui C.C. 1998. Diminished Sonic hedgehog signaling and lack of floor plate differentiation in Gli2 mutant mice. *Development* **125:**2533–2543.

41. Dirks P.B., Harris L., Hoffman H.J., Humphreys R.P., Drake J.M., Rutka J.T. 1996. Supratentorial primitive neuroectodermal tumors in children. *J. Neurooncol.* **29:**75–84.

42. Duffner P.K., Horowitz M.E., Krischer J.P., Friedman H.S., Burger P.C., Cohen M.E., et al. 1993. Postoperative chemotherapy and delayed radiation in children less than three years of age with malignant brain tumors. *N. Engl. J. Med.* **328:**1725–1731.

43. Dunkel I.J., Garvin J.H., Jr., Goldman S., Ettinger L.J., Kaplan A.M., Cairo M., et al. 1998. High dose chemotherapy with autologous bone marrow rescue for children with diffuse pontine brain stem tumors. Children's Cancer Group. *J. Neurooncol.* **37:**67–73.

44. Eberhart C.G., Kepner J.L., Goldthwaite P.T., Kun L.E., Duffner P.K., Friedman H.S., et al. 2002. Histopathologic grading of medulloblastomas: a Pediatric Oncology Group study. *Cancer* **94:**552–560.

45. Eberhart C.G., Tihan T., Burger P.C. 2000. Nuclear localization and mutation of beta-catenin in medulloblastomas. *J. Neuropathol. Exp. Neurol.* **59:**333–337.

46. Finlay J.L., Goldman S., Wong M.C., Cairo M., Garvin J., August C., et al. 1996. Pilot study of high-dose thiotepa and etoposide with autologous bone marrow rescue in children and young adults with recurrent CNS tumors. The Children's Cancer Group. *J. Clin. Oncol.* **14:**2495–2503.

47. Fort D.W., Tonk V.S., Tomlinson G.E., Timmons C.F., Schneider N.R.1994. Rhabdoid tumor of the kidney with primitive neuroectodermal tumor of the central nervous system: associated tumors with different histologic, cytogenetic, and molecular findings. Genes *Chromosomes Cancer* **11:**146–152.

48. Fruhwald M.C., O'Dorisio M.S., Dai Z., Rush L.J., Krahe R., Smiraglia D.J., et al. 2001. Aberrant hypermethylation of the major breakpoint cluster region in 17p11.2 in medulloblastomas but not supratentorial PNETs. *Genes Chromosomes Cancer* **30:**38–47.

49. Garson J.A., Pemberton L.F., Sheppard P.W., Varndell I.M., Coakham H.B., Kemshead J.T. 1989. N-myc gene expression and oncoprotein characterisation in medulloblastoma. *Br. J. Cancer* **59:**889–894.

50. Giangaspero F., Chieco P., Ceccarelli C., Lisignoli G., Pozzuoli R., Gambacorta M., et al. 1991. "Desmoplastic" versus "classic" medulloblastoma: comparison of DNA content, histopathology and differentiation. *Virchows Arch. A. Pathol. Anat. Histopathol.* **418:**207–214.

51. Giangaspero F., Rigobello L., Badiali M., Loda M., Andreini L., Basso G., et al. 1992. Large-cell medulloblastomas. A distinct variant with highly aggressive behavior. *Am. J. Surg. Pathol.* **16:**687–693.

52. Giangaspero F., Perilongo G., Fondelli M.P., Brisigotti M., Carollo C., Burnelli R., et al. 1999. Medulloblastoma with extensive nodularity: a variant with favorable prognosis. *J. Neurosurg.* **91:**971–977.

53. Gilbertson R.J., Clifford S.C., MacMeekin W., Meekin W., Wright C., Perry R.H., et al. 1998. Expression of the ErbB-neuregulin signaling network during human cerebellar development: implications for the biology of medulloblastoma. *Cancer Res.* **58:**3932–3941.

54. Gilbertson R.J., Perry R.H., Kelly P.J., Pearson A.D., Lunec J. 1997. Prognostic significance of HER2 and HER4 coexpression in childhood medulloblastoma. *Cancer Res.* **57:**3272–3280.

55. Gilhuis H.J., Anderl K.L., Boerman R.H., Jeuken J.M., James C.D., Raffel C., et al. 2000. Comparative genomic hybridization of medulloblastomas and clinical relevance: eleven new cases and a review of the literature. *Clin. Neurol. Neurosurg.* **102:**203–209.

56. Giordana M.T., Duo D., Gasverde S., Trevisan E., Boghi A., Morra I., et al. 2002. MDM2 overexpression is associated with short survival in adults with medulloblastoma. *Neuro-oncol.* **4:**115–122.

57. Goodrich, L.V., L. Milenkovic, K.M. Higgins, and M.P. Scott. 1997. Altered neural cell fates and medulloblastoma in mouse patched mutants. *Science* **277:**1109–1113.

58. Gould V.E., Jansson D.S., Molenaar W.M., Rorke L.B., Trojanowski J.Q., Lee V.M., et al. 1990. Primitive neuroectodermal tumors of the central nervous system. Patterns of expression of neuroendocrine markers, and all classes of intermediate filament proteins. *Lab. Invest.* **62:**498–509.

59. Grotzer M.A., Hogarty M.D., Janss A.J., Liu X., Zhao H., Eggert A.,et al. 2001. MYC messenger RNA expression predicts survival outcome in childhood primitive neuroectodermal tumor/medulloblastoma. *Clin. Cancer Res.* **7:**2425–2433.

60. Grotzer M.A., Janss A.J., Phillips P.C., Trojanowski J.Q. 2000. Neurotrophin receptor TrkC predicts good clinical outcome in medulloblastoma and other primitive neuroectodermal brain tumors. *Klin. Padiatr.* **212:**196–199.

61. Hahn W.C., Weinberg R.A. 2002. Modelling the molecular circuitry of cancer. *Nat. Rev. Cancer* **2:**331–341.

62. Hamilton S.R., Liu B., Parsons R.E., Papadopoulos N., Jen J., Powell S.M., et al. 1995. The molecular basis of Turcot's syndrome. *N. Engl. J. Med.* **332:**839–847.

63. Haslam R.H., Lamborn K.R., Becker L.E., Israel M.A. 1998. Tumor cell apoptosis present at diagnosis may predict treatment outcome for patients with medulloblastoma. *J. Pediatr. Hematol. Oncol.* **20:**520–527.

64. He T.C., Sparks A.B., Rago C., Hermeking H., Zawel L., da Costa L.T., et al. 1998. Identification of c-MYC as a target of the APC pathway. *Science* **281:**1509–1512.

65. Herms J., Neidt I., Luscher B., Sommer A., Schurmann P., Schroder T., et al. 2000. C-MYC expression in medulloblastoma and its prognostic value. *Int. J. Cancer* **89:**395–402.

66. Hilden J.M., Watterson J., Longee D.C., Moertel C.L., Dunn M.E., Kurtzberg J., Scheithauer B.W. 1998. Central nervous system atypical teratoid tumor/rhabdoid tumor: response to intensive therapy and review of the literature. *J. Neurooncol.* **40:**265–275.

67. Homfray T.F., Cottrell S.E., Ilyas M., Rowan A., Talbot I.C., Bodmer W.F., Tomlinson I.P. 1998. Defects in mismatch repair occur after APC mutations in the pathogenesis of sporadic colorectal tumours. *Hum. Mutat.* **11:**114–120.

68. Howat A.J., Gonzales M.F., Waters K.D., Campbell P.E. 1986. Primitive neuroectodermal tumour of the central nervous system associated with malignant rhabdoid tumour of the kidney: report of a case. *Histopathology* **10:**643–650.

69. Huang H., Mahler-Araujo B.M., Sankila A., Chimelli L., Yonekawa Y., Kleihues P.,. Ohgaki H. 2000. APC mutations in sporadic medulloblastomas. *Am. J. Pathol.* **156:**433–437.

70. Huang H., Reis R., Yonekawa Y., Lopes J.M., Kleihues P., Ohgaki H. 1999. Identification in human brain tumors of DNA sequences specific for SV40 large T antigen. *Brain Pathology* **9:**33–44.

71. Immaneni A., Lawinger P., Zhao Z., Lu W., Rastelli L., Morris J.H., Majumder S. 2000. REST-VP16 activates multiple neuronal differentiation genes in human NT2 cells. *Nucleic Acids Res.* **28:**3403–3410.

72. Jay V., Squire J., Bayani J., Alkhani A.M., Rutka J.T., Zielenska M. 1999. Oncogene amplification in medulloblastoma: analysis of a case by comparative genomic hybridization and fluorescence in situ hybridization. *Pathology* **31:**337–344.

73. Johnson D.L., McCabe M.A., Nicholson H.S., Joseph A.L., Getson P.R., Byrne J., et al. 1994. Quality of long-term survival in young children with medulloblastoma. *J. Neurosurg.* **80:**1004–1010.

74. Kaatsch P., Rickert C.H., Kuhl J., Schuz J., Michaelis J. 2001. Population-based epidemiologic data on brain tumors in German children. *Cancer* **92:**3155–3164.

75. Kepes J.J., Morantz R.A., Dorzab W.E. 1987. Cerebellar medulloblastoma in a 73-year-old woman. *Neurosurgery* **21:**81–83.

76. Khalili K., Krynska B., Del Valle L., Katsetos C.D., Croul S. 1999. Medulloblastomas and the human neurotropic polyomavirus JC virus. *Lancet* **353:**1152–1153.

77. Kim J.Y., Sutton M.E., Lu D.J., Cho T.A., Goumnerova L.C., Goritchenko L., et al. 1999. Activation of neurotrophin-3 receptor TrkC induces apoptosis in medulloblastomas. *Cancer Res.* **59:**711–719.

78. Kimonis V.E., Goldstein A.M., Pastakia B., Yang M.L., Kase, DiGiovanna J.J., et al. 1997. Clinical manifestations in 105 persons with nevoid basal cell carcinoma syndrome. *Am. J. Med. Genet.* **69:**299–308.

79. Kleihues P., Cavenee W,K. 2000. *Pathology and Genetics Tumours of the Nervous System.* 1st ed. IARC Press, Lyon.

80. Kleihues P., Schauble B., zur Hausen A., Esteve J., Ohgaki H. 1997. Tumors associated with p53 germline mutations: a synopsis of 91 families. *Am. J. Pathol.* 1997. **150:**1–13.

81. Kleihues P., Louis D.N., Scheithauer B.W., Rorke L.B., Reifenberger G., Burger P.C., Cavenee W.K. 2002. The WHO classification of tumors of the nervous system. *J. Neuropathol. Exp. Neurol.* **61:**215–225; discussion 226–229.

82. Klisch J., Husstedt H., Hennings S., von Velthoven V., Pagenstecher A., Schumacher M. 2000. Supratentorial primitive neuroectodermal tumours: diffusion-weighted MRI. *Neuroradiology* **42:**393–398.

83. Koch A., Waha A., Tonn J.C., Sorensen N., Berthold F., Wolter M., et al. 2001. Somatic mutations of WNT/wingless signaling pathway components in primitive neuroectodermal tumors. *Int. J. Cancer* **93:**445–449.

84. Korshunov A., Golanov A., Ozerov S., Sycheva R. 1999. Prognostic value of tumor-associated antigens immunoreactivity and apoptosis in medulloblastomas. An analysis of 73 cases. *Brain Tumor Pathol.* **16:**37–44.

85. Kozmik Z., Sure U., Ruedi D., Busslinger M., Aguzzi A. 1995. Deregulated expression of PAX5 in medulloblastoma. *Proc. Natl. Acad. Sci. USA* **92:**5709–5713.

86. Kraus J.A., Oster C., Sorensen N., Berthold F., Schlegel U., Tonn J.C., et al. 2002. Human medulloblastomas lack point mutations and homozygous deletions of the hSNF5/INI1 tumour suppressor gene. *Neuropathol. Appl. Neurobiol.* **28:** 136–141.

87. Krynska B., Del Valle L., Croul S., Gordon J., Katsetos C.D., Carbone M., et al. 1999. Detection of human neurotropic JC virus DNA sequence and expression of the viral oncogenic protein in pediatric medulloblastomas. *Proc. Natl. Acad. Sci. USA* **96:**11,519–11,524.

88. Krynska B., Otte J., Franks R., Khalili K., Croul S. 1999. Human ubiquitous JCV(CY) T-antigen gene induces brain tumors in experimental animals. *Oncogene* **18:**39–46.

89. Krynska B., Gordon J., Otte J., Franks R., Knobler R., DeLuca A., Giordano A., Khalili K. 1997. Role of cell cycle regulators in tumor formation in transgenic mice expressing the human neurotropic virus, JCV, early protein. *J. Cell Biochem.* **67:**223–230.

90. Laurent J.P., Chang C.H., Cohen M.E. 1985. A classification system for primitive neuroectodermal tumors (medulloblastoma) of the posterior fossa. *Cancer* **56:**1807–1809.

91. Lawinger P., Venugopal R., Guo Z.S., Immaneni A., Sengupta D., Lu W., et al. 2000. The neuronal repressor REST/ NRSF is an essential regulator in medulloblastoma cells. *Nat. Med.* **6:**826–831.

92. Lee D., Kim J.W., Seo T., Hwang S.G., Choi E.-J., Choe J. 2002. SWI/SNF Complex Interacts with Tumor Suppressor p53 and Is Necessary for the Activation of p53-mediated Transcription. *J. Biol. Chem.* **277:**22,330–22,337.

93. Lefkowitz I.B., Packer R.J., Ryan S.G., Shah N., Alavi J., Rorke L.B., et al. 1988. Late recurrence of primitive neuroectodermal tumor/medulloblastoma. *Cancer* **62:**826–830.

94. Lefkowitz I.B., Packer R.J., Siegel K.R., Sutton L.N., Schut L., Evans A.E. 1990. Results of treatment of children with recurrent medulloblastoma/primitive neuroectodermal tumors with lomustine, cisplatin, and vincristine. *Cancer* **65:** 412–417.

95. MacGregor D.N., Ziff E.B. 1990. Elevated c-myc expression in childhood medulloblastomas. *Pediatr. Res.* **28:**63–68.

96. Maleci A., Cervoni L., DelfiniR. 1992. Medulloblastoma in children and in adults: a comparative study. *Acta Neurochir. (Wien)* **119:**62–67.

97. Marec-Berard P., Jouvet A., Thiesse P., Kalifa C., Doz F., Frappaz D. 2002. Supratentorial embryonal tumors in children under 5 years of age: an SFOP study of treatment with postoperative chemotherapy alone. *Med. Pediatr. Oncol.* **38:**83–90.

98. Marino S., Vooijs M., van Der Gulden H., Jonkers J., Berns A. 2000. Induction of medulloblastomas in p53-null mutant mice by somatic inactivation of Rb in the external granular layer cells of the cerebellum. *Genes Dev.* **14:**994–1004.

99. McDonald J.D., Daneshvar L., Willert J.R., Matsumura K., Waldman F., Cogen P.H. 1994. Physical mapping of chromosome 17p13.3 in the region of a putative tumor suppressor gene important in medulloblastoma. *Genomics* **23:**229–232.

100. McNeil D.E., Cote T.R., Clegg L., Rorke L.B. 2002. Incidence and trends in pediatric malignancies medulloblastoma/ primitive neuroectodermal tumor: a SEER update. Surveillance Epidemiology and End Results. *Med. Pediatr. Oncol.* **39:**190–194.

101. Michiels E.M., Weiss M.M., Hoovers J.M., Baak J.P., Voute P.A., Baas F., Hermsen M.A. 2002. Genetic alterations in childhood medulloblastoma analyzed by comparative genomic hybridization. *J. Pediatr. Hematol. Oncol.* **24:**205–210.

102. Mori T., Nagase H., Horii A., Miyoshi Y., Shimano T., Nakatsuru S., et al. 1994. Germ-line and somatic mutations of the APC gene in patients with Turcot syndrome and analysis of APC mutations in brain tumors. *Genes Chromosomes Cancer* **9:**168–172.

103. Morin P.J., Sparks A.B., Korinek V., Barker N., Clevers H., Vogelstein B., Kinzler K.W. 1997. Activation of beta-catenin-Tcf signaling in colon cancer by mutations in beta-catenin or APC. *Science* **275:**1787–90.

104. Morin P.J. 1999. beta-catenin signaling and cancer. *Bioessays* **21:**1021–1030.

105. Moscatello D.K., Holgado-Madruga M., Godwin A.K., Ramirez G., Gunn G., Zoltick P.W., et al. 1995. Frequent expression of a mutant epidermal growth factor receptor in multiple human tumors. *Cancer Research* **55:**5536–5339.

106. Moschovi M., Sotiris Y., Prodromou N., Tsangaris G.T., Constantinidou. Van-Vliet C, Kalpini-Mavrou A.F., Tzortzatou-Stathopoulou F. 1998. Familial medulloblastoma. *Pediatr. Hematol. Oncol.* **15:**421–424.

107. Mullor J.L., Dahmane N., Sun T., Ruiz i Altaba A. 2001. Wnt signals are targets and mediators of Gli function. *Current Biology* **11:**769–773.

108. Nakagawara A. 2001 Trk receptor tyrosine kinases: a bridge between cancer and neural development. *Cancer Lett.* **169:**107–114.

109. Nicholson J.C., Ross F.M., Kohler J.A., Ellison D.W. 1999. Comparative genomic hybridization and histological variation in primitive neuroectodermal tumours. *Br. J. Cancer* **80:**1322–1331.

110. Nishio S., Morioka T., Fukui M. 1998. Primitive neuroectodermal tumors. *Crit. Rev. Neurosurg.* **8:**261–268.

111. Nishizaki T., Harada K., Kubota H., Ozaki S., Ito H., Sasaki K. 1999. Genetic alterations in pediatric medulloblastomas detected by comparative genomic hybridization. *Pediatr. Neurosurg.* **31:**27–32.

112. Olson T.A., Bayar E., Kosnik E., Hamoudi A.B., Klopfenstein K.J., Pieters R.S., Ruymann F.B. 1995. Successful treatment of disseminated central nervous system malignant rhabdoid tumor. *J. Pediatr. Hematol. Oncol.* **17**:71–75.

113. Packer R.J., Biegel J.A., Blaney S., Finlay J., Geyer J.R., Heideman R., et al. 2002. Atypical teratoid/rhabdoid tumor of the central nervous system: report on workshop. *J. Pediatr. Hematol. Oncol.* **24**:337–342.

114. Packer R.J. 1990. Chemotherapy for medulloblastoma/primitive neuroectodermal tumors of the posterior fossa. *Ann. Neurol.* **28**:823–828.

115. Packer R.J., Meadows A.T., Rorke L.B., Goldwein J.L., D'Angio G. 1987. Long-term sequelae of cancer treatment on the central nervous system in childhood. *Med. Pediatr. Oncol.* **15**:241–253.

116. Packer R.J., Cogen P., Vezina G., Rorke L.B. 1999. Medulloblastoma: clinical and biologic aspects. *Neurooncol.* **1**: 232–250.

117. Packer R.J., Sutton L.N., Rorke L.B., Littman P.A., Sposto R., et al. 1984. Prognostic importance of cellular differentiation in medulloblastoma of childhood. *J. Neurosurg.* **61**:296–301.

118. Packer R.J., Sutton L.N., Atkins T.E., Radcliffe J., Bunin G.R., D'Angio G., et al. 1989. A prospective study of cognitive function in children receiving whole-brain radiotherapy and chemotherapy: 2-year results. *J. Neurosurg.* **70**:707–713.

119. Packer R.J., Sposto R., Atkins T.E., Sutton L.N., Bruce D.A., Siegel K.R., et al. 1987. Quality of life in children with primitive neuroectodermal tumors (medulloblastoma) of the posterior fossa. *Pediatr. Neurosci.* **13**:169–175.

120. Packer R.J., Goldwein J., Nicholson H.S., Vezina L.G., Allen J.C., Ris M.D., et al. 1999. Treatment of children with medulloblastomas with reduced-dose craniospinal radiation therapy and adjuvant chemotherapy: A Children's Cancer Group Study. *J. Clin. Oncol.* **17**:2127–2136.

121. Padgett B.L., Walker D.L. 1973. Prevalence of antibodies in human sera against JC virus, an isolate from a case of progressive multifocal leukoencephalopathy. *J. Infect. Dis.* **127**:467–470.

122. Phelan M.L., Sif S., Narlikar G.J., Kingston R.E. 1999. Reconstitution of a core chromatin remodeling complex from SWI/SNF subunits. *Mol. Cell* **3**:247–253.

123. Pietsch T., Waha A., Koch A., Kraus J., Albrecht S., Tonn J.et al. 1997. Medulloblastomas of the desmoplastic variant carry mutations of the human homologue of Drosophila patched. *Cancer Res.* **57**:2085–2088.

124. Pietsch T.,Koch A., Wiestler O.D. 1997. Molecular genetic studies in medulloblastomas: evidence for tumor suppressor genes at the chromosomal regions 1q31-32 and 17p13. *Klin. Padiatr.* **209**:150–155.

125. Pobereskin L., Treip C. 1986. Adult medulloblastoma. *J. Neurol. Neurosurg. Psychiatry* **49**:39–42.

126. Pomeroy S.L., Tamayo P., Gaasenbeek M., Sturla L.M., Angelo M., McLaughlin M.E., et al. 2002. Prediction of central nervous system embryonal tumour outcome based on gene expression. *Nature* **415**:436–442.

127. Reardon D.A., Jenkins J.J., Sublett J.E., Burger P.C., Kun L.K. 2000. Multiple genomic alterations including N-myc amplification in a primary large cell medulloblastoma. *Pediatr. Neurosurg.* **32**:187–191.

128. Reddy A.T., Janss A.J., Phillips P.C., Weiss H.L., Packer R.J. 2000. Outcome for children with supratentorial primitive neuroectodermal tumors treated with surgery, radiation, and chemotherapy. *Cancer* **88**:2189–2193.

129. Redies C., Medina L., Puelles L. 2001. Cadherin expression by embryonic divisions and derived gray matter structures in the telencephalon of the chicken. *J. Comp. Neurol.* **438**:253–285.

130. Reinhardt D., Behnke-Mursch J., Weiss E., Christen H.J., Kuhl J., Lakomek M., Pekrun A. 2000. Rhabdoid tumors of the central nervous system. *Childs Nerv. Syst.* **16**:228–234.

131. Roberts C.W., Galusha S.A., McMenamin M.E., Fletcher C.D., Orkin S.H. 2000. Haploinsufficiency of Snf5 (integrase interactor 1) predisposes to malignant rhabdoid tumors in mice. *Proc. Natl. Acad. Sci. USA* **97**:13,796–13,800.

132. Rorke L.B., Trojanowski J.Q., Lee V.M., Zimmerman R.A., Sutton L.N., Biegel J.A., et al. 1997. Primitive neuroectodermal tumors of the central nervous system. *Brain Pathol.* **7**:765–784.

133. Russo C., Pellarin M., Tingby O., Bollen A.W., Lamborn K.R., Mohapatra G., et al. 1999. Comparative genomic hybridization in patients with supratentorial and infratentorial primitive neuroectodermal tumors. *Cancer* **86**:331–339.

134. Schofield D., West D.C., Anthony D.C., Marshal R., Sklar J. 1995. Correlation of loss of heterozygosity at chromosome 9q with histological subtype in medulloblastomas. *Am. J. Pathol.* **146**:472–480.

135. Schofield D.E., Beckwith J.B., Sklar J. 1996. Loss of heterozygosity at chromosome regions 22q11-12 and 11p15.5 in renal rhabdoid tumors. *Genes Chromosomes Cancer* **15**:10–17.

136. Segal R.A., Goumnerova L.C., Kwon Y.K., Stiles C.D., Pomeroy S.L. 1994. Expression of the neurotrophin receptor TrkC is linked to a favorable outcome in medulloblastoma. *Proc. Natl. Acad. Sci. USA* **91**:12,867–12,871.

137. Shlomit R., Ayala A.G., Michal D., Ninett A., Frida S., Boleslaw G., et al. 2000. Gains and losses of DNA sequences in childhood brain tumors analyzed by comparative genomic hybridization. *Cancer Genet. Cytogenet.* **121**:67–72.

138. Solecki D.J., Liu X.L., Tomoda T., Fang Y., Hatten M.E. 2001. Activated Notch2 signaling inhibits differentiation of cerebellar granule neuron precursors by maintaining proliferation. *Neuron* **31**:557–568.

139. Srinivasan J., Berger M.S., Silber J.R. 1996. p53 expression in four human medulloblastoma-derived cell lines. *Childs Nerv. Syst.* **12**:76–80.

140. Stavrou T., Bromley C.M., Nicholson H.S., Byrne J., Packer R.J., Goldstein A.M., Reaman G.H. 2001. Prognostic factors and secondary malignancies in childhood medulloblastoma. *J. Pediatr. Hematol. Oncol.* **23**:431–436.

141. Steichen-Gersdorf E., Baumgartner M., Kreczy A., Maier H., Fink F.M. 1997. Deletion mapping on chromosome 17p in medulloblastoma. *Br. J. Cancer* **76**:1284–1287.

142. Sussman A., Leviton A., Allred E.N., Aschenbrener C., Austin D.F., Gilles F.H., et al. 1990. Childhood brain tumor: presentation at younger age is associated with a family tumor history. *Cancer Causes Control* **1:**75–79.

143. Tamiya T., Nakashima H., Ono Y., Kawada S., Hamazaki S., Furuta T., et al. 2000. Spinal atypical teratoid/rhabdoid tumor in an infant. *Pediatr. Neurosurg.* **32:**145–149.

144. Taylor M.D., Gokgoz N., Andrulis I.L., Mainprize T.G., Drake J.M., Rutka J.T. 2000. Familial posterior fossa brain tumors of infancy secondary to germline mutation of the hSNF5 gene. *Am. J. Hum. Genet.* **66:**1403–1406.

145. Taylor M.D., Liu L., Raffel C., Hui C.C., Mainprize T.G., Zhang X., et al. 2002. Mutations in SUFU predispose to medulloblastoma. *Nat. Genet.*

146. Thomas P.R., Deutsch M., Kepner V., Boyett J.M., Krischer J., Aronin P., et al. 2000. Low-stage medulloblastoma: final analysis of trial comparing standard-dose with reduced-dose neuraxis irradiation. *J. Clin. Oncol.* **18:**3004–3011.

147. Van Meir E.G. 1998. "Turcot's syndrome": phenotype of brain tumors, survival and mode of inheritance. *Int. J. Cancer* **75:**162–164.

148. Versteege I., Sevenet N., Lange J., Rousseau-Merck M.F., Ambros P., Handgretinger R., et al. 1998. Truncating mutations of hSNF5/INI1 in aggressive paediatric cancer. *Nature* **394:**203–206.

149. Vorechovsky I., Tingby O., Hartman M., Stromberg B., Nister M., Collins V.P., Toftgard R. 1997. Somatic mutations in the human homologue of Drosophila patched in primitive neuroectodermal tumours. *Oncogene* **15:**361–366.

150. Vortmeyer A.O., Stavrou T., Selby D., Li G., Weil R.J., Park W.S., et al. 1999. Deletion analysis of the adenomatous polyposis coli and PTCH gene loci in patients with sporadic and nevoid basal cell carcinoma syndrome-associated medulloblastoma. *Cancer* **85:**2662–2667.

151. Wechsler-Reya R., Scott M.P. 2001. The developmental biology of brain tumors. *Ann. Rev. Neurosci.* **24:**385–428.

152. Weiss E., Behring B., Behnke J., Christen H.J., Pekrun A., Hess C.F. 1998. Treatment of primary malignant rhabdoid tumor of the brain: report of three cases and review of the literature. *Int. J. Radiat. Oncol. Biol. Phys.* **41:**1013–1019.

153. Wetmore C., Eberhart D.E., Curran T. 2000. The normal patched allele is expressed in medulloblastomas from mice with heterozygous germ-line mutation of patched. *Cancer Res.* **60:**2239–2246.

154. Wong A.K., Shanahan F., Chen Y., Lian L., Ha P., Hendricks K., et al. 2000. BRG1, a component of the SWI-SNF complex, is mutated in multiple human tumor cell lines. *Cancer Res.* **60:**6171–6177.

155. Xie J., Johnson R.L., Zhang X., Bare J.W., Waldman F.M., Cogen P.H., et al. 1997. Mutations of the PATCHED gene in several types of sporadic extracutaneous tumors. *Cancer Res.* **57:**2369–2372.

156. Yin X.L., Pang J.C., Ng H.K. 2002. Identification of a region of homozygous deletion on 8p22-23.1 in medulloblastoma. *Oncogene* **21:**1461–1468.

157. Yokota N., Aruga J., Takai S., Yamada K., Hamazaki M., Iwase T., et al. 1996. Predominant expression of human zic in cerebellar granule cell lineage and medulloblastoma. *Cancer Res.* **56:**377–383.

158. Yokota N., Nishizawa S., Ohta S., Date H., Sugimura H., Namba H., Maekawa M. 2002. Role of Wnt pathway in medulloblastoma oncogenesis. *Int. J. Cancer* **101:**198–201.

159. Zeltzer P.M., Boyett J.M., Finlay J.L., Albright A.L., Rorke L.B., Milstein J.M., et al. 1999. Metastasis stage, adjuvant treatment, and residual tumor are prognostic factors for medulloblastoma in children: conclusions from the Children's Cancer Group 921 randomized phase III study. *J. Clin. Oncol.* **17:**832–845.

160. Zhen H.N., Zhang., Bu X.Y., Zhang Z.W., Huang W.J., Zhang P., et al. 1999. Wang, Expression of the simian virus 40 large tumor antigen (Tag) and formation of Tag-p53 and Tag-pRb complexes in human brain tumors. *Cancer* **86:**2124–2132.

161. Zu Rhein G.M. 1983. Studies of JC virus-induced nervous system tumors in the Syrian hamster: a review. *Prog. Clin. Biol. Res.* **105:**205–221.

162. Zuccoli G., Izzi G., Bacchini E., Tondelli M.T., Ferrozzi F., Bellomi M. 1999. Central nervous system atypical teratoid/ rhabdoid tumour of infancy. CT and mr findings. *Clin. Imaging* **23:**356–360.

163. Zupanska A., Kaminska B. 2002. The diversity of p53 mutations among human brain tumors and their functional consequences. *Neurochem. Int.* **40:**637–645.

164. Zurawel R.H., Allen C., Chiappa S., Cato W., Biegel J., Cogen P., de Sauvage F., Raffel C. 2000. Analysis of PTCH/ SMO/SHH pathway genes in medulloblastoma. *Genes Chromosomes Cancer* **27:**44–51.

165. Zurawel R.H., Allen C., Wechsler-Reya R., Scott M.P., Raffel C. 2000. Evidence that haploinsufficiency of Ptch leads to medulloblastoma in mice. Genes Chromosomes *Cancer* **28:**77–81.

166. Zurawel R.H., Chiappa S.A., C. Allen C., Raffel C. 1998. Sporadic medulloblastomas contain oncogenic beta-catenin mutations. *Cancer Res.* **58:**896–899.

II | Mechanisms and Pathways

8

Molecular and Cellular Biology of the Blood–Brain Barrier and Its Characteristics in Brain Tumors

Helga E. de Vries, Lisette Montagne,
Christine D. Dijkstra, and Paul van der Valk

1. FUNCTIONAL CHARACTERISTICS OF THE BLOOD–BRAIN BARRIER

The inner milieu of the central nervous system (CNS) is closely regulated by the blood–brain barrier (BBB). By its unique properties, the BBB restricts the entrance of blood-borne large and hydrophilic compounds into the brain, but also tightly controls cellular entry and the supply of nutrients to the brain. In this chapter, we will address the latest advances in both the cellular and molecular biology of this specialized structure, and discuss its functional characteristics and molecular organization in glioma.

1.1. History and Physiology

The cerebrovasculature differs in a number of properties from perivascular beds. The cerebral capillaries are organized in such a way that they form a continuous cellular barrier that isolates the brain from the general circulation. The function of the BBB is to maintain the homeostasis of the CNS, because serum concentrations of many molecules such as glutamate, potassium, and glycine are toxic to the brain. In essence, the BBB is composed of specialized endothelial cells that are regulated in their function by surrounding cells like astroglia, pericytes, and perivascular macrophages *(11,30)*. The relatively impermeable phenotype of the BBB is thought to exist from the close association between cerebral endothelial cells and astrocyte endfeet touching the basement membrane that surrounds the endothelial lining *(30,44,95)*.

The cerebral endothelium in itself expresses a set of defined characteristics, such as high-electrical-resistance tight junctions (TJs) and specialized transport systems to supply the brain with nutrients. As a result of these features, the BBB has the capacity to actively regulate the passage of solutes from the brain-to-blood and blood-to-brain direction. Molecules may diffuse through the plasma membranes of the brain EC and equilibrate between the blood and brain tissue. In general, transport of compounds across the BBB is dependent on their physicochemical properties like lipid solubility, electrical charge, tertiary structure, their binding to plasma proteins, molecular weight, or extent of ionization. Hydrophilic molecules of around 600 Dalton will be blocked from passage into the brain, whereas more lipid-soluble molecules will readily cross the BBB *(89,90,100)*.

In the late 19th century, Ehrlich *(35)* described the existence of a functional barrier between the blood and the brain, because peripheral injection of the dye Evans Blue stained most tissues but failed to reach the brain and spinal cord. In contrast, injection of a dye into the ventricular system of

From: *Contemporary Cancer Research: Brain Tumors*
Edited by: F. Ali-Osman © Humana Press Inc., Totowa, NJ

the brain produced no peripheral staining *(45)*. Initially, it was believed that the glial endfeet surrounding the brain capillaries formed the barrier. Experiments using the electron dense marker, horseradish peroxidase, indicated that the barrier was in fact localized in the endothelium of the brain *(28,24,102)*. Ultrastructural studies revealed the presence of intercellular TJs of the brain endothelium, thereby creating a continuous barrier in brain capillaries, venules, and arterioles *(101)*.

The BBB is present in 99% of the brain capillaries, but in less than 1% of the brain capillaries; endothelial cells are fenestrated and become more permeable. These leaky vessels are exclusively found in the circumventricular organs such as the pituitary gland, median eminence, area postrema, and subfornical organ *(50)*. In these areas, there is unprotected contact of neurons with blood-molecules, and often endocrine regulatory functions are located there (such as the autonomic nervous system, pituitary functions).

1.2. Cell Types of the Blood–Brain Barrier

Cerebral EC constitute the barrier function of the spinal cord, retina, as well as most areas of the brain and differ from peripheral nervous system. Although the cerebral ECs structurally form the barrier, other cells are required for its proper functioning (for cells of the BBB *see* Fig. 1).

Pericytes that surround the endothelium are considered to act as contractile smooth, muscle-like cells, thereby contributing to the structural integrity of the BBB. Pericytes may also influence the vascular tone of the vessel. Pericytes also have the ability to phagocytose compounds that have crossed the endothelial barrier *(13)* and so limit transport into the CNS parenchyma.

Cells of the macrophage lineage will also contribute to BBB functioning. Perivascular macrophages (PVMs), lying at the interface between the BBB and the CNS parenchyma, may play an important role in monitoring BBB permeability. PVMs are a subset of macrophage that line the vasculature and have been classified variously as clasmatocytes, adventitial cells, perivascular phagocytic cells, Mato cells, etc. PVMs are often referred to as pericytes by many groups in spite of differences between the two cell types. PVMs lie in the perivascular space (Virchow-Robin space), and abut onto the basement membrane of the glia limitans, but they are not surrounded by basement membrane. Capillaries are exclusively surrounded by pericytes and contain no PVM *(77)*, although at the boundary of arterioles and capillaries the two cell types co-exist *(87)*. The PVMs are phagocytic *(2,65)* and play a role in scavenging potential pathogens and macromolecules, and have been suggested to be antigen presenting cells of the CNS *(56)*. Recently, an essential role for these PVMs in cellular trafficking across the BBB under inflammatory conditions has been revealed *(93)*, suggesting that PVMs either by direct contact with the BBB ECs or by the production of soluble molecules influence the permeability of the BBB. Additionally, the other population of resident brain macrophages, the microglia cells, may also influence the cerebral capillaries. PVMs have a distinct phenotype *(48)* and are more activated than microglia *(48,56,70,94)*.

The basal lamina surrounding the brain capillaries is more complex as compared to that of peripheral blood vessels. Blood vessels in the CNS have also been reported to express extracellular matrix molecules laminin 1 and 2 *(62,124)*, which are not detected in blood vessel basement membranes elsewhere and which may be related to their highly specialized structure. Other major components of the basement membrane are collagen (types I, III, and IV), fibronectin, and heparan sulfate proteoglycans *(116,117)*. Both the endothelial cells and astrocytes can produce these constituents. In large vessels, meningothelial cells can also contribute to the basement membrane. Ultrastructurally, two basement membranes can be identified in association with blood vessels in the brain, an endothelial and an astroglial basement membrane. These barriers define the inner and outer limits of the Virchow-Robin perivascular space, which is generally small in the CNS. During CNS inflammation, a separation between the endothelial basement membrane and the parenchymal basement membrane (called glia limitans) is observed in which infiltrated leukocytes have accumulated *(37,115)*. This highly complex extracellular matrix may provide an additional barrier for the diffusion of components into the brain parenchyma.

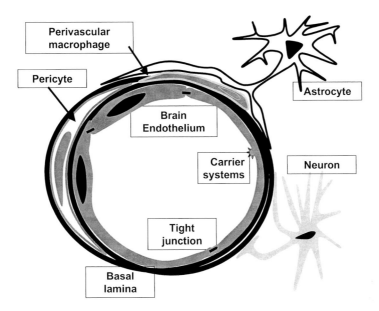

Fig. 1. Cellular composition of the blood–brain barrier. Schematic overview of the cells that form the blood–brain barrier. Cerebral endothelial cells cover the lumen of the brain microvessels and are surrounded by a continuous basal lamina. Pericytes (smooth, muscle-like cells) are also embedded in this lamina. Astrocyte endfeet cover the endothelial monolayer. (Drawing by Ine Vos.)

Astrocytes project their endfeet to this basal lamina and cover more than 95% of the surface of the endothelial cells, thereby forming an interface between the neurons and the endothelium. As a result of this close and abundant contact, astrocytes are believed to influence and conserve the barrier function *(46)*. Transplantation studies revealed that peripheral endothelium has the capacity to form a BBB, because upon the localization in CNS surroundings, these cells develop BBB–EC specific features *(121)*. A number of in vitro experiments also stress the crucial influence of astrocytes to maintain BBB characteristics in brain endothelium in co-culture systems. Astrocytes either by the secretion of soluble factors or direct cell–cell contacts induce high electrical resistance TJs in ECs *(30,95,99,133)*

1.3. Features of the Brain ECs

Although glial elements are required for the barrier function, the fine network of tightly adherent brain ECs in essence forms the BBB. Cerebral EC exhibit functional and morphological differences in comparison with EC derived from peripheral organs. Brain ECs possess a negative anionic charge, lack cellular clefts, fenestrae, a low pinocytotic activity, and an abundance of mitochondria. Caused by this high electrical charge, nonthrombogenic surface, and low expression of adhesion molecules, they repel leukocytes from trafficking into the brain thereby making the CNS an immune-privileged site *(30,54)*. The presence of the continuous seal of TJ complexes between adjacent cells prevents the passage of molecules and ions across the paracellular pathways, the extracellular space between the lateral membranes of neighboring cells. The presence of this TJ defines the polarity of the cell and generating a luminal (apical) and abluminal (basolateral) membrane *(44,60,78,120,133)*.

Functionally, brain ECs have a high metabolic activity caused by the presence of a number of xenobiotic metabolizing enzymes contributing to the protective function of the BBB. Monoamine oxidases, catechol-*O*-methyltransferse, or pseudocholinesterase are capable of degrading neurotransmitters. NADPH cytochrome P450 reductase and glutathion *S*-transferase protect the brain from xenobiotic substances *(6,63)*. Additionally, cerebral EC exhibit a high density of mitochondria, approx 8–11% of the total endothelial cell volume. This allows them to sustain the active transport systems and provides the highly metabolic cells enough energy to maintain TJ integrity.

Although the CNS can control its inner milieu in this way, the existence of a barrier also conveys a necessity for active transport systems to shuttle nutrients to the CNS. The brain endothelium therefore has a number of active transport systems. Brain ECs are actively involved in nutritional supply of the brain by the selective carrier-mediated transport of essential amino acids, glucose, and receptor-mediated transport of insulin, lipoproteins, and transferrin.

Selective carriers exist to actively supply the brain with amino acids, vitamins, free fatty acids, hexoses (especially glucose via the GLUT-1 transporter), nucleic acids/purine bases, and monocarboxylic acid *(10,89)*. Ion transporters such as the potassium/sodium (Na^+/K^+) adenosine triphosphatases (ATPases) aid the passage of charged electrolytes (e.g., Na^+, K^+) across the BBB *(90)*.

Owing to the high expression of P-glycoprotein (Pgp) and other multidrug resistant (MDR) efflux pumps, a number of compounds that on the basis of their physicochemical properties would easily enter the brain are effectively excluded form the CNS. The high expression of Pgp also excludes the brain from compounds that may be beneficial for the treatment of CNS disease, such as brain tumors. Pgp belongs to the adenosine triphosphate (ATP)-binding cassette (ABC) superfamily of active transporters, and so far two different human isoforms of Pgp exist. Although Pgp has been mainly reported in cancerous tissues and cells because of its role in mediating resistance against a wide range of drugs, it is also expressed in several normal tissues including the luminal surface of the endothelial cells comprising the BBB *(21)*. Pgp is associated with MDR in numerous tumors and 6 genes, *MDR-1to MDR-6*, have been identified in humans. So far, *MDR-1, MDR-4, MDR-5*, and *MDR-6* have been reported at the BBB. *MDR-1* is located at the luminal side of brain ECs and functions as an efflux pump for several drugs, e.g., cytostatic drugs (anthracyclines, taxanes) and noncytotoxic drugs (cyclosporin, dexamethasone) *(110,111)*. Recently, genomic studies revealed a set of genes that are specific for the BBB in rats and humans. The brain microvascular endothelium encodes for its unique properties by tissue-specific gene expression within this cell. Currently, studies using a gene microarray approach specific for the BBB revealed 50 gene products specific for BBB endothelium. More than 80% of those were selectively expressed at the BBB; these included novel gene sequences not found in existing databases, and known genes that were not known to be selectively expressed at the BBB. Genes in the latter category include tissue plasminogen activator; insulin-like growth factor-2; myelin basic protein; regulator of G protein signaling 5; utrophin; connexin-45; class I major histocompatibility complex; the rat homolog of the organic anion transporting polypeptide type 2; and transcription factors IκB, hbrm, or EZH1. Identical studies are ongoing for the human BBB and results of these studies may lead to potential new targets for therapy *(72,113)*.

1.4. Molecular Organization of Brain Endothelial Junctions

The highly specialized brain ECs exhibit different metabolic characteristics compared to endothelium of other organs, but also possess well-developed intercellular TJs or so-called zona occludens. In general, brain ECs are not only sealed together by TJs but also by adherent junctions, gap junctions, and desmosomes *(105,118)*.

TJs provide a continuous seal around the apical regions of lateral membranes of the brain ECs. The presence of TJs determine the tightness, and thus the permeability of the brain endothelium by generating a so-called electrical resistance across the brain endothelium, which can be about 1000–1500 Ω/cm^2 *(16)*. In vitro models often monitor this intercellular tightness as a marker for the integrity of the monolayer coupled to diffusion of marker molecules across the endothelial monolayer *(30,95)*. The integrity of the BBB in vitro and in vivo is drastically comprised under inflammatory conditions *(31,96,128)*.

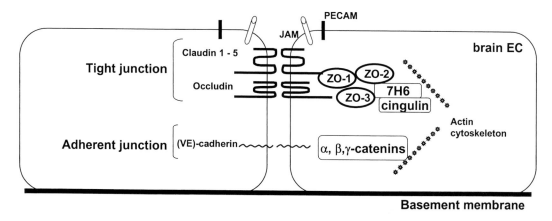

Fig. 2. Molecular organization of brain endothelial cell junctions. Brain endothelial cells express TJs and AJs. Intracellular signaling proteins link the junction proteins to the actin cytoskeleton, thereby influencing the permeability.

Cellular junctions are composed of a network of intracellular and transmembrane proteins that are specific to each type of junction *(26)* (*see* Fig. 2). In epithelial cells, TJs and adherent junctions are clearly separate. In brain ECs there may be a mix of the two junctions in the paracellular cleft *(112)*. Adherent junctions (AJ) molecules, including β catenin, γ catenin and p120, and VE-cadherin, have an important role in controlling paracellular permeability and are a requirement for the successful assembly and integrity of TJs *(20,51)*. The number of TJs in EC inversely relates to the permeability of the endothelial layer, restricting paracellular transport of large and hydrophilic compounds across the brain capillary wall *(30,114)*. So far, two major transmembrane components of the TJ have now been identified, occludin *(43)* and the claudins *(42)*. The phosphoprotein occludin spans the membrane four times with both the amino as well as carboxy terminus located intracellularly. Occludin is thought to be one of the main sealing proteins involved in the TJ *(43,126)*. Occludin is more strongly expressed in brain ECs than peripheral ECs *(58,68)*.

The claudin multi-gene family is comprised of at least 20 members. Structurally, claudins contain two extracellular loops and four transmembrane domains *(42,82,83,126)*. Claudins are believed to be the major transmembrane proteins of the TJ as occludin knock-out mice are still able to form functional TJs *(107)*, whereas claudin knock-out mice are nonviable *(47)*. For brain endothelia, claudin-1 and claudin-5 were found to be expressed *(44,60)*.

Via their carboxy-terminal cytoplasmic tail, occludin and the claudins interact with a number of cytoplasmic zonula occludens proteins (ZO), like ZO-1, ZO-2 and ZO-3 *(39,55)*. These proteins belong to the membrane-associated guanylate kinase (MAGUK) protein family that can interact with other plaque domain molecules such as cingulin. Cingulin *(18)* and 7H6 antigen *(137)*, as well as signaling molecules and cytoskeletal molecules such as cortactin and actin. Other molecules like 7H6, rab3, symplekin, AF-6, and 19B1 have been identified in epithelial TJs, but their role in brain ECs is unknown (for reviews *see* refs. *60,78,120*).

A third transmembrane component of the TJ has recently been described. Junctional adhesion molecule (JAM), a member of the IgSF, is expressed at the TJ. JAM-1 is a member of the immunoglobulin (Ig) superfamily (possessing two variable-region [V]-type Ig domains) and codistributes with TJ components at the apical region of the junction *(7)*. The carboxy-terminal cytoplasmic tail of JAM-1 has been shown to bind the guanylate kinase and/or the acidic domain of occludin, the PSD95/dlg/ZO-1 (PDZ) domain of ZO-1 and cingulin *(7)*. Three members of the JAM family are identified and belong to the Ig superfamilym and are localized at the TJs of both epithelial and endothelial cells *(4,76)*. Recently, an endothelial cell specific adhesion molecule that is a structural equivalent of JAMs was found expressed in the TJ of brain endothelium. This ESAM (or 1G8 antigen) also expresses a PDZ domain, but this did not associate with ZO-1 or with ASIP/PAR3 or AF-6 molecule in contrast to JAM-1 *(86)*.

A number of proteins tightly associate or co-localize with cellular junctions. Platelet endothelial cell adhesion molecule (PECAM-1; CD31) is concentrated at the apical domain of the intercellular junction but not associated with either adherent or TJs *(5)*. PECAM is also a member of the IgSF and is a single chain transmembrane glycoprotein consisting of six extracellular Ig like domains and a cytoplasmic tail. PECAM-1 is involved in cell–cell adhesion through either homophilic interaction *(122)* or heterophilic interaction *(85)* such as with the integrin $\alpha_{\varpi\beta3}$ *(15)*. Recently, altered vascular permeability was detected in PECAM-1 deficient mice, suggesting a role in vascular composition *(49)*. PECAM-1 has also been demonstrated to play a role in several other functions, such as in the transendothelial migration of monocytes across CNS endothelia *(40)*. Besides PECAM, the heavy-glycosylated molecule CD99 was found to be located at the intercellular borders that suggest that this molecule may be present in endothelial junctions *(109)*. Whether this molecule is also present in endothelial cell junction of the brain remains to be established.

Not only the presence of TJ (associated) proteins affect the function or integrity of the junction complex. Several cytoplasmic signaling molecules have been reported to be concentrated at TJs *(78,120)* of which activation may influence the BBB permeability. Two types of heterotrimeric G-proteins $G\alpha_0$ and $G\alpha_{i2}$ localized around TJs were suggested to act as negative regulators for TJ function *(29,106)*. Protein kinase C has also been implicated in the regulation of TJs and is concentrated at TJs *(120)*. TJ proteins are coupled to the actin cytoskeleton and are under the control of a number of intracellular signaling molecules. The small GTPases RhoA, Rac, and Cdc42 are essential mediators of actin reorganization *(53)*. Recently, it was shown that occludin is a target for this GTPase activity and especially that RhoA and its downstream kinase, p160ROCK, are components of a signaling pathway leading to changes in TJ permeability *(59)*.

It has been reported that the degree of tyrosine phosphorylation of junction proteins decreases as TJs become stronger *(69)*. A temporal correlation between phosphorylation of TJ proteins and TJ function was found after incubation of endothelial and epithelial cells with a protein tyrosine phosphatase inhibitor. Treatment of cells with this inhibitor resulted in increased tyrosine phosphorylation of ZO-1 and ZO-2, which paralleled the inhibitor-induced increased permeability *(119)*. Thus, the organization of the TJ complex is under the influence of signaling events that may target directly or indirectly at the TJ, thereby regulating the permeability of the BBB.

Together, the specialized properties of the cerebral endothelium and the surrounding cells will determine whether compounds gain access to the CNS. The BBB is more and more considered to act as a dynamic organ that actively regulates its transport systems or the integrity of its TJs, thereby allowing compounds or cells to enter the CNS.

2. GLIOMA AND THE CEREBROVASCULATURE

The architecture and functioning of the BBB can be drastically altered under neuro-pathological conditions, such as multiple sclerosis, autoimmune deficiency syndrome (AIDS) dementia, or after an ischemic event. The occurrence of tumors in the brain may also induce dramatic changes in the well-organized cerebrovasculature that will be discussed below.

2.1. Glioma Grading

Gliomas make up approx 50% of the primary brain tumors of the CNS in adults, and between 70 and 75% of these tumors are formed by astrocytes. Gliomas may develop *de novo* (primary glioblastomas) or through progression from low-grade or anaplastic astrocytomas (secondary glioblastomas).

Determination of the degree of tissue anaplasia and grade of malignancy of gliomas is based upon qualitative histological features (nuclear pleomorphism, mitoses, endothelial proliferation, and tumor necrosis) *(41)*. This grading procedure is recognized in the revised World Health Organization (WHO) classification of brain tumors for common type astrocytomas *(67)*. Various grades exist to describe the malignancies, benign tumors (grade I), low-grade tumors (grade II), high-grade tumors such as anaplastic astrocytomas (grade III), and gliomablastoma multiforme (grade IV) (for review, *see* ref. *27*).

2.2. Diagnostic Tools

For all glioma entities, the onset of tumor angiogenesis with endothelial proliferation and contrast enhancement in X-ray computed tomography (CT) and magnetic resonance imaging (MRI) seems to be the key criterion indicating tumor progression. Blood perfusion and BBB permeability are of major importance to detect brain tumors using either MRI or CT. Normally, the intact BBB will exclude contrast-enhancing agents from the brain. However, dependent on the neovascularisation within the tumor, a number of diagnostic tools can be used to determine size, location, and the vascularization of brain tumors. CT scans have been routinely used worldwide for the last two decades to diagnose the presence of brain abnormalities. Contrast agents accumulate in the tumor as a result of an increased permeability of the BBB and increased blood volume. Brain tumor microvessels that originate from the neovascularizaton (as observed in high-grade tumors) may be devoid of a BBB, and are thus permeable for the contrast agent. Functional CT scans will provide data to image the BBB permeability and the cerebral blood-volume *(71)*.

Detection of brain tumors is further facilitated by recent developments in MRI techniques. Abnormalities in the vascular structures are readily recognized on MRI and higher contrast resolution will reveal the presence of those tumors that are missed using CT *(27)*. MRI is considered more suitable to detect for low-grade astrocytomas and enables the visualization of skull base tumors. Proper imaging of brain tumors solely based on enhanced BBB permeability as determined by the leakage of contrast agents is difficult because not all brain capillaries are perfused at the same time. Using an animal model, a correlation of the leakage of the contrast agent gadolinium DTPA and growing parameters of the tumor has been made *(129)*, indicating that in the future more advanced MRI techniques may be used as prognostic tools.

So far, CT and MRI still poorly detect small-diameter vessels, which makes it difficult to define tumor angiogenesis. Development of more advanced imaging techniques to monitor cerebrovascular changes may also predict the uptake of anti-cancer drugs in brain tumors.

2.3. Vascular Changes in Glioma

Gliomas are unusual tumors in many aspects. The highly infiltrative growth pattern is one of their characteristics, and tumor cells are capable spreading into the surrounding brain parenchyma over long distances. As a result, these tumors are often unresectable and may remain without neovascularization for at least part of their existence. In low-grade gliomas there is little alteration in the vascular arrangement, and the BBB is intact. However, upon progression tumor cells will cause a distortion of the normal vascular architecture, increasing the distance between vessels, and thus creating hypoxia that in turn triggers angiogenesis.

2.3.1. Angiogenesis, Metastasis, and Matrix Metalloproteinases

One characteristic of angiogenesis is the degradation of the basement membrane and ECM, which are additional physical barriers for cell migration. Angiogenesis, the process of new vessel formation, is a necessary component of malignant tumor progression as rapidly dividing cells require a supply of oxygen and nutrients. However, not all brain tumors depend on angiogenesis, such as low-grade tumors in which the BBB properties still reside in the brain endothelium. In contrast, high-grade tumors are characterized by their angiogenic properties and the BBB properties may be partially lacking. Endothelial cells become hyperplasic with prominent vesicle formation. In addition, vasogenic edema occurs leading to an increase in the cellular content in pinocytotic vesicles, indicating a dysfunction of the BBB. Some capillaries develop fenestrae and have less well-developed sheets of glial endfeet.

During angiogenesis, brain ECs will detach from their ECM, become activated and start to proliferate. In this process, the balance between matrix metalloproteinases (MMPs) and their endogenous inhibitors (TIMPs) is of crucial importance. MMPs are a family of zinc-dependent endopeptidases that are characterized by their ability to degrade various matrix (ECM) components. The family includes collagenases, gelatinases, stromelysins, metalloelastase, and membrane-type metalloproteinases. A major task for MMPs in vivo is the alteration or degradation of ECM molecules to remodel the tissue or assist in the angiogenesis process *(135)*. Upon the activity of MMPs, endothelial cells may be stimulated to migrate to form new vessels. When the normal balance between the proteases and their inhibitors is lost, extensive vessel formation will occur which will result in increased capillary permeability in the newly formed vessels. Pharmaceutical manipulation of the angiogenesis process by influencing MMP activity may suppress the formation of a sufficient vascular bed in the tumor *(136)*, thereby limiting tumor growth.

Consistent with their proteolytic activities, MMPs are also thought to play a role in facilitating tumor cell invasion of the normal brain. Normally released into the extracellular space, MMPs break down the ECM to allow cell growth and to facilitate remodeling. Brain ECs are known to produce MMPs and their activity is regulated by several mediators present in the tumor, like growth factors or inflammatory mediators. For instance, endothelial MMP9 levels are known to increase under the influence of TGFb *(9)*.

Soluble MMPs such as MMP1, 2, 7, 9, are thought to participate in metastasis of tumor cells. In human primary brain tumors, expression of MMP2, MMP3,MMP9, and MMP-14 has been detected, with MMP2, 9, 14 confined to the endothelium *(103,132)*, indicating that the endothelium can contribute to the tumor growth. Both gelatinase-A (MMP2) and gelatinase-B (MMP9) localize in tumor cells, but also in vascular structures in glioma sections *(98)*. An unbalanced MMP-2/TIMP-2 (its inhibitor) ratio in the microenvironment (such as the endothelium) of malignant cells may contribute to their invasive property *(91)*. Pharmaceutically induced changes the endothelial balance in the MMP/TIMP ratio may result in restricting tumor growth by the inhibition of the angiogenesis process, but also influencing the metastasis of tumor cells.

2.3.2. Extracellular Matrix Composition in Gliomas

Not only the breakdown of the ECM will determine the outcome of the angiogenesis in brain tumors, but also its production. In gliomas, an enlargement of the perivascular space surrounding the cerebral blood vessels is observed coupled to an increased thickness of the basement membranes. Structural changes included a thickened, rarefied, and vacuolated lamina *(8,73)*. Dramatic changes in the ECM of high-grade gliomas can be shown (*see* Fig. 3).

Together with the enhanced production of laminin, ahigher deposition of fibronectin, collagen, vitronectin, and tenascin-C was found in a number of gliomas. Recently, a differential gene expression microarray indicated that in low-grade tumors enhanced levels of laminin 9 was found, whereas in high grade tumors the production of the alpha four chain of the ECM molecule laminin-8 was enhanced *(74)*. Formation of this thickened basement membrane around the cerebral capillaries may form an additional barrier for (cytostatic) drugs to enter glioma and thus limit proper treatment.

2.3.4. Growth Factors and Vascular Changes in Gliomas

The angiogenic process is driven by several factors, among which growth factors play a predominant role *(34,127)*. In low-grade brain tumors, growth factor production and the expression of their receptors is limited. In contrast, high-grade gliomas have an abundant expression and production of growth factors and their receptors, to such a degree that angiogenesis runs amok. Endothelial cell

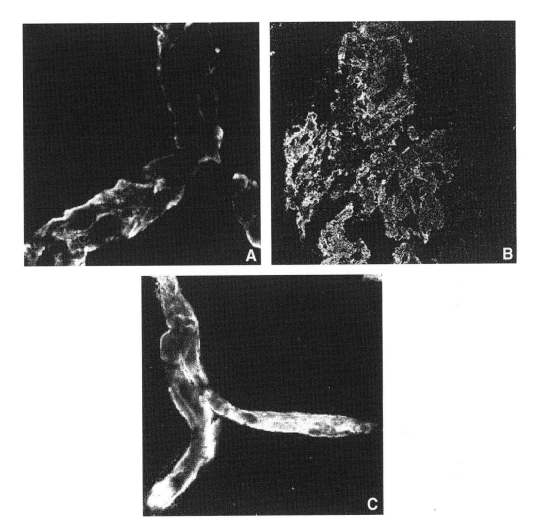

Fig. 3. Changes of the extracellular matrix in glioma. Laminin distribution in type IV astrocytoma as a marker for the organization of the extracellular matrix. **(A)** represents the disorganized distribution of laminin surrounding a vessel. **(B)** shows, that in some areas, laminin is deposited in the surrounding brain parenchyma. **(C)** shows the typical distribution of laminin in control post-mortem tissue. Human brain tissue used in this study was obtained after autopsy with short post-mortem intervals from glioma or control patients. Autopsies were performed under the management of the Netherlands Brain Bank, Amsterdam, The Netherlands. All patients, or their next of kin, had given consent for autopsy and use of their brain tissue for research purposes. Sections were stained and viewed by confocal laser scanning microscopy. Images depicted here are at X63 magnification. (Vos, Montagne. and De Vries, unpublished data).

proliferation by far exceeds migration and tubule formation. As a result, endothelial cells pile up *(12)* and eventually block vessels, causing ischemic necrosis. The endothelial cells of the newly formed vessels do not form a proper BBB, and thus these vessels are leaky *(75)*. This has been demonstrated by the presence of cytostatic drugs within gliomas after intravenous injection of compounds otherwise known for their inability to pass the BBB. Nevertheless, TJ molecules like ZO-1 and occludin are still present in the disordered vessels, suggesting that the microenvironment of the brain still induces expression of these proteins.

The growth factors and growth factor receptors present in gliomas are numerous. These biologically active factors may influence proliferation, tumor cell migration/invasion, angiogenesis, and immune modulation *(34,80,81,92,127)*. Growth factors in gliomas include epidermal growth factor and transforming growth factor β, and also their receptors are known to be induced in brain tumors *(81,84)*. Identically, increased production and expression of other growth factors and their receptors in brain tumors can be detected, like (basic) fibroblast growth factor *(80,127)*: the platelet-derived growth factor isoforms AA, AB, and BB and their receptors *(23,34,127)*; the vascular endothelial growth factors and their receptors flk and flt *(12,17,75,79,134)*; insulin-like growth factor *(57)*; and transforming growth factors *(64,92,131)*. Upon the presence of both the factor and the appropriate receptor, glioma cells can stimulate the tumor cell proliferation and also endothelial cell proliferation *(23,123)*. It is also very likely that the high content of growth factors hinders the normal vessel formation and causes glomeruloid vasculopathy *(12)*.

2.4. Molecular Changes in the Cerebrovasculature in Glioma

2.4.1. Tight Junction Expression in Gliomas

TJs are highly dynamic structures with permeability, assembly, and disassembly characteristics that can be altered by a variety of cellular and metabolic regulators. Reorganization of TJ proteins of the brain endothelium can be found in a number of glioma forms. In the major malignant brain tumor, glioblastoma multiforme, brain microvessels show numerous morphological changes, like formation of fenestrae and endothelial swelling and discontinuous lining.

Recently it was shown that the BBB is molecularly altered in glioblastoma multiforme, revealing a reduced claudin-1 expression in its microvessels. The expression of claudin-5 and occludin were only downregulated in hyperplastic vessels and no apparent changes in the ZO-1 distribution was shown. Changes in the BBB composition results in enhanced permeability of tumor microvessels leading to edema formation associated with a deregulation of TJ proteins *(73)*. Other studies indicate that the TJ protein ZO-1 is still expressed in the endothelial cells in microvessels in astrocytic tumors. However, its expression was weaker in endothelial cells in newly formed microvessels in high-grade tumors compared to normal cerebral capillaries *(108)*. Loss of occludin expression in microvessels and opening of endothelial junctions also occurs in adult human non-neoplastic brain tissue, but different results were obtained in non-neoplastic brain tissue samples, low-grade, and high-grade astrocytomas *(88)*. The expression pattern of TJ proteins ZO-1 and occludin is dramatically altered in high-grade gliomas (*see* Fig. 4).

2.4.2. Growth Factors and Tight Junction Protein Organization

TJ assembly and function can also be modulated during pathological conditions because of the activation of signal transduction pathways. One way that BBB characteristics are lost during glioma formation is the influence of growth factors that are highly produced, like VEGF, on TJs. It is suggested that VEGF induces TJ disassembly and breakdown of the endothelial permeability barrier by altering the organization of TJ proteins. Binding of VEGF to endothelial cell receptors induces receptor dimerization, which then stimulates receptor autophosphorylation and the phosphorylation of downstream signal transduction proteins *(123)*. Upon activation, VEGF receptors are known to phosphorylate several cytoplasmic proteins, including ones that contain receptor phosphotyrosine-binding Src homology 2 (SH2) domains that may be involved in signal transduction, thereby influencing TJ integrity *(52)*. VEGF also induces rapid and transient elevation in cytosolic calcium in several types of cultured peripheral endothelial cells affecting the actin cytoskeleton, which regulates TJ organization *(22)*. TJ s of the BBB are known to be under the control of calcium influx *(14)*, which suggests that VEGF may influence the TJs of the brain endothelium in a similar way.

Recently, a direct effect of VEGF on TJ protein organization has been demonstrated. Studies revealed that VEGF treatment of endothelial monolayers disrupted the distribution of the TJ proteins

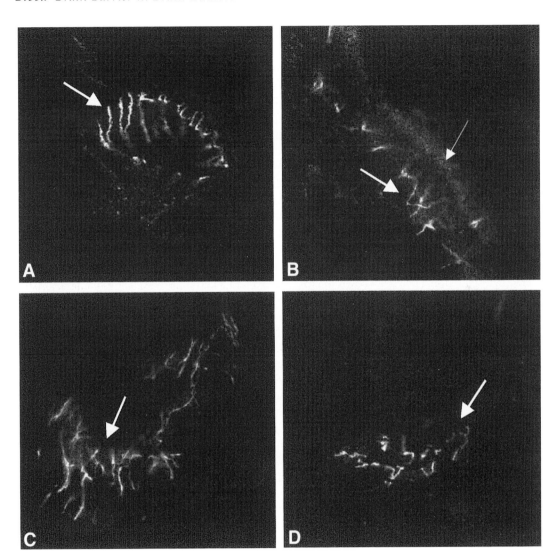

Fig. 4. TJ organization in glioma post-mortem tissue. Sections of high-grade tumors (astrocytoma grade IV) of post-mortem tissue of a glioma patient were stained for the expression of TJ proteins ZO-1 and occludin, and typical examples are shown. In the vessels shown in **(A)**, ZO-1 is clearly expressed as a continuous line (arrow), whereas in another vessel in the glioma, its expression is disorganized (arrow) or has disappeared (thin arrow) **(B)**. Similarly, occludin distribution is disorganized (arrow) **(C)**, whereas in other areas its expression is weaker (arrow) **(D)**. Autopsies were performed under the management of the Netherlands Brain Bank, Amsterdam, The Netherlands. All patients, or their next of kin, had given consent for autopsy and use of their brain tissue for research purposes. Images depicted here are at ×63 magnification. (Vos, Montagne, and De Vries, unpublished data.)

ZO-1 and occludin as well as the actin filaments *(130)*. In vivo, intra-ocular injection of VEGF also caused tyrosine phosphorylation of ZO-1 and occludin phosphorylation as early as 15 min after injection, thereby regulating endothelial paracellular permeability *(1)*. Similarly, VEGF was also found to affect the phosphorylation status of the AJ protein, VE-cadherin *(37)*. Other growth factors present in the tumors may influence the assembly of the TJs. In proximal tubular cells, for instance, TGF-β 1 administration led to loss of cell–cell contact and disassembly of both AJ and TJ complexes *(125)*.

Whether glioma-derived growth factors control the BBB permeability in this way remains to be established. Thus, TJ integrity and BBB function during glioma progression are under the control of a number of factors produced by the surrounding tumor tissue or the endothelium itself.

3. DRUG THERAPY AND THE BLOOD–BRAIN BARRIER

Proper treatment of gliomas is restricted owing to their resistance to chemotherapeutic agents and poor BBB penetration of cytostatic drugs. In high-grade tumors, a number of drugs will reach the brain as a result of the partial dysfunction or complete lack of the presence of the BBB. However, BBB function is still preserved in the low-grade tumors, thereby limiting drug delivery into the CNS. The presence of the BBB will not only limit drug transport into the brain, but more importantly, the high expression of MDR membrane pumps will further limit their transport. A few potential new leads in drug delivery to the CNS will be discussed.

3.1. Current Therapies and the Blood–Brain Barrier

Current therapies are based on the inhibition of tumor cell proliferation by using chemically engineered cytostatic drugs that are known to cross the BBB to a certain extent. The usual noninvasive approach to improve drug delivery to the brain is to "lipidize" the drug, wherein the polar groups on the drug are masked or displaced with lipid groups. The BBB permeability for some cytostatic drugs is thus chemically improved and now drugs such as topoisomerase I inhibitors, oxaliplatin, and temozolomide can readily pass the BBB *(3)*.

Intra-arterial and intrathecal infusion, or intratumoral administration of cytostatic drugs are methods developed to overcome the BBB. Alternatively, active transient BBB disruption is nowadays performed to deliver cytotoxic compounds into the brain. Intra-arterial chemotherapy with osmotic opening of the BBB for the treatment of malignant brain tumors is now used in patients with such tumors *(32)*. The bradykinin B2 receptor agonist, Cereport (RMP-7), selectively increases the permeability of the blood–brain tumor barrier, after which the cytostatic drug carboplatin is efficiently delivered to brain tumors in both animal models and humans *(25)*. Although some of these methods may increase the local concentration-time profile, improvement in clinical outcomes has yet to be definitively established.

More recently, new biological targets are being recognized for treatment, particularly ones that will lead to inhibition of the cellular processes that occur during glioma progression as described earlier. Tumor growth can be inhibited for instance by inhibition of the protein kinase C to limit tumor cell proliferation. Recently, a therapy was developed that inhibits signaling events induced by the activation of growth factor receptors during glioma progression. This tyrosine kinase inhibitor also penetrates the BBB (Gleevec) *(97)*, making it suitable for the treatment of low-grade gliomas. Another class of drugs that inhibits the signaling molecule Ras, a small GTPase, may prove to be successful in limiting tumor progression *(3)*. Becausethese drugs exhibit a wide range of effects, the possibility exists that these compounds not only limit tumor progression but may also inhibit BBB breakdown.

3.2. Trans-Blood–Brain Barrier Delivery Systems

An alternative approach for drug delivery to the CNS is to modify the drug in such a way that the molecule can access one of the endogenous transport systems of the brain endothelium. Experimental therapies now aim to cross the BBB by making use of such delivery factors. The efficacy of a number of CNS delivery systems is predominantly tested in animal models. One strategy to increase CNS entry of a drug is to encapsulate it in liposomes. Liposomes that encapsulate cytostatic drugs like doxorubicin, for instance, are used to improve drug delivery across the BBB *(38)*. CNS delivery systems may also use the intrinsic activity of the BBB to transport compounds via carrier-mediated transport systems, such as, via the glucose and amino acid carriers. Other transport vectors make use of the BBB capacity to actively regulate transport of compounds, for instance, via absorptive-mediated transcytosis, like cationized albumin to which drugs can be conjugated *(89,90)*. Alternatively, drugs can also be transported across the BBB using receptor-mediated transcytosis via the transferrin receptor that is highly expressed on brain endothelium. Liposomes with the anti-transferrin receptor antibody OX-26 incorporated in their lipid layer are thus used to deliver drugs into the CNS *(61)*. This antibody OX-26 alone has also been shown to effectively transcytose conjugated drugs across the cerebral endothelial lining *(90)*. Whether these strategies will be applicable for drug delivery in patients with brain tumors remains to be established.

Pgp, responsible for the drug resistance of the BBB, may restrict the brain entrance or increase the brain clearance of a broad number of therapeutic compounds, including cytotoxic drugs. Few studies have explored the possibilities of structural modification of drugs to bypass MDR *(66)* or co-administration of the drug with Pgp modulators that inhibit the effect of Pgp at the BBB *(19,33)*. Recently, the use of so-called penetratins, serving as drug-conjugated delivery systems, is being explored to circumvent Pgp activity at the BBB. These peptides translocate efficiently through biological membranes and were shown to be successful in the delivery of conjugated doxorubicin into the CNS *(104)*. These peptides have provided the basis for the development of new peptide-conjugated drugs for transport through BBB.

4. CONCLUDING REMARKS

BBB function may be affected severely in gliomas of various grades. A wide range of factors may influence the function of the BBB in gliomas at a molecular level disrupting the intercellular junctions, and at a cellular level affecting BBB selective transport and enzyme systems. In many cases, however, the BBB is still fully or partially functional. Drug delivery to the tumor is therefore restricted and will negatively influence appropriate therapy. In the future, characterization of the features of the BBB in low-grade gliomas by combined genomic or proteomic studies may offer new leads to develop novel BBB-specific delivery factors. Brain drug targeting technology will enable the delivery to cytostatic drugs to the tumors located in the CNS by either circumventing or using the BBB.

REFERENCES

1. Antonetti D.A., Barber A.J., Hollinger L.A., Wolpert E.B., Gardner T.W. 1999. Vascular endothelial growth factor induces rapid phosphorylation of tight junction proteins occludin and zonula occluden 1. A potential mechanism for vascular permeability in diabetic retinopathy and tumors. *J. Biol. Chem.* **274**:23,463–23,467.
2. Angelov D.N., Krebs C., Walther M., Martinez-Portillo F.J., Gunkel A., Lay C.H., et al. 1998. Altered expression of immune-related antigens by neuronophages does not improve neuronal survival after severe lesion of the facial nerve in rats. *Glia* **24**:155–171.
3. Avgeropoulos N.G., Batchelor T.T. 1999. New treatment strategies for malignant glioma. *The Oncologist* **4**:209–224.
4. Aurrand-Lions M., Johnson-Leger C., Wong C., Du Pasquier L., Imhof B.A. 2001. Heterogeneity of endothelial junctions is reflected by differential expression and specific subcellular localization of the three JAM family members. *Blood* **98**:3699–3707.
5. Ayalon O., Sabanai H., Lampugnani M.G., Dejana E., Geiger B. 1994. Spatial and temporal relationships between cadherins and PECAM-1 in cell-cell junctions of human endothelial cells. *J. Cell Biol.* **126**:247–258.
6. Baranczyk-Kuzma A., Audus K.L. 1987. Characteristics of aminopeptidase activity from bovine brain microvessel endothelium. *J. Cereb. Blood Flow Metab.* **7**:801–805.
7. Bazzoni G., Martinez-Estrada O.M., Orsenigo F., Cordenonsi M., Citi S., Dejana E. 2000. Interaction of junctional adhesion molecule with the tight junction components ZO-1, cingulin, and occludin. *J. Biol. Chem.* **275**:20,520–20,526.
8. Bertossi M., Virgintino D., Maiorano E., Occhiogrosso M., Roncali L. 1997. Ultrastructural and morphometric investigation of human brain capillaries in normal and peritumoral tissues. *Ultrastruct. Pathol.* **21**:41–49.
9. Behzadian M.A., Wang X.L., Windsor L.J., Ghaly N., Caldwell R.B. 2001. TGF-beta increases retinal endothelial cell permeability by increasing MMP-9: possible role of glial cells in endothelial barrier function. Invest. Ophthalmol. *Vis. Sci.* **42**:853–859.
10. Betz A.L., Goldstein G.W. 1978. Polarity of the blood–brain barrier: neutral amino acid transport into isolated brain capillaries. *Science* **202**:225–227.

11. Bradbury M.W. 1985. The blood–brain barrier. Transport across the cerebral endothelium. *Circ. Res.* **57:**213–222.

12. Brat D.J., Van Meir E.G. 2001. Glomeruloid microvascular proliferation orchestrated by VPF/VEGF: a new world of angiogenesis research. *Am. J. Pathol.* **158:**1145–1160.

13. Broadwell R.D., Salcman M. 1981. Expanding the definition of the blood–brain barrier to protein. *Proc. Natl. Acad. Sci. USA* **78:**7820–7824.

14. Brown R.C., Davis T.P. 2002. Calcium modulation of adherens and tight junction function: a potential mechanism for blood–brain barrier disruption after stroke. *Stroke* **33:**1706–1711.

15. Buckley C.D., Doyonnas R., Newton J.P., Blystone S.D., Brown E.J., Watt S.M., Simmons D.L. 1996. Identification of alpha v beta 3 as a heterotypic ligand for CD31/PECAM-1. *J. Cell Sci.* **109:**437–445.

16. Butt A.M., Jones H.C., Abbott N.J. 1990. Electrical resistance across the blood–brain barrier in anaesthetized rats: a developmental study. *J. Physiol.* **429:**47–62.

17. Chaudhry I.H., O'Donovan D.G., Brenchley P.E., Reid H., Roberts I.H. 2001. Vascular endothelial growth factor expression correlates with tumor grade and vascularity in gliomas. *Histopathology* **39:**409–415.

18. Citi S., Sabanay H., Kendrick J.J., Geiger B. 1989. Cingulin: characterization and localization. *J. Cell Sci.* **93:**107–122.

19. Colombo T., Zucchetti M., D'Incalci M. 1994. Cyclosporin A markedly changes the distribution of doxorubicin in mice and rats. *J. Pharmacol. Exp. Ther.* **269:**22–27.

20. Corada M., Mariotti M., Thurston G., Smith K., Kunkel R., Brockhaus M., et al. 1999. Vascular endothelial-cadherin is an important determinant of microvascular integrity in vivo. *Proc. Natl. Acad. Sci. USA* **96:**9815–9820.

21. Cordon-Cardo C., O'Brien J.P., Casals D., Rittman-Grauer L., Biedler J.L., Melamed M.R., Bertino J.R. 1989. Multidrug-resistance gene (P-glycoprotein) is expressed by endothelial cells at blood–brain barrier sites. *Proc. Natl. Acad. Sci. USA* **86:**695–698.

22. Criscuolo G.R., Lelkes P.I., Rotrosen D., Oldfield E.H. 1989. Cytosolic calcium changes in endothelial cells induced by a protein product of human gliomas containing vascular permeability factor activity. *J. Neurosurg.* **71:**884–891.

23. Dai. C., Celestino J.C., Okada Y., Louis D.N., Fuller G.N., Holland E.C. 2001. PDGF autocrine stimulation dedifferentiates cultured astrocytes and induces oligodendrogliomas and oligoastrocytomas from neural progenitors and astrocytes in vivo. *Genes Dev.* **15:**1913–1925.

24. Davson H., Oldendorf W.H. 1967. Symposium on membrane transport. Transport in the central nervous system. *Proc. R. Soc. Med.* **60:**326–329.

25. Dean R.L., Emerich D.F., Hasler B.P., Bartus R.T. 1999. Cereport (RMP-7) increases carboplatin levels in brain tumors after pretreatment with dexamethasone. *Neuro-oncol.* **1:**268–274.

26. Dejana E., Corada M., Lampugnani M.G. 1995. Endothelial cell-to-cell junctions. *FASEB J.* **9:**910–918.

27. Del Sole A., Falini A., Ravasi L., Ottobrini D., De Marchis D., Bombardieri E., Lucignani G. 2001. Anatomical and biochemical investigation of primary brain tumours. *Eur. J. Nucl. Med.* **28:**1851–1872.

28. Dempsey E.W., Wislocki G.B. 1955. An electron microscopic study of the blood- brain barrier in the rat, employing silver nitrate as a vital stain. *J. Biophys. Biochem. Cytol.* **1:**245–256.

29. Denker B.M., Saha C., Khawaja S., Nigam S.K. 1996. Involvement of a heterotrimeric G protein alpha subunit in tight junction biogenesis. *J. Biol. Chem.* **271:**25,750–25,753.

30. De Vries H.E., Kuiper J., de Boer A.G., van Berkel T.J.C., Breimer D.D. 1997. The blood–brain barrier in neuroinflammatory diseases (review). *Pharm. Reviews* **49:**143–155.

31. De Vries H.E., Blom-Roosemalen M.C., van Oosten M., de Boer A.G., van Berkel T.J.C., Breimer D.D., Kuiper J. 1996. The influence of cytokines on the integrity of the blood–brain barrier in vitro. *J. Neuroimmunol.* **64:**37–43.

32. Doolittle N.D., Miner M.E., Hall W.A., Siegal T., Jerome E., Osztie E.,et al. 2000. Safety and efficacy of a multicenter study using intraarterial chemotherapy in conjunction with osmotic opening of the blood–brain barrier for the treatment of patients with malignant brain tumors. *Cancer* **88:**637–647.

33. Drion N., Lemaire M., Lefauconnier J.M., Scherrmann J.M. 1996. Role of P-glycoprotein in the blood–brain transport of colchicine and vinblastine. *J. Neurochem.* **67:**1688–1693.

34. Dunn I.F., Heese O., Black P.M. 2000. Growth factors in glioma angiogenesis: FGFs, PDGF, EGF, and TGFs. *J. Neurooncol.* **50:**121–137.

35. Ehrlich P. 1885. *Das Suaerstoffbeduerfnis des Organismus: eine farbenanalystische studie.* Hirschwald, Berlin.

36. Esiri M.M. 1990. Immunological and neuropathological significance of the Virchow-Robin space. *J. Neurol. Sci.* **100:**3–8.

37. Esser S., Lampugnani M.G., Corada M., Dejana E., Risau W. 1998. Vascular endothelial growth factor induces VE-cadherin tyrosine phosphorylation in endothelial cells. *J. Cell Sci.* **111:**1853–1865.

38. Fabel K., Dietrich J., Hau P., Wismeth C., Winner B., Przywara S., et al. 2001. Long-term stabilization in patients with malignant glioma after treatment with liposomal doxorubicin. Cancer **92:**1936–1942.

39. Fanning A.S., Jameson B.J., Jesaitis L.A., Anderson J.M. 1998. The tight junction protein ZO-1 establishes a link between the transmembrane protein occludin and the actin cytoskeleton. *J. Biol. Chem.* **273:**29,745–29,753.

40. Floris S., Ruuls S.R., Wierinckx A., van der Pol S.M.A., Dopp E., van der Meide P.H., et al. 2002. Interferon-beta directly influences monocyte infiltration into the central nervous system. *J. Neuroimmunol.* **127:**69–79.

41. Fuller G.N., Hess K.R., Rhee C.H., Yung W.K., Sawaya R.A., Bruner J.M., ZhangW. 2002. Molecular classification of human diffuse gliomas by multidimensional scaling analysis of gene expression profiles parallels morphology-based classification, correlates with survival, and reveals clinically-relevant novel glioma subsets. *Brain Pathol.* **12**:108–116.

42. Furuse M., Fujita K., Hiiragi T., Fujimoto K., Tsukita S. 1998. Claudin-1 and -2: novel integral membrane proteins localizing at tight junctions with no sequence similarity to occludin. *J. Cell Biol.* **141**:1539–1550.

43. Furuse M., Hirase T., Itoh M., Nagafuchi A., Yonemura S., Tsukita S. 1993. Occludin: a novel integral membrane protein localizing at tight junctions. *J. Cell Biol.* **123**:1777–1788.

44. Gloor S.M., Wachtel M., Bolliger M.F., Ishihara H., Landmann R., Frei K. 2001. Molecular and cellular permeability control at the blood–brain barrier. *Brain Res. Rev.* **36**:258–264.

45. Goldmann E.E. 1909. Die aussere and innere Sekretion des gesundes und kranken Organismus im Lichte der vitalen Farbung. *Beitr. Klin. Chir.* **64**:192–265.

46. Goldstein G.W. 1988. Endothelial cell-astrocyte interactions. A cellular model of the blood–brain barrier. *Ann. N. Y. Acad. Sci.* **529**:31–39.

47. Gow A., Southwood C.M., Li J.S., Pariali M., Riordan G.P., Brodie S.E., et al. 1999. CNS myelin and sertoli cell tight junction strands are absent in Osp/claudin-11 null mice. *Cell* **99**:649–659

48. Graeber M.B., Streit W.J., Kreutzberg G.W. 1989. Identity of ED2-positive perivascular cells in rat brain. *J. Neurosci. Res.* **22**:103–106.

49. Graesser D., Solowiej A., Bruckner M., Osterweil E., Juedes A., Davis S., et al. 2002. Altered vascular permeability and early onset of experimental autoimmune encephalomyelitis in PECAM-1-deficient mice. *J. Clin. Invest.* **109**:383–392.

50. Gross P.M. 1992. Circumventricular organ capillaries. *Prog. Brain Res.* **91**:219–233.

51. Gumbiner B., Lowenkopf T., Apatira D. 1991. Identification of a 160-kDa polypeptide that binds to the tight junction protein ZO-1. *Proc. Natl. Acad. Sci. USA* **88**:3460–3464.

52. Guo D., Jia Q., Song H.Y., Warren R.S., Donner D.B. 1995. Vascular endothelial cell growth factor promotes tyrosine phosphorylation of mediators of signal transduction that contain SH2 domains. Association with endothelial cell proliferation. *J. Biol. Chem.* **270**:6729–6733.

53. Hall A. 1999. RhoGTPases and the actin cytoskeleton. *Science* **279**:509–514.

54. Hardebo J.E., Kahrstrom J. 1985. Endothelial negative surface charge areas and blood–brain barrier function. *Acta Physiol. Scand.* **125**:495–499.

55. Haskins J., Gu L., Wittchen E.S., Hibbard J., Stevenson B.R. 1998. ZO-3, a novel member of the MAGUK protein family found at the tight junction, interacts with ZO-1 and occludin. *J. Cell Biol.* **141**:199–208.

56. Hickey W.F., Kimura H. 1988. Perivascular microglial cells of the CNS are bone marrow-derived and present antigen in vivo. *Science* **239**:290–292.

57. Hirano H., Lopes M.B., Laws E.R. Jr, Asakura T., Goto M., Carpenter J.E., et al. 1999. Insulin-like growth factor-1 content and pattern of expression correlates with histopathologic grade in diffusely infiltrating astrocytomas. *Neurooncol.* **1**:109–119.

58. Hirase T., Staddon J.M., Saitou M., Ando A.Y., Itoh M., Furuse M., et al. 1997. Occludin as a possible determinant of tight junction permeability in endothelial cells. *J. Cell Sci.* **110**:1603–1613.

59. Hirase T., Kawashima S., Wong E.Y., Ueyama T., Rikitake Y., Tsukita S., et al. 2001. Regulation of tight junction permeability and occludin phosphorylation by Rhoa-p160ROCK-dependent and -independent mechanisms. *J. Biol. Chem.* **276**:10,423–10,431.

60. Huber J.D., Egleton R.D., Davis T.P. 2001. Molecular physiology and pathophysiology of tight junctions in the blood–brain barrier. *Trends Neurosci.* **24**:719–725.

61. Huwyler J., Wu D., Pardridge W.M. 1996. Brain drug delivery of small molecules using immunoliposomes. *Proc. Natl. Acad. Sci. USA* **93**:14,164–14,169.

62. Jucker M., Tian M., Ingram D.K. 1996. Laminins in the adult and aged brain. *Mol. Chem. Neuropathol.* **28**:209–218.

63. Kalaria R.N., Harik S.I. 1987. Differential postnatal development of monoamine oxidases A and B in the blood–brain barrier of the rat. *J. Neurochem.* **49**:1589–1594.

64. Kjellman C., Olofsson S.P., Hansson O., Von Schantz T., Lindvall M., Nilsson I., et al. 2000. Expression of TGF-beta isoforms, TGF-beta receptors, and SMAD molecules at different stages of human glioma. *Int. J. Cancer* **89**:251–258.

65. Kida S., Steart P.V., Zhang E.T., Weller R.O. 1993. Perivascular cells act as scavengers in the cerebral perivascular spaces and remain distinct from pericytes, microglia and macrophages. *Acta Neuropathol (Berl)* **85**:646–652.

66. Klopman G., Shi L.M., Ramu A. 1997. Quantitative structure-activity relationship of multidrug resistance reversal agents. *Mol. Pharmacol.* **52**:323–333.

67. Kleihues P., Louis D.N., Scheithauer B.W., Rorke L.B., Reifenberger G., Burger P.C, et al. 2002. The WHO classification of tumors of the nervous system. *J. Neuropathol. Exp. Neurol.* **61**:215–225

68. Kniesel U., Wolburg H. 2000. Tight junctions of the blood–brain barrier. *Cell. Mol. Neurobiol.* **20**:57–76.

69. Lampugnani M.G., Dejana E. 1997. Interendothelial junctions: structure, signaling and functional roles. *Curr. Opin. Cell Biol.* **9**:674–682.

70. Lassmann H., Zimprich F., Vass K., Hickey W.F. 1991. Microglial cells are a component of the perivascular glia limitans. *J. Neurosci. Res.* **28**:236–243.

71. Legget D.A.C., Miles K.A., Kelley B.B. 1999. Blood–brain barrier and blood-volume imaging of cerebral glioma using functional CT: a pictorial view. *Eur. J. Radiol.* **30:**185–190.

72. Li J.Y., Boado R.J., Pardridge W.M. 2001. Blood–brain barrier genomics. *J. Cereb. Blood Flow Metab.* **21:**61–68.

73. Liebner S., Fischmann A., Rascher G., Duffner F., Grote E.H., Kalbacher H., et al. 2000. Claudin-1 and claudin-5 expression and tight junction morphology are altered in blood vessels of human glioblastoma multiforme. *Acta Neuropathol.* **100:**323–331.

74. Ljubimova J.Y., Lakhter A.J., Loksh A., Yong W.H., Riedinger M.S., Miner J.H., et al. 2001. Overexpression of alpha4 chain-containing laminins in human glial tumors identified by gene microarray analysis. *Cancer Res.* **61:**5601–5610.

75. Machein M.R., Kullmer J., Fiebich B.L., Plate K.H., Warnke P.C. 1999. Vascular endothelial growth factor expression, vascular volume, and, capillary permeability in human brain tumors. *Neurosurgery* **44:**732–740.

76. Martìn-Padura I., Lostaglio S., Schneemann M., Williams L., Romano M., Fruscella P., et al. 1998. Junctional adhesion molecule, a novel member of the immunoglobulin superfamily that distributes at intercellular junctions and modulates monocyte transmigration. *J. Cell Biol.* **142:**117–127.

77. Mato M., Ookawara S., Saito-Taki T. 1996. Serological determinants of fluorescent granular perithelial cells along small cerebral blood vessels in rodent. *Acta Neuropathol (Berl).* **72:**117–123.

78. Mitic L.L., Anderson J.M. 1998. Molecular architecture of the tight junction. *Annu. Rev. Physiol.* **60:**121–142.

79. Miyagami M., Tazoe M.,.Nakamura S. 1998. Expression of vascular endothelial growth factor and p53 protein in association with neovascularization in human malignant gliomas. *Brain Tumor Pathol.* **15:**95–100.

80. Miyagi N., Kato S., Terasaki M., Shigemori M., Morimatsu M. 1998. Fibroblast growth factor-2 and –9 regulate proliferation and production of matrix metalloproteinases in human gliomas. *Int. J. Oncol.* **12:**1085–1090.

81. Monaghan M., Mulligan K.A., Gillespie H., Trimble A., Winter P., Johnston P.G., et al. 2000. Epidermal growth factor up-regulates CD44-dependent astrocytmoa invasion in vitro. *J. Pathol.* **192:**519–525.

82. Morita K., Furuse M., Fujimoto K., Tsukita S. 1999a. Claudin multigene family encoding four-transmembrane domain protein components of tight junction strands. *Proc. Natl. Acad. Sci. USA* **96:**511–516.

83. Morita K., Sasaki H., Furuse M., Tsukita S. 1999b. Endothelial claudin: claudin-5/TMVCF constitutes tight junction strands in endothelial cells. *J. Cell Biol.* **147:**185–194.

84. Muleris M., Almeida A., Dutrillaux A.M., Pruchon E., Vega F., Delattre J.Y., et al. 1994. Oncogene amplification in human gliomas: a molecular cytogenetic analysis. *Oncogene* **9:**2717–2722.

85. Muller W.A., Berman M.E., Newman P.J., DeLisser H.M., Albelda S.M. 1992. A heterophilic adhesion mechanism for platelet/endothelial cell adhesion molecule 1 (CD31). *J. Exp. Med.* **175:**1401–1404.

86. Nasdala I., Wolburg-Buchholz K., Wolburg H., Kuhn A., Ebnet K., Brachtendorf G., et al. 2002. A transmembrane tight junction protein selectively expressed on endothelial cells and platelets. *J. Biol. Chem.* **277:**16,294–16,303.

87. Ookawara S., Mitsuhashi U., Suminaga Y., Mato M. 1996. Study on distribution of pericyte and fluorescent granular perithelial (FGP) cell in the transitional region between arteriole and capillary in rat cerebral cortex. *Anat Rec.* **244:** 257–264.

88. Papadopoulos M.C., Saadoun S., Woodrow C.J., Davies D.C., Costa-Martins P., Moss R.F., et al. 2001. Occludin expression in microvessels of neoplastic and non-neoplastic human brain. *Neuropathol. Appl. Neurobiol.* **27:**384–395.

89. PardridgeW.M. 1986. Blood–brain transport of nutrients. *Fed. Proc.* **45:**2047–2049.

90. Pardridge W.M. 2002. Targeting neurotherapeutic agents through the blood–brain barrier. *Arch. Neurol.* **59:**35–40.

91. Planchenault T., Costa S., Fages C., Riche D., Charriere-Bertrand C., Perzelova A., et al. 2001. Differential expression of laminin and fibronectin and of their related metalloproteinases in human glioma cell lines: relation to invasion. *Neurosci Lett* **299:**140–144.

92. Platten M., Wick W., Weller M. 2001. Malignant glioma biology: role for TGF-beta in growth, motility, angiogenesis, and immune escape. *Microsc. Res. Tech.* **52:**401–410.

93. Polfliet M.M.,.Zwijnenburg P.J., van Furth A.M., van der Poll T., Dopp E.A., Renardel de Lavalette C., et al. 2001. Meningeal and perivascular macrophages of the central nervous system play a protective role during bacterial meningitis. *J. Immunol.* **167:**4644–4650.

94. Polfliet M.M., van de Veerdonk F., Dopp E.A., van Kesteren-Hendrikx E.M., van Rooijen N., et al. 2002. The role of perivascular and meningeal macrophages in experimental allergic encephalomyelitis. *J. Neuroimmunol.* **122:**1–8.

95. Prat A., Biernacki K., Wosik K., Antel J.P. 2001. Glial cell influence on the human blood–brain barrier. *Glia* **36:**145–155.

96. QuagliarelloV.J., Wispelwey B., Long W.J., Scheld W.M. 1991. Recombinant human interleukin-1 induces meningitis and blood–brain barrier injury in the rat. Characterization and comparison with tumor necrosis factor. *J. Clin. Invest.* **87:**1360–1366.

97. Radford I.R. 2002. Imatinib. Novartis. *Curr. Opin. Investig. Drugs* **3:**492–499.

98. Raithatha S.A., Muzik H., Rewcastle N.B., Johnston R.N., Edwards D.R., Forsyth P.A. 2000. Localization of gelatinase-A and gelatinase-B mRNA and protein in human gliomas. *Neurooncol.* **2:**145–150.

99. Raub T.J. 1996. Signal transduction and glial cell modulation of cultured brain microvessel endothelial cell tight junctions. *Am. J. Physiol.* **271:**C495–C503.

100. Robinson P.J., Rapoport S.I. 1986. Kinetics of protein binding determine rates of uptake of drugs by brain. *Am. J. Physiol.* **251:**R1212–1220.

101. Reese T.S., Feder N., Brightman M.W. 1971. Electron microscopic study of the blood–brain and blood-cerebrospinal fluid barriers with microperoxidase. *J. Neuropathol. Exp. Neurol.* **30:**137–138.

102. Reese T.S., Karnovsky M.J. 1967. Fine structural localization of a blood–brain barrier to exogenous peroxidase. *J. Cell Biol.* **34:**207–217.

103. Roopraai H.K.,.Van Meter T., Rucklidge G.J., Hudson L., Everal L.P., Pilkington G.J. 1998. Comparative analysis of matrix metalloproteinases by immunocytochemistry, immunohistochemistry and zymography in human primary brain tumours. *Int J Oncol.* **13:**1153–1157.

104. Rousselle C., Clair P., Lefauconnier J.M., Kaczorek M., Scherrmann J.M., Temsamani J. 2000. New advances in the transport of doxorubicin through the blood–brain barrier by a peptide vector-mediated strategy. *Mol. Pharmacol.* **57:**679–686.

105. Rubin L.L. 1992. Endothelial cells: adhesion and tight junctions. *Curr. Opin. Cell Biol.* **4:**830–833.

106. Saha C., Nigam S.K., Denker B.M. 1998. Involvement of Galphai2 in the maintenance and biogenesis of epithelial cell tight junctions. *J. Biol. Chem.* **273:**21,629–21,633.

107. Saitou M, Furuse M., Sasaki H., Schulzke J.D., Fromm M., Takano H., et al. 2000.Complex phenotype of mice lacking occludin, a component of tight junction strands. *Mol. Biol. Cell* **11:**4131–4142.

108. Sawada T., Kato Y., Kobayashi M., Takekekawa Y. 2000. Immunohistochemical study of tight junction-related protein in neovasculature in astrocytic tumor. *Brain Tumor Pathol.* **17:**1–6.

109. Schenkel A.R., Mamdouh Z., Chen X., Liebman R.M., Muller W.A. 2002. CD99 plays a major role in the migration of monocytes through endothelial junctions. *Nat. Immunol.* **3:**143–150

110. Schinkel A.H., Wagenaar E., van Deemter L., Mol C.A., Borst P. 1995. Absence of the mdr1a P-Glycoprotein in mice affects tissue distribution and pharmacokinetics of dexamethasone, digoxin, and cyclosporin A. *J. Clin. Invest* **96:**1698–1705.

111. Schinkel A.H., Mol C.A., Wagenaar E., van Deemter L., Smit J.J., Borst P. 1995b. Multidrug resistance and the role of P-glycoprotein knockout mice. *Eur. J. Cancer* **31A:**1295–1298.

112. Schulze C., Firth J.A. 1993. Immunohistochemical localization of adherens junction components in blood–brain barrier microvessels of the rat. *J. Cell Sci.* **104:**773–782.

113. Shusta E.V.,.Boado R.J., Mathern G.W., Pardridge W.M. 2002. Vascular genomics of the human brain. *J. Cereb. Blood Flow Metab.* **22:**245–252.

114. Simionescu M., Simionescu N. 1986. Functions of the endothelial cell surface. *Ann. Rev. Physiol.* **48:**279–293.

115. Sixt M., Engelhardt B., Pausch F., Hallmann R., Wendler O., Sorokin L.M. 2001. Endothelial cell laminin isoforms, laminins 8 and 10, play decisive roles in T cell recruitment across the blood–brain barrier in experimental autoimmune encephalomyelitis. *J. Cell Biol.* **153:**933–946.

116. Sobel R.A. 1998. The extracellular matrix in multiple sclerosis lesions. *J. Neuropathol. Exp. Neurol.* **57:**205–217

117. Sobel R.A. 2001. The extracellular matrix in multiple sclerosis: an update. *Braz. J. Med. Biol. Res.* **34:**603–609.

118. Staddon J.M., Rubin L.L. 1996. Cell adhesion, cell junctions and the blood–brain barrier. *Curr. Opin. Neurobiol.* **6:**622–627.

119. Staddon J.M., Herrenknecht K., Smales C., Rubin L.L. 1995. Evidence that tyrosine phosphorylation may increase tight junction permeability. *J. Cell Sci.* **108:**609–619.

120. Stevenson B.R., Keon B.H. 1998. The tight junction: morphology to molecules. *Ann. Rev. Cell Dev. Biol.* **14:**89–109.

121. Stewart P.A., Wiley M.J. 1981. Developing nervous tissue induces formation of blood–brain barrier characteristics in invading endothelial cells: a study using quail—chick transplantation chimeras. *Dev. Biol.* **84:**183–192.

122. Sun Q.H., DeLisser H.M., Zukowski M.M., Paddock C., Albelda S.M., Newman P.J. 1996. Individually distinct Ig homology domains in PECAM-1 regulate homophilic binding and modulate receptor affinity. *J. Biol. Chem.* **271:**11,090–11,098.

123. Thomas K.A. 1996. Vascular endothelial growth factor, a potent and selective angiogenic agent. *J. Biol. Chem.* **271:** 603–606.

124. Tian M., Hagg T., Denisova N., Knusel B., Engvall E., Jucker M. 1997. Laminin-alpha2 chain-like antigens in CNS dendritic spines. *Brain Res.* **764:**28–38.

125. Tian Y.C., Phillips A.O. 2002. Interaction between the transforming growth factor-beta type II receptor/Smad pathway and beta-catenin during transforming growth factor-beta1-mediated adherens junction disassembly. *Am. J. Pathol.* **160:**1619–1628.

126. Tsukita S., Furuse M. 1999. Occludin and claudins in tight-junction strands: leading or supporting players? *Trends Cell Biol.* **9:**268–273.

127. Van der Valk P., Lindeman J., Kamphorst W. 1997. Growth factor profiles of human gliomas. Do non-tumour cells contribute to tumour growth in glioma? *Ann.Oncol.* **8:**1023–1029.

128. Van der Goes A., Wouters D., van der Pol S.M.A., Huizinga R., Ronken E., Adamson P., et al. 2001. Reactive oxygen species enhance the migration of monocytes across the blood–brain barrier in vitro. *FASEB J.* **15:**1852–1854.

129. Van der Sanden B.P., Rozijn T.H., Rijken P.F., Peters H.P., Heerschap A., van der Kogel A.J., Bovee W.M. 2000. Noninvasive assessment of the functional neovasculature in 9L-glioma growing in rat brain by dynamic 1H magnetic resonance imaging of gadolinium uptake. *J. Cereb. Blood Flow Metab.* **20:**861–870.

130. Wang W.,.Dentler W.L., Borchardt R.T. 2001. VEGF increases BMEC monolayer permeability by affecting occludin expression and tight junction assembly. *Am. J. Physiol. Heart Circ. Physiol.* **280**:434–440.

131. Wick W., Grimmel C., Wild-Bode C., Platten M., Arpin M., Weller M. 2001. Ezrin-dependent promotion of glioma cell clonogenicity, motility, and invasion mediated by BCL-2 and transforming growth factor-beta2. *J. Neurosci.* **21:** 3360–3368.

132. Wild-Bode C., Weller M., Wick W. 2001. Molecular determinants of glioma cell migration and invasion. *J. Neurosurg.* **94:**978–984.

133. Wolburg H., Neuhaus J., Kniesel U., Krauss B., Schmid E.M, Ocalan M., et al. 1994. Modulation of tight junction structure in blood–brain barrier endothelial cells. Effects of tissue culture, second messengers and cocultured astrocytes. *J. Cell Sci.* **107:**1347–1357.

134. Yao Y.,.Kubota T., Sato K., Kitai R., Takeuchi H., Arishima H. 2001. Prognostic value of vascular endothelial growth factor and its receptors Flt-1 and Flk-1 in astrocytic tumours. *Acta Neurochir. (Wien)* **143:**159–166.

135. Yong V.W.,.Krekoski C.A., Forsyth P.A., Bell R., Edwards D.R. 1998. Matrix metalloproteinases and diseases of the CNS. *Trends Neurosci.* **21:**75–80.

136. Yoshida D., Noha M., Watanabe K., Sugisaki Y., Teramoto A. 2002. SI-27, a novel inhibitor of matrix metalloproteinases with antiangiogenic activity: detection with a variable-pressure scanning electron microscope. *Neurosurgery* **50:** 578–586.

137. Zhong Y., Saitoh T., Minase T., Sawada N., Enomoto K., Mori M. 1993. Monoclonal antibody 7H6 reacts with a novel tight junction-associated protein distinct from ZO-1, cingulin and ZO-2. *J. Cell Biol.* **120:**477–483.

9

Immune Regulation in the Brain

Lessons From Autoimmunity and Implications for Brain Tumor Therapy

Lois A. Lampson

1. INTRODUCTION

This chapter provides a framework for thinking about recent work in brain tumor immunotherapy. The intent is to clarify current goals, aid interpretation of recent findings, and point to the next areas that need attention.

Tumor immunotherapy is a multistep process. Appropriately, the field has focused on the first steps, identifying tumor antigens and developing vaccines against them. As vaccine technology advances, it is time to focus more attention on other aspects of the response. The variety and complexity of immune effector mechanisms, ways of delivering effectors to a brain tumor site, and site-specific differences in immune regulation are stressed below.

In presenting the field, two ideas give perspective. Regarding tumor, the importance of microscopic tumor (micro-tumor) as a target of immunotherapy is stressed. Regarding immune control, the wealth of work in central nervous system (CNS) autoimmune disease is introduced, and implications for brain tumor therapy are brought out.

Emphasis on other aspects of CNS immunology and additional references are found in other articles *(65,67,68,70,85)*, as cited within the text. More detail about the immune response in general can be found in the comprehensive text, *Fundamental Immunology (100)*.

1.1. Important Targets for Immunotherapy

1.1.1. Micro-Tumor as a T-Cell Target

In both animal models and clinical trials, immunotherapy has most often been directed against a discrete tumor mass. Yet, this may not be the most important kind of target nor the most favorable. Increasingly, improvements in conventional therapies are able to image and remove or inactivate a discrete tumor mass (this volume). Conventional therapies may be less effective or appropriate against smaller foci of residual or disseminated tumor (micro-tumor; Fig. 1), which thus becomes more important as a source of tumor recurrence *(12,19,79,92)*.

Some form of micro-tumor is characteristic of most of the tumors that grow in the brain. Although different kinds of tumor have different general patterns of spread, the exact location of disseminated tumor cannot be predicted. The smallest tumor foci may be below the imaging threshold, and safe delivery of therapy is more challenging when tumor is widely disseminated or lies within still-functioning brain tissue.

From: *Contemporary Cancer Research: Brain Tumors*
Edited by: F. Ali-Osman © Humana Press Inc., Totowa, NJ

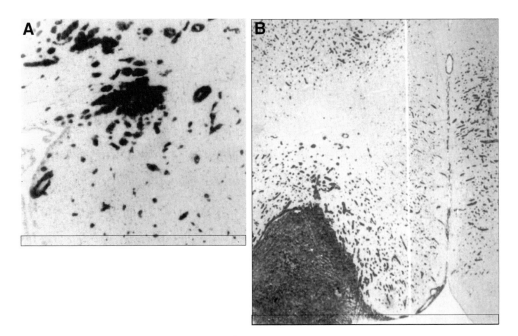

Fig. 1. Disseminated micro-tumor. Tumor cell lines expressing the β-gal marker were implanted in the rat brain, and allowed to grow out from the initial site. Micro-tumor is revealed by histochemical stain for β-gal (Lampson 92). (**A**) Small tumor foci growing near the lateral ventricle. (Ventricle is seen at left edge). (**B**) Widely disseminated micro-tumor. Tumor has spread through the hemisphere of implantation and across the midline (near the right edge). Disseminated micro-tumor is an important and appropriate target for cell-mediated immunotherapy, as discussed in the text. (Panels A and B reprinted with permission from refs. *70,74*, respectively.)

Provocatively, T-cells are adapted to attack tumor with exactly these properties *(65,68,70)*. Activated T-cells can survey the nonlymphoid tissues, including brain, and can selectively attack abnormal targets. The local concentration of tumor-dependent immunosuppressive factors would be less at micro-tumor sites than within a larger tumor mass. The more that is understood about the underlying biology of T-cell traffic (*see* Subheading 5.1), the triggering of T-cell effector functions (*see* Subheading 2.2.1.), and the range of potential effector mechanisms (*see* Subheading 4.3), the more effectively and safely T-cells' potential can be exploited.

1.1.2. Sites of Special Interest

In some cases, even if the tumor can be localized, conventional therapies are problematic. Brainstem glioma is an example. Brainstem glioma is most common in children, for whom radiation and chemotherapy are most dangerous *(29)*. Brainstem surgery has high risk even in adults. Intriguingly, the most aggressive form of brainstem glioma has the infiltrative growth pattern that should be most amenable to immunotherapy (as explained above). Moreover, it may be relatively easy to enhance immune activity in the brainstem, as compared to other brain sites *(85)* (*see* Subheading 2.5.).

1.1.3. Matching Immunotherapy to the Tumor Type and Site

The safest and most effective immunotherapy regimen is likely to vary with the tumor type and site. Different tumors favor different initial locations and different paths of spread. For example, individual tumor cells that infiltrate the brain parenchyma are characteristic of astrocytoma *(62)*. In contrast, blood-borne tumor from other organs first enters the brain as micrometastases in the perivascular space (PVS) *(56)*. Many kinds of metastatic tumor remain within the PVS as they grow, not entering the parenchyma proper. Immune regulation varies from region to region, and also within a region, such as between the PVS and parenchyma proper *(58,68,85)* *(see* Subheading 2.5.). The immune system encompasses a wealth of potential effector cells, mechanisms, and molecular mediators *(see* Subheading 4.). The relative susceptibility to different mechanisms will be different for different tumors *(7,30,35,106)*, and the ease of safely stimulating different effector functions will differ at different sites *(85)* *(see* Subheading 2.5.).

In seeking a more complete and subtle understanding of immune regulation in the tumor-bearing brain, work in other disease contexts is informative. Work in autoimmunity is one rich source of insight, as discussed later.

1.2. Tumor Immunity and Autoimmunity: A Useful Interplay

Recently, there has been a surge of work and interest in brain tumor immunotherapy. Increased understanding of basic immunology and wide availability of new methods and tools have been key factors. The same advances have led to increased understanding of other aspects of CNS immunology, including antiviral responses, graft rejection, and autoimmunity. Insights from each of these areas have important implications for brain tumor immunotherapy. The multiple ways that viruses can escape from immune surveillance *(4)*, and details of the ways that virus is safely cleared are examples *(1)*. Studies of unwanted responses can be just as valuable. The same effector mechanisms that attack CNS grafts should, if properly controlled, be effective against CNS tumors. A particularly fruitful source of insight, not yet wellexploited against tumors, is the extensive literature on CNS autoimmunity.

Even as interest in brain tumor immunotherapy has waxed and waned, there has been a constant focus on the complementary problem of reducing immune activity in autoimmune disease. From the viewpoint of tumor therapy, autoimmunity has been thought of primarily as a source of concern, a side effect to be avoided. But this is to ignore the full potential of the work that has been done. Indeed, many insights about CNS autoimmunity are directly relevant to the challenge of enhancing the response against CNS tumor, as stressed within this chapter.

2. BASIC CONCEPTS AND TERMINOLOGY

In this section, basic features of the immune response are reviewed. For each topic, points relevant to the attack of brain tumor, especially micro-tumor, and lessons from complementary work in autoimmunity are stressed.

2.1. Basic Features of the Immune Response

The immune response reacts to damage or abnormality. Pathogens and damaged, infected, or neoplastic cells can be detected and destroyed. Tumor cells can be recognized if they express abnormal molecules, and many such targets have now been identified *(8,63,98,99)*. (Tumors can also be attacked as a consequence of other kinds of changes, such as over-expression of normal proteins, *see* Subheading 4.1.3.)

2.1.1. Antigen and Fine Specificity

The general term for the object of immune recognition is antigen. The particular part of the antigen that is recognized is referred to as an antigenic determinant or epitope. An epitope is small, just a few amino acids. A single protein can display many different epitopes *(64 65,70)*.

The small epitope size underlies one of the hallmarks of the immune response, its fine specificity. Different pathogens or foreign molecules can be distinguished from each other; even a single amino acid difference can be detected. With respect to tumor, the immune response can distinguish between different tumor types, different tumors of the same type, different parts of the same tumor, and different tumor cells at a single site.

The exquisite fine specificity gives the advantage of selectivity, but has a potential drawback. If the immune response is directed against only one or a few epitopes, tumor variants that can survive without those epitopes may escape immune surveillance *(65,70)*. In a growing tumor such variants may arise spontaneously and then come to predominate under the selective pressure of immuno-therapy.

In the course of a normal response against a complex antigen, the response shifts to encompass new determinants *(epitope spreading) (114,137)*, which may help protect against immune escape. Of course, epitope spreading may also lead to an unwanted response *(73)*. Strategies for immunotherapy differ in the number of antigens targeted initially and the likelihood of epitope spreading *(140)*. In choosing between alternative strategies, balancing the advantages of simplicity vs complexity in the targeted tumor antigen is an important consideration *(68)* (*see* Subheading 7.).

2.1.2. Immune Memory

A second hallmark of the immune response is its capacity for memory. The primary response to a given antigen differs quantitatively and qualitatively from subsequent responses. During the primary response, clones of cells that recognize the antigen are expanded, and the daughter cells display new properties: They display altered migratory behavior, and the requirements for later recognition of the same antigen are less stringent *(26,139)*. Together, these changes make the secondary response faster and more efficient.

Although immune memory and the distinction between primary and secondary responses are classic concepts, many issues are still unresolved *(2,81,107)*. For example, a distinction is often made between two kinds of T-cell progeny: 1) effector T-cells, ready to immediately attack their targets and 2) long-term memory T-cells. However, the lineage relationships between these cells, and even their definitions, are not agreed upon. The role of residual antigen in immune memory is also controversial. One key point that is not disputed, but often overlooked, is that in order to initiate its effector functions, a T-cell must re-recognize its antigen at the tumor site (*see* Subheading 2.2.).

2.1.3. B and T Lymphocytes

The fine specificity and memory of the immune response are mediated by lymphocytes. Each lymphocyte clone has a characteristic receptor. The immune response to a given tumor or pathogen reflects the net activity of all the individual lymphocyte clones whose receptors have been stimulated by its antigens.

Different subsets of lymphocytes have different functions. B lymphocytes (B-cells) mediate a humoral response. In the effector phase, differentiated cells in the B-cell lineage (activated B-cells and plasma cells) secrete antibody, a protein of the immunogloblin class, that specifically binds to the antigen. T lymphocytes (T-cells) mediate a response that is both cell-mediated and cell-directed. T-cells recognize antigen on a cell surface (*see* Subheading 3.1.1.). In the effector phase, T-cells may lyse their targets by mechanisms that require cell-to-cell contact. T-cells can also secrete molecules that directly attack cellular targets, or attract or activate other cells to do so (*see* Subheading 4.3.). Unlike antibodies, the effector molecules secreted by T-cells are not specific for their targets. Instead, their specificity comes from their local concentration. The local concentration is achieved by the T-cell's juxtaposition to its target, hence, a cell-mediated response.

2.2. How the Response Unfolds

2.2.1. Priming vs Effector Function

Upon their first exposure to antigen in the secondary lymphoid tissues (lymph nodes, spleen), naive lymphocytes can be stimulated or primed. The stimulated cells undergo clonal expansion, pro-ducing daughter cells with the same antigen specificity, but with other properties altered in ways that make subsequent stimulation by the same antigen more efficient (*see* Subheading 2.1.2.).

Among the changes, the daughters of stimulated T-cells preferentially survey the nonlymphoid tissues, including the brain *(68,139)*. If a daughter T-cell re-recognizes the stimulating antigen at the tumor site *(39,52)*, it can be triggered to carry out its effector functions. One source of confusion in the brain tumor literature is that the requirement for two separate antigen recognition steps, one at the site of priming and one at the tumor site, is often blurred.

2.2.2. Sites of Priming

Lymphocytes are primed most efficiently in organized secondary lymphoid tissue (lymph nodes, spleen) *(148)*. One reason is that trapping of antigen is facilitated. Free antigen is trapped by local phagocytes, and migratory cells that have previously ingested antigen are arrested. The coming together of the different cell types needed for successful initiation of an immune response is also facilitated. The participating cells may include phagocytes that can ingest, process, and present antigen, and different lymphocyte subpopulations that stimulate and regulate each other *(1)* (*see* Subheading 4.4.1.).

To give a specific example that is relevant to current vaccine strategies: skin dendritic cells (DC) take up antigen in the skin, then carry it to the draining lymph nodes where they can present it to passing lymphocytes. Naive T-cells recirculate among the secondary lymphoid tissues. If the appropriate antigen is presented, a naive T-cell can be arrested and primed. Successful priming leads to clonal expansion of the responding T-cell, producing daughter cells that preferentially survey the nonlymphoid tissues, including the brain *(68,139)*. If a daughter cell re-recognizes its antigen at a brain tumor site, it can be triggered to carry out its effector functions.

2.2.3. Interpreting Some Recent Studies

For the reasons given above, one would not expect to efficiently initiate an immune response within the brain itself. At the same time, animals have been successfully immunized following injection of material directly into the brain or into a brain tumor site *(33,128)*. However, this does not necessarily mean that the response was initiated in the brain. Rather, antigen may be carried from the brain, via the CSF or other known pathways *(18,54,70)*, to organized lymphoid tissue. The cervical lymph nodes that act as draining nodes for the brain, may be a particularly favorable site for initiating a response to CNS antigen *(46,40)*. The response would then develop as described earlier: naive, antigen-specific cells would be arrested and stimulated in the draining nodes. Following clonal expansion, antigen-specific daughter cells would enter the circulation, preferentially surveying the nonlymphoid tissues, including brain. Migrant T-cells that re-recognized their antigen within the brain could be triggered to carry out their effector functions at that site.

2.2.4. Summary

For T-cells to attack tumor in the brain, three steps must occur (Fig. 2); first, naive T-cells must be stimulated (for example, by means of a vaccine). This happens most efficiently in organized lymphoid tissue. Second, daughters of the stimulated T-cells must migrate to tumor sites within the brain (*see* Subheading 5.1.). Third, at the tumor site, the T-cells must be triggered by recall recognition of the original tumor antigen.

2.3. Other Kinds of Responses

2.3.1. Inflammation

The inflammatory response also reacts to damage or abnormality. It differs from the immune response because it lacks fine specificity and memory. Instead, broad classes of pathogens or general tissue damage are recognized. The inflammatory response is mediated by a combination of endogenous phagocytes and other resident cells plus blood-borne leukocytes, using receptors such as pattern recognition molecules (PRM) that recognize broad categories of insults *(28)*. For example, phagocytes respond to Gram-negative bacteria as a class, whereas the immune system can distinguish between different Gram-negative bacteria *(42)*.

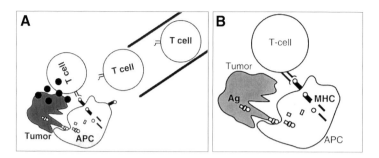

Fig. 2. Important steps for T-cell-mediated immunotherapy. (**A**) Overview of some key steps. Step 1. Activation. In secondary lymphoid tissues, T-cells are activated against tumor antigen and undergo clonal expansion (not shown). Step 2. Migration. The daughter cells survey the tissues. If they bind to appropriate adhesion molecules on brain vessels, they can extravasate. (T-cells within the vasculature are depicted at upper right; extravasation, at lower left.) Step 3. Triggering effector function. To carry out its effector functions, a T-cell must be triggered by recall recognition of tumor antigen (lower left). The indirect pathway, which allows presentation of ingested antigen, is shown: Tumor antigen (white shapes) has been ingested by an antigen-presenting cell (APC) and processed to peptides within the APC. Peptides are then complexed with the APC's class II MHC proteins (dark rectangles), for presentation on the surface of the APC. The recall presentation triggers the T-cell to secrete TNF-α and other factors (dark discs) that directly attack the tumor, or attract and activate other cells to do so. (**B**) Enlarged view of indirect pathway. Because it does not depend on MHC expression or processing by the tumor cell itself, the indirect pathway deserves more emphasis, as discussed in the text. (Figure modified with permission from ref. *70*.)

In practice, the immune and inflammatory responses are inextricably intertwined *(70)*. Phagocytes can present antigen to lymphocytes *(see* Subheading 2.3.1). Conversely, a major effector pathway of lymphocytes involves the attraction and activation of phagocytes *(see* Subheading 4.4.2). Phagocytes and lymphocytes share attack mechanisms, and secrete and respond to many of the same regulatory molecules. The common current terminology, referring to the inflammatory and immune responses as innate and adaptive immunity, respectively, emphasizes their inter-relationships *(48)* although it does blur their differences.

2.3.2. Completing the Picture

The body is protected from infection and neoplasia by additional defense mechanisms that don't fall neatly into the traditional framework. Natural killer (NK) cells recognize abnormal cells in a way that complements T-cell recognition *(1,10,135)*. Molecular mediators of the immune and inflammatory responses can be made by other cells as well, and can serve both protective functions and other functions.

For example, tumor necrosis factor (TNF)-α is made by many cell types, including T-cells and macrophages, and neurons. TNF-α can kill tumor cells directly, and can attack tumor indirectly by attracting and activating other cells *(see* Subheading 4.3.). In many neurologic disorders, TNF-α or other inflammatory mediators are thought to exacerbate disease. The source of the mediators can be endogenous cells or blood-borne inflammatory cells, with the relative importance of each different in different disorders *(70)*. Its multifaceted role as an inflammatory mediator is not the only function TNF-α can play in the brain. It can also act as a neurotransmitter *(9)*.

The variety and complexity of normal protective mechanisms are relevant to brain tumor therapy in two ways. The more that is understood about the different cell types and molecular mediators, the better they can be exploited against tumor. More subtly, appreciation of the multifunctional nature of individual molecules should permit both greater safety and novel strategies of immune control *(85)* *(see* Subheading 2.5.).

2.4. The Brain vs Other Organs

2.4.1. "Privilege" as Misnomer

Until recently, it was widely believed that immune surveillance excluded the brain (immune privilege). In fact, this idea was not justified by the original work, which showed rather that initiation of some kinds of immune responses can be relatively inefficient in the brain; it was clear that the effector phase could be active in the CNS *(3)*. For example, it is more efficient to initiate an immune response to a tissue graft or tumor placed under the skin, than if the same graft or tumor is placed in the brain. However, once the response has been initiated, grafts and tumor in the brain can be attacked *(3)*. The most recent work reconfirms the potential efficacy of immune effector mechanisms in the CNS, and extends insight into the subtleties of immune control.

Several anatomical features of the CNS that were once thought to contribute to immune privilege can now be seen in a different light *(70)*. Although the physical blood-brain barrier does indeed exclude large proteins, including antibodies, from the brain it does not prevent the entry of metabolically active cells *(see* Subheading 5.1.3.) *(68)*. Although the brain does not have a conventional lymphatic drainage, antigen can be carried out of the brain in the cerebrospinal fluid (CSF) or by other routes *(18,54,68,70)*. Although the major histocompatibility complex (MHC) proteins that mediate antigen presentation are not normally detected in most brain cells *(see* Subheading 3.2.), neither are they detected in normal parenchymal cells of many other tissues, such as skeletal muscle (Fig. 3). Moreover, in brain as in other tissues, MHC expression is under regulatory control *(see* Subheading 3.2.1.; Fig. 4). Finally, although overwhelming inflammation cannot be tolerated within the confines of the skull, this is not a necessary sequel to immune activity. On the contrary, immune activity can be under tight regulatory control (Fig. 5; *see* Subheading 4.2.).

More recently appreciated features of the immune response can also be seen as examples of general regulatory mechanisms, rather than immune privilege. Anterior chamber-associated immune deviation (ACAID) refers to a characteristic balance of immune effector mechanisms that is seen in the anterior chamber of the eye *(121)*. The balance is thought to protect against uncontrolled inflammation, which is as harmful in the eye as in the brain *(122)*. However, despite its name, this deviation may be seen as an example of the more general concept of regional immunity *(121)*. For a given antigen, the balance of immune effector mechanisms differs between tissues and organs, and even with an organ *(see* Subheading 2.5.).

2.4.2. Fas–FasL in the Brain

Another phenomenon that may be interpreted in terms of balance, rather than privilege, is Fas–FasL-mediated apoptosis. In the simplest case, Fas ligand (FasL) on an activated T-cell interacts with Fas on an antigen-bearing target cell, and this leads to apoptotic death of the target. However, the developing picture of Fas–FasL distribution and function is far more complex.

T-cells can express Fas, which enables them to kill tumor, but can also express FasL, which means that they themselves can be targets. Brain tumor cells can express FasL, which makes them potential targets, but can also express Fas *(145)*. Thus, they can kill each other, and can also kill T-cells. Fas is also expressed on cells of the normal brain. In response to these findings, it has been suggested that Fas on brain tumors protects them from T-cell attack, and that Fas in normal brain contributes to immune privilege by causing the apoptosis of entering T-cells *(106,110)*. However, a broader view gives a different perspective.

The Fas–FasL system also serves more general immune control, not limited to the brain or its tumors *(13,116)*. Non-CNS tissues and tumors can also express Fas and FasL *(7,77,118)*. Although clonal expansion is a key element of the T-cell response to antigen *(see* above), the expansion must be controlled, and the accumulation of T-cells and other inflammatory cells must also be controlled. One control mechanism is through death of activated T-cells (activation-induced cell death), and this can indeed be mediated by Fas–FasL interaction *(78)*. However, control of T-cell proliferation and

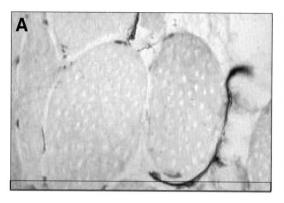
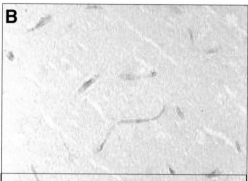

Fig. 3. Immune quiescence in non-lymphoid tissues. **(A)** In normal human skeletal muscle, strong MHC antigen expression (black after antibody staining) is seen in endothelial cells, but not in muscle fibers themselves, and few inflammatory cells are seen. (High power view, D.I.C. [Nomarski] optics.) **(B)** Similarly, in normal brain, MHC antigen expression is seen in endothelial cells but not neural cells, and few inflammatory cells are seen. (Low power view.) (Panels A and B taken from work reported in refs. *73, 65*, respectively.)

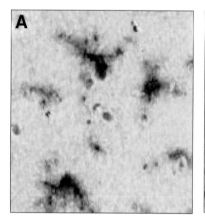
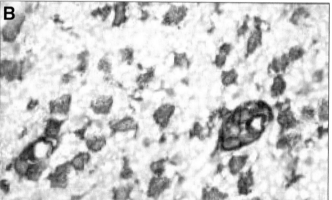

Fig. 4. A stereotyped pattern of MHC upregulation in the CNS. In many experimental and pathological conditions, the strongest MHC antigen expression in the brain or spinal cord is the class II MHC expression of microglia and other phagocytes. In the same tissue, endothelial cells appear class I+ and other endogenous cells (neurons, astrocytes, oligodendrocytes) appear MHC-negative. **(A)** Class II+ microglia in rat brain after intracerebral injection of the MHC-upregulating cytokine, IFN-γ. Note strong class II expression in cells with the characteristic morphology of activated microglia; surrounding tissues appears negative. **(B)** Class II+ phagocytes, foamy after the ingestion of myelin debris, in human spinal cord, taken at autopsy from the affected area in the neurodegenerative disorder, amyotrophic lateral sclerosis (ALS). The strong class II MHC expression is localized to phagocytes, not other neural cells. In both panels, tissue has been stained with monoclonal antibody to class II MHC proteins. (Panel A reprinted with permission from ref. *65*; panel B with permission from ref. *73*.)

accumulation is not only important in the brain; control is essential even in the lymphoid tissues *(82,123,126,133)*.

At the same time, there is ample evidence that T-cells can carry out their effector functions in the brain and elsewhere *(70)*. Thus, if FasL in the brain (or other tissues) does cause the death of entering T-cells, there must still be time for the T-cells to carry out their effector functions *(27)*.

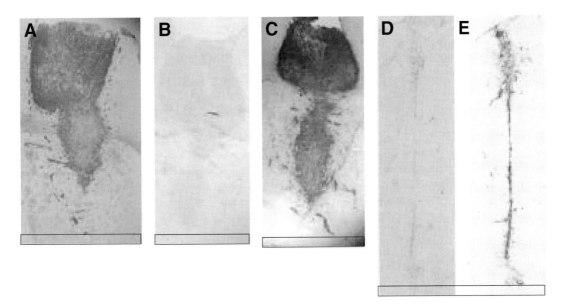

Fig. 5. Controlled response to tumor. **(A)** In a rat model, a tumor cell line grows in a stereotyped pattern in an untreated control rat. In the figure, cells bearing the tumor marker, β-gal protein, appear dark grey, after histochemical stain for β-gal. **(B)** In a different rat, which received immunotherapy, hypercellularity is seen in the same pattern (light grey, after hematoxylin counterstain), but the cells do not bear the tumor marker. **(C)** Instead, responding cells—including T-cells and phagocytes—appear in the same stereotyped pattern seen in the control **(A)**, as if the tumor had been replaced by responding cells. In the figure, activated phagocytes, stained with antibody, appear dark grey. **(D)** In another experiment, when therapy is farther advanced, all that remains is some hypercellularity along the needle track (light grey, after hematoxylin). Staining sections adjacent to the one shown in D reveals that the area is occupied by responding cells (stained dark in **[E]** after antibody stain for phagocytes), not tumor cells. (Panels A and B reprinted with permission from refs. *70,74*, respectively.)

Yet, another layer of complexity is added by functional heterogeneity. Activated T-cells can be killed through the Fas–FasL pathway, but at some points in their differentiation, T-cells can be resistant to attack *(104,116)*; tumor cells can also be resistant *(7,30,106)*. Indeed, in some circumstances Fas–FasL interactions may cause cell proliferation, rather than cell death *(116)*.

2.4.3. Some General Principles

The developing picture of Fas–FasL distribution and function is consistent with general principles stressed throughout this chapter: The molecules are multifunctional and affect many cell types. Their immune function contributes to a complex regulatory balance rather than privilege. Although the brain's low immune background helps to reveal subtle effects, the findings are relevant to other tissues as well not unique to the brain.

2.5. Local Heterogeneity Within the Brain

2.5.1. Site-Specific Immune Control

Typically, immune regulation is studied and thought of at the level of the whole organ: brain, lung, etc. More recent work draws attention to local differences within organs *(47,80)*, and the contribution of local regulatory molecules to site-specific control *(85,86)*. In seeking the most efficient and benign regimen for tumor in still-functioning brain tissue, the principle of site-specific control is important to bear in mind.

2.5.2. Evidence for Site-Specific Control

At sufficiently high doses, immunoactive cytokines can be broadly active in the CNS. As the cytokine dose is lowered, more subtle effects are seen. Work illustrating these points in a rat model, using IFN-γ as the cytokine, is described below.

Local exposure to IFN-γ can enhance two key aspects of T-cell surveillance. It can enhance T-cell accumulation *(58,102)*. It can also increase the number of activated APC available to trigger T-cell effector functions. In the rat, a single intrastriatal injection of 10,000 U IFN-γ activates microglia throughout the brain *(115)*. Experimentally, one measure of microglial activation is the upregulation of the class II MHC proteins that mediate indirect T-cell triggering *(see* Subheading 2.3.1.; Fig. 2B). When lower IFN-γ doses are injected into different local sites, site-specific effects are revealed. For example, IFN-γ action is relatively efficient in the brainstem, and much less efficient in the hippocampus *(103)*. When the effect of IFN-γ on T-cell accumulation is measured, the same hierarchy is seen *(102)*.

2.5.3. A Role for Local Neurochemicals

Many factors can contribute to site-specific cytokine effects. The bulk flow path of injected drug and the local density of potential target cells are obvious possibilities, ones that would also be relevant in human patients. However, in the work described above, these factors could not fully account for the results *(86,102,103)*.

An attractive alternative was suggested by the multifunctional nature of many regulatory molecules *(64,86)*. This led to the hypothesis that, in addition to their neurobiological functions, local neurochemicals might also influence local immune control. More specific predictions followed from the known anatomical distribution of some prominent neurochemicals, and their known effects outside the brain or in vitro *(86):* It was predicted that substance P (SP), which is abundant in the brainstem and immune-activating in other contexts, might contribute to the efficiency of IFN-γ action at that site. This prediction was supported experimentally as shown in Fig. 6: SP binds to the NK-1 receptor. In the brainstem, local injection of an NK-1 receptor antagonist (Spantide I) prevented IFN-γ action, implicating endogenous SP in the IFN-γ effects. Moreover, injection of exogenous SP enhanced IFN-γ action above what was achieved with IFN-γ alone *(86)*.

In further studies, it was shown that SP did not have a similar effect in the hippocampus. In contrast (and as predicted), a role was shown for glutamate, acting through the NMDA receptor: In the hippocampus, the NMDA receptor antagonist, MK-801, did enhance IFN-γ activity; MK-801 did not have a similar effect in the brainstem *(86)*.

Thus, cytokine action was site-specific at two levels. There were site-specific differences in the response to IFN-γ alone. In addition, there were site-specific differences in the relative importance of two widely distributed neurochemicals, SP and glutamate, on the IFN-γ effects.

2.5.4. Implications of Site-Specific Control

Site-specific immune control, and the role of local neurochemicals, have important implications. Clinically, site-specific control may contribute, among many factors, to the anatomic localization of many CNS disorders. Therapeutically, local neurochemicals may offer a novel target for immune control *(85,86)*. To give a specific example in a tumor context: new therapies are urgently needed for brainstem glioma *(see* Subheading 1.1.2). The relative ease of immune activation suggests that the brainstem may be a favorable site for immunotherapy. The influence of SP (Fig. 6) suggests a novel way of enhancing immune activity at that site.

2.5.5. How Can Selective Regulation Be Achieved?

SP may well contribute to immune regulation in the brainstem *(see* above), but it also influences pain and many essential neurobiological brainstem functions. How could one gain selective control, modifying only immune activity? Work in other contexts does suggest opportunities for selective

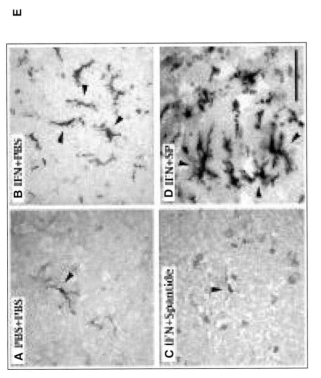

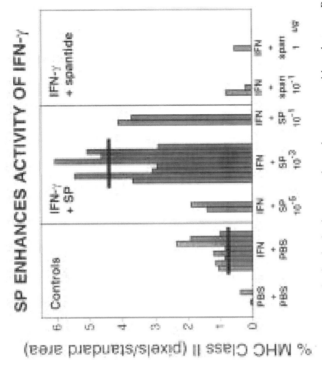

Fig. 6. Local neurochemicals contribute to site-specific immune control. Figure shows results in the brainstem, where the neuropeptide substance P (SP) enhances the microglial-activating activity of IFN-γ. (**A–D**) Local injection of 300 U IFN-γ activates microglia throughout the brainstem, causing them to enlarge and to upregulate their class II MHC expression. Activated microglia appear black in the figure, after antibody staining for class II MHC protein. (**A**) Minimal class II upregulation is seen after control injections of PBS. (**B**) Some activation is seen after IFN-γ followed by PBS. (**C**) The activation shown in B is blocked when IFN-γ is followed by Spantide I, an antagonist for the NK-1 receptor (which is used by SP). (**D**) Activation is increased by injecting SP immediately after IFN-γ. E. To obtain quantitative data, image analysis was used to measured dark pixels per standard area from Subheadings such as those shown in A–D. For each rat, a constant-sized region of optimal staining was measured. Each vertical bar shows data from one rat. (Panels reprinted with permission from ref. 86.)

185

control. For example, (a) Microglia or other cells may have variant SP receptors *(6,83)*; (b) the dose-response curves for different effects are likely to differ *(58)*; (c) the neurobiological effects of SP are exquisitely localized, and may cancel each other out when a larger area is involved *(25,146)*; (d) SP agonists and antagonists have been safely used in rodents (citations above); and (e) SP antagonists, aimed at blocking SP action in the CNS, have been safely used in clinical trials (not related to immune control) *(59)*.

2.5.6. A General Principle

More generally, the multifunctional nature of SP is not unique. On the contrary, most regulatory molecules are multifunctional *(64)*. Among examples mentioned in this chapter, TNF-α and nitric oxide (NO) can each mediate target attack in the immune and inflammatory responses, but can also act as neurotransmitters *(9,136)*. Fas–FasL interactions can cause target apoptosis but also T-cell apoptosis (*see* Subheading 2.4.2.). Thus, whichever molecular mediators are exploited for brain tumor therapy, there is a general need to find strategies for selective control.

3. HOW T-CELLS RECOGNIZE THEIR ANTIGEN

In the cell-mediated immune response, special requirements for antigen recognition affect both T-cell priming and effector triggering. Implications for effector triggering are discussed below.

3.1. T-Cells and MHC Restriction

3.1.1. What Is Recognized

In a B-cell, the receptor for antigen is a membrane-associated form of the same antibody that the B-cell is able to secrete. The B-cell can bind directly to its antigen. The antigen can be cell-bound or free.

For a T-cell, recognition of antigen is less direct. A protein antigen must first be processed to peptides. A peptide must then be presented, bound to another protein, on a cell surface. The presenting protein must be one of a family of proteins that are coded in the MHC. The T-cell receptor recognizes the peptide–MHC complex. This phenomenon is called MHC restriction.

The apparent complexity of T-cell/antigen interaction actually magnifies the flexibility of the T-cell response. Any tumor component, including cytoplasmic or nuclear proteins or proteins destined to be secreted, can be processed and presented to T-cells. Variations in the pathway allow for presentation of antigen by a tumor cell itself, and presentation of antigen that has been ingested by other cells (Fig. 2B; *see* Subheading 3.2.2.). Thus, T-cells are able to respond to any kind of tumor-associated abnormality. Tumor antigens are not limited to cell-surface proteins, as had long been assumed.

MHC restriction has several implications for tumor therapy in general, and brain tumor therapy in particular, as described in the following Subheadings. Many of the implications follow from the structure of the MHC proteins, which is reviewed first.

3.1.2. Major Histocompatibility Complex Proteins

The MHC contains a family of multi-gene families, several of which are essential to the immune response. Antigen presentation is mediated by the class I and class II MHC proteins. In humans, there are three classical class I proteins (HLA-A, B, C molecules) and three class II proteins (HLA-DP, DQ, DR). Each of these proteins is polymorphic and co-dominantly expressed *(93,143)*. Thus, a given individual may express as many as 12 different HLA proteins (two HLA-A alleles, two HLA-B alleles, etc.).

The class I and class II MHC proteins can fold to form a peptide-binding groove *(24)*. For a given peptide and MHC protein, the match between the peptide side-chains and the contact residues of the groove determines the binding energy. Although the peptide-binding grooves differ somewhat for class I vs class II MHC proteins, the effective size of an antigenic determinant is always just a few (8–12) amino acids, that is, small compared to the size of most proteins.

Two factors increase the likelihood that a given foreign protein can be recognized by a given individual. First, the small size of an antigenic determinant means that the protein may contain many potential determinants (epitopes). Second, the complex MHC phenotype (6 HLA molecules, co-dominantly expressed) increases the likelihood that one of the potential epitopes will fit in one of the MHC grooves with high enough binding energy to stimulate a response. Although it is unlikely for two unrelated individuals to have identical MHC phenotypes, some alleles, such as HLA-A2, are relatively common. In seeking to identify new tumor antigens, antigens that bind to the most common alleles are of special interest.

3.1.3. Clinical Consequences of Major Histocompatibility Complex Restriction

Many of the consequences of MHC restriction are tied to the polymorphic nature of the MHC proteins. Because the MHC proteins are polymorphic, a given antigen is recognized by different individuals in different ways *(96)*. Different epitopes will be important, and, even for the same epitope, the binding energies will be different when the peptide is displayed in the grove of different MHC proteins. This is one reason why some strains of mice or rats respond to a given antigen with a vigorous immune response, and others respond more weakly or not at all. It is the reason that much effort has been spent in asking whether particular diseases are associated with particular MHC phenotypes. In terms of autoimmunity, MHC polymorphism can help explain why only some individuals develop a given autoimmune disease, such as multiple sclerosis (MS), and why MS patients show different levels of disease severity. In terms of tumor, MHC polymorphism can help explain heterogeneity in the response of different patients to their brain tumors, even if the tumors express shared antigens, and to tumor vaccines.

Another consequence of MHC polymorphism is that T-cells are not easily shared between patients. The polymorphic MHC proteins are major targets of graft rejection (which is how they were originally discovered, and explains their name). The complexity of the MHC phenotype makes it difficult to match unrelated individuals. If T-cells from one patient were used to treat a second patient, the T-cells would be subject to graft rejection.

Ultimately, it may be possible to turn the consequences of MHC incompatibility to advantage. For example, some degree of graft/host interaction can enhance the anti-tumor response *(33,60,61,109)*. In whatever way MHC restriction is to be exploited, the local distribution and regulation of the MHC proteins are key considerations, as reviewed below.

3.2. Major Histocompatibility Complex Distribution and Its Implications in the Brain

3.2.1. Major Histocompatibility Complex Distribution

Perceptions about the distribution of the MHC proteins and the implications have been in flux. The class II MCH proteins are expressed primarily by phagocytes and other antigen-presenting cells (APCs). Class I MHC proteins are often described as ubiquitous, with the brain as an exception. Indeed, lack of MHC expression has been thought to contribute to immune privilege of the CNS.

However, much work now supports a different view: It is now more widely appreciated that class I MHC proteins have a heterogeneous distribution within most tissues and organs *(36,66)*; the brain is not unique. For example, class I MHC proteins are not detected in most cells of the normal brain, but, using the same methods, are also not detected in normal skeletal muscle *(73)* (Fig. 3). Moreover, MHC expression, for both class I and class II MHC proteins, is under regulatory control. In brain as in muscle, MHC expression is increased in many pathological and experimental settings *(66,73)*.

The class I and II MHC proteins are regulated independently. When brain Subheadings are stained with antibodies to class I or class II MHC proteins, a stereotyped pattern is seen under many circumstances: among parenchymal cells, the strongest staining is the class II MHC expression displayed by activated microglia and other phagocytes (Fig. 4). Weaker class I MHC expression can also be detected in these cells. Endothelial cells are class I⁺ and inflammatory cells can be class I⁺ or class II⁺, according to the cell type. However, under ordinary staining conditions, neurons, astrocytes, oligodendrocytes, and also many tumor cells, appear MHC-negative *(23,65,66,72)*.

As described earlier, T-cell-mediated attack of tumor requires two antigen recognition steps. Initial recognition occurs during priming in organized lymphoid tissue. Recall recognition is needed to trigger effector function at the tumor site (*see* Subheading 2.2.). The MHC expression pattern described above has important implications for effector triggering in the brain. The most common pattern of expression, with class II⁺ phagocytes predominating, favors indirect antigen presentation to class II-restricted T-cells, as described below.

3.2.2. Direct vs Indirect Antigen Presentation

Cells that express MHC proteins, and can carry out the necessary processing steps, may present their own antigen to T-cells (direct pathway). The class I MHC proteins are considered most important for this pathway. For appropriate targets, this is one pathway by which T-cells can directly attack infected or neoplastic cells. However, many potential targets *(101,125)*, including many brain tumor cells *(67,72)*, show at best weak MHC expressionor may be defective at other steps *(97,101,125)*.

Fortunately, there is also an indirect pathway. In that case, APCs use their own MHC proteins to present antigen that they have ingested and degraded (Fig. 2B). The class II MHC proteins are considered most important for this pathway. Potential APCs in the brain include endogenous microglia, perivascular phagocytes, and blood-borne monocytes. At least in vitro all of these cell types can serve as APCs presenting ingested antigen to trigger previously-activated T-cells *(21,23,113)*. An especially attractive feature of the indirect pathway is its flexibility. A tumor-adjacent APC can present ingested tumor antigen, even if the tumor cell itself is unable to do so.

3.2.3. Implications for Brain Tumor Therapy

In the brain, the most common pattern of MHC expression is well-suited to the indirect pathway. In tumor-bearing brains, as well as in many other conditions, the most prominent MHC expression is the class II MHC expression of potential APC. In the same slides, tumor cells themselves can appear MHC-negative *(23,72,142)*. In a rat model, even after multiple intratumoral injections of the MHC-upregulating cytokine IFN-γ, this dichotomy was maintained *(142)*.

To date, work in tumor immunotherapy has stressed effector functions that require direct T-cell/tumor interaction. The greater flexibility of indirect antigen presentation, plus the characteristic MHC distribution pattern in the CNS, suggest that greater attention to effector triggering by the indirect pathway may be especially fruitful for brain tumor immunotherapy *(65,68,70)*.

3.2.4. Current Questions

The different alternatives for antigen presentation (direct or indirect; different potential APC) contribute to the flexibility of the immune response. Not surprisingly, the same variety has made it difficult to determine the most important pathways in particular contexts. For example, although it has long been known that oligodendrocytes are damaged in MS, the pathway by which this occurs is still controversial: To what extent do oligodendrocytes present their own antigen to activated T-cells (direct pathway)? What is the relative importance of presentation of ingested antigen by APCs (indirect pathway)? If the indirect pathway is indeed important, which of the potential APCs of the CNS (microglia, blood-borne monocytes, perivascular phagocytes) is most important? If more than one pathway or APC is involved, do they all play the same role? Alternatively, does some of the presented antigen trigger attack functions, whereas other presented antigen triggers T-cell anergy, regulatory T-cell functions, or T-cell death *(27,84)* (*see* Subheading 4.1.)?

Such basic questions about CNS antigen presentation are directly applicable to brain tumor therapy. It is well known that class II⁺ mononuclear phagocytes can be abundant in and near CNS tumors *(23,67,72)*. However, class II⁺ mononuclear phagocytes can originally be derived from parenchymal microglia, perivascular phagocytes, or recentlyarrived blood-borne monocytes. All of these cell types can assume the same macrophage morphology; once this has happened, there is usually no simple way to determine the origin.

Mononuclear phagocytes can present antigen to trigger T-cell effector functions, but can also induce tolerance or regulatory functions (*see* Subheading 4.1.). They can also influence tumor independently of their potential function as APCs. They can directly attack tumor (*55,57*), but can also secrete growth factors (*53,89,111*). In teasing out the contributions of the different subpopulations, studies in autoimmunity and tumor immunity should complement and reinforce each other.

3.2.5. Summary and Implications for Brain Tumor Therapy

To trigger anti-tumor effector function, activated T-cells must re-recognize their antigen at the tumor site. The antigen must be presented in a complex with an MHC protein. The antigen can be presented by the tumor cell itself, or by a tumor-adjacent APC. Presentation of ingested antigen, by tumor-adjacent APCs, is of special interest for tumor in the brain. To date, most work in tumor immunotherapy has focused on direct presentation by tumor cells themselves. Giving more emphasis to indirect antigen presentation should be fruitful.

The complexities of antigen presentation are but one facet of the fully-developed immune response. A comparable variety is seen in immune effector functions, as discussed below.

4. THE VARIETY AND COMPLEXITY OF IMMUNE ACTIVITY

An anti-tumor response can include a variety of T-cell-mediated functions, other immune effectors, and also other kinds of cells and mediators, each with its feedback controls. Some of the many possibilities, stressing alternative T-cell functions, are discussed below. First, however, alternatives to attack function are reviewed.

4.1. Alternatives to Target Attack

4.1.1. Regulation and Tolerance

The immune response is normally thought of in terms of attack functions: successful attack of tumor or pathogens and unwanted attack of neural grafts, in neurodegeneration, or in autoimmune disease. Yet, progression to target attack is just one of the possible outcomes of the interaction between a lymphocyte and its antigen.

The immune response depends on the capacity of lymphocytes to recognize antigen. Each clone of lymphocytes has a characteristic antigen receptor. The energy with which the antigen (or antigen-MHC complex) binds the receptor determines the outcome. If the binding energy is too low, there will be no effect (immune ignorance). If it is high enough to stimulate the lymphocyte, the consequence may be one of the possible forms of immune tolerance: the lymphocyte may be killed (clonal deletion), or it may be made unresponsive to further stimulation (anergy). Alternatively, the lymphocyte may be stimulated into a regulatory pathway (*see* Subheading 4.6.3.). Thus, stimulation into an attack pathway is but one among many alternatives.

4.1.2. Factors That Affect the Outcome

The outcome of antigen binding to a lymphocyte receptor depends on the lymphocyte itself, the antigen-bearing cell, and the regulatory environment. T-cells recognize cell-bound antigen I in the form of a peptide-MHC complex (*see* Subheading 3.1.1.). To be primed successfully, a naive T-cell must also recognize other molecules, co-stimulatory molecules, on the antigen-bearing cell. The role of co-stimulation in triggering effector function is less clear. Co-stimulation can increase the efficiency of re-stimulation, but may not be required (*26*).

4.1.3. A Regulatory Continuum

Although the immune system is often described as distinguishing between "self" and "non-self," the discrimination is more complex than these terms imply (*117*). Tolerance can indeed be established against self-antigens, either during development or later. However, tolerance is not an all-or-nothing phenomenon. Tolerance to self-antigen can be broken. Tolerance can also be induced to foreign antigen, including tumor antigen *(118)*.

The consequences of auto-recognition are subtle; it is not necessarily harmful. Immune ignorance and tolerance do indeed protect against harmful self-reactivity (autoimmune disease). At the same time, the immune response can safely target normal proteins in appropriate circumstances. In particular, it is possible to safely target normal proteins as tumor antigens *(20,96,119,138)*. The normal proteins may be over-represented in tumor cells, as compared to normal cells. Alternatively, normal cells that share the target antigen may be expendable; the immunoglobulin idiotype is the classic example of this kind of tumor antigen *(65,70,75,124)*.

More generally, recognition of self-determinants can contribute to immune regulation and homeostasis *(32,117,147)*. Even when immune attack is most desirable, against tumor or infection, the regulatory function is still as important as the attack function. Fas-FasL interactions (*see* Subheading 2.4.2.), activation-induced cell death (*see* Subheading 2.4.2.), and the Th1/Th2 counterbalance (*see* Subheading 4.6.3.) are three specific examples of immune feedback controls discussed in the text.

4.1.4. Conclusions

Tumor immunity and autoimmunity may be seen as parts of a continuum, rather than separate processes. Normal proteins can serve as practically useful tumor antigens, and a response to normal proteins can contribute to feedback control. Further insight into the importance of feedback controls comes from work in autoimmunity, as discussed below.

4.2. A Lesson From Autoimmunity: The Strength of Feedback Controls

4.2.1. A Basic Model of Central Nervous System Autoimmunity

Among the most widely studied autoimmune diseases are MS and the animal model of CNS autoimmunity, experimental autoimmune encephalomyelitis (EAE). Although there are many questions about how well EAE mimics MS, there is no doubt that it has provided much basic understanding of immune regulation in the CNS.

EAE can be initiated by sensitizing (immunizing) a susceptible rodent strain (mouse, rat, guinea pig) with a component of myelin. In one common protocol, Lewis (LEW) rats are sensitized with myelin basic protein (MBP) that has been emulsified in complete Freund's adjuvant (CFA) and injected into one hind footpad. No further manipulations are made. Within several days, the rats show ascending neurologic symptoms, first a limp tail, hind limb paralysis next. Ultimately, surviving rats recover and are now refractory to further challenge with MPB *(34)*.

4.2.2. Implications for Tumor Therapy

There is great concern that successful brain tumor immunotherapy may lead to autoimmunity against normal CNS antigens. The experience from EAE models gives a different perspective. In practice, it can be difficult to induce EAE and still more difficult to maintain it *(34)*. Indeed, experience with EAE suggests that just the opposite concern may be more pertinent: Strong feedback controls protect against autoimmune disease. To what extent do these same feedback controls also make it difficult to achieve and maintain an effective response against tumor? Anti-tumor responses can show reduced efficacy with time *(94,149)*. The same feedback controls that protect against autoimmunity are likely to play a role.

Understanding of feedback controls, how they can go awry, and how they can be manipulated, is a key aspect of current research. For tumor therapy, a conservative goal is the most benign response that will successfully attack residual or disseminated tumor that cannot be reached or attacked by other means. The variety of possible attack functions and combinations is reviewed next.

4.3. Attack Functions Mediated by T-Cells

4.3.1. Direct Attack by the T-Cell Itself

If an MHC$^+$ infected or neoplastic cell presents its own antigen to an effector T-cell, attack mechanisms that require cell-to-cell contact are possible. One major pathway is initiated by interaction between FasL on the T-cell and Fas on the target cell (*see* Subheading 2.4.2.); downstream signaling ultimately leads to apoptosis of the target cell. The second major pathway requiring cell-cell contact involves the pore-forming protein, perforin. In this case, the T-cell inserts perforin into the membrane of the target cell. Granzymes, degradative enzymes made by the T-cell, are then inserted through the pore. The granzymes initiate a signaling sequence that leads to death of the target *(41)*.

T-cells can also attack their targets by secreted factors, such as TNF-α *(70)*. This form of attack can be used whether the tumor antigen is presented by the tumor cell itself (direct pathway), or by a tumor-adjacent APCs (indirect pathway) (*see* Subheading 3.2.2.).

4.3.2. T-Cell Attack Via Phagocytes and Other Secondary Cells

T-cells can kill tumor targets directly, as described above. At least in vitro, a single T-cell can kill more than one target *(31)*. However, a more efficient way to attack a multicellular, growing target is for the T-cell to amplify its own response, attracting and activating phagocytes and other cells that can contribute to target attack *(113)*. In this case, the fundamental contributions of the T-cell are to reach the target (migration; *see* Subheading 5), recognize that the target is present (recall recognition of tumor antigen; *see* Subheading 2.2.1.), and then secrete factors that initiate an attack cascade. The general model for this type of response is the delayed-type hypersensitivity (DTH) response.

The list of possible attack molecules that can be secreted by activated phagocytes includes cytokines such as TNF-α or IFN-γ; *NO* and other reactive nitrogen intermediates (RNI); and reactive oxygen intermediates (ROI). As explained above, none of these molecules is specific for the target. Instead, specificity comes from the local concentration at the tumor site. Tumor cells or normal cells are attacked as bystanders, according to their relative vulnerability to the local mix of secreted factors. Toxins, growth factors, and other molecules secreted by phagocytes, tumor cells, blood-borne cells, and endogenous cells can all contribute to the net effect.

4.3.3. A Specific Example

The sequence leading to phagocyte-mediated attack is well-documented in EAE models (*see* Subheading 4.2.1.). After immunization with CNS antigen, T-cells that enter the CNS and re-recognize their antigen can initiate an attack cascade, attracting and activated both local cells (microglia, astrocytes, resident phagocytes) and blood-borne inflammatory cells. If the initiating T-cells are marked, relatively few are seen in the tissue; most local T-cells have been attracted as part of the cascade *(17)*. The bulk of the final tissue damage is thought to be caused by phagocytes, attracted or activated as the response unfolds. If their activity is blocked, disease is prevented or reduced *(5,11,129)*.

4.4. T-Cell Nomenclature

Two different nomenclatures are commonly used to describe T-cells. The basic definitions, and how they are currently combined are reviewed below.

4.4.1. Cytotoxic T Lymphocytes vs Th

In the traditional, function-based nomenclature, T-cells are classified according to whether they directly lyse their targets (cytotoxic T lymphocytes [CTL]), or release regulatory molecules (helper/inducer T-cells, Th). In the initiation of the immune response, Th are necessary for the full stimulation of both B-cells and CTL. Different Th subpopulations that secrete different cytokines, play complementary roles. Th1 are important for activating CTL, and Th2 are important for activating B-cells. Th1 and Th2 can also play complementary roles in the effector phase (*see* Subheading 4.6.3.).

The second major T-cell demarcation refers to the MHC restricting element. Characteristic accessory proteins are also taken into account, as described below.

4.4.2. Class I-Restricted/CD8+ vs Class II-Restricted/CD4+ T-Cells

T-cell recognize antigen that has been complexed to MHC proteins (*see* Subheading 3.1.). For each T-cell clone, the T-cell receptor specifies not only the antigen specificity, but also whether the antigen must be presented by class I or class II MHC proteins. In practice, class I-restricted T-cells are often identified by their expression of the CD8 accessory protein that binds to a nonpolymorphic determinant on class I molecules. Similarly, class II-restricted T-cells are often identified by their expression of the CD4 accessory protein that binds to class II MHC proteins.

Although the functional demarcation, CTL or Th, was once thought to imply the MHC restricting element, this is no longer the case. Rather, the two nomenclatures can complement each other, as reviewed below.

4.4.3. Traditional Emphasis on Cytotoxic T Lymphocytes

The ability of T-cells to act as CTL, lysing their targets through cell-cell contact, is the effector mechanism most often stressed for tumor therapy. Class I-restricted CTL are usually emphasized, for two interlocking reasons: 1) more cell type express class I than class II MHC proteins and 2) the class I pathway is the main path for presentation of antigen made by a tumor cell itself (*see* Subheading 3.2.2.). Thus, most tumor studies have aimed to exploit class I-restricted CTL. For class II-expressing target cells, class II-restricted T-cells can also act as CTL.

4.4.4. Attractive Features of Th

T-cells can also attack their targets without making direct contact. Acting as Th, T-cells can secrete factors that directly lyse tumor targets or attract and activate other cells to do so (*see* Subheading 4.3.2.). This pathway is more general than the CTL pathway, because it does not depend upon the tumor cell presenting its own antigen. Rather, ingested tumor antigen can be presented to the Th by tumor-adjacent APCs (*see* Subheading 3.2.2.). The class II-restricted pathway is the most important path for presentation of ingested antigen.

Increasing attention is now being paid to the attack potential of class II-restricted T-cells *(37,43,44)*. The characteristic MHC distribution patterns in the brain, with class II+ APC predominating (*see* Subheading 3.2.2.), make class II-restricted T-cells of special interest at that site *(65,68,70)*.

4.4.5. Summary

T-cells are subdivided according to whether they recognize antigen in the context of class I or class II MHC proteins. Whether they are class I-restricted or class II-restricted, T-cells may act as CTL, attacking their targets via cell–cell contacts, or as Th, attacking via secreted factors *(1,65)*. Most work to date has focused on class I-restricted CTL. Because of their flexibility, class II-restricted Th merit more attention, especially against tumor in the CNS.

4.5. Antibody-Mediated Attack

The binding of antibody does not, by itself, kill a tumor target. The antibody-target interaction must be amplified. The amplification depends on a general structural feature of antibody molecules. Different populations of B-cells produce different antibody classes (isotypes, IgM, IgG, IgA), with somewhat different structures. Within each isotype, the antibody proteins have a common constant region and an antigen-binding variable region. The variable region binds specifically to the target. Attack of a cellular target is amplified through the constant region.

Isotypes that bind complement can initiate an enzymatic cascade that kills the target cell *(35)*. Alternatively, antibody constant regions can be recognized by Fc receptors on macrophages or NK cells. The antibody can then act as a bridge between the effector cell (which recognizes the constant region) and the target cell (which is recognized by the variable region). Formation of the bridge activates the effector to secrete toxic factors, so that the target is killed as a bystander. The term for this mechanism is antibody-dependent cell-mediated cytotoxicity (ADCC) *(35)*.

4.6. A Multifaceted Response

4.6.1. Comparing Mechanisms

Different effector mechanisms offer complementary advantages. To give but a few examples, taken from within this chapter: metabolically active T-cells can migrate to tumor sites; they are not blocked by the physical blood–brain barrier. Because they recognize processed antigen, T-cells can detect internal tumor antigens. T-cells can kill tumor cells through cell–cell contact, but this requires the tumor cell to present its own antigen. T-cells can also kill tumor cells indirectly, but normal cells may be attacked as bystanders. Blood-borne monocytes can participate in T-cell-mediated attack. Monocytes can also enter the brain and respond to tumor without the participation of lymphocytes, but the fine specificity of the immune response is sacrificed. In practice, each of these mechanisms can contribute to the fully developed immune response.

4.6.2. The Interplay of Multiple Mechanisms

Although it is useful to explain the different attack mechanisms one by one, they are not likely to work in isolation. T-cells can attack targets by cell-to-cell contact and by secreted factors, and can activate phagocytes. Bystander killing can be mediated by T-cells, activated phagocytes, or NK cells, using overlapping sets of secreted factors. Striking examples of the impact of combining mechanisms are seen in EAE.

In a widely used variant of the basic EAE model described above (*see* Subheading 4.2.1.), Th1 from sensitized animals are used to transfer EAE to naive hosts. Although Th alone, and even a single Th1 clone, can transfer disease, the final pathology is seen to reflect a cascade of events: The original Th1 travel through the blood and some extravasate at the cerebral vessels; those that recognize their antigen in the CNS are triggered to carry out their effector functions; the triggered cells secrete factors that attract and activate blood-borne inflammatory cells and local phagocytes (*see* Subheading 4.3.2.).

In addition to the general inflammatory activation, different specific immune effector functions can also contribute to tissue damage. Although EAE can be transferred by class II-restricted Th1, class I-restricted/CD8+ T-cells can also mediate tissue damage *(45)*. Although EAE is usually described as a T-cell-mediated disease, antibodies to CNS antigen can exacerbate damage. Indeed, the pathology more closely resembles that of MS when an antibody response is included *(17,88,120)*.

The immune response is dynamic, and not all of the components are destructive. As the response unfolds, different subpopulations, functions, and molecular mediators predominate. Local attack functions are dampened by feedback controls, to be followed by tissue repair.

4.6.3. The Th1/Th2 Counterbalance

Yet another facet of immune regulation is its context dependence. The Th1/Th2 counterbalance provides a specific example. Th1 and Th2 are alternative differentiation states for cytokine-secreting Th (*see* Subheading 4.4.1). The Th1 pathway is characterized by production of IL-2, a T-cell growth factor; and of TNF-α and IFN-γ, two cytokines that can mediate both direct and indirect target attack. The complementary Th2 pathway is characterized by production of IL-4 and IL-10, two cytokines that down-regulate Th1 responses.

The functional consequences of a particular Th1/Th2 balance are context dependent. In the setting of a T-cell-mediated response to tumor, Th1 cells would be expected to mediate tumor attack and Th2 cells would be expected to modulate that response *(111)*. The Th2 modulation can be desirable, preventing an over-exuberant response. Alternatively, too great a Th2 contribution may suppress anti-tumor activity.

In other contexts, the optimal Th1/Th2 balance may be different. In one animal model, brain tumor attack was mediated by eosinophils *(127)*. In that setting, IL-4, which is a Th2 product, enhanced the mast cell attack.

4.6.4. Implications

The complex, context-dependent nature of the immune response mandates care in interpreting the results of experimental or clinical studies. In terms of the example given above: in eosinophil-mediated attack, IL-4 secreting Th2 cells act as anti-tumor effectors *(127)*. In CTL-mediated attack Th1 cells are the effectors and Th2 act as regulators.

Experimentally, the balance of functions will vary with the tumor model. Results in vitro will not necessarily predict the net balance of functions in vivo *(130)*. In vivo, the balance of functions can vary with the animal species and strain, the tumor type, and the local site. Identifying the most important effector function for a particular model may be of most value for the basic understanding it can give *(69)*. The particular function that shows efficacy in a given tumor model won't necessarily be the most favorable for human patients, and, in any case, a mix of functions may be preferable.

5. DELIVERY OF EFFECTOR FUNCTION TO THE TUMOR SITE

In seeking to exploit the full complexity of the immune response, it is important to consider the paths in organized lymphoid tissue (*see* Subheading 2.2.2.), but tumor must be attacked in each tissue where it grows. For this to be possible, immune effectors must leave the organized lymphoid tissue and come into contact with their tumor targets. The potential for immune effectors to reach tumor is of special interest for tumor that is too small to be imaged, widely disseminated, or not readily accessed by conventional means (such as tumor in the brainstem). The delivery of T-cell-mediated and B-cell-mediated effector function to brain tumor sites is reviewed later.

5.1. T-Cells

5.1.1. General Patterns of T-Cell Traffic

T-cells effect a cell-mediated response; the T-cell itself must be adjacent to its target (*see* Subheading 2.1.3.). This is facilitated because priming alters the T-cell migration pattern. Naive T-cells preferentially enter organized lymphoid tissues, where they are most likely to be effectively stimulated (*see* Subheading 2.2.1.). Following activation and clonal expansion, the traffic pattern of the daughter cells is shifted towards surveillance of the nonlymphoid tissues *(139)*, including the brain *(68)*. The combination of random and specific factors that dictate T-cell traffic is discussed below.

5.1.2. How T-Cells Reach Their Targets

If vaccination is successful activated tumor-specific T-cells will enter the blood. If the cells recognize appropriate adhesion molecules on the cerebral vessels they may leave the blood at that point. If they encounter tumor—and if they are triggered by the activating tumor antigen—they can carry out their effector functions at the tumor site.

It is important to stress how many of the post-vaccination steps are not antigen-specific. T-cells move through the vasculature with the general blood flow; they do not home to the CNS (although that term is often used). T-cells extravasate if they recognize appropriate adhesion molecules on the cerebral endothelial cells. The same adhesion molecules mediate extravasation in other nonlymphoid tissues. Brain-specific or brain tumor-specific adhesion molecules have not been identified.

Some steps can be influenced by the presence of tumor. Tumor-dependent changes may activate tumor-adjacent vessels, making it more likely that T-cells will bind and extravasate. Movement through edema fluid at tumor sites, changes in the extracellular matrix in the vicinity of tumor, or tumor-dependent chemo-attractants can increase the likelihood of T-cell–tumor interactions. However, each of these factors would have the greatest impact after the T-cell had entered the local vasculature.

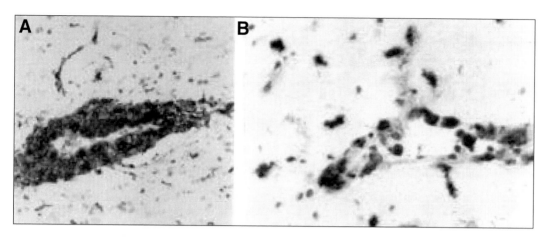

Fig. 7. Migration to perivascular space vs. brain proper. Blood-borne inflammatory cells (T-cells, monocytes, etc.) can accumulate as cuffs in the perivascular space (PVS) (**A**), or move into the brain parenchyma proper (**B**). The most important site for immunotherapy depends upon the tumor type. Blood-borne metastases of most nonlymphoid tumors accumulate in the PVS. Infiltration of the parenchyma is a hallmark of astrocytoma. CNS lymphoma is found at both sites. In seeking to enhance T-cell surveillance, the optimal regimen may vary with the tumor type and site. (Panels A and B reprinted with permission from refs. *71,65*, respectively.)

5.1.3. T-Cells and the Blood–Brain Barrier

T-cell surveillance of the brain is often discussed in terms of crossing the blood–brain barrier (BBB). This terminology is misleading, for two reasons; 1) it gives a false impression of how cell migration is controlled and 2) it implies that T-cells do not normally enter the brain.

Regarding control of migration, the physical BBB (endothelial tight junctions and glial endfeet) does indeed stop the passive entry of large proteins, but does not stop the entry of metabolically active cells. Instead, entry of T-cells (and other inflammatory cells) is controlled by the profile of adhesion molecules on the cerebral endothelial cells. If the appropriate signals are presented, the inflammatory cells are arrested and can begin the multi-step process leading to extravasation *(139)*. Entry of inflammatory cells need not compromise the physical BBB; even as blood-borne cells pass into the brain, the physical barrier to protein entry can remain *(68,70)*.

5.1.4. Perivascular Space vs Parenchyma Proper

After leaving the blood, migrant cells pass into the perivascular space (PVS). The migrants may remain in the PVS as perivascular cuffs, or may pass into the brain parenchyma proper (Fig. 7). This is true for T-cells and other inflammatory cells, and also for some tumors, such as CNS lymphoma. The controlling steps are not well understood, but physical crowding is not the limiting factor. T-cells or other migrants can form large cuffs, or the same cell types may move into the brain proper (Fig. 7).

The distinction between cuffing and infiltration of the brain parenchyma merits attention when planning immunotherapy. Metastases of most nonlymphoid tumors remain as perivascular cuffs, at least initially, but CNS lymphoma can be found in both the PVS and the brain proper. Of course, primary brain tumors do grow in the brain proper, and infiltration of the parenchyma is a hallmark of astrocytoma. If one aims to enhance immune surveillance of CNS tumor, the optimal regimen is likely to vary with the tumor type and site (*see* Subheading 1.1.3.).

5.1.5. Overview

T-cell/tumor juxtaposition is necessary, but not sufficient, for antigen-specific attack. Once a T-cell has made contact with tumor, its effector functions must be triggered by recall recognition of its antigen. The antigen can be presented by a tumor-adjacent APC that has ingested it; it need not be presented by the tumor cell itself. Effector triggering is an additional step, but it is what gives the response its specificity and thus contributes to its safety.

Lest the full sequence of required steps seem improbable, it is important to stress that T-cells can be effective in the CNS. They can cure tumor, clear virus, and also cause unwanted destruction of grafts or autoimmune disease *(70)*. In each case, the challenge is to safely modify the response in the desired direction.

5.2. Antibodies and B-Cells

5.2.1. How Antibodies Reach Their Targets

Antibody-forming cells (activated B-cells and plasma cells) can secrete their antibody into the serum, which gives it access to most organs and tissues. The brain is a well-known exception. Antibody molecules are too large to cross the intact BBB. The barrier may be broken or abnormal within a tumor mass, but this is less likely at micro-tumor sites. Even within a tumor mass, delivery of drugs can be inefficient within the chaotic tumor vasculature *(134)*.

One general strategy has been to modify the antibody protein, making it smaller but still retaining the antigen-binding site *(141)*. To make the antibody smaller, it is necessary to sacrifice or truncate at least one of the features that contribute to its efficacy: its multivalent structure, or its constant region. One complementary strategy is to join the antibody fragment to a separate effector molecule, such as a radionuclide or toxin *(141)* (this volume). Detailed knowledge of antibody structure and function, plus the growing ease of protein engineering, make it likely that some form of antibody can be used to successfully attack tumor *(124)*, including tumor in the brain (this volume).

5.2.2. Migration of the B-Cells Themselves

A complementary approach, focused on delivery of B-cells rather than secreted antibody, may also be fruitful. Because B-cells mediate a humoral response, the traffic of B-cells themselves is not usually emphasized in a tumor context. However, B-cells do have characteristic traffic patterns. Antibody-forming cells lodge in preferred sites from which they secrete their antibody *(38)*. Provocatively, antibody-forming cells can lodge in the CNS, and can secrete antibody there for prolonged periods *(91,131)*. Immunoglobulin is found in the CSF in MS and many other neurologic disorders, and antibody-forming cells can be found in the perivascular spaces, the choroid plexus, or brain parenchyma *(17,105,144)*.

The underlying mechanisms that favor localization of antibody-forming cells to the CNS are not well understood, and may repay more attention. On the one hand, this may give insight into the underlying biology of primary CNS lymphoma. Most often a B-cell lymphoma, CNS lymphoma is the major CNS tumor of AIDS, and is increasing in the general population, especially among the elderly.

In terms of brain tumor therapy, focus on delivery of B-cells themselves may be a productive complement to focus on delivery of modified antibody protein. The goal would be to cause activated, tumor-specific B-cells to lodge in the brain and secrete their antibody, or engineered alternatives, directly into the CSF, or even into the PVS at tumor sites.

5.3. Other Effectors

Although this chapter stresses T-cells and antibody, other effectors can also travel to a brain tumor site, or be made to do so. Blood-borne monocytes have multiple potential roles in tumor therapy. These short-lived cells are continually replenished from the bone marrow. Once they enter the tissue, they can differentiate into macrophages, which are long-lived and cannot divide. Monocytes and macrophages can serve as APCs, presenting ingested antigen to trigger T-cell effector function at a tumor site (*see* Subheading 3.2.2.). In turn, a key T-cell effector function is to attract and activate monocytes or other mononuclear phagocytes to attack nearby tumor (*see* Subheading 4.3.2.). Increasing monocyte traffic to tumor sites might thus serve two complementary goals: monocytes may serve as a source of fresh APC, not yet suppressed by the tumor micro-environment. Increasing monocyte traffic might also be a way of amplifying the T-cells' effector functions. The potential importance of monocytes and macrophages in tumor destruction, as well as the need for careful control, is strongly supported by complementary experience in EAE (*see* Subheading 4.3.3.).

Yet a third approach is to exploit the anti-tumor activity of monocytes and macrophages directly *(55)*, independent of T-cell function. These three goals are not mutually exclusive. For each, it is important to gain better understanding of monocyte traffic and of the multiple functions that monocytes and macrophages can serve. Points of current interest include the different possible consequences of antigen presentation (stimulation, anergy, etc.) (*see* Subheading 4.1.1.), and the balance between secretion of tumor-killing toxins and secretion of factors that might promote tumor growth *(53,89,111)*.

An alternative to cellular effectors is to introduce drugs directly into the blood or CSF. Traditional limitations have been a short half-life in vivo, toxicity at tumor-free sites, and, for CNS tumors, the need to cross the BBB. As novel delivery systems are developed *(14,50,108)*, it is useful to compare their advantages and limitations to those of migratory cells.

6. ENHANCING IMMUNE SURVEILLANCE: TUMOR VACCINES AND BEYOND

The discussion above provides a foundation for understanding the rationale behind current approaches to immunotherapy. The discussion below serves as a summary of the points that have been covered, and illustrates how some of the post-vaccine steps can be enhanced.

6.1. Step 1: Tumor Vaccines

6.1.1. For a Pathogen (Bacterium or Virus), Vaccines Are Prophylactic

If the patient is later exposed to the same pathogen, the relatively efficient secondary response is triggered (*see* Subheading 2.1.2.). For tumor patients, the context for vaccination is rather different. When detected, a brain tumor is already growing, it may already be widely disseminated within the CNS, and may have already modified the patient's immune response. The patient may have become tolerant to tumor antigens *(118)*, and may display more generalized immunosuppression as well *(87,90)*, both locally and systemically. Breaking tolerance to tumor antigen may be an essential step in tumor therapy. Insight into possible strategies can come from work in the complementary context of autoimmunity.

6.1.2. Lessons From Autoimmunity

As with tumor, it is likely that autoimmune activity will already have been established when vaccination is initiated. Inverting the goals for tumor, the aim of immune manipulation is to restore or establish tolerance, or to favor regulatory functions over attack functions. Generalized immunosuppression is not attractive because it lacks specificity; the patient is made more vulnerable to tumor and infection. A more directed strategy is to delete the unwanted clones of responding cells. In practice, this has been difficult because of the heterogeneity of the response, and its feedback controls. If dominant clones are eliminated, other clones can become prominent. An alternative strategy is to cause the autoantigen to be presented in a form, or via a route, that is expected to shift the regulatory balance. Efforts to induce oral tolerance in MS and EAE exemplify this approach *(49)*. Although the goal is inverted, all of this work is relevant to brain tumor therapy. Against tumor, specific (rather than general) immune activation is preferable; activating a small number of tumor-specific T-cell clones is not likely to be sufficient; and the same variables that can favor a regulatory response can also be adjusted to favor tumor attack.

6.1.3. The Next Steps for Brain Tumor Therapy

To date, work in brain tumor therapy has focused, appropriately, on stimulating a strong response against tumor antigen. As vaccine strategies become successful, it is timely to consider what mix of effector functions might be most desirable (*see* Subheading 4.), how one might safely enhance delivery of effectors, and, for T-cell-mediated functions, what might safely enhance effector triggering at the tumor site. Some examples are given below.

6.2. Step 2: Enhancing Extravasation

T-cell extravasation can be increased by activating the T-cell and by activating the cerebral vessels *(71)*. T-cell activation can be achieved by immunization (vaccination). Activation of cerebral vessels can be achieved by intracerebral injection of cytokines such as IFN-γ or TNF-α *(58,71)*. Intracerebral injection concentrates the cytokine in the region of interest, and avoids systemic toxicities. In tumor-free rats, the two steps, immunization to activate the T-cells and intracerebral cytokine to activate the vessel, were found to be at least additive *(71)*. In tumor-bearing rats, IFN-γ retained its ability to enhance T-cell extravasation *(112)*.

A striking facet of the enhanced T-cell accumulation was its tight control. In tumor-free rats, the number of T-cells per field, and the sizes of perivascular cuffs, remained moderate *(71)*. In tumor-bearing rats, T-cells were concentrated in tumor areas. Foci of inflammation were not seen distant from the tumor site *(23,70)* (Fig. 5).

6.3. Step 3: Enhancing Antigen Presentation

APCs are normally quiescent in the CNS, but are readily activated, for example, by exposure to cytokines *(66)*. The indirect pathway of triggering T-cell effector function, in which ingested tumor antigen is presented by class II⁺ APC, is of special interest in the brain (*see* Subheading 3.2.3.). In tumor-free rats, intracerebral injection of IFN-γ upregulates class II MHC expression in APC at all potential sites of tumor spread, including the parenchyma proper (both grey matter and white matter), the perivascular space, and the periventricular area *(70,71)*.

In more recent work, a panel of glioma cell lines with different immune behaviors was evaluated to extend the analysis to tumor-bearing rats.. The panel included tumors that had been judged nonimmunogenic or immunosuppressive by other criteria. Implanted cells were allowed to grow for up to three weeks. For all the tumors, even when tumor had grown to fill half the hemisphere of implantation, the ability of IFN-γ to upregulate class II MHC expression of potential APC was retained *(23)*.

6.4. Conclusion

Although tumors are known to be immunosuppressive, suppression need not be equal for all functions or at all sites. The robust ability of IFN-γ to enhance T-cell accumulation and to upregulate class II MHC expression by APC is encouraging. What additional steps may be required to achieve tumor control, and how the findings can best be translated to human patients, must now be pursued. In evaluating different regimens, site-specific effects, and the effect of manipulating local neurochemicals will be of interest *(85,86)*, (*see* Subheading 2.5.3.).

7. BROADER ISSUES

7.1. Alternative Philosophies

The combination of new basic understanding and new tools has enormously increased the potential power of immunotherapy. It is not yet clear how this power can best be used. To what extent should one aim for subtle shifts in the normal regulatory balance, taking advantage of the full complexity of normal effector mechanisms and feedback controls? To what extent should one aim for a synthetic response, using immune effectors, or perhaps just the underlying principles, in new ways?

In addressing these broad questions, as well as many others, the appropriate use of small animal models is an important concern.

7.2. Small Animal Models

7.2.1. Need for New Models

Understandably, most clinical and experimental work in brain tumor immunotherapy has focused on larger tumor masses. Larger tumors can be readily visualized and measured, and present the most urgent clinical problem. However, as explained above (*see* Subheading 1.1.), larger tumor masses may not be the most appropriate targets for immunotherapy. Rather, smaller foci of residual or disseminated tumor, especially tumor that is distributed within still-functioning brain tissue, may be the most important and most favorable targets.

Traditionally, small animal models have not been well-suited to micro-tumor study. In many cases, tumor cell lines have been grown as masses under the skin, where they can be most easily followed, but the anatomic and pharmacologic complexity of the CNS is lost. In intracerebral models, a tumor cell line is typically implanted in the striatum, and then grows out from the implantation site as an expanding mass. When tumor does spread away from the main mass, spread though the PVS and by other routes may be seen *(76)*, but true infiltration of the parenchyma proper is usually not observed. To permit study of human tumors, human cells are often grown in immunodeficient mice or rats, which precludes study of the normal immune response.

7.2.2. Some Solutions

More recently, small animal models have been developed that are better suited to study of brain micro-tumor and micro-tumor immunotherapy. Causing tumor cell lines to constitutively express the lacZ reporter gene product, *E. coli*-β-galactosidase (β-gal) is useful in several ways. The β-gal protein is produced as a cell-filling cytoplasmic protein. A simple histochemical stain allows identification of even single tumor cells in tissue Subheadings (Fig. 1) *(76)*. The intensely colored reaction product facilitates quantitative image analysis (Fig. 1) *(65)*. Complementing its value as a marker, the β-gal protein also serves as a well-defined surrogate tumor antigen *(74)*, one whose immunologic properties have been well-studied in other contexts.

Although tumor cell lines are typically implanted in the striatum, this is not necessary. Cell lines expressing the β-gal marker can be used study tumor, including micro-tumor, in most locations. Examples include tumor that has disseminated through the brainstem and cerebellum, after implantation in the pons *(112)*; tumor that has spread through the periventricular area *(51)* (Fig. 1A); tumor that has seeded the CSF *(76)*; and blood-borne micro-metastases in the PVS *(51)*.

Marked tumor cell lines can be used to study many paths of tumor spread within the CNS *(76)*. However, most rodent glioma cell lines do not show the infiltrative spread that is characteristic of human astrocytoma. In the newest small animal models, defined genetic manipulations cause mice to spontaneously develop brain tumors that mimic genetic features of human glioma, and may also show infiltrative growth *(15,22,132)*. Taken together, the different types of current small animal models offer complementary advantages *(69)*. The genetic models are better mimics of human disease, but the implantation models are more practical for appropriate questions.

7.2.3. Remaining Problems

Some problems are not readily solved even in the newest models *(69)*. Small animal models are necessary for ethical, logistic, and financial reasons. However, the spatial and temporal scales are not well matched to human patients, and species differences, both biochemical and anatomical, can influence results at many levels. In the specific case of immunotherapy, small animal models provide less time for a tumor to affect its immune environment, and less time for autoimmunity or other potential side effects to develop, as compared to human patients.

Although many of the problems inherent in using small animal models are not easily circumvented, it is essential to acknowledge them, and to search for others. Awareness of the problems need not invalidate the models, but can rather guide the way questions are framed and results are interpreted *(69)*. Brain tumor researchers come under much pressure to show efficacy and cures in preclinical studies. Human immunotherapy trials have often been disappointing. Greater emphasis on identifying problems and stressing the models may contribute to more successful translation to human patients.

7.3. Summary and Conclusions

Brain tumor vaccines are an important first step toward brain tumor immunotherapy. This chapter has stressed the many other steps that also deserve attention. Topics have included the variety and complexity of possible effector mechanisms, the need to deliver effectors to the tumor, and the need to trigger T-cell effector function at the tumor site. Bringing out subtleties of immune regulation, the effect of the local neuroregulatory environment, and the need to match immunotherapy to the tumor type and site, are stressed. Giving perspective, the appropriateness of micro-tumor as a T-cell target is emphasized. As the beauty and complexity of the immune response are increasingly revealed, lessons from other clinical contexts, complemented by thoughtful use of small animal models, should aid in finding the most favorable applications to brain tumor therapy.

ACKNOWLEDGMENTS

Work from the author's laboratory was funded by NIMH, The American Brain Tumor Association (ABTA), The American Cancer Society (ACS), the Elsa U. Pardee Foundation, the National Multiple Sclerosis Society (NMSS), the U.S. Army Medical Research and Material Command DOD 1999 Breast Cancer Research Program, and the generosity of private donors. The many contributions of recent trainees, especially Tanya Dutta, Yoichi Kondo, M.D., Ph.D., Lynnette Phillips McCluskey, Ph.D., and Rupa Kapoor are acknowledged with pleasure.

REFERENCES

1. Armstrong W.S., Lampson L.A. 1997. Direct cell-mediated responses in the nervous system: CTL vs. NK activity, and their dependence upon MHC expression and modulation, in *Immunology of the Nervous System* (Keane R.W., Hickey W.F., eds), Oxford. pp. 493–547.
2. Bachmann M.F., Barner M., Viola A., Kopf M. 1999. Distinct kinetics of cytokine production and cytolysis in effector and memory T cells after viral infection. *Eur. J. Immunol.* **29**:291–299.
3. Barker C.F., Billingham R.E. 1977. Immunologically privileged sites. *Adv. Immunol.* **25**:1–54.
4. Barrett J.W., Cao J.X., Hota-Mitchell S., McFadden G. 2001. Immunomodulatory proteins of myxoma virus. *Semin. Immunol.* **13**:73–84.
5. Bauer J., Ruuls S.R., Huitinga I., Dijkstra C.D. 1996. The role of macrophage subpopulations in autoimmune disease of the central nervous system. *Histochem. J.* **28**:83–97.
6. Beaujouan J.C., Saffroy M., Torrens Y., Glowinski J. 2000. Different subtypes of tachykinin NK(1) receptor binding sites are present in the rat brain. *J. Neurochem.* **75**:1015–26.
7. Becher B., D'Souza S.D., Troutt A.B., Antel J.P. 1998. Fas expression on human fetal astrocytes without susceptibility to fas-mediated cytotoxicity. *Neuroscience.* **84**:627–634.
8. Boon T., Cerottini J.C., Van den Eynde B., et al. 1994. Tumor antigens recognized by T lymphocytes. *Annu. Rev. Immunol.* **12**:337–365.
9. Breder C.D., Hazuka C., Ghayur T., et al. 1994. Regional induction of tumor necrosis factor-a expression in the mouse brain after systemic lipopolysaccharide administration. *Neurobiology.* **91**:11,393–11,397.
10. Brooks A.G., Boyington J.C., Sun P.D. 2000. Natural killer cell recognition of HLA class I molecules. *Rev. Immunogenet.* **2**:433–48.
11. Brosnan C. F., Bornstein M.B., Bloom B.R. 1981. The effects of macrophage depletion on the clinical and pathologic expression of experimental allergic encephalomyelitis. *J. Immunol.* **126**:614–620.
12. Burger P.C. 1990. Classification, grading, and patterns of spread of malignant gliomas, in *Malignant Cerebral Glioma* (Apuzzo M.L.J., ed.). Park Ridge, IL, American Association of Neurological Surgeons, pp 3–17.
13. Chappell D.B., Restifo N.P. 1998. T cell-tumor cell: a fatal interaction? *Cancer Immunol. Immunother.* **47:** 65–71.

14. Chen M.Y., Lonser R.R., Morrison P.F., Governale L.S., Oldfield E.H. 1999. Variables affecting convection-enhanced delivery to the striatum: a systematic examination of rate of infusion, cannula size, infusate concentration, and tissue cannula sealing time. *J. Neurosurg.* **90:** 315–320.

15. Corcoran R.B., Scott M.P. 2001. A mouse model for medulloblastoma and basal cell nevus syndrome. *J. Neuro-Oncol.* **53:**307–311.

16. Cross A.H., Cannella B., Brosnan C.F., Raine C.S. 1990. Homing to central nervous system vasculature by antigen-specific lymphocytes. I. Localization of 14C-labeled cells during acute, chronic, and relapsing experimental allergic encephalomyelitis. *Lab. Invest.* **63:**162–70.

17. Cross A.H., Trotter J.L., Lyons J. 2001. B cells and antibodies in CNS demyelinating disease. *J. Neuroimmunol.* **112:** 1–14.

18. Cserr H.F., Harling-Berg C., Ichimura T., Knopf P.M.,Yamada S. 1990. Drainage of cerebral extracellular fluids into cervical lymph: an afferent limb in brain/immune system interactions, in *Pathophysiology of the blood-brain barrier* (Johansson B.B., Owman C.H., Widner H., eds.) Elsevier.

19. Daumas-Duport C., Scheithauer B.W., Kelly P.J. 1987. A histologic and cytologic method for the spatial definition of gliomas. *Mayo Clin. Proc.* **62:** 435–449.

20. DeLeo A.B. 1998. p53-based immunotherapy of cancer. *Crit. Rev. Immunol.* **18:** 29–35.

21. Dhib-Jalbut S., Gogate N., Jiang H., Eisenberg H., Bergey G. 1996. Human microglia activate lymphoproliferative responses to recall viral antigens. *J. Neuroimmunol.* **65:** 67–73.

22. Ding H., Guha A. 2001. Mouse astrocytoma models: embryonic stem cell mediated transgenesis. *J. Neuro-Oncol.* **53:** 289–299.

23. Dutta T., Lampson L.A. 1998. MHC-expression and IFN-mediated enhancement in the presence of growing brain tumor in situ. *Cancer Res.* **58:** abst #4454.

24. Eckels D.D. 2000. MHC: function and implication on vaccine development. *Vox Sang.* **78(Suppl 2):**265–267.

25. Elliott P., Paris J., Mitsushio H., Lorens S. 1990. Neuronal sites mediating locomotor hyperactivity following central neurokinin agonist administration. *Pharm. Biochem. Behav.* **37:**329–333.

26. Flynn K., Mullbacher A. 1996. Memory alloreactive cytotoxic T cells do not require costimulation for activation in vitro. Immunol. *Cell. Biol.* **74:**413–420.

27. Ford A.L., Foulcher E., Lemckert F.A., Sedgwick J.D. 1996. Microglia induce CD4 T lymphocyte final effector function and death. *J. Exp. Med.* **184:**1737–1745.

28. Fraser I.P., Koziel H., Ezekowitz R.A.B. 1998. The serum mannose-binding protein and the macrophage mannose receptor are pattern recognition molecules that link innate and adaptive immunity. *Immunology* **10:**363–372.

29. Freeman C.R., Bourgouin P.M., Sanford R.A., Cohen M.E., Friedman M.E., Kun L.E. 1996. Long term survivors of childhood brain stem gliomas treated with hyperfractionated radiotherapy. *Cancer* **77:**555–562.

30. Frost P., Bonavida B. 2000. Circumvention of tumor cell escape following specific immunotherapy. *Cancer Biother. Radiopharm.* **15:**141–152.

31. Garcia-Penarrubia P., Bankhurst A.D. 1989. Kinetic analysis of effector cell recycling and effector-target binding capacity in a model of cell-mediated cytotoxicity. *J. Immunol.* **143:**2101–2111.

32. George J., Levy Y., Shoenfeld Y. 1996. Immune network and autoimmunity. *Intern. Med.* **35:**3–9.

33. Glick R.P., Lichtor T., Mogharbel A., Taylor C.A., Cohen E.P. 1997. Intracerebral versus subcutaneous immunization with allogeneic fibroblasts genetically engineered to secrete interleukin-2 in the treatment of central nervous system glioma and melanoma. *Neurosurgery* **41:**898–906.

34. Gordon F.L., Nguyen K.B., White C.A., Pender M.P. 2001. Rapid entry and downregulation of T cells in the central nervous system during the reinduction of experimental autoimmune encephalomyelitis. *J. Neuroimmunol.* **112:** 15–27.

35. Gorter A., Meri S. 1999. Immune evasion of tumor cells using membrane-bound complement regulatory proteins. *Immunol. Today* **20:**576–582.

36. Grabowska A., Lampson L.A. 1995. MHC expression in nonlymphoid tissues of the developing embryo: Strongest class I or class II expression in separate populations of potential antigen-presenting cells in the skin, lung, gut and inter-organ connective tissue. *Dev. Comp. Immunol.* **19:**425–450.

37. Greenberg P. 1991. Adoptive T cell therapy of tumors: mechanisms operative in the recognition and elimination of tumor cells. *Adv. Immunol.* **49:**281–355.

38. Grossi CE, Ciccone E., Tacchetti C., Santoro G., Anastasi G. 2000. Anatomy of the immune system: facts and problems. *Ital. J. Anat. Embryol.* **105:**97–124.

39. Guilloux Y., Bai X.F., Liu X., Zheng P., Liu Y. 2001. Optimal induction of effector but not memory antitumor cytotoxic T lymphocytes involves direct antigen presentation by the tumor cells. *Cancer Res.* **61:**1107–1112.

40. Harling-Berg C., Knopf P.M., Merriam J., Cserr H.F. 1989. Role of cervical lymph nodes in the systemic humoral immune response to human serum albumin microinfused into rat cerebrospinal fluid. *J. Neuroimmunol.* **25:**185–193.

41. Henkart P.A. 1999. Cytotoxic T lymphocytes, in *Fundamental Immunology* 4th Ed. (Paul W.E.) Lippincott-Raven, Philadelphia, PA, pp. 1021–1049.

42. Hiernaux J., Bona C.A. 1982. Shared idiotypes among monoclonal antibodies specific for different immunodominant sugars of lipopolysaccharide of different Gram-negative bacteria. *Proc. Natl. Acad. Sci.USA* **79:**1616–1620.

43. Hu H.M., Winter H., Urba W.J., Fox B.A. 2000. Divergent roles for CD4+ T cells in the priming and effector/memory phases of adoptive immunotherapy. *J. Immunol.* **165:**4246–4253.

44. Hung K.,Hayashi R.,Lafond-Walker A.,Lowenstein C., Pardoll D., Levitsky H. 1998. The central role of CD4(+) T cells in the antitumor immune response. *J. Exp. Med.* **188:**2357–2368.

45. Huseby E.S., Liggitt D., Brabb T., Schnabel B., Ohlen C., Goverman J. 2001. A pathogenic role for myelin-specific CD8(+) T cells in a model for multiple sclerosis. *J. Exp. Med.* **194:**669–676.

46. Inoue M., Plautz G.E., Shu S. 1996. Treatment of intracranial tumors by systemic transfer of superantigen-activated tumor-draining lymph node T cells. *Cancer Res.* **56:**4702–4708.

47. James S. P., Kwan W.C., Sneller M.C. 1990. T cells in inductive and effector compartments of the intestinal mucosal immune system of nonhuman primates differ in lymphokine mRNA expression, lymphokine utilization, and regulatory function. *J. Immunol.* **144:**1251–1256.

48. Janeway, Jr., C. A. 2001. How the immune system works to protect the host from infection: a personal view. *Proc. Natl. Acad. Sci. USA* **98:**7461–7468.

49. Jewell S.D.,Gienapp I.E., Cox K.L., Whitacre C.C. 1998. Oral tolerance as therapy for experimental autoimmune encephalomyelitis and multiple sclerosis: demonstration of T cell anergy. *Immunol. Cell. Biol.* **76:**74–82.

50. Joki T., Machluf M., Atala A., Zhu J., Seyfried N.T., Dunn I.F., et al. 2001. Continuous release of endostatin from microencapsulated engineered cells for tumor therapy. *Nature Biotechnol.* **9:**35–39.

51. Kapoor R., Durham J., Kondo Y., Lampson. 2002 L.A. Distribution of brain-metastasizing mammary carcinoma after intracarotid artery delivery in the rat. AACR Annual Meeting.

52. Ke Y., Ma H., Kapp J.A. 1998. Antigen is required for the activation of effector activities, whereas interleukin 2 Is required for the maintenance of memory in ovalbumin- specific, CD8+ cytotoxic T lymphocytes. *J. Exp. Med.* **187:**49–57.

53. Kerschensteiner M., Gallmeier E., Behrens L., Leal V.V., Misgeld T., Klinkert W.E., et al. 1999. Activated human T cells, B cells, and monocytes produce brain-derived neurotrophic factor in vitro and in inflammatory brain lesions: a neuroprotective role of inflammation? *J. Exp. Med.* **189:**865–870.

54. Kida S., Weller R.O., Zhang E-T., et al. 1995. Anatomical pathways for lymphatic drainage of the brain and their pathological significance. *Neuropathol. App. Neurobiol.* **21:**181–184.

55. Killion J.J., Fidler I.J. 1998. Therapy of cancer metastasis by tumoricidal activation of tissue macrophages using liposome-encapsulated immunomodulators. *Pharmacol. Ther.* **78:**141–154.

56. Kindt G.W. 1964. The pattern of location of cerebral metastatic tumors. *J. Neurosurg.* **21:**54–57.

57. Kirsch M., Fischer H., Schackert G. 1994. Activated monocytes kill malignant brain tumor cells in vitro. *J. Neuro-Oncol.* **20:**35–45.

58. Kondo Y., Lampson L.A. 2000. Enhancing T cell surveillance of brain micro-tumor: Different drugs optimize T cell entry to grey or white matter. Proc. AACR. **41:**192.

59. Kramer M.S., Cutler N., Feighner J., et al. 1998. Distinct mechanism for antidepressant activity by blockade of central substance P receptors. *Science.* **281:**1640–1645.

60. Kruse C.A., Lillehei K.O., Mitchell D.H., Kleinschmidt-DeMasters B., Bellgra D. 1990. Analysis of interleukin 2 and various effector cell populations in adoptive immunotherapy of 9L rat gliosarcoma: allogeneic cytotoxic T lymphocytes prevent tumor take. *Proc. Natl. Acad. Sci. USA* **87:**9577–9581.

61. Kruse C.A., Cepeda L., Owens B., Johnson S.D., Stears J., Lillehei K.O. 1997. Treatment of recurrent glioma with intracavitary alloreactive cytotoxic T lymphocytes and interleukin-2. *Cancer Immunol. Immunother.* **45:**77–87.

62. Kupsky W.J., Schoene W.C. 1993. Classification and pathology of astrocytomas, in *Astrocytomas: Diagnosis, Treatment and Biology* (Black P. McL., Schoene W. C., Lampson, L.A., eds.) Blackwell Scientific, pp. 3–25.

63. Kurpad S.N., Zhao X.G., Wikstrand C.J., et al. 1994. Tumor antigens in astrocytic gliomas. *Glia* 15: 244–256.

64. Lampson L.A. 1984. Molecular bases of neuronal individuality: Lessons from anatomical and biochemical studies with monoclonal antibodies, in *Monocolonal Antibodies and Functional Cell Lines: Progress and Applications* (Kennett R.H., et al., eds.) Plenum Press, pp. 153–189.

65. Lampson L.A. 1993. Cell-mediated immunotherapy directed against disseminated tumor in the brain, in *Astrocytomas: Diagnosis, Treatment and Biology* (Black P. McL., Schoene W.C., Lampson L.A., eds.) Blackwell Scientific, pp. 261–289.

66. Lampson L.A. 1995. Interpreting MHC class I expression and class I/class II reciprocity in the CNS: Reconciling divergent findings. *Micros. Res. Tech.* **32:** 267–285.

67. Lampson L.A. 1997. Immunobiology of brain tumors: Antigens, effectors, and delivery to sites of microscopic tumor in the brain, in *Cancer of the Nervous System* (Black P. McL., Loeffler J.S., eds.), Blackwell, pp. 874–906.

68. Lampson L.A. 1998. Beyond Inflammation: Site-directed Immunotherapy. *Immunol. Today* **19:**17–22.

69. Lampson L.A. 2001. New animal models to probe brain tumor biology, therapy, and immunotherapy: advantages and remaining concerns. *J. Neuro-Oncol.* **53:** 275–287.

70. Lampson L.A. 2002. Basic Principles of CNS immunology, in *Youman's Neurological Survey, 5th ed.*, (Winn H.R., ed.), Saunders, W.B., in press.

71. Lampson, L.A., A. Chen, A.O. Vortmeyer, A.E. Sloan, Z. Ghogawala, L. Kim. 1994. Enhanced T cell migration to sites of microscopic CNS disease: Complementary treatments evaluated by 2- and 3-D image analysis. *Brain Pathol.* **4:**125–134.

72. Lampson L.A., Hickey W.F. 1986. Monoclonal antibody analysis of MHC expression in human brain biopsies: Tissue ranging from "histologically normal" to that showing different levels of glial tumor involvement. *J. Immunol.* **136:** 4054–4062.

73. Lampson L.A., Kushner P.D., Sobel R.A. 1990. Major histocompatibility antigen expression in the affected tissues in amyotrophic lateral sclerosis. *Ann. Neurol.* **28:**365–372.

74. Lampson L.A., Lampson M.A., Dunne A.D. 1993. Exploiting lacZ reporter gene for quantitative analysis of disseminated tumor growth in the brain: Use of lacZ gene product as tumor antigen, to evaluate antigenic modulation, and to facilitate image analysis. *Cancer Res.* **53:**176–182.

75. Lampson L.A., Levy R. 1979. A role for clonal antigens in cancer diagnosis and therapy. *J. Natl. Cancer Inst.* **62:**217–219.

76. Lampson L.A., Wen P., Roman V.A., Morris J.H., Sarid J. 1992. Disseminating tumor cells and their interactions with leukocytes visualized in the brain. *Cancer Res.* **52:**1008–1025.

77. Lee S.H., Shin M.S., Park W.S., Kim S.Y., Dong S.M., Lee H.K, et al. 1999. Immunohistochemical analysis of Fas ligand expression in normal human tissues. *APMIS* **107:**1013–1019.

78. Lenardo M., Chan K.M., Hornung F., McFarland H., Siegel R., Wang, J., Zheng L. 1999. Mature T lymphocyte apoptosis— immune regulation in a dynamic and unpredictable antigenic environment. *Annu. Rev. Immunol.* **17:**221–253.

79. Loeffler J.S., Alexander III E., Hochberg F.H., et. al. 1990. Clinical patterns of failure following stereotactic interstitial irradiation for malignant gliomas. *Int. J. Radiat. Oncol. Biol. Phys.* **19:**1455–1462.

80. Luettig B., Kaiser M., Bode U., Bell E.B., Sparshott S.M., Bette M., Westermann J. 2001. Naive and memory T cells migrate in comparable numbers through the normal rat lung: only effector T cells accumulate and proliferate in the lamina propria of the bronchi. *Am. J. Respir. Cell Mol. Biol.* **25:**69–77.

81. Manjunath N., Shankar P., Wan J., Weninger W., Crowley M.A., Hieshima K., et al. 2001. Effector differentiation is not prerequisite for generation of memory cytotoxic T lymphocytes. *J. Clin. Invest.* **108:**871–878.

82. Marrack P., Bender J., Hildeman D., Jordan M., Mitchell T., Murakami M., et al. 2000. Homeostasis of alpha beta TCR+ T cells. *Nat. Immunol.* **1:**107–111.

83. Martin F.C., Anton P.A., Gornbein J.A., Shanahan F., Merrill J.E. 1993. Production of interleukin-1 by microglia in response to substance P: role for a non-classical NK-1 receptor. *J. Neuroimmunol.* **42:**53–60.

84. Matyszak M.K.,Denis-Donini S.,Citterio S.,Longhi R., Granucci P., Ricciardi-Castagnoli F. 1999. Microglia induce myelin basic protein-specific T cell anergy or T cell activation, according to their state of activation. *Eur. J. Immunol.* **29:**3063–76.

85. McCluskey L.P., Lampson L.A. 2000. Local neurochemicals and site-specific immune regulation in the CNS. *J. Neuropathol. Exp. Neurol.* **59:**177–187.

86. McCluskey LP., Lampson L.A. 2001. Local immune regulation in the central nervous system by substance P vs. glutamate. *J. Neuroimmunol.* **116:**136–146.

87. McVicar D.W., Davis D.F., Merchant R.E. 1992. In vitro analysis of the proliferative potential of T cells from patients with brain tumor: glioma-associated immunosuppression unrelated to intrinsic cellular defect. *J. Neurosurg.* **76:**251–260.

88. Meeson A.P., Piddlesden S., Morgan B.P., et al. 1994. The distribution of inflammatory demyelinated lesions in the central nervous system of rats with antibody-augumented demyelinating experimental allergic encephalomyelitis. *Exp. Neurol.* **129:**299–310.

89. Moalem G., Leibowitz-Amit R., Yoles E., et al. 1999. Autoimmune T cells protect neurons from secondary degeneration after central nervous system axotomy. *Nature Med.* **5:**49–55.

90. Morford L.A., Elliott L.H., Carlson S.L., et al. 1997. T cell receptor-mediated signaling is defective in T cells obtained from patients with primary intracranial tumors. *J. Immunol.* **159:**4415–4425.

91. Moskophidis D., Lohler J., Lehmann-Grube F. 1987. Antiviral antibody-producing cells in parenchymatous organs during persistent virus infection. *J. Exp. Med.* **165:**705–719.

92. Nakagawa K., Aoki Y., Fujimaki T., Tago M., Terahara A., Karasawa K., et al. 1998. High-dose conformal radiotherapy influenced the pattern of failure but did not improve survival in glioblastoma multiforme. *Int. J. Radiat. Oncol. Biol. Phys.* **40:**1141–1149.

93. Navarrete C.V. 2000. The HLA system in blood transfusion. *Baillieres Best Pract. Res. Clin. Haematol.* **13:**511–532.

94. North R.J., Awwad M., Dunn P.L. 1989. The immune response to tumors. *Transplant. Proc.* **21:**575–577.

95. O'Connell J., Bennett M.W., O'Sullivan G.C., Collins J.K., Shanahan F. 1999. The Fas counterattack: cancer as a site of immune privilege. *Immunol. Today* **20:**46–52.

96. Offringa R., van der Burg S.H., Ossendorp F., Toes R.E., Melief C.J. 2000. Design and evaluation of antigen-specific vaccination strategies against cancer. *Curr. Opin. Immunol.* **12:**576–582.

97. Pamer E., Cresswell P. 1998. Mechanisms of MHC class I-restricted antigen processing. *Annu. Rev. Immunol.* **16:** 323–358.

98. Pardoll D.M. 1994. Tumour antigens. A new look for the 1990's. *Nature* **369:**357–358.

99. Parmiani, G. 2001. Melanoma antigens and their recognition by T cells. *Keio J. Med.* **50:**86–90.

100. Paul W.E. 1999. *Fundamental Immunology* 4th ed., Lippincott-Raven, Philadelphia, PA. pp. 1021–1049.

101. Pawelec G., Heinzel S., Kiessling R., Muller L., Ouyang Q., Zeuthen J. 2000. Escape mechanisms in tumor immunity: a year 2000 update. *Crit. Rev. Oncog.* **11:**97–133.

102. Phillips L.M., Lampson L.A. 1999. Site-specific control of T cell traffic in the brain: T cell entry to brain stem vs. hippocampus after local injection of IFN-γ. *J. Neuroimmunol.* **96:**218–227.

103. Phillips L.M., Simon P., Lampson L.A. 1999. Site-specific immune regulation in the brain: differential modulation of MHC proteins in brainstem vs. hippocampus. *J. Comp. Neurol.* **405:**322–333.

104. Pilling D., Akbar A.N., Shamsadeen N., Scheel-Toellner D., Buckley C., Salmon M. 2000. High cell density provides potent survival signals for resting T-cells. *Cell. Mol. Biol.* **46:**163–74.

105. Prineas J.W., Wright R.G. 1978. Macrophages, lymphocytes, and plasma cells in the perivascular compartment in chronic multiple sclerosis. *Lab. Invest.* **38:**409–421.

106. Saas P., Walker P.R., Hahne M., Quiquerez A.L., Schnuriger V., Perrin G., et al. 1997. Fas ligand expression by astrocytoma in vivo: maintaining immune privilege in the brain? *J. Clin. Invest.* **99:**1173–1178.

107. Sallusto F., Lenig D., Forster R., Lipp M, Lanzavecchia A. 1999. Two subsets of memory T lymphocytes with distinct homing potentials and effector functions. *Nature* **401:**708–712.

108. Santini J.T., Cima M.J., Langer R. 1999. A controlled release microchip. *Nature* **397:** 335–338.

109. Schleuning M. 2000. Adoptive allogeneic immunotherapy—history and future perspectives. *Transfus.Sci.* **23:**133–150.

110. Schmied M., Breitschopf H., Gold R., Zischler H., Rothe G., Wekerle H., Lassmann H. 1993. Apoptosis of T lymphocytes in experimental autoimmune encephalomyelitis. Evidence for programmed cell death as a mechanism to control inflammation in the brain. *Am. J. Pathol.* **143:**446–452.

111. Schreiber H., Wu T.H., Nachman J., Rowley D.A. 2000. Immunological enhancement of primary tumor development and its prevention. *Semin. Cancer Biol.* **10:**351–357.

112. Seabrook T.J., Lampson L.A. 2002. IFN-γ increases the entry of T cells at micro-tumors in a rat model of brainstem glioma. AAI Annual Mtg, New Orleans, MI.

113. Sedgwick J.D., Ford A.L., Foulcher E., Airriess R. 1998. Central nervous system microglial cell activation and proliferation follows direct interaction with tissue-infiltrating T cell blasts. *J. Immunol.* **160:**5320–5330.

114. Sercarz E.E. 1986. Hierarchies of epitope preference and the problem of Ir gene control. *Concepts Immunopathol.* **3:** 61–73.

115. Sethna M.P., Lampson L.A. 1991. Immune modulation within the brain: Recruitment of inflammatory cells and increased major histocompatibility antigen expression following intracerebral injection of IFN-γ. *J. Neuroimmunol.* **34:**121–132.

116. Siegel R. M., Chan F.K., Chun H.J., Lenardo M.J. 2000. The multifaceted role of Fas signaling in immune cell homeostasis and autoimmunity. *Nat. Immunol.* **1:**469–474.

117. Silverstein A.M., Rose N.R. 2000. There is only one immune system! The view from immunopathology. *Semin. Immunol.* **12:** 173–178.

118. Sotomayor E.M., Borrello I., Levitsky H.I. 1996. Tolerance and cancer: a critical issue in tumor immunology. *Crit. Rev. Oncog.* **7:** 433–456.

119. Stauss H.J. 2001. Benign autoimmunity to combat malignancy. *Clin. Exp. Immunol.* **125:**1–2.

120. Stefferl A., Brehm U., Storch M., Lambracht-Washington D., Bourquin C., Wonigeit K., et al. 1999. Myelin oligodendrocyte glycoprotein induces experimental autoimmune encephalomyelitis in the "resistant" Brown Norway rat: disease susceptibility is determined by MHC and MHC-linked effects on the B cell response. *J. Immunol.* **163:**40–49.

121. Streilein J.W. 1999. Immunoregulatory mechanisms of the eye. *Prog. Retin. Eye Res.* **18:**357–370.

122. Streilein J.W., Stein-Streilein J. 2000. Does innate immune privilege exist? *J. Leukoc. Biol.* **67:**479–487.

123. Surh C. D., Sprent J. 2000. Homeostatic T cell proliferation: how far can T cells be activated to self-ligands? *J. Exp. Med.* **192:**F9–F14.

124. Syrengelas A. D., Levy R. 1999. DNA vaccination against the idiotype of a murine B cell lymphoma: mechanism of tumor protection. *J. Immunol.* **162:**4790–4795.

125. Tait B.D. 2000. HLA class I expression on human cancer cells. Implications for effective immunotherapy. *Hum. Immunol.* **61:**158–165.

126. Tanchot C., Fernandes H.V., Rocha B. 2000. The organization of mature T-cell pools. *Philos.Trans. R. Soc. Lond. B Biol.Sci.* **355:**323–328.

127. Tepper R.I., Coffman R.L., Leder P. 1992. An eosinophil-dependent mechanism for the antitumor effect of interleukin-4. *Science.* **257:**548–551.

128. Todo T., Rabkin S.D., Sundaresan P., Wu A., Meehan K.R., Herscowitz H.B., Martuza R.L. 1999. Systemic antitumor immunity in experimental brain tumor therapy using a multimutated, replication-competent herpes simplex virus. *Hum. Gene Ther.* **10:**2741–2755.

129. Tran E. H., Hoekstra K., van Rooijen N., Dijkstra C.D., Owens T. 1998. Immune invasion of the central nervous system parenchyma and experimental allergic encephalomyelitis, but not leukocyte extravasation from blood, are prevented in macrophage-depleted mice. *J. Immunol.* **161:**3767–3775.

130. Turner W.J.D., Chatten J., Lampson L.A. 1990. Human neuroblastoma cell growth in xenogeneic hosts: Comparison of T cell-deficient and NK-deficient hosts, and subcutaneous or intravenous injection routes. *J. Neuro-Oncol.* **8:**121–132.

131. Tyor W.R., Wesselingh S., Levine B., Griffin D.E. 1992. Long term intraparenchymal Ig secretion after acute viral encephalitis in mice. *J. Immunol.* **149:**4016–4020.

132. Uhrbom L., Holland E.C. 2002. Modeling gliomagenesis with somatic cell gene transfer using retroviral vectors. *J. Neuro-Oncol.* **53:**297–330.

133. Upham J.W., Strickland D.H., Robinson B.W., Holt P.G. 1997. Selective inhibition of T cell proliferation but not expression of effector function by human alveolar macrophages. *Thorax* **52:**786–795.

134. Vajkoczy P., Menger M.D. 2000. Vascular microenvironment in gliomas. *J. Neuro-Oncol.* **50:**99–108.

135. Vales-Gomez M., Reyburn H., Strominger J. 2000. Molecular analyses of the interactions between human NK receptors and their HLA ligands. *Hum. Immunol.* **61:**28–38.

136. Valtschanoff J.G., Weinberg R.J., Kharazia V.N. 1993. Neurons in rat hippocampus that synthesize nitric oxide. *J. Comp. Neurol.* **331:**111–121.

137. Vanderlugt C.L., Begolka W.S., Neville K.L., et al. 1998. The functional significance of epitope spreading and its regulation by co-stimulatory molecules. *Immunol. Rev.* **164:**63–72.

138. Vierboom M., Nijman H.W., Offringa R., et al. 1997. Tumor eradication by wild-type p53-specific cytotoxic T lymphocytes. *J. Exp. Med.* **186:**695–704.

139. von Andrian U.H., Mackay C.R. 2000. T-cell function and migration. Two sides of the same coin. *N. Engl. J. Med.* **343:**1020–1034.

140. Voskuhl R.R., Farris R.W., Nagasato K., McFarland H.F., Dalcq M.D. 1996. Epitope spreading occurs in active but not passive EAE induced by myelin basic protein. *J. Neuroimmunol.* **70:**103–111.

141. Weiner L.M., Adams G.P. 2000. New approaches to antibody therapy. *Oncogene* **19:**6144–6151.

142. Wen P., Lampson M.A., Lampson L.A. 1992. Effects of gamma interferon on major histocompatibility complex expression and lymphocytic infiltration in the 9L gliosarcoma brain tumor model: Implications for strategies of immunotherapy. *J. Neuroimmunol.* **36:**57–68.

143. Williams T.M. 2001. Human leukocyte antigen gene polymorphism and the histocompatibility laboratory. *J. Mol. Diagn.* **3:**98–104.

144. Williamson R.A., Burgoon M.P., Owens G.P., Ghausi O., Leclerc E., Firme L., et al. 2001. Anti-DNA antibodies are a major component of the intrathecal B cell response in multiple sclerosis. *Proc. Natl. Acad. Sci. USA* **98:**1793–1798.

145. Yang B.C., Wang Y.S., Liu H.S., Lin S.J. 2000. Ras signaling is involved in the expression of Fas-L in glioma. *Lab. Invest.* **80:**529–537.

146. Yeomans D., Proudfit H. 1992. Antinociception induced by microinjection of substance P into the A7 catecholamine cell group in the rat. *Neuroscience* **49:**681–691.

147. Zanelli E., Breedveld F.C, de Vries R.R. 2000. HLA association with autoimmune disease: a failure to protect? *Rheumatology* **39:**1060–1066.

148. Zinkernagel R.M. 2001. Immunity against solid tumors? *Int. J. Cancer* **93:**1–5.

149. Zou J.P., Shimizu J, Ikegame K., et al. 1992. Tumor-bearing mice exhibit a progressive increase in tumor antigen-presenting cell function and a reciprocal decrease in tumor antigen-responsive CD4+ T cell activity. *J. Immunol.* **148:**648–655.

10

Genetic Pathways in the Evolution of Gliomas

Hiroko Ohgaki and Paul Kleihues

During the past decade, a wealth of data has accumulated on somatic mutations in human gliomas. These include, as in tumors of other organs, amplification and overexpression of oncogenes and inactivation of tumor-suppressor genes. These genetic alterations do not occur randomly, but in patterns and combinations that correspond to clinically and histopathologically defined entities. For some gliomas, in particular those of oligodendroglial lineage, genetic profiling appears to be more precise than histological typing for prediction of response to chemotherapy and clinical outcome.

1. ASTROCYTIC TUMORS

Tumors of astrocytic origin are divided into two different types: 1) the pilocytic astrocytoma of children and adolescents, and 2) the diffuse astrocytomas that manifest predominantly in adults. These neoplasms differ with respect to location, age distribution, biological behavior, and genetic alterations. This chapterfocuses on diffuse astrocytomasthat share the following characteristics: they may arise at any site in the central nervous system (CNS), preferentially in the cerebral hemispheres of adults; have a wide range of histopathological features and biological behavior, diffusely infiltrating adjacent and distant brain structures, largely irrespective of histological grade; and have an inherent tendency to progress to a more malignant phenotype *(18)*. The most malignant endpoint in this progression is the glioblastoma. Rather than dealing with low-grade and anaplastic astrocytomas separately, they are dealt with in the context of the genetic pathway to secondary glioblastoma.

1.1. Primary and Secondary Glioblastoma

Glioblastomas (World Health Organization [WHO] grade IV) are the most frequent and malignant human brain tumors, accounting for 12–15% of all intracranial neoplasms and 50–60% of all astrocytic tumors *(45)*. The majority of glioblastomas develop very rapidly without clinical, radiological, or morphological evidence of a less malignant precursor lesion. These glioblastomas are termed primary or *de novo* glioblastomas. Patients with primary glioblastoma have a short clinical history (less than 3 mo in most cases), and typically present with large tumors which on magnetic resonance imaging (MRI) show central necrosis and extensive perifocal edema. This terminology refers to the lack of an identifiable precursor lesion rather than to the assumption that this lesion results from a single-step malignant transformation.

Other glioblastomas develop slowly through progression from low-grade diffuse astrocytoma (WHO grade II) or anaplastic astrocytoma (WHO grade III) and are termed secondary glioblastomas. Although this is a commonplace experience in the clinical setting, the designations primary and secondary glioblastoma have been conceptual, rather than being used as diagnostic terms, mainly because both glioblastoma types share similar histological features *(12,98,100)*. This has also made it difficult to estimate the relative frequency at which both subsets of glioblastoma occur, but it is

From: *Contemporary Cancer Research: Brain Tumors*
Edited by: F. Ali-Osman © Humana Press Inc., Totowa, NJ

undisputed that the primary glioblastoma is the prevailing type and probably accounts for more than 80% of glioblastoma cases *(22)*.

Data on the survival of patients with primary and secondary glioblastomas are still scarce. Scherer *(100)* stated that a more favorable clinical outcome is one of the characteristics of the secondary glioblastoma, and this is supported by a study of 188 glioblastoma cases, in which patients with prior low-grade glioma had significantly longer survival, the median survival being 40.5 mo *(132)*. In contrast, a recent clinical epidemiology study showed no significant difference in prognosis *(22)*. A recent population-based study on the survival of glioma patients in the Canton of Zürich, Switzerland, showed similar survival rates for patients with primary and secondary glioblastomas *(15)*.

1.2. Age and Sex Distribution

Primary glioblastomas tend to develop in older patients (mean, 55–60 yr), whereas secondary glioblastomas are typically diagnosed at around age 40 yr *(22,125)* (Fig. 1). The male/female ratio tends to be higher for primary than secondary glioblastomas *(122,125)*, and this is consistent with the finding in unselected series of glioblastomas that lesions with *TP53* mutations occur more frequently in women and in younger patients *(57,86,122)*.

1.3. Dynamics of Astrocytoma Progression

Low-grade diffuse astrocytomas are well differentiated tumors that typically develop in young adults. They grow slowly, diffusely infiltrate the surrounding normal brain, and show an intrinsic tendency to progress to more malignant histological types, i.e., anaplastic astrocytoma and, eventually, glioblastoma (secondary glioblastoma) *(94)*. The time course of progression from low-grade astrocytoma to glioblastoma varies considerably, with intervals ranging from less than 1 yr to more than 10 yr *(79)*. The mean time for progression from low-grade astrocytoma is approx 4–5 yr *(126)*. Anaplastic astrocytoma is considered a lesion of intermediate malignancy in the progression of low-grade astrocytomas to glioblastoma. However, an alternative pathway circumventing the anaplastic astrocytoma has also been proposed *(115)*.

1.4. Genetic Alterations

We have carried out genetic analyses of glioblastomas that were selected on the basis of stringent criteria *(7,8,28,67–70,96,112,125)*. A short clinical history and the presence of the histological features of a full-blown glioblastoma at the first biopsy are essential criteria for the diagnosis of a primary glioblastoma. Conversely, the definition of secondary glioblastoma requires clinical (neuro-imaging) and/or histological evidence of evolution from a less malignant precursor lesion, i.e., low-grade or anaplastic astrocytoma. In our study, primary glioblastomas were included if the clinical history was less than 3 mo and histopathological features of glioblastoma were present at the first biopsy. The possibility exists that primary glioblastomas may have a significantly longer preoperative history, but in order to clearly distinguish between the two subsets, the window of eligibility was deliberately kept small. The diagnosis of secondary glioblastoma required at least two biopsies taken at an interval of more than 6 mo, to avoid sampling error, and clinical as well as histopathological evidence of progression from low-grade or anaplastic astrocytoma.

1.4.1. TP53/MDM2/p14^{ARF} Pathway

Dysregulation of the $G_1 \rightarrow S$ cell-cycle checkpoint is one of the most important mechanisms in the carcinogenic process. The *TP53* tumor-suppressor gene is a key regulator of the $G_1 \rightarrow S$ cell-cycle checkpoint, apoptosis, and DNA repair *(3,111)*. Following DNA damage, TP53 is activated and induces the transcription of a large number of genes, including *p21$^{Waf1/Cip1}$*, which is capable of silencing the cyclin-dependent kinases (CDKs) that are essential for $G_1 \rightarrow S$ transition *(3,103,117)*. MDM2 protein binds to TP53 and induces degradation and transactivational silencing of TP53 *(64,80)*. p14^{ARF} acts by binding directly to MDM2, resulting in stabilization of both TP53 and MDM2 *(42,82,109,134)*.

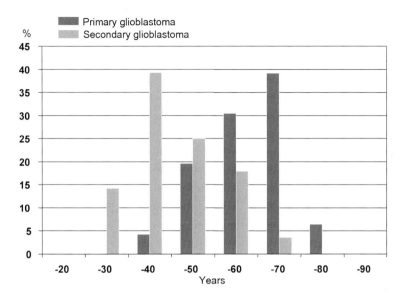

Fig. 1. Age distribution of patients with primary and secondary glioblastomas. Primary glioblastomas develop in older patients (mean age, 58.7 + 1.4 yr), whereas secondary glioblastomas occur in younger patients (mean age, 40.6 + 2.2 yr). Data are based on 46 primary glioblastomas and 28 secondary glioblastomas used for genetic analyses in our laboratory.

Thus, inactivation of the *TP53* pathway may result from *TP53* mutation, *MDM2* amplification, or loss of *p14^{ARF}* expression.

TP53 mutations were among the first genetic alterations identified in astrocytic brain tumors *(73)*. In unselected series of glioblastomas, the reported frequency varies considerably, with a mean of 25–30% *(55,78)*. A different picture emerges if primary and secondary glioblastomas are analyzed separately. *TP53* mutations are rare in primary glioblastomas (<10%), whereas secondary glioblastomas have a high incidence of *TP53* mutations (>65%), of which approx 90% are already present in the first biopsy *(124,125)*. Accumulation of *TP53* protein is more frequently observed than *TP53* mutations *(50,57,72,124)*, but is also significantly more common in secondary (>90%) than in primary glioblastomas (<35%) *(125)*. The percentage of glioma cells with TP53 protein accumulation appears to increase from the first biopsy to recurrent tumors *(93,124)*. The time till progression to anaplastic astrocytoma or glioblastoma was somewhat shorter for low-grade astrocytomas carrying a *TP53* mutation *(124)*. Progression of low-grade astrocytoma to anaplastic astrocytoma or glioblastoma appears to occur at a similar frequency in lesions with (79%) and without (63%) *TP53* mutations, indicating that this genetic alteration is associated with tumor recurrence but is not predictive of progression to a more malignant phenotype *(124)*.

Amplification of *MDM2* is present in less than 10% of glioblastomas *(91)* and these all appear to be primary glioblastomas that lack a TP53 mutation *(7,91)*. Overexpression of MDM2 was observed immunohistochemically in more than 50% of primary glioblastomas *(7,48,71)*. In contrast, less than 10% of secondary glioblastomas showed MDM2 overexpression. Thus, MDM2 overexpression with or without gene amplification is a genetic hallmark of the primary glioblastoma that typically lacks a *TP53* mutation. The majority of glioblastomas (approx 70%) contain short forms of alternatively spliced *MDM2* transcripts that lack a region including the TP53 binding domain *(61)*.

Loss of *p14^{ARF}* expression was observed in the majority of glioblastomas (76%), and this correlated with the gene status, i.e., homozygous deletion or promoter methylation *(67)*. There was no significant difference in the overall frequency of *p14^{ARF}* alterations between primary and secondary glioblastomas, but there was a tendency toward more frequent *p14^{ARF}* methylation in secondary glioblastomas than in primary glioblastomas *(67)*. The analysis of multiple biopsies from the same patients revealed methylation of p14^{ARF} even in one-third of low-grade astrocytomas *(67)*.

1.4.2. p16^{INK4a}/CDK4/RB1 Pathway

p16^{INK4a} binds to CDK4 and inhibits the CDK4/cyclin D1 complex *(37,102,103)*. This complex phosphorylates RB1 protein (pRb), thereby inducing the release of the E2F transcript factor that activates genes involved in the late G$_1$ and S phases *(37,102,103)*. The *p15^{INK4b}* gene on the *CDKN2B* locus of chromosome 9p21 is structurally highly homologous to *p16^{INK4a}* *(31)*. Like p16^{INK4a}, p15^{INK4b} binds to CDK4 and CDK6, resulting in inhibition of the RB1-mediated G$_1$→S transition *(31,102)*. Disruption of the RB1 pathway, with subsequent dysregulation of progression into S phase, may therefore be caused by loss of p16^{INK4a}/p15^{INK4b} expression, *CDK4* amplification, or loss of pRb expression.

Homozygous *p16^{INK4a}* deletions were more frequent in primary than in secondary glioblastomas *(8,67)*, and the majority of glioblastomas with *EGFR* amplification show a *p16^{INK4a}* deletion *(32)*. However, there was no significant difference in the overall frequency of *p16^{INK4a}* alterations (homozygous deletion and promoter methylation) between primary and secondary glioblastomas *(67)*.

Sequencing of all 27 exons of the *RB1* gene has revealed inactivating mutations in 5–12% of unselected glioblastomas *(33,39,40,114)*. Like *RB1* mutations in retinoblastomas *(34)*, most *RB1* mutations in glioblastomas result in a truncated pRB protein *(33,114)* that does not enter the nucleus. Homozygous deletions in the *RB1* locus have been reported in a small fraction of glioblastomas (3/120, 3%) *(40)*. Loss of *RB1* expression was detected by immunohistochemistry in 5–27% of glioblastomas *(8,16,33,114)*. There was a clear correlation between loss of *RB1* expression and promoter methylation of the *RB1* gene, suggesting that promoter methylation is the major mechanism underlying loss of *RB1* expression in glioblastomas *(70)*. Promoter methylation was found significantly more frequently in secondary (43%) than in primary glioblastomas (14%). In patients with multiple biopsies, methylation of the *RB1* promoter was not detectable in low-grade diffuse and anaplastic astrocytoma, indicating that loss of *RB1* expression as a result of promoter methylation is a late event during astrocytoma progression *(70)*.

In unselected and selected series of glioblastomas, *p16^{INK4a}* deletion and *RB1* alterations were found to be mutually exclusive *(8,16,114)*.

Epidermal growth factor receptor *(EGFR)* gene is involved in control of cell proliferation and is amplified and overexpressed in more than one-third of glioblastomas, sometimes in a truncated and rearranged form *(18,24,53,66,133)*. The most common alteration is a deletion of exons 2–7 from the extracellular domain, resulting in a truncated mutant receptor *(24,74,110,133)*. This mutant EGFR confers enhanced tumorigenicity on human glioblastoma cells by increasing proliferation and reducing apoptosis *(65)*, apparently through the *Ras-Shc-Grb2* pathway *(83)*. Glioblastomas with *EGFR* amplification typically show simultaneous loss of chromosome 10 *(119)*. In unselected series of glioblastomas, *EGFR* amplification has been reported to occur at a frequency of approx 30–40% *(56,78)*. In a study in our laboratory, *EGFR* amplification was present in approx 40% of primary glioblastomas but in none of the secondary glioblastomas analyzed *(112)*. EGFR immunoreactivity was also much more frequent in primary glioblastomas (> 60%) than in secondary glioblastomas (<10%) *(125)*. All primary glioblastomas with *EGFR* amplification showed *EGFR* overexpression, and 11 of 15 (73%) of those with *EGFR* overexpression showed *EGFR* amplification *(112)*.

1.4.3. LOH no. 10 and the PTEN Tumor-Suppressor Gene

The majority of glioblastomas appear to have lost an entire copy of chromosome 10 *(29,41,58, 85,116)*. In glioblastomas with partial LOH no. 10, at least three common deletions have been identified, i.e., 10p14-pter *(41,43,44,47,107,116)*, 10q23-24 *(1,29,41,43,58,85,107)*, and 10q25-qter

(1,29,41,43,58,85,107), suggesting the presence of several tumor-suppressor genes. LOH no. 10 has been detected at similar frequencies in primary (47%) and secondary glioblastomas (54%) *(28)*. The majority (88%) of primary glioblastomas with LOH no. 10 showed LOH at all informative markers, suggesting loss of the entire chromosome 10, whereas secondary glioblastomas with LOH no. 10 showed partial or complete loss of chromosome 10q but no loss of 10p *(28)*.

The *PTEN* tumor-suppressor gene on chromosome 10q23.3 *(52,108)* is mutated in approx 30% of unselected glioblastomas *(10,23,87,123)*. Our study shows that *PTEN* mutations occur almost exclusively in primary glioblastomas (32%) and rarely (4%) in secondary glioblastomas *(112)*. *TP53* and *PTEN* mutations in glioblastomas were mutually exclusive in selected and unselected glioblastomas *(87,112)*.

1.4.4. LOH 1p

LOH on chromosome 1p has also been found in approx 25% of low-grade diffuse astrocytomas, approx 20% of anaplastic astrocytomas, and approx 10% of glioblastomas *(4,49,59,118)*. Recent mappings have narrowed down the common deletion on chromosome 1p to the 1p36.3 and 1p34-35 regions *(38,104)*, but tumor-suppressor genes at these loci have not yet been identified. LOH no. 1q was detected in 12% of primary and 15% of secondary glioblastomas *(69)*.

1.4.5. LOH 19q

LOH on chromosome 19q occurs in approx 40% of anaplastic astrocytomas and approx 20% of unselected glioblastomas *(120,121)*. LOH on chromosome 19q has frequently been found in secondary glioblastomas (54%) but rarely in primary glioblastomas (6%) *(69)*. The common deletion was located at 19q13.3. These results suggest that tumor-suppressor gene(s) located on chromosome 19q are frequently involved in the progression from low-grade astrocytoma to secondary glioblastoma, but do not play a major role in the evolution of primary glioblastomas.

1.4.6. LOH 13q

LOH on chromosome 13q has been found in 25–45% of unselected glioblastomas *(16,33,40,114)*. LOH on 13q was detected in 12% of primary and 38% of secondary glioblastomas, and typically included the *RB1* locus *(69)*. The fact that LOH on 13q and on 19q is largely mutually exclusive in glioblastomas suggests that tumor-suppressor genes on 13q and 19q may be functionally related *(69)*.

O^6-Alkylguanine-DNA alkyltransferase (MGMT) is a repair protein that specifically removes promutagenic alkyl groups from the O^6 position of guanine in DNA. Therefore, MGMT protects cells against carcinogenesis induced by alkylating agents, and it has been reported that MGMT activity is inversely correlated with tissue-specific tumorigenesis induced by alkylating agents in rats *(30,60)*. In tumor cells, repair of O^6-alkylguanine adducts by tumor cells has been implicated in drug resistance, because it reduces the cytotoxicity of alkylating chemotherapeutic agents. Loss of *MGMT* expression is caused by methylation of promoter CpG islands *(84,131)* and has been observed in a variety of human cancers, including gliomas *(25)*. *MGMT* methylation was detected in 75% of secondary glioblastomas, significantly more than in primary glioblastomas (36%) *(68)*. Approximately 50% of low-grade astrocytomas already showed *MGMT* methylation, and this was significantly associated with the presence of *TP53* mutations, in particular G:C→A:T mutations at CpG sites *(68)*.

1.4.7. Genetic Pathways

The genetic pathways leading to the evolution of primary and secondary glioblastoma are shown in Fig. 2. Despite some overlap, the pathogenesis of these two subtypes of glioblastomas is quite different, suggesting that they constitute different diseases, on the basis of both their clinical and genetic profiles. It should, however, be noted that these data were generated mostly from cohorts of patients carefully selected on the basis of clinical history and, in the case of secondary glioblastoma, multiple biopsies in the same patient. Although glioblastoma biopsies from patients with histologi-

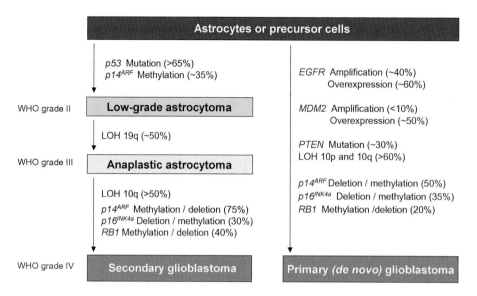

Fig. 2. Genetic pathways leading to primary and secondary glioblastomas.

cally proven progression from low-grade astrocytoma typically contain a *TP53* mutation, this does not allow the conclusion that *all* glioblastomas with a *TP53* mutation have progressed from a prior low-grade glioma. Similarly, primary glioblastomas with a very short clinical history typically contain *EGFR* amplification/overexpression and LOH on the entire chromosome 10, but data are not available showing that *all* glioblastomas with these genetic alteration developed *de novo*. More subtypes of glioblastoma exist with intermediate clinical and genetic profiles. This is exemplified by rare glioblastoma subtypes, the gliosarcoma, and giant cell glioblastoma.

Gliosarcomas comprise approx 2% of all glioblastomas *(75)* and are characterized by a biphasic tissue pattern with areas displaying glial and mesenchymal differentiation *(75)*. Gliosarcomas are clinically and genetically close to primary glioblastomas, except for the absence of *EGFR* amplification *(75,95)* (Table 1). Analyses in gliomatous and sarcomatous components showed identical genetic alterations, including *TP53* and *PTEN* mutations, *p16INK4a* deletions and co-amplification of *MDM2* and *CDK4* in both tumor areas *(6,95)*. This strongly supports the concept of a monoclonal origin of gliosarcomas and evolution of the sarcomatous component as a result of aberrant mesenchymal differentiation in a highly malignant astrocytic neoplasm.

Giant-cell glioblastomas are characterized by a predominance of bizarre (monstrous) multinucleated giant cells and, on occasion, an abundant stromal reticulin network *(77)*. This glioblastoma variant accounts for less than 1% of all brain tumors and up to 5% of glioblastomas *(77)*. Giant-cell glioblastoma develops clinically *de novo* after a short clinical history and tends to be macroscopically well delineated with a somewhat better prognosis than the ordinary glioblastoma. It frequently contains *TP53* mutations (75–90%) *(62,77,81)* and *PTEN* mutations (approx 30%), but rarely shows *p16INK4a* homozygous deletion, *EGFR* amplification, or *MDM2* amplification. Thus, giant-cell glioblastomas occupy a hybrid position, sharing with primary glioblastomas a short clinical history, the absence of a less malignant precursor lesion, and frequent *PTEN* mutations. With secondary glioblastomas, they have in common a younger patient age at manifestation and a high frequency (>70%) of *TP53* mutations (Table 1).

Table 1
Genetic Profiles of Glioblastoma Subtypes

	Primary glioblastoma	Gliosarcoma	Giant cell glioblastoma	Secondary glioblastoma
Clinical onset	*de novo*	*de novo*	*de novo*	Secondary
Preoperative history	1.7 mo	2 mo	1.6 mo	>25 m
M/F ratio	1.4	1.4	1.7	0.8
Age at diagnosis	59 yr	56 yr	42 yr	41 yr
PTEN mutation	30%	37%	33%	5%
p16^{INK4a} deletion	36%	37%	0%	4%
TP53 mutation	11%	26%	78%	67%
MDM2 amplification	7%	5%	0%	0%
EGFR amplification	39%	0%	6%	0%

1.5. Phenotype vs Genotype Correlation in Primary and Secondary Glioblastomas

Since primary and secondary glioblastomas are usually histologically indistinguishable, at least one genetic alteration should be common, if the phenotype is a reflection of genotype. Neuro-pathologists occasionally observe an abrupt transition from low-grade or anaplastic astrocytoma to glioblastoma, suggesting the emergence of a new tumor clone. We microdissected such glioblastoma foci and compared the chromosome 10 status with that of the respective low-grade or anaplastic astrocytoma areas of the same biopsy. In glioblastoma foci, deletions were typically detected distal from *PTEN* at 10q25-qter, covering the *DMBT1* and *FGFR2* loci *(27)*. This suggests that the acquisition of a highly malignant glioblastoma phenotype is associated with loss of a putative tumor-suppressor gene on 10q25-qter. The *DMBT1* gene on chromosome 10q25-26 has been considered a candidate tumor suppressor *(63)*. It is deleted in >50% of glioblastomas, i.e., at a frequency similar to that of LOH 10q *(63,106)*, but there has been no report so far that this gene is mutated in human neoplasms.

In one study, the majority (67%) of glioblastomas composed of small, densely packed tumor cells showed *EGFR* amplification, whereas 32% of glioblastomas with both small and nonsmall cell areas and only 9% of glioblastomas without small cell areas showed *EGFR* amplification. This suggests that *EGFR* amplification is associated with a small-cell glioblastoma phenotype and that small-cell glioblastomas constitute a major component of primary glioblastomas *(13)*.

The presence of necrosis is a histological hallmark of glioblastomas and is an essential criterion for distinguishing glioblastomas from anaplastic astrocytomas. Two types of necrosis are typically encountered in glioblastomas *(14,51)*. One consists of multiple small, irregularly shaped, band-like or serpiginous necrotic foci, surrounded by radially orientated, densely packed, small fusiform glioma cells in a "pseudopalisading" pattern. Pseudopalisading necrosis occurs at a similar frequency in primary and secondary glioblastomas *(113)*. The second type consists of large areas of geographic necrosis containing necrotic vessels and tumor cells. This type of necrosis is apparently a result of insufficient blood supply, and is therefore considered ischemic in nature *(51)*. Such large necrosis is observed in 100% of primary glioblastomas, but in only half of secondary glioblastomas *(113)*. This correlates well with reports indicating that the absence of necrosis is associated with a younger age of patients and a more favorable prognosis *(2,11)*. Expression of Fas/APO-1 (CD95), an apoptosis-mediating cell membrane protein, is predominantly observed in glioma cells surrounding large ischemic necrosis, and thus significantly more frequent in primary than in secondary glioblastomas, suggesting that these subtypes of glioblastoma differ in both the extent and mechanism of necrogenesis *(113)*.

1.6. Gene Expression Profiles

Use of cDNA microarrays has revealed significant changes in gene expression already at the stage of low-grade astrocytomas *(35,54,99)*. In unselected glioblastomas, up- or down-regulation in comparison to normal brain tissues was found in significantly larger numbers of genes in glioblastomas than in low-grade or anaplastic astrocytomas *(54,99)*. One study using an 11,000-gene microarray showed that approx 3000 genes were up-or down-regulated in glioblastomas in comparison to control tissues (corpus callosum) *(54)*. These cDNA array analyses led to the interesting observation that an α4 chain-containing laminin isoform, laminin-8 (α4β1γ1), was overexpressed mainly in blood vessel walls of glioblastomas, whereas another α4 chain-containing laminin isoform, laminin-9 (α4β2γ1), was expressed in low-grade astrocytomas and normal brain *(54)*. One study using array-based comparative genomic hybridization showed significant amplification of the *CDK4, GLI, MYCN, MYC, MDM2*, and *PDGFRA* genes in glioblastomas *(36)*. Another study using an oligonucleotide microarray showed that of approx 6800 genes that were analyzed, a set of 360 genes provided a molecular signature that distinguished between glioblastomas and pilocytic astrocytomas *(97)*.

2. OLIGODENDROGLIOMAS

Oligodendrogliomas account for approx 4% of all primary brain tumors and represent 5–18% of all gliomas. Oligodendroglioma WHO grade II is a well differentiated and diffusely infiltrating glioma manifesting in adults, that is composed predominantly of cells resembling oligodendroglia. Histologically, it is composed of tumor cells with rounded, homogeneous nuclei and on paraffin sections, a swollen, clear cytoplasm (honeycomb appearance). Microcalcifications, mucoid/cystic degeneration, and a chicken-wire vascular pattern are additional features of oligodendrogliomas. Anaplastic oligodendrogliomas WHO grade III show focal or diffuse histological features of malignancy, such as increased cellularity, marked nuclear atypia, and marked mitotic activity. Microvascular proliferation and necrosis may be present in anaplastic oligodendrogliomas.

2.1. Genetic Alterations

Oligodendrogliomas are genetically characterized by LOH on chromosomes 1p and 19q in up to 90% of cases *(5,9,49,59,90,92,104,118)*. LOH on 1p and 19q has been identified as a predictor of prolonged overall survival of patients with oligodendrogliomas (WHO grade II) *(105)*. *TP53* mutations occur in 5–15% of oligodendrogliomas *(9,59,76,118)* and approx 20% of oligodendrogliomas show *p14^{ARF}* methylation *(129)*.

Anaplastic oligodendrogliomas (WHO grade III) share with oligodendroglioma WHO grade II frequent LOH on 1p and 19q, and this is associated with sensitivity to PCV (procarbazine, CCNU, vincristine) chemotherapy and with longer survival of patients *(17)*. Anaplastic oligodendrogliomas in addition carry several genetic alterations, including LOH on chromosome 9p (20–50%), LOH on chromosome 10 (15–40%) and gain of chromosome 7 (10–40%) *(88)*. In anaplastic oligodendrogliomas, the RB1/CDK4/p16^{INK4a}/p15^{INK4b} pathway was disrupted in 13 of 20 (65%) cases, by either *RB1* alteration, *CDK4* amplification, or *p16^{INK4a}/p15^{INK4b}* homozygous deletion or promoter hypermethylation. Furthermore, 50% of anaplastic oligodendrogliomas showed alterations in the TP53 pathway through promoter hypermethylation or homozygous deletion of the *p14^{ARF}* gene and, less frequently, through *TP53* mutation or *MDM2* amplification. It was notable that concurrent disruption of the RB1/CDK4/p16^{INK4a}/p15^{INK4b} and the TP53/p14^{ARF}/MDM2 pathways occurs in 45% of anaplastic oligodendrogliomas *(128,129)*. A small fraction of anaplastic oligodendrogliomas show *EGFR* amplification, *MYC* amplification and *VEGF* overexpression *(88)*. The genetic pathway to oligodendrogliomas and anaplastic oligodendrogliomas is summarized in Fig. 3.

A recent study with hierarchical clustering of gene expression profiling using an oligonucleotide microarray showed distinct gene expression patterns in WHO grade II and III oligodendrogliomas *(130)*.

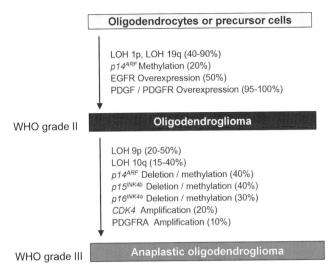

Fig. 3. Genetic pathways to oligodendrogliomas.

3. PHENOTYPE VS GENOTYPE IN THE DIAGNOSIS OF OLIGODENDROGLIOMA AND LOW-GRADE ASTROCYTOMA

In a substantial fraction of cases, histological distinction of low-grade astrocytomas from oligoastrocytomas and oligodendrogliomas may be subjective and shows high inter-observer variability, even among neuropathologists applying the criteria of the new WHO classification *(46)*. This particularly true for tumors that contain small areas of oligodendroglial differentiation. These tumors are variably diagnosed as low-grade diffuse astrocytomas, oligoastrocytomas, or even oligodendrogliomas.

Histological hallmarks of oligodendrogliomas include a perinuclear halo, which may produce a honeycomb or fried egg appearance, and a dense network of branching capillaries resembling chicken-wire. Based on these classical histological criteria, the frequency of oligodendrogliomas has been estimated as amounting to 5–18% of all gliomas *(98,101)*. Since the diagnosis of oligodendroglioma has favorable prognostic implications, there is a recent tendency to expand the histological criteria of oligodendrogliomas to include features such as nuclear regularity and roundness, often accompanied by a thin, eccentric rim of eosinophilic cytoplasm and an apparent lack of cell processes *(19,20,26)*. Oligodendrogliomas diagnosed based on such criteria may represent 25–33% of all glial tumors *(19,21,26)*.

However, expanding the diagnostic criteria may be misleading. The majority of oligodendrogliomas >90%) with the typical perinuclear halo in over 50% of tumor cells and with a chicken-wire vascular pattern showed LOH on 1p/19q *(127)*, whereas most oligodendrogliomas with a perinuclear halo in over 50% of tumor cells lacked LOH 1p/19q, but carried a *TP53* mutation. Because LOH on 1p/19q is a significant predictor of chemosensitivity in anaplastic oligodendrogliomas *(17)* and increased survival of patients with oligodendrogliomas and anaplastic oligodendrogliomas *(17,105)*, oligodendrogliomas with the classical histological features are likely to be chemosensitive, whereas those diagnosed with less stringent criteria are not likely to have better prognosis.

Oligoastrocytomas are defined as neoplasms with a conspicuous mixture of two distinct cell types resembling neoplastic oligodendrocytes and astrocytes *(89)*. Approximately 30–50% of oligoastrocytomas show LOH on 1p/19q *(49,59,92,118)*, and approx 30% contain *TP53* mutations and/or LOH on chromosome 17p *(59,92,118)*. Oligoastrocytomas with *TP53* mutations and/or LOH on chromosome 17p do not show LOH on 1p/19q, and vice versa *(59,92)*. Oligoastrocytomas with LOH on 1p/19q typically have predominant features of oligodendroglioma, whereas those with *TP53* mutations are more often astrocytoma-predominant *(59)*. In a recent study, a subset (approx 20%) of tumors diagnosed as low-grade astrocytomas contained small areas with oligodendroglial features but this was not predictive regarding the presence of either *TP53* mutations or LOH on chromosomes 1p/19q, suggesting that the presence of small oligodendroglial foci in low-grade diffuse astrocytomas does not necessarily reflect the presence of an oligodendroglial genotype, and therefore does not predict sensitivity to chemotherapy *(127)*.

In contrast to the occasional histological ambiguity, *TP53* mutations and LOH 1p/19q were mutually exclusive in oligodendrogliomas, low-grade astrocytomas, and oligoastrocytomas *(59,89,127)*, and therefore genetic typing of low-grade astrocytomas, oligoastrocytomas, and oligodendrogliomas may be helpful to predict prognosis of patients.

4. CONCLUSIONS AND SUMMARY

Glioblastomas may develop *de novo* (primary glioblastomas) or through progression from low-grade or anaplastic astrocytoma (secondary glioblastomas). These subtypes of glioblastoma constitute distinct disease entities that affect patients at different ages, evolve through different genetic pathways, and are likely to differ in prognosis and response to therapy. Primary glioblastomas develop in older patients and typically show *EGFR* amplification (approx 40%), EGFR overexpression (approx 60%), p16 homozygous deletion (approx 30%), LOH on the entire chromosome 10 (>60%), and *PTEN* mutations (approx 30%). Secondary glioblastomas develop in younger patients and often contain *TP53* mutations (>65%) and *p14^ARF* methylation (approx 35%) as the earliest detectable alterations. Additional genetic alterations in the pathway leading to secondary glioblastomas include LOH on 19q (approx 50%) and 10q (>50%) and *RB1* methylation (approx 40%). These characteristics are largely derived from patients selected on the basis of clinical history and sequential biopsies. More subtypes of glioblastoma may exist with intermediate clinical and genetic profiles. This is exemplified by the genetic profile of two glioblastoma variants, giant cell glioblastoma and gliosarcoma.

In contrast to astrocytic tumors, oligodendrogliomas are more susceptible to chemotherapy and have better prognosis; this correlates with the presence of LOH on 1p/19q which occurs in up to 90% of oligodendrogliomas. A small subset of oligodendrogliomas contains *TP53* mutations (5–15%) and *p14^ARF* methylation (approx 20%). Anaplastic oligodendrogliomas (WHO grade III) share with oligodendroglioma WHO grade II frequent LOH on 1p and 19q, but often carry additional genetic alterations, including LOH on chromosomes 9p (20–50%) and 10 (15–40%), gain of chromosome 7 (10–40%) and concurrent disruption of the RB1/CDK4/p16^INK4a/p15^INK4b and TP53/p14^ARF/MDM2 pathways (45%).

Histological distinction between low-grade astrocytomas, oligoastrocytomas, and oligodendrogliomas may be difficult, with high inter-observer variability. The majority of oligodendrogliomas (>90%) with typical perinuclear halos in over 50% of tumor cells show LOH on 1p/19q, whereas oligodendrogliomas with a perinuclear halo in less than 50% of tumor cells typically lack LOH on 1p/19q, but may carry a *TP53* mutation. Foci with oligodendroglial features in otherwise typical low-grade astrocytomas are not predictive for LOH on 1p/19q, and therefore do not predict sensitivity to chemotherapy.

REFERENCES

1. Albarosa R., Colombo B.M., Roz L., Magnani I., Pollo B., Cirenei N., et al. 1996. Deletion mapping of gliomas suggests the presence of two small regions for candidate tumor-suppressor genes in a 17-cM interval on chromosome 10q. *Am. J. Hum. Genet.* **58:**1260–1267.
2. Barker F.G., Davis R.L., Chang S.M., Prados M.D. 1996. Necrosis as a prognostic factor in glioblastoma multiforme. *Cancer* **77:**1161–1166.

3. Bartek J., Lukas J. 2001. Pathways governing G1/S transition and their response to DNA damage. *FEBS Lett.* **490:** 117–122.

4. Bello M.J., Leone P.E., Nebreda P., de Campos J.M., Kusak M.E., Vaquero J., et al. 1995. Allelic status of chromosome 1 in neoplasms of the nervous system. *Cancer Genet.Cytogenet.* **83:**160–164.

5. Bello M.J., Leone P.E., Vaquero J., de Campos J.M., Kusak M.E., Sarasa J.L., et al. 1995. Allelic loss at 1p and 19q frequently occurs in association and may represent early oncogenic events in oligodendroglial tumors. *Int. J. Cancer* **64:**207–210.

6. Biernat W., Aguzzi A., Sure U., Grant J.W., Kleihues P., Hegi M.E. 1995. Identical mutations of the p53 tumor suppressor gene in the gliomatous and the sarcomatous components of gliosarcomas suggest a common origin from glial cells. *J. Neuropathol. Exp. Neurol.* **54:**651–656.

7. Biernat W., Kleihues P., Yonekawa Y., Ohgaki H. 1997. Amplification and overexpression of MDM2 in primary (*de novo*) glioblastomas. *J. Neuropathol. Exp. Neurol.* **56:**180–185.

8. Biernat W., Tohma Y., Yonekawa Y., Kleihues P., Ohgaki H. 1997. Alterations of cell cycle regulatory genes in primary (*de novo*) and secondary glioblastomas. *Acta. Neuropathol.* **94:**303–309.

9. Bigner S.H., Matthews M.R., Rasheed B.K., Wiltshire R.N., Friedman H.S., Friedman A.H., et al. 1999. Molecular genetic aspects of oligodendrogliomas including analysis by comparative genomic hybridization. *Am. J. Pathol.* **155:** 375–386.

10. Boström J., Cobbers J.M.J.L., Wolter M., Tabatabai G., Weber R.G., Lichter P., et al. 1998. Mutation of the *PTEN (MMAC1)* tumor suppressor gene in a subset of glioblastomas but not in meningiomas with loss of chromosome arm 10q. *Cancer Res.* **58:**29–33.

11. Burger P.C., Green S.B. 1987. Patient age, histologic features, and length of survival in patients with glioblastoma multiforme. *Cancer* **59:**1617–1625.

12. Burger P.C., Kleihues P. 1989. Cytologic composition of the untreated glioblastoma with implications for evaluation of needle biopsies. *Cancer* **63:**2014–2023.

13. Burger P.C., Pearl D.K., Aldape K., Yates A.J., Scheithauer B.W., Passe S.M., et al. 2001. Small cell architecture—A histological equivalent of EGFR amplification in glioblastoma multiforme? *J. Neuropathol. Exp. Neurol.* **60:**1099–1104.

14. Burger P.C., Scheithauer B.W. 1994. *Tumors of the Central Nervous System.* Armed Forces Institute of Pathology, Washington, D.C.

15. Burkhard C., Schüler G., Di Patre P.L., Schüler D.L.U., Kleihues P., Ohgaki H. A population-based study on the incidence of survival of glioma patients in Switzerland not yet decided, in press.

16. Burns K.L., Ueki K., Jhung S.L., Koh J., Louis D.N. 1998. Molecular genetic correlates of p16, cdk4, and pRb immunohistochemistry in glioblastomas. *J. Neuropathol. Exp. Neurol.* **57:**122–130.

17. Cairncross J. G., Ueki K., Zlatescu M.C., Lisle D.K., Finkelstein D.M., Hammond R.R., et al. 1998. Specific genetic predictors of chemotherapeutic response and survival in patients with anaplastic oligodendrogliomas. *J. Natl. Cancer Inst.* **90:**1473–1479.

18. Cavenee W.K., Furnari F.B., Nagane M., Huang H.J.S., Newcomb E.W., Bigner D.D., et al. 2000. Diffusely infiltrating astrocytomas, in *Pathology and Genetics of Tumours of the Nervous System* (Kleihues P., Cavenee W.K., eds.), IARC Press, Lyon, pp. 10–21.

19. Coons S.W., Johnson P.C., Scheithauer B.W., Yates A.J., Pearl D.K. 1997. Improving diagnostic accuracy and interobserver concordance in the classification and grading of primary gliomas. *Cancer* **79:**1381–1393.

20. Daumas-Duport C., Varlet P., Tucker M.L., Beuvon F., Cervera P., Chodkiewicz J.P. 1997. Oligodendrogliomas. Part I: patterns of growth, histological diagnosis, clinical and imaging correlations: a study of 153 cases. *J. Neurooncol.* **34:** 37–59.

21. Donahue B., Scott C.B., Nelson J.S., Rotman M., Murray K.J., Nelson D.F., et al. 1997. Influence of an oligodendroglial component on the survival of patients with anaplastic astrocytomas: a report of Radiation Therapy Oncology Group 83-02. *Int. J. Radiat. Oncol. Biol. Phys.* **38:**911–914.

22. Dropcho E.J., Soong S.J. 1996. The prognostic impact of prior low grade histology in patients with anaplastic gliomas: a case-control study. *Neurology* **47:**684–690.

23. Duerr E.M., Rollbrocker B., Hayashi Y., Peters N., Meyer-Puttlitz B., Louis D.N., et al. 1998. *PTEN* mutations in gliomas and glioneuronal tumors. *Oncogene* **16:**2259–2264.

24. Ekstrand A.J., Sugawa N., James C.D., Collins V.P. 1992. Amplified and rearranged epidermal growth factor receptor genes in human glioblastomas reveal deletions of sequences encoding portions of the N- and/or C-terminal tails. *Proc. Natl. Acad. Sci.USA* **89:**4309–4313.

25. Esteller M., Hamilton S.R., Burger P.C., Baylin S.B., Herman J.G. 1999. Inactivation of the DNA repair gene *O⁶-methylguanine-DNA methyltransferase* by promoter hypermethylation is a common event in primary human neoplasia. *Cancer Res.* **59:**793–797.

26. Fortin D., Cairncross G.J., Hammond R.R. 1999. Oligodendroglioma: an appraisal of recent data pertaining to diagnosis and treatment. *Neurosurgery* **45:**1279–1291.

27. Fujisawa H., Kurrer M., Reis R.M., Yonekawa Y., Kleihues P., Ohgaki H. 1999. Acquisition of the glioblastoma phenotype during astrocytoma progression is associated with LOH on chromosome 10q25-qter. *Am. J. Pathol.* **155:**387–394.

28. Fujisawa H., Reis R.M., Nakamura M., Colella S., Yonekawa Y., Kleihues P., Ohgaki H. 2000. Loss of heterozygosity on chromosome 10 is more extensive in primary *(de novo)* than in secondary glioblastomas. *Lab. Invest.* **80:**65–72.

29. Fults D., Pedone C.A., Thompson G.E., Uchiyama C.M., Gumpper K.L., Iliev D., et al. 1998. Microsatellite deletion mapping on chromosome 10q and mutation analysis of *MMAC1, FAS,* and *MXI1* in human glioblastoma multiforme. *Int. J. Oncol.* **12:**905–910.

30. Goth R., Rajewsky M.F. 1974. Persistence of O6-ethylguanine in rat-brain DNA: correlation with nervous system-specific carcinogenesis by ethylnitrosourea. *Proc. Natl. Acad. Sci. USA* **71:**639–643.

31. Hannon G.J., Beach D. 1994. p15INK4B is a potential effector of TGF-beta-induced cell cycle arrest. *Nature* **371:** 257–261.

32. Hayashi Y., Ueki K., Waha A., Wiestler O.D., Louis D.N., von Deimling A. 1997. Association of *EGFR* gene amplification and *CDKN2 (p16/MTS1)* gene deletion in glioblastoma multiforme. *Brain Pathol.* **7:**871–875.

33. Henson J.W., Schnitker B.L., Correa K.M., von Deimling A., Fassbender F., Xu H.J, et al. 1994. The retinoblastoma gene is involved in malignant progression of astrocytomas. *Ann. Neurol.* **36:**714–721.

34. Hogg A., Bia B., Onadim Z., Cowell J.K. 1993. Molecular mechanisms of oncogenic mutations in tumors from patients with bilateral and unilateral retinoblastoma. *Proc. Natl. Acad. Sci. USA* **90:**7351–7355.

35. Huang H., Colella S., Kurrer M., Yonekawa Y., Kleihues P., Ohgaki H. 2000. Gene expression profiling of low-grade diffuse astrocytomas by cDNA arrays. *Cancer Res.* **60:**6868–6874.

36. Hui A.B., Lo K.W., Yin X.L., Poon W.S., Ng H.K. 2001. Detection of multiple gene amplifications in glioblastoma multiforme using array-based comparative genomic hybridization. *Lab. Invest.* **81:**717–723.

37. Huschtscha L.I., Reddel R.R. 1999. p16^{INK4a} and the control of cellular proliferative life span. *Carcinogenesis* **20:** 921–926.

38. Husemann K., Wolter M., Buschges R., Bostrom J., Sabel M., Reifenberger G. 1999. Identification of two distinct deleted regions on the short arm of chromosome 1 and rare mutation of the CDKN2C gene from 1p32 in oligodendroglial tumors. *J. Neuropathol. Exp. Neurol.* **58:**1041–1050.

39. Ichimura K., Bolin M.B., Goike H.M., Schmidt E.E., Moshref A., Collins V.P. 2000. Deregulation of the p14^{ARF}/MDM2/p53 pathway is a prerequisite for human astrocytic gliomas with G_1-S transition control gene abnormalities. *Cancer Res.* **60:**417–424.

40. Ichimura K., Schmidt E.E., Goike H.M., Collins V.P. 1996. Human glioblastomas with no alterations of the *CDK2A* (*p16 ^{INK4A}, MTS1*) and *CDK4* genes have frequent mutations of the retinoblastoma gene. *Oncogene* **13:**1065–1072.

41. Ichimura K., Schmidt E.E., Miyakawa A., Goike H.M., Collins V.P. 1998. Distinct patterns of deletion on 10p and 10q suggest involvement of multiple tumor suppressor genes in the development of astrocytic gliomas of different malignancy grades. *Genes Chromosomes Cancer* **22:**9–15.

42. Kamijo T., Weber J.D., Zambetti G., Zindy F., Roussel M.F., Sherr C.J. 1998. Functional and physical interactions of the ARF tumor suppressor with p53 and Mdm2. *Proc. Natl. Acad. Sci. USA* **95:**8292–8297.

43. Karlbom A.E., James C.D., Boethius J., Cavenee W.K., Collins V.P., Nordenskjöld M., Larsson C. 1993. Loss of heterozygosity in malignant gliomas involves at least three distinct regions on chromosome 10. *Hum. Genet.* **92:**169–174.

44. Kimmelman A.C., Ross D.A., Liang B.C. 1996. Loss of heterozygosity of chromosome 10p in human gliomas. *Genomics* **34:**250–254.

45. Kleihues P., Burger P.C., Collins V.P., Newcomb E.W., Ohgaki H., Cavenee W.K. 2000. Glioblastoma in *Pathology and Genetics of Tumours of the Nervous System* (Kleihues P., Cavenee W.K., eds.), IARC Press, Lyon, pp. 29–39.

46. Kleihues P., Cavenee W.K. 2000. *Pathology and Genetics of Tumours of the Nervous System.* International Agency for Research on Cancer, Lyon.

47. Kon H., Sonoda Y., Kumabe T., Yoshimoto T., Sekiya T., Murakami Y. 1998. Structural and functional evidence for the presence of tumor suppressor genes on the short arm of chromosome 10 in human gliomas. *Oncogene* **16:**257–263.

48. Korkolopoulou P., Christodoulou P., Kouzelis K., Hadjiyannakis M., Priftis A., Stamoulis G., et al. 1997. MDM2 and p53 expression in gliomas: a multivariate survival analysis including proliferation markers and epidermal growth factor receptor. *Br. J. Cancer* **75:**1269–1278.

49. Kraus J.A., Koopmann J., Kaskel P., Maintz D., Brandner S., Schramm J., et al. 1995. Shared allelic losses on chromosomes 1p and 19q suggest a common origin of oligodendroglioma and oligoastrocytoma. *J. Neuropathol. Exp. Neurol.* **54:**91–95.

50. Lang F.F., Miller D.C., Koslow M., Newcomb E.W. 1994. Pathways leading to glioblastoma multiforme: a molecular analysis of genetic alterations in 65 astrocytic tumors. *J. Neurosurg.* **81:**427–436.

51. Lantos P.L., VandenBerg S.R., Kleihues P. 1996. Tumours of the nervous system in *Greenfield's Neuropathology,* vol. 2. (Graham D.I., Lantos P.L., eds.), Arnold, London, pp. 583–879.

52. Li J., Yen C., Liaw D., Podsypanina K., Bose S., Wang S.I., et al. 1997. *PTEN,* a putative protein tyrosine phosphatase gene mutated in human brain, breast, and prostate cancer. *Science* **275:**1943–1947.

53. Libermann T.A., Nusbaum H.R., Razon N., Kris R., Lax I., Soreq H., et al. 1985. Amplification, enhanced expression and possible rearrangement of EGF receptor gene in primary human brain tumours of glial origin. *Nature* **313:**144–147.

54. Ljubimova J.Y., Lakhter A.J., Loksh A., Yong W.H., Riedinger M.S., Miner J.H., et al. 2001. Overexpression of α4 chain-containing laminins in human glial tumors identified by gene microarray analysis. *Cancer Res.* **61:**5601–5610.

55. Louis D.N. 1994. The p53 gene and protein in human brain tumors. *J. Neuropathol. Exp. Neurol.* **53:**11–21.

56. Louis D.N., Gusella J.F. 1995. A tiger behind many doors: multiple genetic pathways to maligant glioma. *TIG* **11:** 412–415.

57. Louis D.N., von Deimling A., Chung R.Y., Rubio M.P., Whaley J.M., Eibl R.H., et al. 1993. Comparative study of p53 gene and protein alterations in human astrocytic tumors. *J. Neuropathol. Exp. Neurol.* **52:**31–38.

58. Maier D., Comparone D., Taylor E., Zhang Z., Gratzl O., Van Meir E.G., et al. 1997. New deletion in low-grade oligodendroglioma at the glioblastoma suppressor locus on chromosome 10q25-26. *Oncogene* **15:**997–1000.

59. Maintz D., Fiedler K., Koopmann J., Rollbrocker B., Nechev S., Lenartz D., et al. 1997. Molecular genetic evidence for subtypes of oligoastrocytomas. *J. Neuropathol. Exp. Neurol.* **56:**1098–1104.

60. Margison G.P., Kleihues P. 1975. Chemical carcinogenesis in the nervous system. Preferential accumulation of O6-methylguanine in rat brain deoxyribonucleic acid during repetitive administration of N-methyl-N-nitrosourea. *Biochem. J.* **148:**521–525.

61. Matsumoto R., Tada M., Nozaki M., Zhang C.L., Sawamura Y., Abe H. 1998. Short alternative splice transcripts of the mdm2 oncogene correlate to malignancy in human astrocytic neoplasms. *Cancer Res.* **58:**609–613.

62. Meyer-Puttlitz B., Hayashi Y., Waha A., Rollbrocker B., Bostrom J., Wiestler O.D., et al. 1997. Molecular genetic analysis of giant cell glioblastomas. *Am. J. Pathol.* **151:**853–857.

63. Mollenhauer J., Wiemann S., Scheurlen W., Korn B., Hayashi Y., Wilgenbus K.K., et al. 1997. *DMBT1*, a new member of the SRCR superfamily, on chromosome 10q25.3-26.1 is deleted in malignant brain tumours. *Nat. Genet.* **17:**32–39.

64. Momand J., Zambetti G.P., Olson D.C., George D., Levine A.J. 1992. The mdm-2 oncogene product forms a complex with the p53 protein and inhibits p53-mediated transactivation. *Cell* **69:**1237–1245.

65. Nagane M., Coufal F., Lin H., Bogler O., Cavenee W.K., Huang H.J. 1996. A common mutant epidermal growth factor receptor confers enhanced tumorigenicity on human glioblastoma cells by increasing proliferation and reducing apoptosis. *Cancer Res.* **56:**5079–5086.

66. Nagane M., Lin H., Cavenee W.K., Huang H.J. 2001. Aberrant receptor signaling in human malignant gliomas: mechanisms and therapeutic implications. *Cancer Lett.* **162**(Suppl)**:**S17–S21.

67. Nakamura M., Watanabe T., Klangby U., Asker C.E., Wiman K.G., Yonekawa Y., et al. 2001. *P14* [Arf] deletion and methylation in genetic pathways to glioblastomas. *Brain Pathol.* **11:**159–168.

68. Nakamura M., Watanabe T., Yonekawa Y., Kleihues P., Ohgaki H. 2001. Promoter hypermethylation of the DNA repair gene *MGMT* in astrocytomas is frequently associated with G:C—A:T mutations of the *TP53* tumor suppressor gene. *Carcinogenesis* **22:**1715–1719.

69. Nakamura M., Yang F., Fujisawa H., Yonekawa Y., Kleihues P., Ohgaki H. 2000. Loss of heterozygosity on chromosome 19 in secondary glioblastomas. *J. Neuropathol. Exp. Neurol.* **59:**539–543.

70. Nakamura M., Yonekawa Y., Kleihues P., Ohgaki H. 2001. Promoter hypermethylation of the *RB1* gene in glioblastomas. *Lab. Invest.* **81:**77–82.

71. Newcomb E.W., Cohen H., Lee S.R., Bhalla S.K., Bloom J., Hayes R.L., Miller D.C. 1998. Survival of patients with glioblastoma multiforme is not influenced by altered expression of p16, p53, EGFR, MDM2 or Bcl-2 genes. *Brain Pathol.* **8:**655–667.

72. Newcomb E.W., Madonia W.J., Pisharody S., Lang F.F., Koslow M., Miller D.C. 1993. A correlative study of p53 protein alteration and p53 gene mutation in glioblastoma multiforme. *Brain Pathol.* **3:**229–235.

73. Nigro J.M., Baker S.J., Preisinger A.C., Jessup J.M., Hostetter R., Cleary K., et al. 1989. Mutations in the p53 gene occur in diverse human tumour types. *Nature* **342:**705–708.

74. Nishikawa R., Ji X.D., Harmon R.C., Lazar C.S., Gill G.N., Cavenee W.K., Huang H.J. 1994. A mutant epidermal growth factor receptor common in human glioma confers enhanced tumorigenicity. *Proc. Natl. Acad. Sci. USA* **91:**7727–7731.

75. Ohgaki H., Biernat W., Reis R., Hegi M., Kleihues P. 2000. Gliosarcoma in *Pathology and Genetics of Tumours of the Nervous System* (Kleihues P., Cavenee W.K., eds.), IARC Press, Lyon, pp. 42–44.

76. Ohgaki H., Eibl R.H., Wiestler O.D., Yasargil M.G., Newcomb E.W., Kleihues P. 1991. p53 mutations in nonastrocytic human brain tumors. *Cancer Res.* **51:**6202–6205.

77. Ohgaki H., Peraud A., Nakazato Y., Watanabe K., von Deimling A. 2000. Giant cell glioblastomain *Pathology and Genetics of Tumours of the Nervous System* (Kleihues P., Cavenee W.K., eds.), International Agency for Research on Cancer, Lyon, pp. 40–41.

78. Ohgaki H., Schauble B., zur Hausen A., von Ammon K., Kleihues P. 1995. Genetic alterations associated with the evolution and progression of astrocytic brain tumours. *Virchows Arch.* **427:**113–118.

79. Ohgaki H., Watanabe K., Peraud A., Biernat W., von Deimling A.,Yasargil G., Yonekawa Y., Kleihues P. 1999. A case history of glioma progression. *Acta Neuropathol.* **97:**525–535.

80. Oliner J.D., Pietenpol J.A., Thiagalingam S., Gyuris J., Kinzler K.W., Vogelstein B. 1993. Oncoprotein MDM2 conceals the activation domain of tumour suppressor p53. *Nature* **362:**857–860.

81. Peraud A., Watanabe K., Schwechheimer K., Yonekawa Y., Kleihues P., Ohgaki H. 1999. Genetic profile of the giant cell glioblastoma. *Lab. Invest.* **79:**123–129.

82. Pomerantz J., Schreiber-Agus N., Liegeois N.J., Silverman A., Alland L., Chin L., et al. 1998. The *Ink4a* tumor suppressor gene product, p19[Arf], interacts with MDM2 and neutralizes MDM2's inhibition of p53. *Cell* **92:**713–723.

83. Prigent S.A., Nagane M., Lin H., Huvar I., Boss G.R., Feramisco J.R., et al. 1996. Enhanced tumorigenic behavior of glioblastoma cells expressing a truncated epidermal growth factor receptor is mediated through the Ras-Shc-Grb2 pathway. *J. Biol. Chem.* **271:**25,639–25,645.

84. Qian X.C., Brent T.P. 1997. Methylation hot spots in the 5′ flanking region denote silencing of the O^6-methylguanine-DNA methyltransferase gene. *Cancer* Res. **57:**3672–3677.

85. Rasheed B.K., McLendon R.E., Friedman H.S., Friedman A.H., Fuchs H.E., Bigner D.D., Bigner S.H. 1995. Chromosome 10 deletion mapping in human gliomas: a common deletion region in 10q25. *Oncogene* **10:**2243–2246.

86. Rasheed B.K., McLendon R.E., Herndon J.E., Friedman H.S., Friedman A.H., Bigner D.D., Bigner S.H. 1994. Alterations of the *TP53* gene in human gliomas. *Cancer Res.* **54:**1324–1330.

87. Rasheed B.K., Stenzel T.T., McLendon R.E., Parsons R., Friedman A.H., Friedman H.S., et al. 1997. *PTEN* gene mutations are seen in high-grade but not in low-grade gliomas. *Cancer Res.* **57:**4187–4190.

88. Reifenberger G., Kros J.M., Burger P.C., Louis D.N., Collins V.P. 2000. Anaplastic oligodendroglioma in *Pathology and Genetics of Tumours of the Nervous System* (Kleihues P., Cavenee W.K., eds.), IARC Press, Lyon, pp. 62–64.

89. Reifenberger G., Kros J.M., Burger P.C., Louis D.N., Collins V.P. 2000. Oligoastrocytoma in *Pathology and Genetics of Tumours of the Nervous System* (Kleihues P., Cavenee W.K., eds.), IARC Press, Lyon, pp. 65–67.

90. Reifenberger G., Kros J.M., Burger P.C., Louis D.N., Collins V.P. 2000. Oligodendrogliomain *Pathology and Genetics of Tumours of the Nervous System* (Kleihues P., Cavenee W.K., eds.), IARC Press, Lyon, pp. 56–61.

91. Reifenberger G., Liu L., Ichimura K., Schmidt E.E., Collins V.P. 1993. Amplification and overexpression of the MDM2 gene in a subset of human malignant gliomas without p53 mutations. *Cancer Res.* **53:**2736–2739.

92. Reifenberger J., Reifenberger G., Liu L., James C.D., Wechsler W., Collins V.P. 1994. Molecular genetic analysis of oligodendroglial tumors shows preferential allelic deletions on 19q and 1p. *Am. J. Pathol.* **145:**1175–1190.

93. Reifenberger J., Ring G.U., Gies U., Cobbers L., Oberstrass J., An H.X., et al. 1996. Analysis of p53 mutation and epidermal growth factor receptor amplification in recurrent gliomas with malignant progression. *J. Neuropathol. Exp. Neurol.* **55:**822–831.

94. Reis R.M., Herva R., Koivukankas J., Mironov N., Bär W., Kleihues P., Ohgaki H. 2000. Second primary glioblastoma. *J. Neuropathol. Exp. Neurol.* **60:**208–215.

95. Reis R.M., Konu-Lebleb021cioglu D., Lopes J.M., Kleihues P., Ohgaki H. 2000. Genetic profile of gliosarcomas. *Am. J. Pathol.* **156:**425–432.

96. Reyes-Mugica M., Rieger-Christ K., Ohgaki H., Ekstrand B.C., Helie M., Kleinman G., et al. 1997. Loss of *DCC* expression and glioma progression. *Cancer Res.* **57:**382–386.

97. Rickman D.S., Bobek M.P., Misek D.E., Kuick R., Blaivas M., Kurnit D.M., et al. 2001. Distinctive molecular profiles of high-grade and low-grade gliomas based on oligonucleotide microarray analysis. *Cancer Res.* **61:**6885–6891.

98. Russel, D.S., Rubinstein L.J. 1989. *Pathology of Tumours of the Nervous System.* Edward Arnold, London.

99. Sallinen S.L., Sallinen P.K., Haapasalo H.K., Helin H.J., Helen P.T., Schraml P., et al. 2000. Identification of differentially expressed genes in human gliomas by DNA microarray and tissue chip techniques. *Cancer Res.* **60:**6617–6622.

100. Scherer H.J. 1940. Cerebral astrocytomas and their derivatives. *Am. J. Cancer* **40:**159–198.

101. Schiffer D. 1997. *Brain Tumors. Biology, Pathology, and Clinical References.* Springer, Berlin.

102. Sherr C.J. 1996. Cancer cell cycles. *Science* **274:**1672–1677.

103. Sherr C.J., Roberts J.M. 1999. CDK inhibitors: positive and negative regulators of G_1–phase progression. *Genes Dev.* **13:**1501–1512.

104. Smith J.S., Alderete B., Minn Y., Borell T.J., Perry A., Mohapatra G., et al. 1999. Localization of common deletion regions on 1p and 19q in human gliomas and their association with histological subtype. *Oncogene* **18:**4144–4152.

105. Smith J.S., Perry A., Borell T.J., Lee H.K., O'Fallon J., Hosek S.M., et al. 2000. Alterations of chromosome arms 1p and 19q as predictors of survival in oligodendrogliomas, astrocytomas, and mixed oligoastrocytomas. *J. Clin. Oncol.* **18:**636–645.

106. Somerville R.P.T., Shoshan Y., Eng C., Barnett G., Miller D., Cowell J.K. 1998. Molecular analysis of two putative tumour suppressor genes, *PTEN* and *DMBT*, which have been implicated in glioblastoma multiforme disease progression. *Oncogene* **17:**1755–1757.

107. Sonoda Y., Murakami Y., Tominaga T., Kayama T., Yoshimoto T., Sekiya T. 1996. Deletion mapping of chromosome 10 in human glioma. *Jpn. J. Cancer Res.* **87:**363–367.

108. Steck P.A., Pershouse M.A., Jasser S.A., Yung W.K., Lin H., Ligon A.H., et al. 1997. Identification of a candidate tumour suppressor gene, *MMAC1*, at chromosome 10q23.3 that is mutated in multiple advanced cancers. *Nat.Genet.* **15:**356–362.

109. Stott F.J., Bates S., James M.C., McConnell B.B., Starborg M., Brookes S., et al. 1998. The alternative product from the human *CDKN2A* locus, p14^{ARF}, participates in a regulatory feedback loop with p53 and MDM2. *EMBO J.* **17:** 5001–5014.

110. Sugawa N., Ekstrand A.J., James C.D., Collins V.P. 1990. Identical splicing of aberrant epidermal growth factor receptor transcripts from amplified rearranged genes in human glioblastomas. *Proc. Natl. Acad. Sci. USA* **87:**8602–8606.

111. Taylor W.R., Stark G.R. 2001. Regulation of the G2/M transition by p53. *Oncogene* **20:**1803–1815.

112. Tohma Y., Gratas C., Biernat W., Peraud A., Fukuda M., Yonekawa Y., et al. 1998. *PTEN (MMAC1)* mutations are frequent in primary glioblastomas (de novo) but not in secondary glioblastomas. *J. Neuropathol. Exp. Neurol.* **57:** 684–689.

113. Tohma Y., Gratas C., Van Meir E.G., Desbaillets I., Tenan M., Tachibana O., et al. 1998. Necrogenesis and Fas/APO–1(CD95) expression in primary (*de novo*) and secondary glioblastomas. *J. Neuropathol. Exp. Neurol.* **57:**239–245.

114. Ueki K., Ono Y., Henson J.W., Efird J.T., von Deimling A., Louis D.N. 1996. CDKN2/p16 or RB alterations occur in the majority of glioblastomas and are inversely correlated. *Cancer Res.* **56:**150–153.

115. van Meyel D.J., Ramsay D.A., Casson A.G., Keeney M., Chambers A.F., Cairncross J.G. 1994. p53 mutation, expression, and DNA ploidy in evolving gliomas: evidence for two pathways of progression. *J. Natl. Cancer Inst.* **86:**1011–1017.

116. Voesten A.M.J., Bijleveld E.H., Westerveld A., Hulsebos T.J.M. 1997. Fine mapping of a region of common deletion on chromosome arm 10p in human glioma. *Genes Chromosomes Cancer* **20:**167–172.

117. Vogelstein B., Lane D., Levine A.J. 2000. Surfing the p53 network. *Nature* **408:**307–310.

118. von Deimling A., Fimmers R., Schmidt M.C., Bender B., Fassbender F., Nagel J., et al. 2000. Comprehensive allelotype and genetic anaysis of 466 human nervous system tumors. *J. Neuropathol. Exp. Neurol.* **59:**544–558.

119. von Deimling A., Louis D.N., von Ammon K., Petersen I., Hoell T., Chung R.Y., et al. 1992. Association of epidermal growth factor receptor gene amplification with loss of chromosome 10 in human glioblastoma multiforme. *J. Neurosurg.* **77:**295–301.

120. von Deimling A., Louis D.N., von Ammon K., Petersen I., Wiestler O.D., Seizinger B.R. 1992. Evidence for a tumor suppressor gene on chromosome 19q associated with human astrocytomas, oligodendrogliomas, and mixed gliomas. *Cancer Res.* **52:**4277–4279.

121. von Deimling A., Nagel J., Bender B., Lenartz D., Schramm J., Louis D.N., Wiestler O.D. 1994. Deletion mapping of chromosome 19 in human glioimas. *Int. J. Cancer* **57:**676–680.

122. von Deimling A., von Ammon K., Schoenfeld D., Wiestler O.D., Seizinger B.R., Louis D.N. 1993. Subsets of glioblastoma multiforme defined by molecular genetic analysis. *Brain Pathol.* **3:**19–26.

123. Wang S.I., Puc J., Li J., Bruce J.N., Cairns P., Sidransky D., Parsons R. 1997. Somatic mutations of *PTEN* in glioblastoma multiforme. *Cancer Res.* **57:**4183–4186.

124. Watanabe K., Sato K., Biernat W., Tachibana O., von Ammon K., Ogata N., et al. 1997. Incidence and timing of *p53* mutations during astrocytoma progression in patients with multiple biopsies. *Clin. Cancer Res.* **3:**523–530.

125. Watanabe K., Tachibana O., Sato K., Yonekawa Y., Kleihues P., Ohgaki H. 1996. Overexpression of the EGF receptor and *p53* mutations are mutually exclusive in the evolution of primary and secondary glioblastomas. *Brain Pathol.* **6:** 217–224.

126. Watanabe K., Tachibana O., Yonekawa Y., Kleihues P., Ohgaki H. 1997. Role of gemistocytes in astrocytoma progression. *Lab. Invest.* **76:**277–284.

127. Watanabe T., Nakamura M., Kros J.M., Yonekawa Y., Kleihues P., Ohgaki H. 2000. Phenotype *versus* genotype correlation in oligodendrogliomas and low–grade diffuse astrocytomas *Acta Neuropathol.*103:267–275.

128. Watanabe T., Nakamura M., Yonekawa Y., Kleihues P., Ohgaki H. 2001. Promoter hypermethylation and homozygous deletion of the *p14* ^ARF^ and *p16* ^INK4a^ genes in oligodendrogliomas. *Acta Neuropathol.* **101:**185–189.

129. Watanabe T., Yokoo H., Yokoo M., Yonekawa Y., Kleihues P., Ohgaki H. 2001. Concurrent inactivation of RB1 and TP53 pathways in anaplastic oligodendrogliomas. *J. Neuropathol. Exp. Neurol.* **60:**1181–1189.

130. Watson M.A., Perry A., Budhjara V., Hicks C., Shannon W.D., Rich K.M. 2001. Gene expression profiling with oligonucleotide microarrays distinguishes World Health Organization grade of oligodendrogliomas. *Cancer Res.* **61:**1825–1829.

131. Watts G.S., Pieper R.O., Costello J.F., Peng Y.M., Dalton W.S., Futscher B.W. 1997. Methylation of discrete regions of the O^6–methylguanine DNA methyltransferase (MGMT) CpG island is associated with heterochromatinization of the MGMT transcription start site and silencing of the gene. *Mol. Cell Biol.* **17:**5612–5619.

132. Winger M.J., Macdonald D.R., Cairncross J.G. 1989. Supratentorial anaplastic gliomas in adults. The prognostic importance of extent of resection and prior low–grade glioma. *J. Neurosurg.* **71:**487–493.

133. Wong A.J., Ruppert J.M., Bigner S.H., Grzeschik C.H., Humphrey P.A., Bigner D.S., Vogelstein B. 1992. Structural alterations of the epidermal growth factor receptor gene in human gliomas. *Proc. Natl. Acad. Sci. USA* **89:**2965–2969.

134. Zhang Y., Xiong Y., Yarbrough W.G. 1998. ARF promotes MDM2 degradation and stabilizes p53: ARF–INK4a locus deletion impairs both the Rb and p53 tumor suppression pathways. *Cell* **92:**725–734.

DNA Damage and Repair in the Therapeutic Response of Tumors of the Central Nervous System

Henry S. Friedman, M. Eileen Dolan, and Francis Ali-Osman

1. CHEMOTHERAPY OF CENTRAL NERVOUS SYSTEM TUMORS

1.1. Malignant Glioma

Glioblastoma multiforme (GBM) is one of the most refractory of all human malignancies with a median survival of 8–12 mo following diagnosis (46). Conventional treatment options, specifically surgery, radiotherapy, and chemotherapy have produced only trivial increases in survival of patients with GBM. Although newer chemotherapeutic strategies have been identified, such as the activity of CPT-11 against recurrent GBM (58), locally implanted BCNU wafers (111), or the O^6-benzylguanine-mediated depletion of O^6-alkylguanine-DNA alkyltransferase to restore sensitivity to nitrosoureas or methylators (57,54). New strategies, including modulation or reversal of resistance to chemotherapy, will be needed to dramatically enhance survival of patients with GBM.

1.2. Medulloblastoma

Considerable progress has been made in understanding the phenotype, genotype, clinical course, and treatment of medulloblastoma (59). Identification of adverse prognostic features, including metastases (M1-4), or substantial (>1.5 cm^2) residual tumor post-surgery have clarified the need for precise tumor staging and intensification of therapy for high-risk patients. Newly defined molecular parameters that may prove critical for identification of high-risk medulloblastoma in future clinical trials include loss of heterozygosity for 17p (12). Therapeutic achievements include the cure of the majority (approx 70%) of children with standard-risk medulloblastoma using surgery, radiotherapy, and adjuvant chemotherapy, (43,81,103) and increased survival of young children with medulloblastoma using neo-adjuvant (pre-radiotherapy) chemotherapy (39).

1.3. Chemotherapy of Glioma: Nitrosoureas

The role of chemotherapy in the treatment of high-grade glioma has remained controversial. Although several small studies suggested a benefit from chemotherapy (61,117), BTCG 7201 was the first large study to demonstrate a possible additive effect of BCNU with radiation (128). The addition of post-radiation BCNU (80 mg/m^2 × 3 d every 8 wk) produced a median survival of 51 wk compared to 36 wk for radiotherapy alone. The difference in survival was not statistically significant, but provocative enough to provide the foundation of BTCG 7501. This study treated all patients with whole brain radiotherapy and then randomized them to treatment on one of four arms including high-dose methylprednisone, with or without BCNU or procarbazine (65). Patients treated on the BCNU

From: *Contemporary Cancer Research: Brain Tumors*
Edited by: F. Ali-Osman © Humana Press Inc., Totowa, NJ

or procarbazine arms had a significant increase in median survival over treatment of the high-dose methylprednisone arm (50 vs 40 wk). Although the BTCG concluded that BCNU or procarbazine in the post-radiation setting benefited patients with high-grade glioma, it is important to realize that it is possible that the patients on no-chemotherapy high-dose methylprednisone "control" suffered a high number of steroid-induced complications reducing median survival compared to the BCNU or procarbazine arm *(46)*.

Data was generated from NCDG trial 6G61, which randomized patients with high-grade glioma to whole brain radiotherapy with hydroxyurea, plus either BCNU or PCV (procarbazine, CCNU, vincristine) *(84)*. The analysis of all patients revealed that there was a nonstatistically significant increase in survival favoring PCV *(86)*. However, a subgroup analysis by Levin et al. *(85)* revealed that patients with anaplastic astrocytoma survived nearly twice as long when treated with PCV compared to BCNU (151.1 vs 82.1 wk, respectively). Based on this report, PCV became the standard, post-radiation treatment for patients with anaplastic astrocytoma. More recently, reanalysis of this data failed to confirm an advantage of PCV over BCNU.

1.4. Chemotherapy of Malignant Glioma: Temozolomide

Preliminary phase I and II trials in England initially demonstrated the activity of temozolomide in patients with recurrent high-grade glioma *(101)*. Subsequent multi-institutional trials have demonstrated activity of temozolomide in patients with recurrent anaplastic astrocytoma and glioblastoma multiforme *(137,138)*. These earlier trials, coupled with the marked activity of temozolomide against a panel of central nervous system (CNS) tumor xenografts growing in athymic nude mice *(51)*, provided the foundation for a trial evaluating temozolomide in the treatment of patients with newly diagnosis malignant glioma. Thirty-three patients with newly diagnosed GBM and five patients with newly diagnosed anaplastic astrocytoma were treated with temozolomide at a starting dose of 200 mg/m^2/d for 5 consecutive days with repeat dosing every 28 d following the first daily dose *(57)*. Of the 33 GBM patients, complete responses (CR) were seen in 3 patients; partial responses (PR) were seen in 14 patients; stable disease (SD) was seen in 4 patients; and 12 patients developed progressive disease (PD). Toxicity included infrequent grade 3/4 myelosuppression, constipation, nausea, and vomiting.

1.5. Chemotherapy of Medulloblastoma: Alkylators

The activity of alkylating agents in the treatment of medulloblastoma has been defined in both laboratory and clinical studies. Initial work demonstrated the potential role of the oxazophosphorine cyclophosphamide in the treatment of medulloblastoma *(10,48,49,53,55)*. Additional studies documented the activity of a series of classical bifunctional alkylating agents in the treatment of a panel of human medulloblastoma continuous cell lines and transplantable xenografts. These led directly to a successful phase II trial of melphalan for recurrent medulloblastoma *(49,56)*, and a Duke trial for patients with newly diagnosed and recurrent high-risk brain tumors, including medulloblastoma *(52)*. The phase III trials, which have demonstrated adjuvant chemotherapy-mediated increased survival of children with high-risk medulloblastoma, all include substantial reliance on alkylating agents *43,81,103,120)*. In summary, the identification of the activity of alkylators is the foundation for the chemotherapy-induced improvements in treatment of medulloblastoma.

Cyclophosphamide is the most active alkylating agent identified to date in the treatment of medulloblastoma, with a response rate approaching 90% *(82,99)*. Following confirmation of the activity and acceptable toxicity of cyclophosphamide in multidrug regimens for recurrent high-risk medulloblastoma *(53,100)* national studies are evaluating the efficacy of cyclophosphamide-based chemotherapy in children with high-risk (CCG protocol 9L31) medulloblastoma. Furthermore, a cyclophosphamide-based regimen is being used in a randomized national study designed to decrease the dose of neuraxis radiotherapy (POG/CCG Protocol A9961). The prodigious activity, aldehyde dehydrogenase-mediated sparing of hematopoeitic stem cells *(73)* and intestinal mucosal cells *(24)*, and successful dose escalation with concomitant use of cytokines such as GM-CSF *(82,99)*, support further use and study of cyclophosphamide in the treatment of medullo-blastoma.

2. CHEMOTHERAPY MECHANISMS OF ACTION AND RESISTANCE

2.1. Chloroethylnitrosoureas: Mechanisms of Action

The CENUs have a broad spectrum of activity, including activity against melanoma, Hodgkin's disease, and non-Hodgkin's lymphoma, as well as CNS tumors including malignant glioma and medulloblastoma. CENUs include BCNU (N,N^1-*bis*[2-chloroethyl]-*N*-nitrosourea), CCNU (*N*-[2-chloroethyl]-*N*-cyclohexyl-*N*-nitrosourea), and methyl CCNU. Each of these agents produce 92% N^7G mono-adducts, 4% N^7G-N^7G interstrand crosslinks, and 4% N^3C-N^1G interstrand crosslinks *(124,125)*. Initial reaction of a CENU with the O^6 position of guanine is followed by an intermolecular rearrangement forming an intramolecular N^1, O^6-ethanoguanine adduct. Ultimately, the exocyclic C-O bond is cleaved and reaction with the N3 position of cytosine in the complementary strand results in the N^3C-N^1G diadduct *(64,91)*, which appears to be the cytotoxic molecular lesion *(6,23, 44,75,76,78)*.

2.2. Temozolomide: Mechanisms of Action

The methylation of DNA seems to be the principal mechanism responsible for the cytotoxicity of temozolomide to malignant cells. Among the lesions produced in DNA after treatment of cells with temozolomide, the most common is methylation at the N^7 position of guanine, followed by methylation at the O^3 position of adenine and the O^6 position of guanine *(28)*. Although both the N^7-methylguanine and O^3-methyladenine adducts probably contribute to the antitumor activity of temozolomide in some if not all sensitive cells, their role is controversial *(20,27,89)*. The O^6-methylguanine adduct (which accounts for 5% of the total adducts formed by temozolomide) *(28)* probably plays a critical role in the antitumor activity of the agent. This is supported by the correlation between the sensitivity of tumor cell lines to temozolomide and the activity of the DNA repair protein O^6-alkylguanine-DNA alkyltransferase (AGT), which specifically removes alkyl groups at the O^6 position of guanine. Cell lines that have low levels of AGT are sensitive to the cytotoxicity of temozolomide, whereas cell lines that have high levels of this repair protein are much more resistant to this drug *(31,130,132)*. This correlation has also been observed in human glioblastoma xenograft models *(51,108,131)*. The correlation of sensitivity to the drug with the ability to repair the O^6-alkylguanine lesion also have been seen with procarbazine, DTIC, and the chloroethylating agents BCNU and CCNU *(25,31,34)*.

The cytotoxic mechanism of temozolomide appears to be related to the failure of the DNA MMR system to find a complementary base for methylated guanine. This system involves the formation of a complex of proteins that recognize, bind to, and remove mismatch bases *(38,87,104)*. The proposed hypothesis is that when this repair process is targeted to the DNA strand opposite the O^6-MG, it cannot find a correct partner, thus resulting in long-lived nicks in the DNA *(70)*. These nicks accumulate and persist into the subsequent cell cycle, where they ultimately inhibit initiation of replication in the daughter cells, blocking the cell cycle at the G_2-M boundary *(70,71,72,121)*. In both murine *(121)* and human *(122)* leukemia cells, sensitivity to temozolomide correlates with increased fragmentation of DNA and apoptotic cell death.

2.3. Cyclophosphamide: Mechanisms of Action

The toxic effect of the nitrogen mustards and related compounds such as cyclophosphamide is directly related to the production of DNA interstrand crosslinks via formation of mono-adducts at the N^7 position of guanine in DNA *(19,24,47,66,75–77,79,83,90,94,95,97,127,141)*.

2.4. Chloroethylnitrosoureas and Temozolomide: Mechanisms of Resistance

2.4.1. O^6-Alkylguanine-DNA Alkyltransferase

The major mechanism of resistance to alkylnitrosourea and methylator therapy is the DNA repair protein AGT *(106)*. AGT removes chloroethylation or methylation damage from the O^6 position of guanine prior to cell injury and death.

The history of studies relating AGT to alkylator resistance goes back to the late 1970swhen an inducible repair system in E. coli for reversing the effects of alkylating agents was described by Samson and Cairns *(112)*. This "adaptive response" proved to be due in part to the function of the enzyme AGT allowing repair of O^6-alkylguanine residues prior to DNA replication. Day et al. *(26)* and Sklar and Strauss *(116)* subsequently demonstrated that 30% of human tumor cell lines could not repair O^6-alkylguanine and demonstrated increased sensitivity to alkylating agents—these tumor cell lines were designated Mer- or Mex-. Subsequent studies demonstrated the absence of AGT in cell-free extracts of Mer- cells, unlike the presence of this enzyme in virtually all others, including non-malignant mammalian cell extracts *(16,107,133,135)*. Erickson et al. *(41)* reported that Mer- cell lines displayed increased DNA–DNA crosslinking and cell kill when treated with chloroethyl-nitrosoureas. Bodell et al. *(15)* subsequently demonstrated that human glioma-derived cell lines that are capable of repairing the O^6-alkyl lesions (hence Mer+) were more resistant to the cytotoxic effects of the nitrosoureas in cell culture. Furthermore, resistance to the nitrosoureas was highly specific, because cross-resistance was not seen to cisplatinum or nitrogen mustard *(2)*. Brent et al. *(18)* demonstrated the inverse relationship between AGT and sensitivity to MeCCNU in human rhab-domyosarcoma xenografts.

The high incidence of AGT activity in human CNS tumors *(133)*, as well as the inverse relationship between procarbazine activity and alkyltransferase levels in human brain tumor xenografts *(114)*, supported a role for this protein in mediating resistance to nitrosoureas in patients with CNS tumors and provided an approach for reversal of drug resistance. Recent clinical trials have shown an inverse relationship between survival and AGT levels in patients with malignant glioma who receive BCNU therapy *(14,42,68,69)*, thus providing a strong rationale for strategies designed to deplete tumor AGT levels before therapy with BCNU.

Immunohistochemistry for the detection of the human DNA mismatch repair proteins MSH2 and MLH1 and AGT was performed with monoclonal antibodies and characterized with respect to percent cellular reactivity for patients treated on the Duke phase 2 trial of temozolomide. MSH2 was detected in > 60% of cells in 32 of 38 subjects (84.2%). The response rate in these patients was 50% as compared to a response rate of 33.3% among those in whom MSH2 was detected in ≤ 60% of cells. This difference was not statistically significant at $p = 0.66$. Similarly, MLH1 was detected in > 60% of cells in 34 of 38 subjects (89.5%). The response rate in these patients (high-level status) was 47% as compared to a response rate of 50% among those in whom MLH1 was detected in ≤ 60% of cells (low-level status). This difference was not statistically significant at $p > 0.9$. These results showed the limited prognostic value afforded to analysis of MSH2 and MLH1 status, at least by immunohis-tochemical techniques, in predicting response to temozolomide. However, the prognostic value of immunohistochemical analysis of AGT status was far more important. AGT was detected in ≥ 20% of cells in 11 of 36 subjects (30.5%). The response rate was 9.1% in these patients (high-level status) as compared to a response rate of 60.0% in the 25 patients in whom AGT was detected in < 20% of cells (low-level status). These results indicate that although the patients with partial and complete responses are virtually all in a category predictive for "favorable" results (i.e., high percentage of cells staining for MSH2 and MLH1 and low percentage of cells staining for AGT) a prior knowledge of these parameters only predicts approx 66% of the responses no doubt reflecting, among other possibilities, alternative mechanisms of resistance. Eleven patients whose tumors had high percentage of cells stain-ing for AGT reveals different results, with 1 PR, 2 SD, and 8 PD. These results clearly suggest that definition of AGT status can identify the majority of patients who will not respond to temozolomide.

2.4.2. Non-O⁶-Alkylguanine-DNA Alkyltransferase

An additional mechanism of resistance to chloroethyl nitrosoureas is glutathione-mediated quenching of the mono-adduct *(5,8,9)*. However, the mono-adduct is not susceptible to either AGT removal or glutathione quenching *(9,106)*. Additional mechanisms of resistance must be operational and repair of the DNA interstrand crosslink is a possible mechanism to be considered *(7)*. Indeed, several investigators have demonstrated repair of BCNU-induced DNA interstrand crosslink although the cellular pathways remain undefined *(4,7,119)*.

An additional mechanism of resistance to temozolomide in CNS tumors was recently identified after our laboratory established a methylator-resistant human GBM xenograft by serially treating the parent xenograft with procarbazine *(52)*. A deficiency of DNA mismatch repair from the absence of a functional hMSH2, was noted in the resistant xenograft. Additional work has demonstrated temozolomide resistance mediated by mismatch repair deficiency in cell lines *(88,130)*. Although mismatch repair deficiency has been associated with human tumor cell resistance to methylators *(74,80)*, this observation that serial in vivo methylator treatment produced acquired mismatch repair deficiency suggests that this may be clinically relevant.

2.5. Cyclophosphamide: Mechanisms of Resistance

The recognition of the frequency and consequences of alkylator resistance in the therapy of medulloblastoma (and indeed in the entire spectrum of human malignancies) has fueled a plethora of studies designed to identify and theoretically bypass or reverse the mechanisms mediating this resistance. Resistance to alkylating agents, including cyclophosphamide, is multifactorial with a diverse spectrum of mechanisms observed in murine and human neoplasia, including increased aldehyde dehydrogenase activity *(67)*, increased GST activity *(92,123)*, and elevated levels of GSH *(1)*.

Repair of DNA interstrand crosslinks is increasingly being correlated to cellular resistance of tumor cells to these agents. A diverse spectrum of approaches quantitating repair in whole cells, including evaluation of unscheduled DNA synthesis, rate of adduct or crosslink removal, and expression and survival of damaged plasmids have shown enhanced DNA repair in resistant (to nitrogen mustards or cisplatin) tumor cells *(11,13,17,21,22,40,60,62,67,77,93,105,115,126,129,136,140)*.

Resistance of medulloblastoma to cyclophosphamide is similarly multifactorial, with increased aldehyde dehydrogenase activity *(50)*, elevated glutathione content *(50)*, and repair of DNA interstrand crosslinks *(37)* demonstrated in a panel of cell lines with clinically acquired or laboratory-generated resistance. The consequences of cyclophosphamide resistance, in conjunction with the therapeutic value of this agent in the treatment of medulloblastoma, make it critical to understand the mechanisms of this resistance.

3. MODULATION OF O⁶-ALKYLGUANINE-DNA ALKYLTRANSFERASE TO ENHANCE ALKYLATOR AND METHYLATOR ACTIVITY

3.1. Inhibition of O⁶-Alkylguanine-DNA Alkyltransferase

Depletion of AGT, either by methylating agents that generate O⁶-methylguanine residues in DNA *(3,29,31–35,63,98,134,139)*, renders cells more sensitive to chloroethylnitrosourea and methylator-induced cytotoxicity, presumably by way of increased formation of interstrand cross-links or initiation of a lethal cycle of mismatch repair. The role of AGT inhibitors in modulating temozolomide or chloroethylnitrosourea activity in clinical trials will be limited by the magnitude of demonstrable AGT activity in patients' tumors as well as the toxicity to normal tissue produced by inhibition of repair activity. Although approx 30% of human tumor cell lines are AGT deficient, the majority of primary tumor samples demonstrate the presence of this enzyme and may be appropriate targets for combination therapy. Methylating agents such as streptozocin or temozolomide can decrease AGT activity by the introduction of O⁶-methylguanine moieties into DNA that are subsequently repaired by AGT. Nevertheless, the dose of methylating agent required for appreciable enzyme inhibition can be associated with significant toxicity *(98)*. Furthermore, methylating agents may present the risk of introducing promutagenic lesions, with a potential for the development of new malignancies *(106)*. O^6-alkylguanines are direct, specific substrates for AGT and produce inhibition by "suicide" inactivation. Although O^6-methylguanine increased nitrosourea activity in vitro, the substantial doses required in vivo (reflecting its low affinity for AGT), coupled with the limited solubility of this agent, renders it ineffective in vivo *(30)*.

3.2. O^6-Benzylguanine

O^6-Benzylguanine, which demonstrates greater affinity for the alkyltransferase protein compared with O^6-methylguanine, effectively enhances nitrosourea activity both in vitro and in vivo. Early studies *(33,98)* have demonstrated cessation of growth but no tumor regressions using combination therapy with O^6-benzylguanine plus a nitrosourea. Later studies demonstrated substantial growth delays of human medulloblastoma and glioma xenografts growing subcutaneously and intracranially in athymic nude mice, and were the first to demonstrate complete and partial tumor regressions in almost all the tumors treated with BCNU plus O^6-benzylguanine. Furthermore, no additional toxicity was seen using reduced doses of BCNU *(45,50)*.

3.3. Phase I Trial of O^6-Benzylguanine

Early phase evaluation of anticancer agents has traditionally used toxicity to establish dosing schedules. However, because BG is a biochemical modulatory agent, the dose of BG required to deplete AGT activity in tumor was considered in its clinical development. We conducted a phase 1 trial of pre-surgery O^6-benzylguanine in patients with malignant glioma, which was designed to define the dose required for depletion of tumor AGT activity *(57)*. Patients were treated approx 18 h prior to craniotomy at doses ranging between 40–100 mg/m^2 intravenously over 1 h. Resected tumor was snap frozen in liquid nitrogen and AGT activity analyzed using a biochemical assay measuring removal of O^6-methylguanine from a methylated DNA substrate. Cohorts of up to 14 patients were treated at a specific dose of O^6-BG, with a target endpoint of $\geq 11/14$ patients with undetectable tumor AGT levels (defined as < 10 fmol/mg protein). Thirty patients with malignant gliomas were enrolled, with 11/11 patients treated at 100 mg/m^2 O^6-benzylguanine demonstrating undetectable tumor AGT levels. No toxicity was noted. These results indicate that 100 mg/m^2 of O^6-benzylguanine can maintain tumor AGT levels < 10 fmol/mg protein for at least 18 h after treatment, a time interval in which BCNU-induced adducts are converted into interstrand crosslinks. In a separate study using needle biopsies from patients with systemic tumors, Spiro et al. *(118)* determined the dose required to reduce AGT activity to undetectable levels 18 h post-BG treatment as 120 mg/m^2. The difference in the biochemical modulatory dose between these studies could reflect differences in the site of the tumor (glioma vs systemic tumors), the limitations in assaying small needle biopsies vs surgical biopsies or random variation.

3.4. Phase I Trials of O^6-Benzylguanine Plus BCNU

Three academic centers (Duke University, University of Chicago, and Case Western Reserve) conducted phase I trials combining O^6-benzylguanine with BCNU to define the toxicity and maximum tolerated dose (MTD) of BCNU in conjunction with the preadministration of O^6-benzylguanine in patients with cancer *(36,54,113,118)*. The Duke study focused on recurrent or progressive malignant glioma *(54)*, whereas the other studies evaluated patients with systemic tumors. Patients were treated with O^6-BG at a dose of 100 mg/m^2 followed 1 h later by BCNU. Cohorts of 3 to 6 patients were treated with escalating doses of BCNU, and patients were observed for at least 6 wk before being considered assessable for toxicity. Twenty-three patients were treated (22 with glioblastoma multiforme and one with anaplastic astrocytoma). Four dose levels of BCNU (13.5, 27, 40, and 55 mg/m²) were evaluated, with the highest dose level being complicated by grade 3 or 4 thrombocy-topenia and neutropenia. These results indicate that the MTD of BCNU, when given in combination with O⁶-BG at a dose of 100 mg/m², is 40 mg/m² administered at 6-wk intervals. This study provided the foundation for a phase II trial of O⁶-BG plus BCNU in nitrosourea-resistant malignant glioma.

3.5. Phase II Trial of O⁶-Benzylguanine Plus BCNU

We ultimately treated 18 patients with nitrosourea-resistant GBM with BCNU plus O⁶-benzyl-guanine using the doses detailed in the phase 1 trial summarized earlier *(110)*. No responses were seen and 8 patients displayed grade 3/4 hematopoeitic toxicity. These results indicate that either additional mechanisms of resistance to nitrosoureas are operational or more likely the dose of BCNU, limited by toxicity, was too low to produce anti-tumor activity. This provides rationale for tumor (as opposed to bone marrow) specific AGT depletion.

In total, these results indicate the failure of BCNU plus O⁶-benzylguanine to restore sensitivity to patients whose GBMs are BCNU resistant and the reduction of the BCNU dose that can be given as a result of hematopoeitic toxicity. The reduced dose of BCNU may explain the failure to see tumor responses although alternative mechanisms of resistance are potentially operational. This strongly supports our efforts to utilize regional administration of AGT inhibitors in combination with systemic or regional chemotherapy to increase the therapeutic index.

3.6. Phase I Trial of O⁶-Benzylguanine Plus Temozolomide

We are conducting a phase I trial of temozolomide plus O⁶-BG to define the MTD of temozolomide along with the toxicity and activity of this drug combination in the treatment of adults with progressive or recurrent, World Health Organization (WHO) grade 3 or greater astrocytoma, oligodendro-glioma, or mixed glial tumor *(110)*. Patients are treated with IV O⁶-BG and a 48-h infusion of O⁶-BG. Following demonstration of the dose of O⁶-BG (120 mg/m² over 1 h followed by the 48 h infusion of 30 mg/m²/d) that depletes tumor AGT levels, we started temozolomide at a single dose of 100 mg/m² given at the end of the IV push of O⁶-BG. Temozolomide doses are escalated in cohorts of 3 to 6 patients. Treatment cycles are repeated at 28-d intervals. Radiographic response criteria were utilized to evaluate activity using T₁-weighted, enhanced MRI images. Twenty-one patients have been treated to date, 15 with glioblastoma multiforme (GBM), 5 with anaplastic astrocytoma (AA), and 1 with anaplastic oligodendroglioma (AO). Seven patients received temozolomide at 100 mg/m², 7 received 200 mg/m², 6 received 267 mg/m², and 1 received 355 mg/m². Toxicities observed thus far have been limited to 1 patient with grade-3 neutropenia, and 1 patient with grade-3 alanine amino-transferase (ALT) elevation. Stable disease has been observed in 4 patients; 2 after one cycle and 2 after two cycles. A patient who previously failed temozolomide has shown a near complete response while completing six cycles of this drug combination. Further enrollment will continue to determine the MTD and toxicity of this drug combination and result in a phase 2 trial of O⁶-BG plus temozolomide in patients with temozolomide-resistant malignant glioma.

REFERENCES

1. Ahmad S., Okine L., Le B., et al. 1987. Elevation of glutathione in phenylalanine mustard-resistant murine L1210 leukemia cells. *J. Biol. Chem.* **262**:15048–15053.
2. Aida T., Bodell W.J. 1987. Cellular resistance to chloroethylnitrosoureas, nitrogen, mustard, and cisdiammine dichloroplatinum (II) in human glial-derived lines. *Cancer Res.* **47**:1361–1366.
3. Aida T., Cheitlin R.A., Bodell W.J. 1987. Inhibition of O⁶-alkylguanine-DNA alkyltransferase activity potentiates cytoxicity and induction of SCE's in human glioma cells resistant to 1,3-bis(2-chloroethyl)-1-nitrosourea. *Carcinogenesis* **8**:1219–1223.
4. Ali-Osman F., Berger M.S., Rajagopa S., Spence A., Livingston R.B. 1993. Topoisomeras II inhibition and altered kinetics of formation and repair of nitrosourea and cisplatin induced DNA interstrand crosslinks and cytotoxicity in human glioblastoma cells. *Cancer Res.* 53:5663.

5. Ali-Osman F., Caughlan J., Gray G.S. 1989. Decreased DNA interstrand crosslinking and cytotoxicity induced in human brain tumor cells by 1,3-bis(2-chloroethyl)-1-nitrosourea after in vitro reaction with glutathione. *Cancer Res.* **49:**5954–5958.

6. Ali-Osman F., Giblin J., Berger M., Murphy M.J., Jr., Rosenblum M.L. 1985. Chemical structure of carbamoylating groups and their relationship to bone marrow toxicity and antiglioma activity of bifunctionally alkylating and carbamoylating nitrosoureas. *Cancer Res.* 45:4185–4191.

7. Ali-Osman F., Rairkar A., Young P. 1995. Formation and repair of 1,3-bis-(2-chloroethyl)-1-nitrosourea and cisplatin induced total genomic DNA interstrand crosslinks in human glioma cells. *Cancer Biochem. Biophys.* **14:**231–241.

8. Ali-Osman F Stein D.E., Renwick A. 1990. Glutathione content and glutathione-S-transferase expression in 1,3-bis(2-chloroethyl)-1-nitrosourea-resistant human malignant astrocytoma cell lines. *Cancer Res.* 6976–6980.

9. Ali-Osman F. 1989. Quenching of DNA crosslink precursors of chloroethylnitrosoureas and attenuation of DNA interstrand crosslinking by glutathione. *Cancer Res.* **49:**5258–5261.

10. Allen J.C., Helson L. 1981. High-dose cyclophosphamide chemotherapy for recurrent CNS tumors in children. *J. Neurosurg.* **55:**749–756.

11. Batist G., Torres-Garcia S., Demuys J.-M., et al. 1989. Enhanced DNA cross-link removal: the apparent mechanism of resistance in a clinically relevant melphalan-resistant human breast cancer cell line. *Mol. Pharmacol.* **36:**224–230.

12. Batra S.K., McLendon R.E., Koo J.S., Castelino-Prabhu S., Fuchs H.E., Krischer J.P., et al. 1995. Prognostic implications of chromosome 17p deletions in human medulloblastomas. *J. Neurooncol.* **24:**39–45.

13. Bedford P., Fichtinger-Schepman A., Shellard S., et al. 1988. Differential repair of DNA adducts in human bladder and testicular tumour continuous cell lines. *Cancer Res.* **48:**3019–3024.

14. Belanich M., Pastor M., Randall T., et al. 1996. Retrospective study of the correlation between the DNA repair protein alkyltransferase and survival of brain tumor patients treated with carmustine. *Cancer Res.* **56:**783–788.

15. Bodell W.J., Aida T., Berger M.S., Rosenblum M. 1986. Increased repair of O6-alkylguanine-DNA alkyltransferase in glioma-derived human cells resistant to the cytotoxic and cytogenetic effects of 1,3-bis(2-chloroethyl)-1-nitrosourea. *Carcinogenesis* **6:**879–883.

16. Bogden J.M., Eastman A., Bresnick E. 1981. A system in mouse liver for the repair of O6-methylguanine lesions in methylated DNA. *Nucleic Acids Res.* **9:**3089–3103.

17. Bramson J., McQuillan A., Panasci L.C. 1995. DNA repair enzyme expression in chronic lymphocytic leukemia via-a-vis nitrogen mustard drug resistance. *Cancer Lett.* **90:**139–148.

18. Brent T.P., Houghton P.J., Houghton J. 1985. O^6-alkylguanine-DNA alkyltransferase activity correlates with the therapeutic response of human rhabdomyosarcoma xenografts to 1-(2-chloroethyl)-3-(trans-4-methylcyclohexyl)-1-nitrosoures. *PNAS* **82:**2985–2989.

19. Brookes P., Lawley P.D. 1961. The reaction of mono- and di-functional alkylating agents with nucleic acids. *Biochem. J.* 80:496–503.

20. Catapano C.V., Broggini M., Erba E., Ponti M., Mariani L. Citti L., D'Incalci M. 1987. *In vitro* and *in vivo* methazolastone-induced DNA damage and repair in L-1210 leukemia sensitive and resistant to chloroethylnitrosoureas. *Cancer Res.* **47:**4884–4889.

21. Chao C., Lee Y., Cheng P., Lin-Chao S. 1991. Enhanced host cell reactivation of damaged plasmid DNA in HeLa cells resistant to *cis*-diamminedichloroplatinum(II). *Cancer Res.* **51:**601–605.

22. Chao C., Lee Y., Lin-Chao S. 1990. Phenotypic reversion of cisplatin resistance in human cells accompanies reduced host cell reactivation or damaged plasmid. *Biochem. Biophys. Res. Commun.* **170:**851–859.

23. Colvin M., Brundrett R.B., Cowens W. Jardine I., Ludlum D.B. 1976. A chemical basis for the antitumor activity of chloroethylnitrosoureas. *Biochem. Pharmacol.* **25:**695–699.

24. Colvin M., Chabner B.A. 1990. Alkylator agents, In Cancer Chemotherapy Principles and Practice (Chabner, B.A., Colins, J.M., eds.), J.P. Lippincott, Philadelphia, PA, pp. 276–313.

25. D'Atri S., Piccioni D., Castellano A., Tuorto V., Franchi A., Lu K., et al. 1995. Chemosensitivity to triazene compounds and O6-alkylguanine-DNA alkyltransferase levels: studies with blasts of leukaemic patients. *Ann. Oncol.* **6:**389–393.

26. Day R.S., Ziolowski C.H.J., Scudiero D.A., Meyer S.A., Lubiniecki A.J., Girardi S.M., et al. 1980. Defective repair of alkylated DNA by human tumor and SV40-transformed human cell stains. *Nature* **288:**724–727.

27. Deans B., Tisdale M.J. 1992.Antitumor imidazotetrazines XXVIII 3-methyladenine DNA glycosylase activity in cell lines sensitive and resistant to temozolomide. *Cancer Lett.* **63:**151–157.

28. Denny B.J., Wheelhouse R.T., Stevens M.F.G., Tsang L.L.H., Slack J.A. 1994.A NMR and molecular modeling investigation of the mechanism of activation of the antitumor drug temozolomide and its interaction with DNA. *Biochem.* **33:**9045–9051.

29. Dolan M.E., Corsico C.D., Pegg A.E. 1985. Exposure of HeLa cells to O^6-alkylguanines increases sensitivity to the cytotoxic effects of alkylating agents. *Biochem. Biophys. Res. Comm.* **132:**1778–1785.

30. Dolan M.E., Larkin G.L., English H.F., et al. 1989. Depletion of O^6-alkylguanine-DNA alkyltransferase activity in mammalian tissues and human tumor xenografts in nude mice by treatment with O^6-methylguanine. *Cancer Chemother. Pharmacol.* **25:**103–108.

31. Dolan M.E., Mitchell R.B., Mummert C., et al. 1991. Effect of O⁶-benzylguanine analogues on sensitivity of human tumor cells to the cytotoxic effects of alkylating agents. *Cancer Res.* 51:3367–3372.

32. Dolan M.E., Morimoto K., Pegg A.E. 1985. Reduction of O⁶-alkylguanine-DNA alkyltransferase activity in HeLa cells treated with O⁶-alkylguanines. *Cancer Res.* **45**:6413–6417.

33. Dolan M.E., Moschel R.C., Pegg A.E. 1990. Depletion of mammalian O⁶-alkylguanine-DNA alkyltransfererse activity by O⁶-benzylguanine provides a means to evaluate the role of this protein in protection against carcinogenic and therapeutic alkylating agents. Proc. Natl. Acad. Sci. USA 87:5368–5372.

34. Dolan M.E. Stine L., Mitchell R.B., et al. 1990. Modulation of mammalian O⁶-alkylguanine-DNA alkyltransferase in vivo by O⁶-benzylguanine and its effect on the sensitivity of human glioma tumor to 1-(2-chloroethyl)-3-(4-methyl-cyclohexyl)-1 nitrosourea. *Cancer Commun.* **2**:371–377.

35. Dolan M.E., Young G.S., Pegg A.E. 1986. Effect of O⁶-alkylguanine pretreatment on the sensitivity of human colon tumor cells to the cytotoxic effects of chloroethylating agents. *Cancer Res.* 46:4500–4504.

36. Dolan M.E., Roy S.K., Fasanmade A.A., Paras P.R., Schilsky R.L., Ratain M.J. 1998. O⁶-benzylguanine in humans: metabolic, pharmacokinetic, and pharmacodynamic findings. *J. Clin. Oncol.* **16**:1803–1810.

37. Dong, Q., Bullock, N., Ali-Osman, F., Colvin, O.M., Bigner, D.D., Friedman, H.S. 1996. Repair analysis of 4-hydroperoxycyclophosphamide-induced DNA interstrand crosslinking in the c-myc gene in 4-hydroperoxycyclophosphamide-sensitive and –resistant medulloblastoma cell lines. *Cancer Chemother. Pharmcol.* **37**:242–246.

38. Drummond J.T., Li G.M., Longley M.J., Modrich P. 1995. Isolation of an hMSH2-p160 heterodimer that restores DNA mismatch repair to tumor cells. *Science (Washington, DC)* **268**:1909–1912.

39. Duffner P.K., Horowitz M.E., Krischer J., Friedman H.S., Burger P.C., Cohen M.E., et al. 1993. Post‚Ä'operative chemotherapy and delayed radiation in children less than 3 years of age with malignant brain tumors: a Pediatric Oncology Group study. *New Engl. J. Med.* **328**:1725–1731.

40. Eastman A., Schulte N. 1988. Enhanced DNA repair as a mechanism of resistance to *cis*-diamminedichloroplatinum(II). *Biochem.* **27**:4730–4734.

41. Erickson L.C., Laurent G., Sharkey N.A., Kohn K. 1980 DNA cross-linking and monoadduct repair in nitrosourea—treated human tumor cells. *Nature* **288**:727–729.

42. Esteller M., Garcia-Foncillas J., Andion E., Goodman S.N., Hidalgo O.F., Vanaclocha V., et al. 2000. Inactivation of the DNA-repair gene MGMT and the clinical response of gliomas to alkylating agents. *New Engl. J. Med.* **243**:1350–1354.

43. Evans A.E., Jenkin R.D.T., Sposto R., et al. 1990. The treatment of medulloblastoma. Results of a prospective randomized trial of radiation therapy with and without CCNU, vincristine and prednisone. *J. Neurosurg.* **72**:572–582.

44. Ewig R.A., Kohn K.W. 1977. DNA damage and repair in mouse leukemia L1210 cells treated with nitrogen mustard. 1,3-bis(2-chloroethyl)-1-nitrosourea and other nitrosoureas. *Cancer Res.* **37**:2114–2122.

45. Felker G.M., Friedman H.S., Dolan M.E., Moschel R.C., Schold C. 1993. Treatment of subcutaneous and intracranial brain tumor xenografts with O⁶-benzylguanine and 1,3 bis(2-chloroethyl)-1-nitrosourea. *Cancer Chemother. Pharmacol.* **32**:471–476.

46. Fine, H.A. 1994. The basis for current treatment recommendations for malignant gliomas. *J. Neuro-Oncol.* **20**:111–120.

47. Fram R.J., Sullivan J., Marinus M.G. 1986. Mutagenesis and repair of DNA damage caused by nitrogen mustard, N,N'-bis(2-chloroethyl)-N-nitrosourea (BCNU), streptozotocin, and mitomycin C in E. coli. *Mutat. Res.* **166**:229–242.

48. Friedman H.S., Bigner S.H., McComb R.D., et al. 1983. A model for human medulloblastoma: growth, morphology and chromosomal analysis in vitro and in athymic mice. J. *Neuropathol. Ex. Neurol.* **42**:485–503.

49. Friedman H.S., Colvin O.M., Ludeman S.M., et al. 1986. Experimental chemotherapy of human medulloblastoma with classical alkylators. *Cancer Res.* **46**:2827–2833.

50. Friedman H.S., Dolan M.E., Moschel R.C., Pegg A.E., Felker GM, Rich J, et al. 1992. Enhancement of nitrosourea activity in medulloblastoma and glioblastoma multiforme. *JNCI* **84**:1926–1931.

51. Friedman H.S., Dolan M.E., Pegg A.E., Marcelli S., Keir S., Catino J.J., et al. 1995. Activity of temozolomide with or without O⁶,Ä'benzylguanine in the treatment of central nervous system tumor xenografts. *Cancer Res.* **55**:2853–2857.

52. Friedman H.S., Johnson S.P., Dong Q., Schold S.C., Rasheed B.K.A., Bigner S.H., et al. 1997. Methylator resistance mediated by mismatch repair deficiency in a glioblastoma multiforme xenograft. *Cancer Res.* **57**:2933–2936.

53. Friedman H.S., Mahaley M.S. Jr, Schold S.C. Jr, et al. 1986 Efficacy of vincristine and cyclophosphamide in the therapy of recurrent medulloblastoma. *Neurosurgery* **18**:335–340.

54. Friedman H.S., Pluda J., Quinn J.A., Ewesuedo R.B., Long L., Friedman A.H., et al. 2000. Phase I trial of carmustine plus O⁶-benzylguanine for patients with recurrent or progressive malignant glioma. *J. Clin. Oncol.* **18**:3522–3528.

55. Friedman H.S., Schold S.C. Jr, Bigner D.D. 1986. Chemotherapy of subcutaneous and intracranial human medulloblastoma xenografts in athymic nude mice. *Cancer Res.* **46**:224–228.

56. Friedman H.S., Schold S.C., Mahaley M.S., Colvin O.M., Oakes W.J., Vick N.A., et al. 1989. Phase II treatment of medulloblastoma and pineoblastoma with melphalan: clinical therapy based on experimental models of human medulloblastoma. *J. Clin. Oncol.* **7**:904–911.

57. Friedman, H.S., Kokkinakis, D.M., Pluda, J., Friedman, A.H., Cokgor, I., Haglund, M.M., et al. 1998. Phase I trial of O⁶-benzylguanine for patients undergoing surgery for malignant glioma. *J. Clin. Oncol.* **16**:3570–3575.

58. Friedman, H.S., Petros, W.P., Friedman, A.H., Schaaf, L.J., Kerby, T., Lawyer, J., et al. 1999. Irinotecan therapy in adults with recurrent or progressive malignant glioma. *J. Clin. Oncol.* **17:**1516–1525.

59. Friedman H.S., Oakes W.J., Bigner, S.H., et al. 1991. Medulloblastoma: tumor biological and clinical perspectives. *J. Neurooncol.* **11:**1–15.

60. Futscher B.W., Pieper R.O., Dalton W.S., et al. 1992. Gene-specific DNA interstrand cross-links produced by nitrogen mustard in the human tumor cell line Colo320HSR. *Cell Growth Differ.* 3:217–223.

61. Garrett M.J., Hughes H.J., Freeman L.S. 1978. A comparison of radiotherapy alone with radiotherapy and CCNU in cerebral glioma. *Clin. Oncol.* **4:**71–76.

62. Geleziunas R., McQuillan A., Malapetsa A., et al. 1991. Increased DNA synthesis and repair-enzyme expression in lymphocytes from patients with chronic lymphocytic leukemia resistant to nitrogen mustards. *J. Natl. Cancer Inst.* **83:** 557–564.

63. Gerson S.L., Trey J.E., Miller K. 1988. Potentiation of nitrosourea cytotoxicity in human leukemic cells by inactivation of O6-alkylguanine-DNA alkyltransferase. *Cancer Res.* **48:**1521–1527.

64. Gonzaga P.E., Potter P.M., Niu T.Q., Yu D., Ludlum D.B., Rafferty J.A., et al. Identification of the crosslink between human O^6-methylguanine-DNA methyltransferase and chloroethylnitrosourea-treated DNA. *Cancer Res.* **52:** 6052–6058.

65. Green S.B., Byar D.P., Walker M.D., Pistenmaa D.A., Alexander E., Jr. Batzdorf U., et al. 1983. Comparison of carmustine, procarbazine, and high-dose methylprednisolone as additions to surgery and radiotherapy for the treatment of malignant glioma. *Cancer Treat. Rep.* **67:**121–132.

66. Hansson J. Lewensohn R., Ringborg U., et al. 1987. Formation and removal of DNA cross-links induced by melphalan and nitrogen mustard in relation to drug-induced cyotoxicity in human melanoma cells. *Cancer Res.* **47:**2631–2637.

67. Hilton J. 1984. Deoxyribonucleic acid crosslinking by 4-hydroperoxycyclophosphamide in cyclophosphamide-sensitive and –resistant L1210 cells. *Biochem. Pharmacol.* 33:1867–1872.

68. Hotta T., Saito T., Fujita H., Mikami T. Kurisu K., Kiya K., et al. 1994. O^6-alkylguanine-DNA alkyltransferase activity of human malignant glioma and its clinical implications. *J. Neuro-Oncol.* **21:**135–140.

69. Jaeckle, K.A., Eyre, H.J., Townsend, J.J., Schulman, S., Knudson, H.M., Belanich, M., et al. 1998. Correlation of tumor O6 methylguanine-DNA methyltransferase levels with survival of malignant astrocytoma patients treated with bis-chloroethylnitrosourea: a Southwest Oncology Group study, *J. Clin. Oncol.* **16:**3310–3315.

70. Karran P., Macpherson P., Ceccotti S., Dogliotti E., Griffin S., Bignami M. 1993. O^6-methylguanine residues elicit DNA repair synthesis by human cell extracts. *J. Biol. Chem.* **268:**15,878–15,886.

71. Karran P., Hampson R. 1996. Genomic instability and tolerance to alkylating agents. *Cancer Surv.* **28:**69–85.

72. Karran P., Bignami M. 1992. Self-destruction and tolerance in resistance of mammalian cells to alkylation damage. *Nucleic Acids Res.* **20:**2933–2940.

73. Kastan M.B., Schlaffer E., Russo J.E., et al. 1990. Direct demonstration of elevated aldehyde dehydrogenase in human hematopoietic progenitor cells. *Blood* **75:**1947–1950.

74. Kat A., Thilly W.G., Fang W.H., Longley M.J., Li G.M., Modrich P. 1993. An alkylation-tolerant, mutator human cell line is deficient in strand-specific mismatch repair. *Proc. Natl. Acad. Sci. USA* **90:**6424–6428.

75. Kohn K.W., Erickson L.C., Laurent G., Incore J., Sharkey N., Ewig R.A.1981. DNA crosslinking and the origin of sensitivity to chloroethylnitrosoureas, in *Nitrosoureas* (Prestayko A.W., Crooke S.T., Baker L.H., Carter S.K., Schein P.S., eds.), Academic Press, New York, pp. 69–83.

76. Kohn K.W., Ewig R.A.G., Erikson L.C., et al. 1981. Measurement of strand breaks and crosslinks by alkaline elution, in *DNA Repair: A Laboratory Manual of Research Procedures* (Friedberg E.C., Hanawalt P.C., eds.), Marcel Dekker, Inc., New York, pp. 379–401.

77. Kohn K.W., Spears C.L., Doty P. 1966. Interstrand cross-linking of DNA by nitrogen mustard. *J. Mol. Biol.* **19:**266–288.

78. Kohn K.W. 1977. Interstrand crosslinking of DNA by 1,3-bis(2-chloroethyl)-1-nitrosourea and other 1-(2-haloethyl)-1-nitrosourea. *Cancer Res.* **37:**1450–1454.

79. Kohn K.W., Hartley J.A., Mattes W.B. 1987. Mechanisms of DNA sequence selectivity of guanine-N7 positions by nitrogen mustards. *Nucleic Acids Res.* **15:**10,531–10,549.

80. Koi M., Umar A., Chauhan D.P., Cherian S.P., Carethers J.M., Kunkel T.A., Boland C.R. 1994. Human chromosome 3 corrects mismatch repair deficiency and microsatellite instability and reduces N-methyl-N'-nitro-N-nitrosoguanidine tolerance in colon tumor cells with homozygous hMLH1 mutation (Published erratum appears in Cancer Res. 55:201, 1995). *Cancer Res.* **54:**4308–4312.

81. Krischer J.D., Ragab A.H., Kun L., et al. 1991. Nitrogen mustard, vincristine, procarbazine and prednisone as adjuvant chemotherapy in the treatment of medulloblastoma: A POG study. *J Neurosurg.* **74:**905–909.

82. Lachance, D.H., Oette, D., Schold, S.C., Jr., Brown, M., Kurtzberg, J., Graham, M.L., et al. 1995. Dose escalation trial of cyclophosphamide with sagramostim in the treatment of central nervous system (CNS) neoplasms. *Med. Pediatr. Oncol.* 24:241–247.

83. Lawley P.D., Brookes P. 1967. Interstrand cross-linking of DNA by bifunctional alkylating agents. *J. Mol. Biol.* **25:** 143–160.

84. Levin V.A. 1985. Chemotherapy of primary brain tumors.*Neurol. Clin.* **3**:855–866.

85. Levin V.A., Silver P., Hannigan J., Wara W.M., Cotin P.H., Davis R.L., Wilson C.B. 1990. Superiority of post-radio-therapy adjuvant chemotherapy with CCNU, procarbazine, and vincristine (PCV) over BCNU for anaplastic gliomas. *Int. J. Radiation Oncol. Biol. Phys.* **18**:321–324.

86. Levin V.A., Wara W.M., Davis R.L., et al. 1986.NCOG protocol 6G91: seven-drug chemothearpy and irradiation for patients with glioblastoma multiforme. *Cancer Treat. Rep.* **70**:739–744.

87. Li, G.M., Modrich P. 1995. Restoration of mismatch repair to nuclear extracts of H6 colorectal tumor cells by a heterodimer of human MutL homologs. *Proc. Am. Assoc. Cancer Res.* **92**:1950–1954.

88. Liu L., Markowitz, S., Gerson S.L. 1996. Mistmach repair mutations override alkyltransferase in conferring resistance to temozolomide but not to 1,3-bis(2-chloroethyl)nitrosourea. *Cancer Res.* **56**:5375–5379.

89. Liu L., Taverna P., Whitacre C.M., Chatterjee S., Gerson S.L. 1999.Pharmacologic disruption of base excision repair sensitizes mismatch repair-deficient and –proficient colon cancer cells to methylating agents. *Clin. Cancer Res.* **5**:2908–2917.

90. Maccubbin A.E., Cabailes L., Riordan J.M., Huang D.H., Gurto H.L. 1991. A cyclophosphamide/DNA phosphoester adduct formed in vitro and in vivo. *Cancer Res.* **51**:886–892.

91. MacFarland J.G., Kirk M.C., Ludlum D.B. 1990. Mechanism of action of the nitrosoureas-IV. Synthesis of the 2-haloethylnitrosourea-induced DNA crosslink 1-(3-cytosinyl),2-(1-guanl)ethane. *Biochem. Pharmacol.* **39**:33–36.

92. McGown A.T., Fox B.W. 1986. A proposed mechanism of resistance to cyclophosphamide and phosphoramide mustard in a Yoshida cell line in vitro. *Cancer Chemother. Pharmacol.* **17**:223–226.

93. Masuda H., Ozols R., Lai J., et al. 1988. Increased DNA repair as a mechanism of acquired resistance to cis-diamminedchloroplatinum(II) in human ovarian cancer cell lines. *Cancer Res.* **48**:5713–5719.

94. Mattes W.B., Hartley J.A., Kohn K.W. 1986. DNA sequence selectivity of guanine-N7 alkylation by nitrogen mustards. *Nucleic Acids Res.* **14**:2971–2987.

95. Mattes W.B., Hartley J.A., Kohn K.W. 1986. Mechanism of DNA strand breakage by piperidine at sites of N7-alkylguanines. *Biochem. Biophys. Acta.* **868**:71–76.

96. Mattes W.B., O'Connor T.R. 1993. Recognition and repair by the E.coli Alk A protein of DNA adducts induced by nitrogen mustards. *Environ. Mol. Mutagen* **21**:46.

97. Mehta J.R., Przybylski M., Ludlum D.B. 1980. Alkylation of guanosine and deoxyguanosine by phosphoramide mustard. *Cancer Res.* **40**:4183–4186.

98. Mitchell R.B., Moschel R.C., Dolan M.E. 1992. Effect of O^6-benzylguanine on the sensitivity of human tumor xenografts to 1,3-bis(2-chloroethyl)-1-nitrosourea and on DNA interstrand cross-link formation. *Cancer Res.* **52**:1171–1175.

99. Moghrabi A., Fuchs H., Brown M., Schold Jr., S.C., Graham M., Kurtzberg J., et al. 1995. Cyclophosphamide in combination with sargramostim for treatment of recurrent medulloblastoma. *Med. Pediatr. Oncol.* **25**:190–196.

100. Mosijczuk A.D., Nigro M.A., Thomas P.R.M., Burger P.C., Krischer J.P., Morantz R., et al. 1993. Pre-radiation che-motherapy in advanced medulloblastoma: a Pediatric Oncology Group pilot study. *Cancer* **72**:2755–2762.

101. Newlands E.S., Backledge G.P., Slack J.A., Rustin G.J.S., Smith D.B., Stuart N.S.A., et al. 1992. Phase I trial of temozolomide (CCRG 81045: M&B 39831: NSC 362856). *Br. J. Cancer* **65**:287–291.

102. O'Reilly S.M., Newlands E.S., Glaser M.G., Bramptom M., Rice-Edwards J.M., Illingworth R.D., et al. 1993. Temozolomide: a new oral cytoxic chemotherapeutic agent with promising activity against primary brain tumours. *Eur. J. Cancer* **29A**:940–942.

103. Packer R.J., Goldwein J., Nicholson H.S., Vezina L.G., Allen J.C., Ris M.D., et al. 1999. Treatment of children with medulloblastomas with reduced-dose craniospinal radiation therapy and adjuvant chemotherapy: a Children's Cancer Group Study. *J. Clin. Oncol.* **17**:2127–2136.

104. Palombo F., Gallinari P., Iaccarino I., Lettieri T., Hughes M., D'Arrigo A., et al. 1995. GTBP, a 160-kilodalton protein essential for mismatch-binding activity in human cells. *Science (Washington, DC)* **268**:1912–1914.

105. Panasci L., Henderson D., Torres-Garcia S.J., Skalski V., Caplan S., Hutchinson M. 1988. Transport, metabolism, and DNA interaction of melphalan in lymphocytes from patients with chronic lymphocytic leukemia. *Cancer Res.* **48**:1972–1976.

106. Pegg A.E. 1990.Mammalian O^6-alkylguanine-DNA alkyltransferase: regulation and importance in response to alkylat-ing carcinogenetic and therapeutic agents. *Cancer Res.* **50**:6119–6129.

107. Pegg A.E., Wiest L., Foote R.S., Mitra S., Perry W. 1983. Purification and properties of O^6-methylguanine-DNA transmethylase from rat liver. *J. Biol. Chem.* 258:2327–2333.

108. Plowman J., Waud W.R., Koutsoukos A.D., Rubinstein L.V., Moore T.D., Grever MR. 1994. Preclinical antitumor activity of temozolomide in mice: efficacy against human brain tumor xenografts and synergism with 1,3-bis(2-chloroethyl)-1-nitrosourea. *Cancer Res.* 54:3793–3799.

109. Quinn J.A., Pluda J., Dolan M.E., Delaney S., Kaplan R., Rich J.N., et al. 2002. Phase II Trial of carmustine plus O^6-benzylguanine for patients with nitrosourea-resistant recurrent or progressive malignant glioma. *J. Clin. Oncol.* **20**:2277–2283.

110. Quinn J.A., Friedman A.H., Reardon D.A., Rich J.N., Sampson J.H., Evans B., et al. 2002. Phase II trial of Temodar in patients with progressive or recurrent low grade glioma. *J. Clin. Oncol.*, submitted.

111. Rhines L.D., Sampath P., Dolan M.E., Tyler B.M., Brem H., Weingart J. 2000. O^6-benzylguanine potentiates the antitumor effect of locally delivered carmustine against an intracranial rat glioma. *Cancer Res.* **60:**6307–6310.

112. Samson L., Cairns J. 1977. A new pathway for DNA repair in *E. Coli. Nature* **267:**281–284.

113. Schilsky R L, Dolan ME, Bertucci D, Ewesuedo RB, Vogelzang NJ, Mani S, et al. 2000. Phase I clinical and pharmacological study of O6-benzylguanine followed by carmustine in patients with advanced cancer. *Clin. Cancer Res.* **6:**3025–3031.

114. Schold S.C. Jr, Brent T.P., von Hofe E., et al. 1989. O^6-alkylguanine-DNA alkyltransferase and sensitivity to procarbazine in human brain tumor xenografts. *J. Neurosurg.* **70:**573–577.

115. Sheibani N., Jennerwein M., Eastman A. 1989. DNA repair in cells sensitive and resistant to *cis*-diamminedichloroplatinum(II): host cell reactivation of damaged plasmid DNA. *Biochemistry* **28:**3120.

116. Sklar R., Strauss B. 1981. Removal of O^6-methylguanine from DNA of normal and xeroderma pigmentosum-derived lymphoblastoid cells. *Nature* **289:**417–420.

117. Solero C.L., Monfardini S., Brambilla C., et al. 1979. Controlled study with BCNU vs CCNU as adjuvant chemotherapy following surgery plus radiotherapy for glioblastoma multifome. *Cancer Clin. Trials* **1979:**43–48.

118. Spiro T. P., Gerson, S. L., Liu L., Majka S., Haaga J., Hoppel C. L., et al. 1999. O6-benzylguanine: a clinical trial establishing the biochemical modulatory dose in tumor tissue for alkyltransferase-directed DNA repair. *Cancer Res.* **59:**2402–2410.

119. Sriram R., Ali-Osman F. 1990. S1-nuclease enhancement of the ethidium bromide binding assay of drug-induced DNA interstrand crosslinking in human brain tumor cells. *Biochem.* **187:**345–348.

120. Tait D.M., Thornton-Jones H., Bloom H.J.G., et al. 1990. Adjuvant chemotherapy for medulloblastoma: The first multi-centre control trial of the International Society of Paediatric Oncology (SIOP I). *Eur. J. Cancer.* **26:**464–469.

121. Taverna P., Catapano C.V., Citti L., Bonfanti M., D'Incalci M. 1992. Influence of O^6-methylguanine on DNA damage and cytotoxicity of temozolomide in L1210 mouse leukemia sensitive and resistant to chloroethylnitrosoureas. *Anticancer Drugs* **3:**401–405.

122. Tentori L., Graziani G., Gilberti S., Lacal P.M., Bonmassar E., D'Atri S. 1995. Triazene compounds induce apoptosis in O$_6$-alkylguanine-DNA alkyltransferase deficient leukemia cell lines. *Leukemia* **9:**1888–1895.

123. Tew K.D., Clapper M.L. 1988. Glutathione-*S*-transferases and anticancer drug resistance, in Mechanisms of Drug Resistance in Neoplastic Cells (Woolley, P.V., Tew K.D., eds.), Academic Press, NY, pp. 141–160.

124. Tong W.P., Kirk M.C., Ludlum D.B. 1982. Formation of the crosslink (deoxycytidyl-deoxyguanosinyl) ethane in DNA treated with BCNU. *Cancer Res.* 42:**3102**–3105.

125. Tong W.P., Kohn K.W., Ludlum D.B. 1982. Modification of DNA by different haloethylnitrosoureas. *Cancer Res.* **42:**4460–4464.

126. Torres-Garcia S.J., Cousineau L., Caplan S., et al. 1989. Correlation of resistance to nitrogen mustards in chronic lymphocytic leukemia with enhanced removal of melphalan-induced DNA cross-links. *Biochemical. Pharm.* **38:**3122–3123.

127. Vu V.T., Fenselau C.C., Colvin O.M. 1981. Identification of three alkylated nucleotide adducts from the reaction of guanosine 5'-monophosphate with phosphoramide mustard. *J. Am. Chem. Soc.* **103:**7362–7364.

128. Walker M.D., Green S.B., Byar D.P., et al. 1980. Randomized comparisons of radiotherapy and nitrosoureas for the treatment of malignant gliomas after surgery. *N. Engl. J. Med.* **303:**1323–1329.

129. Wassermann K., Kohn K.W., Bohr V.A. 1990. Heterogeneity of nitrogen mustard-induced DNA damage and repair at the level of the gene in chinese hamster ovary cells. *J. Biol. Chem.* **265:**13,906–13,913.

130. Wedge S.R., Porteous J.K., Newlands E.S. 1996. 3-aminobenzamide and/or O^6-benzylguanine evaluated as an adjuvant to temozolomide or BCNU treatment in cell lines of variable mismatch repair status and O^6-alkylguanine-DNA alkyltransferase activity. *Br. J. Cancer* 74:**1030**–1036.

131. Wedge S.R., Porteous J.K., Newlands E.S. 1997. Effect of single and multiple administration of an O^6-benzylguanine/temozolomide combination: an evaluation in a human melanoma xenograft model. *Cancer Chemother. Pharmacol.* **40:**266–272.

132. Wedge S.R., Porteous J.K., May B.L., Newlands E.S. 1996. Potentiation of temozolomide and BCNU cytotoxicity by O6-benzylguanine: a comparative study *in vitro. Br. J. Cancer* **71:**482–490.

133. Wiestler O., Kleihues P., Pegg A.E. 1984. O^6-alkylguanine-DNA alkyltransferase activity in human brain and brain tumors. *Carcinogenesis* **5:**121–124.

134. Yarosh D.B., Hurst-Calderone S., Babich M.A., et al. 1986. Potentiation of O^6-methylguanine-DNA methyltransferase and sensitization of human tumor cells to killing by chloroethylnitrosourea by O^6-methylguanine as a free base. *Cancer Res.* **46:**1663–1668.

135. Yarosh D.B. 1985. The role of O^6-methylguanine DNA methyltransferase in cell survival, mutagenesis and carcinogenesis. *Mutation Res.* **145:**1–16.

136. Yen L., Woo A., Christopoulopoulos G., Batist G., Panasci L., Roy R., et al. 1995. Enhanced host cell reactivation capacity and expression of DNA repair genes in human breast cancer cells resistant to bi-functional alkylating agents. *Mutat. Res.* **337:**179–189.

137. Yung, A., Levin, V.A., Brada, M., Friedman, H., Osoba, D., Olson, J., et al. 2000. Randomized, multicenter, open-label, Phase II, comparative study of temozolomide and procarbazine in the treatment of patients with glioblastoma multiforme at first relapse. *Br. J. Cancer* **83:**588–593.

138. Yung, A., Prados M., Poisson M., Rosenfeld S., Brada M., Friedman H.,et al. 1999. for the Temodal Brain Tumor Group: Multicenter Phase II trial of temozolomide in patients with malignant astrocytoma at first relapse. *J. Clin. Oncol.* **17:**2762–2769.

139. Zlotogorski C., Erickson L.C. 1984. Pretreatment of human colon tumor cells with DNA methylating agents inhibits their activity to repair chloroethyl monoadducts. *Carcinogenesis* **5:**83–87.

140. Zwelling L., Anderson T., Kohn K. 1979. DNA protein and DNA interstrand cross-linking by *cis-* and *trans-*platinum(II) diamminedichloride in L1210 mouse leukemia cells and relation to cytotoxicity. *Cancer Res,* **39:**365.

141. Zwelling L.A., Michaels S., Scharwtz H., et al. 1981. DNA cross-linking as an indicator of sensitivity and resistance of mouse L1210 leukemia to cis-diamminedichloroplatinum (II) and L-phenylalanine mustard. *Cancer Res.* **41:**640–649.

12

Role of Urokinase-Type Plasminogen Activator Receptor in Human Glioma Invasion

Sanjeeva Mohanam and Jasti S. Rao

1. INTRODUCTION

Tumor invasion results from a coordinated interaction between proteolytic enzymes that degrade basement membranes and extracellular matrix (ECM), and adhesive proteins that participate in cell attachment and migration. Degradation of the ECM is accomplished through the integrated action of several enzyme systems, including the activation of plasminogen through the urokinase pathway to generate plasmin. Plasminogen activators (PAs) released from cancer cells also aid in generating plasmin, thereby facilitating the invasion of those cells into the surrounding tissue *(22)*. The two types of PAs, urokinase-type plasminogen activator (uPA) and tissue-type plasminogen activator (tPA), are considered to be independent gene products with distinctive structural and functional properties. Although their protein and cDNA sequences are quite different, uPA and tPA share a major substrate (plasminogen) and specific serpin-class inhibitors, the plasminogen-activator inhibitors (PAIs). uPA is secreted as a single pro-uPA zymogen that has little plasminogen-activating activity, is independent of fibrin, and is largely receptor-bound, whereas the single-chain form of tPA is catalytically active, fibrin-dependent, and primarily intravascular. Plasmin generated by either tPA or uPA directly degrades several protein constituents of the ECM, as well as activating certain other protease zymogens and latent growth factors and releasing growth factors from their ECM binding sites *(57)*. Of these two profibrinolytic enzymes, uPA has been studied more thoroughly in relation to tumor invasion.

2. UROKINASE-TYPE PLASMINOGEN ACTIVATOR RECEPTOR

The receptor for the urokinase-type plasminogen activator (uPAR), also called CD87, is related to members of the human CD59 and the mouse Ly-6 family *(89)*. The uPAR gene has been mapped to chromosome 19q13.2 and is composed of seven exons, separated by six introns, and occupies about 21.23 kb *(85)*. The expression of the uPAR gene can be regulated via the Sp1, AP-2, NFκB, and AP-1 transcription factors by specific motifs contained within the first 188 bp upstream of the transcriptional start site *(63,86)*. The messenger ribonucleic acid (mRNA) for uPAR also contains another specific sequence within the coding region (nucleotides 195–246) that can destabilize mRNA upon binding to an unidentified protein *(72)*. Human uPAR is encoded as a 1.4-kb mRNA transcript *(69)*. Primer extension experiments have demonstrated that the transcription start site is located 50 bp upstream of the translation start site of the human uPAR gene *(85)*.

The uPAR is expressed on the surface of many normal cell types, including circulating blood leukocytes, endothelial and vascular smooth muscle cells, fibroblasts, and bone marrow cells, as well

From: *Contemporary Cancer Research: Brain Tumors*
Edited by: F. Ali-Osman © Humana Press Inc., Totowa, NJ

as on a variety of neoplastic cells *(4)*. Recently, Montuori et al. *(54,55)* reported that uPA upregulates the cell surface expression of its own receptor, independently of its enzymatic activity, in several cell types. In contrast, uPA-mediated induction of uPAR in Beas2B lung epithelial cells is not accomplished through its receptor and requires enzyme activity *(73)*. The expression of the uPAR gene is influenced by tumor promoters, growth factors, cytokines, hormones, atherogenic lipoproteins, and hypoxia at both the transcriptional and post-transcriptional levels. Both extracellular signaling-regulated kinase (ERK) and C-jun *N*-terminal kinase (JNK) seem to be involved in the full induction of uPAR by phorbol myristate acetate (PMA) *(28,40)*. The constitutive and inducible expression of the uPAR requires a jun-D and a c-jun binding AP-1 motif *(41)*.

The uPAR is synthesized as a 313-amino acid polypeptide that is folded through disulfide bonding into three homologous repeats known as domains 1, 2, and 3. A heavily glycosylated protein, uPAR contains five potential glycosylation sites. Its hydrophobic carboxy-terminal domain is processed during biosynthesis and substituted by a glycosylphosphatidylinositol (GPI) anchor that targets the receptor to the outer leaflet of the plasma membrane bilayer. At the cell surface, uPAR exists in both a three-domain form that is capable of binding uPA and a two-domain form (devoid of domain 1) that does not bind uPA *(15)*. Formation of the uPAR–uPA complex with high affinity seems to require that residues located at equivalent positions in uPAR domains 1 and 3 be in close physical proximity to each other *(64)*. Pro-uPA, di-isopropyl fluorophosphate (DFP)-inactivated uPA, uPA, and the amino-terminal fragment of uPA all bind with the same affinity to uPAR. The interaction of uPA with its receptor exhibits some species specificity; human uPA does not bind to murine uPAR, and murine uPA does not recognize human uPAR. The amino acids Asn22, Asn27, His29, and Trp30 in human uPA have been identified as being key determinants in the species-specific binding of uPA to uPAR *(67)*. Four regions within the uPAR sequence have been found to bind directly to uPA: two distinct regions in uPAR domain 1 containing amino acids 13–20 and amino acids 74–84, and two regions in the putative loop 3 of domains 2 and 3, uPAR (154–176) and uPAR (247–276) *(42)*.

GPI-anchored uPAR is susceptible to glycolytic and lipolytic enzymes, the action of which releases the entire protein moiety or parts of it from the cell surface. uPA is capable of cleaving GPI-anchored uPAR in the linker region between domains 1 and 2; this region is also sensitive to cleavage by other proteases. Recent studies have shown that purified full-length GPI-anchored uPAR was more susceptible to uPA-mediated cleavage than was recombinant truncated soluble uPAR (suPAR) *(31)*. Anchorless, soluble forms of uPAR and uPAR fragments D1 and D2–D3 have been identified in conditioned medium from various cell lines *(58,75)*, and in body fluids from cancer patients *(45,58,82)*; these fragments may arise by differential splicing, proteolysis, or phospholipase C cleavage of the GPI anchor. The uPAR is shed from the surface of uPAR-expressing cells, most of which do not have an intact glycolipid anchor either constitutively or in response to certain soluble stimuli. Recombinant suPAR fragments have strong and specific chemotactic activity in several different cell types in vitro *(17,80)*. Use of cellular and soluble uPAR and mutant receptors has shown that D1 plays a crucial role in the ability of uPAR to mediate cellular binding to vitronectin (VN) *(74)*. In vitro, the soluble uPA–uPAR complex can be harbored by cell-surface and ECM-bound VN *(10)*; this harboring would result in redistribution and enhancement of uPA-dependent plasminogen activation at sites distant from the location of uPAR production *(8)*. Spliced uPAR cDNAs that lack the sequence encoding the GPI attachment site also have been detected in mouse, rat, and human tissues *(4,50)*.

The uPAR is essential for the cell-surface-associated plasminogen activation mediated by its ligand uPA. Binding of uPA to uPAR regulates uPA activity, accelerating its conversion from prouPA to the active form. Receptor-bound uPA that is complexed to its inhibitor, plasminogen activator inhibitor-1 (PAI-1), is internalized by low-density lipoprotein receptor-related protein (LRP) and degraded in lysosomes *(18)*. Recently, Czekay et al. *(14)* showed that binding of uPAR to LPR is essential for clearance of uPA–PAI-1 complexes, regeneration of unoccupied uPAR, and plasmin generation at the cell surface. In vivo, the uPAR can function independently of uPA. For example, injection of a fusion protein (a growth factor domain of murine uPA conjugated to human immunoglobulins [IgG]) impaired the influx of neutrophils into the lung in response to a chemotactic agent in wild-type and uPA-null mice, but not in uPAR-null mice *(84)*. This impairment was related to uPAR occupancy and not to disruption of uPAR-mediated proteolysis, indicating that uPAR has protease-independent functions in vivo *(84)*. In another study, mice deficient in uPAR (uPAR–/–) were shown to have diminished neutrophil recruitment in response to *Pseudomonas aeruginosa* infection compared with neutrophil recruitment in wild-type mice, indicating that this function is independent of uPA activity *(29)*.

3. TUMOR CELL INVASION

The expression level of uPAR on cells strongly correlates with their migratory and invasive potential, although proteolytic activity of uPA is not always required for cell migration. Also, high expression of uPA is linked to poor prognosis in patients with one of several tumor types *(71,95)*. uPAR-dependent cell-surface plasminogen activation contributes to the invasiveness and metastatic behavior of tumor cells. On the one hand, inhibition of uPAR expression has been shown to inhibit tumor cell invasiveness, prevent metastasis, reverse invasive behavior, and increase the tumor latency period *(2,4,39,49,97)*. Conversely, overexpression of uPAR in human tumor cells resulted in increased invasiveness and tumorigenicity both in vivo and in vitro *(50)*. Bacteriophage peptides that inhibit the uPA–uPAR interaction have been shown to inhibit angiogenesis and primary tumor growth in syngeneic mice *(46)*. For some tumor types (e.g., colorectal carcinoma, breast cancer, and squamous cell lung carcinoma), the presence of high levels of uPAR seems to indicate poor prognosis *(25,71,95)*. Patients with lung, ovarian, breast, or colorectal cancer have also been shown to have higher plasma levels of suPAR than do healthy individuals *(59)*. In another study by the same investigators, suPAR levels correlated with number of circulating tumor cells in patients with acute myeloid leukemia. Moreover, given that suPAR levels decreased rapidly during chemotherapy in these patients, the elevated plasma suPAR was thought to have been produced by circulating tumor cells *(58)*. Another group found that serum suPAR levels were greatly elevated in the majority of patients with benign prostate hyperplasia and prostate cancer but not in normal individuals, suggesting that suPAR may be useful as a diagnostic marker or an indicator of prognosis in patients with prostate cancer *(45)*.

4. CELL ADHESION AND SIGNALING

The expression of uPAR on the surface of different cells varies. In contrast to normal cells, malignant tumor cells usually overexpress uPAR *(4,15,52)*. Many lines of evidence support the notion that uPAR also takes part in multiple lateral protein-protein interactions, relevant not only to proteolysis *(98)* but also to cell adhesion and signal transduction *(36)*, where uPAR serves as a cell-surface molecule that interacts with many potential ligands *(15)*. The uPAR has been reported to have three unrelated extracellular protein ligands—uPA, VN *(30)*, and kininogen *(13)*. Additional nonintegrin co-receptors such as gp 130, mannose-6-phosphate-receptor/insulin-like growth factor-II receptor, LRP, or uPAR-associated protein (uPARAP/Endo 180) have been found in physical association with uPAR in vitro *(7,23,35,61,87)*. Cell motility (such as that associated with chemotaxis or cell migration) stimulated by active uPA can involve plasmin generation and subsequent degradation of ECM proteins or proteolytic "trimming" of cell surface components, including adhesion receptors and uPAR itself. The latter process refers to the generation of truncated uPAR; truncated soluble uPAR seems to mimic uPA in stimulating chemotaxis in rat smooth muscle cells *(17)*. The binding of uPA to uPAR induces cell adhesion, migration, proliferation, and maintenance of differentiation programs that are preceded by a signaling event and activation of genes, suggesting that uPAR undergoes a conformational change to initiate signaling. In one study, two forms of uPA, the wild-type form and a mutant form in which 24 amino acids at the amino-terminus had been substituted with a random sequence of amino acids, showed similar binding to uPAR, but only the wild-type uPA induced cell migration *(77)*. Chemotaxis of THP-1 monocytes can be induced not only by uPA or its amino-terminus fragment but also by the two-domain D2–D3 form of uPAR, whereas suPAR did not induce chemotaxis *(24,68)*. A synthetic peptide containing the sequence of the linker region that connecting domains 1 and 2 in intact uPAR could stimulate chemotaxis of THP-1 monocylic cells, uPAR-deficient macrophages, and NIH3T3 fibroblasts *(24)*. In MCF-7 breast carcinoma cells, by contrast, both the connecting peptide and the intact suPAR induced cell migration *(60)*.

The uPAR domains 2 and 3 are also important in VN binding *(30)*. Multimeric rather than mono-meric, VN is the predominant high-affinity ligand for uPAR. Because overlapping binding sites for uPAR, PAI-1, and kininogen are present along the amino-terminal domain of VN *(66)*, uPAR and PAI-1 compete for binding to VN *(19)* in addition to VN binding to uPAR *(9,83)*. Through these differential interactions, uPAR and αv integrin-mediated cell adhesion to VN can be competed for by PAI-1 and kininogen, respectively. A two-chain, high molecular weight form of kininogen devoid of its component vasodilator peptide bradykinin has been shown to bind uPAR in a zinc-dependent manner, to compete with VN for binding to uPAR, and to dissociate cell-bound VN from uPAR *(9)*. The activities of uPA and PAI-1 contribute to the dual functionality (proteolysis and cell adhesion) of the uPAR system in cellular interactions. VN has been shown to concentrate the uPA–suPAR complex to cell surfaces and ECM sites, which leads to the accumulation of plasminogen activator activity required for cell migration and tissue remodeling. uPA and VN promote direct interactions between uPAR and the integrins as well as modulating both uPAR and integrin function. However, even though the effects of VN and uPA on cell migration are additive, the signaling pathways that mediate these effects are different in rat aortic smooth muscle cells *(16)*. In human melanoma cells, blocking the VN receptor with immobilized antibodies induced a rapid, up to 4.5-fold increase in uPAR mRNA levels and resulted in a significant increase in cell-surface-associated plasmin, which coincided with an increase in cell invasion *(33)*. Moreover, uPAR fragments can promote uPAR-dependent cell adhesion on VN; to do so, fragment (154–176) in D2 requires the presence of uPA, but fragment (247–276) in D3 does not *(42)*.

uPAR has also been associated with several members of the β1, β2, and β3-integrin families, indicating the strong involvement of uPAR in cell adhesion and migration as well as supporting the concept that integrins may function as signal transducers for plasminogen activation. The coexistence of uPAR with specific integrins at different cellular locations is a prerequisite for the regulation of integrin function by the uPAR *(81)*. In leukocytes, uPAR interacts with various β2 integrins, and consequently the inhibition or removal of uPAR will result in integrin dysfunction. In an in vivo study, the β2 integrin-dependent recruitment of leukocytes to the inflamed peritoneum of uPAR-deficient mice was significantly reduced relative to that in wild-type animals *(44)*, indicating that both β2 integrin-mediated leukocyte–endothelial cell interactions and their recruitment to inflamed areas require the presence of uPAR. The association between uPAR and the β2 integrins have been clearly shown to initiate a variety of direct and indirect regulatory mechanisms for both adhesive and proteolytic processes *(65)*.

The uPAR forms "*cis*"-interactions with integrins as an associated protein and thereby transduces proliferative or migratory signals to cells upon binding of uPA. Binding of suPAR to α4β1 and αvβ3 is blocked by known soluble ligands and by mutated integrin that inhibits ligand binding, suggesting that uPAR is an integrin ligand in addition to being an integrin-associated protein *(79)*. In addition, GPI-anchored uPAR on the cell surface specifically binds to integrins on contiguous cells, suggesting that uPAR–integrin interactions may mediate cell-to-cell interactions ("*trans*"-interactions) *(79)*. In nonhematopoietic cells that do not express β2 integrins, the uPAR seems to interact with β1 and β3 integrins *(90)*. uPAR specifically associates with certain members of the β1 and β3 integrin families on adherent tumor cells, and ECM components induce specific integrin–uPAR associations to enable directional proteolysis by which tumor cells can migrate and invade *(62,65,90)*. In recent experiments, a peptide homologous to integrin sequences suspected of being a uPAR binding site was identified and shown to disrupt uPAR–integrin interactions *(76)*. Several studies point to the possibility that the level of caveolin influences the outcome of uPAR–integrin interactions *(88)*. However, results obtained with the tumorigenic carcinoma cells HEp3, which do not contain caveolin, indicate that the density with which uPAR is expressed and the association of uPAR with respective integrins determines the state of integrin activation *(2)*.

Substantial evidence supports the concept that uPA–uPAR–integrin interactions activate signaling pathways and adhesion or migration events. Co-immunoprecipitation of cell lysates with anti-uPAR antibodies has identified a multitude of signaling cascades, among them several Src protein tyrosine kinase cascades. Src pathways have been implicated in the chemotaxis of THP-1 and smooth muscle cells *(17,24)*. Treatment with uPA or its amino-terminal fragment has been shown to regulate the switch between active and inactive states of Hck and Fgr protein tyrosine kinases in myeloid cells *(11)*. In HEp3 cells, uPA binding to uPAR induces a strong, persistent, fibronectin-dependent activation of ERK signaling *(3)*. In that study, when uPAR was downregulated or the uPAR–integrin interaction was disrupted in HEp3 cells, the ERK pathway became deactivated, the cells arrested in G0/G1, and tumors became dormant. uPA is involved in the activation of focal adhesion kinase (FAK) and p130cas in the prostate cancer cell line (LNCaP) *(96)* and endothelial cells *(78)*, but the mechanism through which uPAR is activated is not known. Several other signaling pathways have been identified as a result of uPA binding to uPAR or uPAR aggregation through specific cross-linking antibodies. Studies have shown that uPAR is an activator of the Jak/Stat signaling and transcription pathway in both tumor epithelial and vascular smooth muscle cells *(20,21,35)*. Current studies suggest that the uPA–uPAR–integrin complex mediates signaling through the MEK-ERK pathway, with upstream feeding signals derived from Src, Src-like kinases, and FAK, and activation of these pathways produces different biological outcomes such as differentiation, migration, and growth in various tumor cells.

5. UROKINASE-TYPE PLASMINOGEN ACTIVATOR RECEPTOR AND ITS ROLE IN GLIOMAS

Gliomas, the most common of the primary brain tumors, extensively invade the surrounding normal brain tissue and are extremely refractory to therapy. Proteolytic degradation of the ECM *(70)* is thought to be the initial step in the process of glioma tumor cell invasion and neovascularization. The roles of uPA and its receptor in this process have attracted a great deal of research attention. An increase in uPA activity has been found in the more malignant astrocytoma cell lines in vitro *(51,53)*, and in malignant human brain tumors in vivo *(38,92)*; in the latter situation, the presence of high uPA levels was associated with poor prognosis *(6,32)*. The invasive capability of tumor cells is facilitated by the expression of uPAR on the tumor cell surface *(43)*. uPAR-mediated pericellular proteolysis or the interaction of uPAR with adhesion molecules results in variable adhesion or detachment events and is pivotal for the control of cell migration and invasion.

We found that the expression of uPAR in human glioblastoma cell lines could contribute to their invasive capability *(26,53)*. uPAR expression was significantly higher in anaplastic astrocytoma and glioblastoma cells than in normal brain tissues or in low-grade gliomas, and uPAR tended to be found in the greatest amounts at the leading edges of the tumors *(26,93)*. In U251MG glioblastoma cells, uPAR was found to be localized at the cell–ECM focal contacts, together with the $\alpha v \beta 3$ integrin *(26)*. Other studies indicated that LRP was overexpressed in malignant astrocytomas, especially in glioblastomas, and that the increased expression of LRP seemed to correlate with the expression of uPAR and the malignancy of the astrocytomas *(91)*. The addition of basic fibroblast growth factor (bFGF) or transforming growth factor (TGF)-α to human glioma cells produced increases in cellular mRNA levels of uPAR and uPA, and the addition of anti-uPAR monoclonal antibodies to these cells significantly inhibited their bFGF- or TGF-α-induced invasiveness *(56)*. We also found that uPAR promoter activity was upregulated in high-grade glioblastoma cell lines, a finding that suggests that increased transcription is likely to be the mechanism underlying the increase in uPAR expression in high-grade gliomas *(5)*.

Selective inhibition of the uPA–uPAR interaction is considered a feasible approach for the treatment of malignant brain tumors. Downregulation of uPAR expression in glioblastoma cells by expression of an antisense-uPAR vector significantly decreased the migration and invasiveness of those cells *(48,49)*. Furthermore, glioblastoma cells expressing antisense-uPAR complementary deoxyribonucleic acid (cDNA), or cells in which uPAR has been downregulated by the addition of an adenoviral Ad-uPAR construct formed significantly smaller tumors when they were injected into the cerebra of nude mice *(27,47)*. Moreover, injection of the Ad-uPAR construct into previously established subcutaneous U87MG tumors in nude mice caused regression of those tumors *(47)*, a finding that supports the therapeutic potential of targeting the uPA–uPAR system for the treatment of gliomas. Antisense-mediated downregulation of uPAR expression in glioblastoma cells has been shown to increase expression of integrin $\alpha3\beta1$, but not that of integrin $\alpha5\beta1$, in vitro *(12)*. In our experiments, reducing the expression of uPAR in human glioma cells led to morphologic changes, decreased spreading, and cytoskeletal disorganization, suggesting that coordinated expression of uPAR and integrins may be involved in the spreading of glioma cells *(12)*. Stable antisense-uPAR transfectants of glioblastoma cells undergo apoptosis when injected intracerebrally in nude mice or grown on fibronectin or VN-coated tissue culture plates in vitro. The increase in apoptotic cell death in vitro was associated with increased expression of the apoptotic protein Bax in uPAR-downregulated glioblastoma cells *(34)*. We also found that the antisense-uPAR stable transfectants had a loss in mitochondrial transmembrane potential, a corresponding release of cytochrome C from mitochondria, and a subsequent activation of caspase-9 in stable uPAR-antisense transfectants relative to the behavior of the parental cells *(94)*. Moreover, antisense-uPAR-transfected glioblastoma cells exhibited higher levels of the tumor necrosis factor-α-related apoptosis-inducing ligand (TRAIL) receptors DR4 and DR5 than did parental cells, rendering the transfectants susceptible to apoptotic stimuli such as TRAIL *(37)*. These findings suggest that downregulation of uPAR expression in human glioblastoma cells inhibits the invasiveness of these cells and enhances their susceptibility to apoptotic stimuli.

The tumor suppressor gene p16 is frequently inactivated in gliomas. Recent reports indicate that restoration of p16 protein inhibited $\alpha v\beta3$ integrin-mediated cell spreading on VN *(1)*. We hypothesized that downregulation of uPAR and overexpression of p16 may cause downregulation of $\alpha v\beta3$ integrin and integrin-mediated signaling between VN and tumor cells. To test this hypothesis, we used replication-deficient adenovirus vectors containing a bicistronic construct in which both antisense-uPAR and sense-p16 expression cassettes (Ad-uPAR-p16) were inserted in the E1-deleted region of the vector. We demonstrated that infecting malignant glioblastoma cells with this Ad-uPAR-p16 vector in the presence of VN resulted in decreased $\alpha v\beta3$ integrin expression and integrin-mediated biological effects, including reductions in adhesion, migration, proliferation, and survival *(1)*. These results support the concept that downregulation of the expression of integrin $\alpha v\beta3$, and the biological effects that depend on integrin-mediated signaling, in glioma cells through adenovirus-mediated transfer of the antisense-uPAR and sense-p16 genes may have therapeutic potential for treating human gliomas.

6. SUMMARY

In general, the role of uPAR seems to be to integrate different cellular events, such as focused proteolysis, dynamic multiple interactions between uPA, uPAR, PAI-1, ECM proteins, integrins and endocytosis receptors, cytoskeletal reorganization, and changes in gene expression. The uPAR has several potential ligands and seems to activate several signal transduction pathways, thus modulating cell attachment and chemotaxis by mechanisms independent of uPA's catalytic function or secondary to its uPA- or plasmin-mediated proteolysis. Investigations in cancer patients indicate that uPAR expression can be valuable as a marker of prognosis. Overexpression of uPAR in established glioblastoma cell lines and in brain tumor tissues suggests that uPAR may play a role in tumor invasiveness and malignancy, which in turn indicates that uPAR is a candidate for targeted gene therapy. Downregulation of uPAR expression in human glioblastoma cells through the use of an antisense approach has been shown to decrease tumor formation in nude mice and to induce apoptotic cell death. In this context, interfering with uPAR expression may offer an effective therapeutic strategy against malignant glioma in humans.

ACKNOWLEDGMENTS

This work was supported in part by NCI grant CA 75557 (to J.S.R.).

REFERENCES

1. Adachi Y., Lakka S.S., Chandrasekar N., Yanamandra N., Gondi C.S., Mohanam S., et al. 2001. Down-regulation of integrin αvβ3 expression and integrin-mediated signaling in glioma cells by adenovirus-mediated transfer of antisense urokinase-type plasminogen activator receptor (uPAR) and sense p16 genes. *J. Biol. Chem.* **276:**47,171–47,177.
2. Aguirre Ghiso J.A., Kovalski K., Ossowski L. 1999. Tumor dormancy induced by downregulation of urokinase receptor in human carcinoma involves integrin and MAPK signaling. *J. Cell Biol.* **147:**89–104.
3. Aguirre-Ghiso J.A., Liu D., Mignatti A., Kovalski K., Ossowski L. 2001. Urokinase receptor and fibronectin regulate the ERK^MAPK to p38 ^MAPK activity ratios that determine carcinoma cell proliferation or dormancy in vivo. *Mol. Biol. Cell* **12:**863–879.
4. Andreasen P.A., Egelund R., Petersen H.H. 2000. The plasminogen activation system in tumor growth, invasion, and metastasis. *Cell. Mol. Life Sci.* **57:**25–40.
5. Bhattacharya A., Lakka S.S., Mohanam S., Boyd D., Rao J.S. 2001. Regulation of the urokinase-type plasminogen activator receptor gene in different grades of human glioma cell lines. *Clin. Cancer Res.* **7:**267–276.
6. Bindal A.K., Hammoud M., Shi W.M., Wu S.Z., Sawaya R., Rao J.S. 1994. Prognostic significance of proteolytic enzymes in human brain tumors. *J. Neuro-Oncol.* **22:**101–110.
7. Behrendt N., Jensen O.N., Engelholm L.H., Mortz E., Mann M., Dano K. 2000. A urokinase receptor-associated protein with specific collagen binding properties. *J. Biol. Chem.* **275:**1993–2002.
8. Carriero M.V., Del Vecchio S., Franco P., Potena M.I., Chiaradonna F., Botti G., et al. 1997. Vitronectin binding to urokinase receptor in human breast cancer. *Clin. Cancer. Res.* **3:**1299–1308.
9. Chavakis T., Kanse S.M., Lupu F., Hammes H.P., Muller-Esterl W., Pixley R.A., et al. 2000. Different mechanisms define the antiadhesive function of high molecular weight kininogen in integrin- and urokinase receptor-dependent interactions. *Blood* **96:**514–522.
10. Chavakis T., Kanse S.M., Yutzy B., Lijnen H.R., Preissner K.T. 1998. Vitronectin concentrates proteolytic activity on the cell surface and extracellular matrix by trapping soluble urokinase receptor-urokinase complexes. *Blood* **91:**2305–2312.
11. Chiaradonna F., Fontana L., Iavarone C., Carriero M.V., Scholz G., Barone M.V., Stoppelli M.P. 1999. Urokinase receptor-dependent and -independent p56/59(hck) activation state is a molecular switch between myelomonocytic cell motility and adherence. *EMBO J.* **18:**3013–3023.
12. Chintala S.K., Mohanam S., Go Y., Venkaiah B., Sawaya R., Gokaslan Z.L., Rao J.S. 1997. Altered in vitro spreading and cytoskeletal organization in human glioma cells by downregulation of urokinase receptor. *Mol. Carcinogenesis* **20:**355–365.
13. Colman R.W., Pixley R.A., Najamunnisa S., Yan W., Wang J., Mazar A., McCrae K.R. 1997. Binding of high molecular weight kininogen to human endothelial cells is mediated via a site within domains 2 and 3 of the urokinase receptor. *J. Clin. Invest.* **100:**1481–1487.
14. Czekay R.P., Kuemmel T.A., Orlando R.A., Farquhar M.G. 2001. Direct binding of occupied urokinase receptor (uPAR) to LDL receptor-related protein is required for endocytosis of uPAR andregulation of cell surface urokinase activity. *Mol. Biol. Cell* **12:**1467–1479.
15. Dear A.E., Medcalf R.L. 1998. The urokinase-type-plasminogen-activator receptor (CD87) is a pleiotropic molecule. *Eur. J. Biochem.* **252:**185–193.
16. Degryse B., Orlando S., Resnati M., Rabbani S.A., Blasi F. 2001. Urokinase/urokinase receptor and vitronectin/αvβ3 integrin induce chemotaxis and cytoskeleton reorganization through different signaling pathways. *Oncogene* **20:**2032–2043.
17. Degryse B., Resnati M., Rabbani S.A., Villa A., Fazioli F., Blasi F. 1999. Src-dependence and pertussis-toxin sensitivity of urokinase receptor-dependent chemotaxis and cytoskeleton reorganization in rat smooth muscle cells. *Blood* **94:**649–662.

18. Degryse B., Sier C.F., Resnati M., Conese M., Blasi F. 2001. PAI-1 inhibits urokinase-induced chemotaxis by internalizing the urokinase receptor. *FEBS Lett.* **505:**249–254.

19. Deng G., Curriden S.A., Hu G., Czekay R.P., Loskutoff D.J. 2001. Plasminogen activator inhibitor-1 regulates cell adhesion by binding to the somatomedin B domain of vitronectin. *J. Cell. Physiol.* **189:**23–33.

20. Dumler I., Kopmann A., Wagner K., Mayboroda O.A., Jerke U., Dietz R., et al. 1999. Urokinase induces activation and formation of Stat4 and Stat1-Stat2 complexes in human vascular smooth muscle cells. *J. Biol. Chem.* **274:**24,059–24,065.

21. Dumler I., Weis A., Mayboroda O.A., Maasch C., Jerke U., Haller H., Gulba D.C. 1998. The Jak/Stat pathway and urokinase receptor signaling in human aortic vascular smooth muscle cells. *J. Biol. Chem.* **273:**315–321.

22. Ellis V, Murphy G. 2001. Cellular strategies for proteolytic targeting during migration and invasion. *FEBS Lett.* **506:**1–5.

23. Engelholm L.H., Nielsen B.S., Dano K., Behrendt N. 2001. The urokinase receptor associated protein (uPARAP/endo180): a novel internalization receptor connected to the plasminogen activation system. *Trends Cardiovasc. Med.* **11:**7–13.

24. Fazioli F., Resnati M., Sidenius N., Higashimoto Y., Appella E., Blasi F. 1997. A urokinase-sensitive region of the human urokinase receptor is responsible for its chemotactic activity. *EMBO J.* **16:**7279–7286.

25. Foekens J.A., Peters H.A., Look M.P., Portengen H., Schmitt M., Kramer M.D, et al. 2000. The urokinase system of plasminogen activation and prognosis in 2780 breast cancer patients. *Cancer Res.* **60:**636–643.

26. Gladson C.L., Pijuan-Thompson V., Olman M.A., Gillespie G.Y., Yacoub I.Z. 1995. Up-regulation of urokinase and urokinase receptor genes in malignant astrocytoma. *Am. J. Pathol.* **146:**1150–1160.

27. Go Y., Chintala S.K., Mohanam S., Gokaslan Z., Venkaiah B., Bjerkvig R.,et al. 1997. Inhibition of in vivo tumorigenicity and invasiveness of a human glioblastoma cell line transfected with antisense uPAR vectors. *Clin. Exp. Metastasis* **15:**440–446.

28. Gum R., Juarez J., Allgayer H., Mazar A., Wang Y., Boyd D. 1998. Stimulation of urokinase-type plasminogen activator receptor expression by PMA requires JNK1-dependent and –independent signaling modules. *Oncogene* **17:**213–225.

29. Gyetko M.R., Sud S., Kendall T., Fuller J.A., Newstead M.W., Standiford T.J. 2000. Urokinase receptor-deficient mice have impaired neutrophil recruitment in response to pulmonary Pseudomonas aeruginosa infection. *J. Immunol.* **165:**1513–1519.

30. Hoyer-Hansen G., Behrendt N., Ploug M., Dano K., Preissner K.T. 1997. The intact urokinase receptor is required for efficient vitronectin binding: receptor cleavage prevents ligand interaction. *FEBS Lett.* **420:**79–85.

31. Hoyer-Hansen G., Pessara U., Holm A., Pass J., Weidle U., Dano K., Behrendt N. 2001. Urokinase-catalysed cleavage of the urokinase receptor requires an intact glycolipid anchor. *Biochem. J.* **358:**673–679.

32. Hsu D.W., Efird J.T., Hedley-Whyte E.T. 1995. Prognostic role of urokinase-type plasminogen activator in human gliomas. *Am. J. Pathol.* **147:**114–123.

33. Khatib A.M., Nip J., Fallavollita L., Lehmann M., Jensen G., Brodt P. 2001. Regulation of urokinase plasminogen activator/plasmin-mediated invasion of melanoma cells by the integrin vitronectin receptor $\alpha v\beta 3$. *Int. J. Cancer* **91:**300–308.

34. Kin Y., Chintala S.K., Go Y., Sawaya R., Mohanam S., Kyritsis A.P., Rao J.S. 2000. A novel role for the urokinase-type plasminogen activator receptor in apoptosis of malignant gliomas. *Int. J. Oncol.* **17:**61–65.

35. Koshelnick Y., Ehart M., Hufnagl P., Heinrich P.C., Binder B.R. 1997. Urokinase receptor is associated with the components of the JAK1/STAT1 signaling pathway and leads to activation of this pathway upon receptor clustering in the human kidney epithelial tumor cell line TCL-598. *J. Biol. Chem.* **272:**28,563–28,567.

36. Koshelnick Y., Ehart M., Stockinger H., Binder B.R. 1999. Mechanisms of signaling through urokinase receptor and the cellular response. *Thromb. Haemostasis* **82:**305–311.

37. Krishnamoorthy B., Darnay B., Aggarwal B., Dinh D.H., Kouraklis G., Olivero W.C., et al. 2001. Glioma cells deficient in urokinase plaminogen activator receptor expression are susceptible to tumor necrosis factor -α-related apoptosis-inducing ligand-induced apoptosis. *Clin. Cancer Res.* **7:**4195–4201.

38. Lakka S.S., Bhattacharya A., Mohanam S., Boyd D., Rao J.S. 2001. Regulation of the uPA gene in various grades of human glioma cells. *Int. J. Oncol.* **18:**71–79.

39. Lakka S.S., Rajagopal R., Rajan M.K., Mohan P.M., Adachi Y., Dinh D.H, et al. 2001. Adenovirus-mediated antisense urokinase-type plasminogen activator receptor gene transfer reduces tumor cell invasion and metastasis in non-small cell lung cancer cell lines. *Clin. Cancer Res.* **7:**1087–1093.

40. Lengyel E., Wang H., Gum R., Simon C., Wang Y., Boyd D. 1997. Elevated urokinase-type plasminogen activator receptor expression in a colon cancer cell line is due to a constitutively activated extracellular signal-regulated kinase-1-dependent signaling cascade. *Oncogene* **14:**2563–2573.

41. Lengyel E., Wang H., Stepp E., Juarez J., Wang Y., Doe W., et al. 1996. Requirement of an upstream AP-1 motif for the constitutive and phorbol ester-inducible expression of the urokinase-type plasminogen activator receptor gene. *J. Biol. Chem.* **271:**23,176–23,184.

42. Liang O.D., Chavakis T., Kanse S.M., Preissner K.T. 2001. Ligand binding regions in the receptor for urokinase-type plasminogen activator. *J. Biol. Chem.* **276:**28,946–28,953.

43. MacDonald T.J., DeClerck Y.A., Laug W.E. 1998. Urokinase induces receptor mediated brain tumor cell migration and invasion. *J. Neuro-Oncol.* **40:**215–226.

44. May A.E.,, Kanse S.M., Lund L.R., Gisler R.H., Imhof B.A., Preissner K.T. 1998. Urokinase receptor (CD87) regulates leukocyte recruitment via β2 integrins in vivo. *J. Exp. Med.* **188:**1029–1037.

45. McCabe N.P., Angwafo F.F., Zaher A., Selman S.H., Kouinche A., Jankun J. 2000. Expression of soluble urokinase plasminogen activator receptor may be related to outcome in prostate cancer patients. *Oncol. Rep.* **7:**879–882.

46. Min H.Y., Doyle L.V., Vitt C.R., Zandonella C.L., Stratton-Thomas J.R., Shuman M.A., Rosenberg S. 1996. Urokinase receptor antagonists inhibit angiogenesis and primary tumor growth in syngeneic mice. *Cancer Res.* **56:**2428–2433.

47. Mohan P.M., Chintala S.K., Mohanam S., Gladson C.L., Kim E.S., Gokaslan Z.L., et al. 1999. Adenovirus-mediated delivery of antisense gene to urokinase-type plasminogen activator receptor suppresses glioma invasion and tumor growth. *Cancer Res.* **59:**3369–3373.

48. Mohan P.M., Lakka S.S., Mohanam S., Kin Y., Sawaya R., Kyritsis S.P., Nicolson G.L., Rao J.S. 1999. Downregulation of the urokinase-type plasminogen activator receptor through inhibition of translation by antisense oligonucleotide suppresses invasion of human glioblastoma cells. *Clin. Exp. Metastasis* **17:**617–621.

49. Mohanam S., Chintala S,K., Go Y., Bhattacharya A., Venkaiah B., Boyd D., et al. 1997. In vitro inhibition of human glioblastoma cell line invasiveness by antisense uPA receptor. *Oncogene* **14:**1351–1359.

50. Mohanam S., Gladson C.L., Rao C.N., Rao J.S. 1999. Biological significance of the expression of urokinase-type plasminogen activator receptors (uPARs) in brain tumors. *Front. Biosci.* **4:**D178–D187.

51. Mohanam S., Jasti S.L., Kondraganti S.R., Chandrasekar N., Kin Y., Fuller G.N., et al. 2001. Stable transfection of urokinase-type plasminogen activator antisense construct modulates invasion of human glioblastoma cells. *Clin. Cancer Res.* **7:**2519–2526.

52. Mohanam S., Go Y., Sawaya R., Venkaiah B., Mohan P.M., Kouraklis G.P., et al. 1999. Elevated levels of urokinase-type plasminogen activator and its receptor during tumor growth in vivo. *Int. J. Oncol.* **14:**169–174.

53. Mohanam S., Sawaya R., McCutcheon I., Ali-Osman F., Boyd D., Rao J.S. 1993. Modulation of in vitro invasion of human glioblastoma cells by urokinase-type plasminogen activator receptor antibody. *Cancer Res.* **53:**4143–4147.

54. Montuori N., Mattiello A., Mancini A., Santoli M., Taglialatela P., Caputi M., Rossi G., Ragno P. 2001. Urokinase-type plasminogen activator up-regulates the expression of its cellular receptor through a post-transcriptional mechanism. *FEBS Lett.* **508:**379–384.

55. Montuori N., Salzano S., Rossi G., Ragno P. 2000. Urokinase-type plasminogen activator up-regulates the expression of its cellular receptor. *FEBS Lett.* **476:**166–170.

56. Mori T., Abe T., Wakabayashi Y., Hikawa T., Matsuo K., Yamada Y., Kuwano M., Hori S. 2000. Up-regulation of urokinase-type plasminogen activator and its receptor correlates with enhanced invasion activity of human glioma cells mediated by transforming growth factor-alpha or basic fibroblast growth factor. *J. Neuro-Oncol.* **46:**115–123.

57. Murphy G., Gavrilovic J. 1999. Proteolysis and cell migration: creating a path? *Curr. Opin. Cell. Biol.* **11:**614–621.

58. Mustjoki S., Sidenius N., Sier C.F., Blasi F., Elonen E., Alitalo R., Vaheri A. 2000. Soluble urokinase receptor levels correlate with number of circulating tumor cells in acute myeloid leukemia and decrease rapidly during chemotherapy. *Cancer Res.* **60:**7126–7132.

59. Mustjoki S., Sidenius N., Vaheri A. 2000. Enhanced release of soluble urokinase receptor by endothelial cells in contact with peripheral blood cells. *FEBS Lett.* **486:**237–242.

60. Nguyen D.H., Webb D.J., Catling A.D., Song Q., Dhakephalkar A., Weber M.J., et al. 2000. Urokinase-type plasminogen activator stimulates the Ras/Extracellular signal-regulated kinase (ERK) signaling pathway and MCF-7 cell migration by a mechanism that requires focal adhesion kinase, Src, and Shc. Rapid dissociation of GRB2/Sps-Shc complex is associated with the transient phosphorylation of ERK in urokinase-treated cells. *J. Biol. Chem.* **275:** 19,382–19,388.

61. Nykjaer A., Christensen E.I., Vorum H., Hager H., Petersen C.M., Roigaard H., et al. 1998. Mannose 6-phosphate/insulin-like growth factor-II receptor targets the urokinase receptor to lysosomes via a novel binding interaction. *J. Cell Biol.* **141:**815–828.

62. Ossowski L., Aguirre-Ghiso J.A. 2000. Urokinase receptor and integrin partnership: coordination of signaling for cell adhesion, migration and growth. *Curr. Opin. Cell Biol.* **12:**613–620.

63. Park I.K., Lyu M.A., Yeo S.J., Han T.H., Kook Y.H. 2000. Sp1 mediates constitutive and transforming growth factor beta-inducible expression of urokinase type plasminogen activator receptor gene in human monocyte-like U937 cells. *Biochim. Biophys. Acta.* **1490:**302–310.

64. Ploug M. 1998. Identification of specific sites involved in ligand binding by photoaffinity labeling of the receptor for the urokinase-type plasminogen activator. Residues located at equivalent positions in uPAR domains I and III participate in the assembly of a composite ligand-binding site. *Biochemistry* **37:**16,494–16,505.

65. Preissner K.T., Kanse S.M., May A.E. 2000. Urokinase receptor: a molecular organizer in cellular communication. *Curr. Opin. Cell. Biol.* **12:**621–628.

66. Preissner K.T., Seiffert D. 1998. Role of vitronectin and its receptors in haemostasis and vascular remodeling. *Thromb. Res.* **89:**1–21.

67. Quax P.H.A., Grimbergen J.M., Lansink M., Bakker A.H.F., Belin D., van Hinsbergh V.W.M., Varheijen J.H. 1998. Binding of human urokinase-type plasminogen activator to its receptor. Residues involved in species specificity and binding. *Arterioscler. Throm. Vasc. Biol.* **18:**693–701.

68. Resnati M., Guttinger M., Valcamonica S., Sidenius N., Blasi F., Fazioli F. 1996. Proteolytic cleavage of the urokinase receptor substitutes for the agonist-induced chemotactic effect. *EMBO J.* **15**:1572–1582.

69. Roldan A.L., Cubellis M.V., Masucci M.T., Behrendt N., Lund L.R., Dano K., et al. 1990. Cloning and expression of the receptor for human urokinase plasminogen activator, a central molecule in cell surface, plasmin-dependent proteolysis. *EMBO. J.* **9**:467–474.

70. Rooprai H.K., McCormick D. 1997. Proteases and their inhibitors in human brain tumours: a review. *Anticancer Res.* **17**:4151–4162.

71. Schmitt M., Harbeck N., Thomssen C., Wilhelm O., Magdolen V., Reuning U., et al. 1997. Clinical impact of the plasminogen activation system in tumor invasion and metastasis: prognostic relevance and target for therapy. *Thromb. Haemostasis* **78**:285–296.

72. Shetty S., Idell S. 1998. A urokinase receptor mRNA binding protein from rabbit lung fibroblasts and mesothelial cells. *Am. J. Physiol.* **274**:L871–L882.

73. Shetty S., Idell S. 2001. Urokinase induces expression of its own receptor in Beas2B lung epithelial cells. *J. Biol. Chem.* **276**:24,549–24,556.

74. Sidenius N., Blasi F. 2000. Domain 1 of the urokinase receptor (uPAR) is required for uPAR-mediated cell binding to vitronectin. *FEBS Lett.* **470**:40–46.

75. Sidenius N., Sier C.F., Blasi F. 2000. Shedding and cleavage of the urokinase receptor (uPAR): identification and characterisation of uPAR fragments in vitro and in vivo. *FEBS Lett.* **475**:52–56.

76. Simon D.I., Wei Y., Zhang L., Rao N.K., Xu H., Chen A., et al. 2000. Identification of a urokinase receptor-integrin interaction site. Promiscuous regulator of integrin function. *J. Biol. Chem.* **275**:10,228–10,234.

77. Stepanova V., Mukhina S., Kohler E., Resink T.J., Erne P., Tkachuk V.A. 1999. Urokinase plasminogen activator induces human smooth muscle cell migration and proliferation via distinct receptor-dependent and proteolysis-dependent mechanisms. *Mol. Cell. Biochem.* **195**:199–206.

78. Tang H., Kerins D.M., Hao Q., Inagami T., Vaughan D.E. 1998. The urokinase-type plasminogen activator receptor mediates tyrosine phosphorylation of focal adhesion proteins and activation of mitogen-activated protein kinase in cultured endothelial cells. *J. Biol. Chem.* **273**:18,268–18,272.

79. Tarui T., Mazar A.P., Cines D.B., Takada Y. 2001. Urokinase-type plasminogen activator receptor (CD87) is a ligand for integrins and mediates cell-cell interaction. *J. Biol. Chem.* **276**:3983–3990.

80. Trigwell S., Wood L., Jones P. 2000. Soluble urokinase receptor promotes cell adhesion and requires tyrosine-92 for activation of p56/59(hck). *Biochem. Biophys. Res. Commun.* **278**:440–446.

81. van der Pluijm G., Sijmons B., Vloedgraven H., van der Bent C., Drijfhout J.W., Verheijen J, et al. 2001. Urokinase-receptor/integrin complexes are functionally involved in adhesion and progression of human breast cancer in vivo. *Am. J. Pathol.* **159**:971–982

82. Wahlberg K., Hoyer-Hansen G., Casslen B. 1998. Soluble receptor for urokinase plasminogen activator in both full-length and a cleaved form is present in high concentration in cystic fluid from ovarian cancer. *Cancer Res.* **58**:3294–3298.

83. Waltz D.A., Natkin L.R., Fujita R.M., Wei Y., Chapman H.A. 1997. Plasmin and plasminogen activator inhibitor type 1 promote cellular motility by regulating the interaction between the urokinase receptor and vitronectin. *J. Clin. Invest.* **100**:58–67.

84. Waltz D.A., Fujita R.M., Yang X., Natkin L., Zhuo S., Gerard C.J., et al. 2000. Nonproteolytic role for the urokinase receptor in cellular migration in vivo. *Am. J. Respir. Cell. Mol. Biol.* **22**:316–322.

85. Wang Y. 2001. The role and regulation of urokinase-type plasminogen activator receptor gene expression in cancer invasion and metastasis. *Med. Res. Rev.* **21**:146–170.

86. Wang Y., Dang J., Wang H., Allgayer H., Murrell G.A., Boyd D. 2000. Identification of a novel nuclear factor-kappaB sequence involved in expression of urokinase-type plasminogen activator receptor. *Eur. J. Biochem.* **267**: 3248–3254.

87. Webb D.J., Nguyen D.H., Gonias S.L. 2000. Extracellular signal-regulated kinase functions in the urokinase receptor-dependent pathway by which neutralization of low density lipoprotein receptor-related protein promotes fibrosarcoma cell migration and matrigel invasion. *J. Cell Sci.* **113**:123–134.

88. Wei Y., Yang X., Liu Q., Wilkins J.A., Chapman H.A. 1999. A role for caveolin and the urokinase receptor in integrin-mediated adhesion and signaling. *J. Cell Biol.* **144**:1285–1294.

89. Witz I.P. 2000. Differential expression of genes by tumor cells of a low or a high malignancy phenotype: the case of murine and human Ly-6 proteins. *J. Cell. Biochem. Suppl.* **34**:61–66.

90. Xue W., Mizukami I., Todd III, R.F., Petty H.R. 1997. Urokinase-type plasminogen activator receptors associate with beta1 and beta3 integrins of fibrosarcoma cells: dependence on extracellular matrix components. *Cancer Res.* **57**:1682–1689.

91. Yamamoto M., Ikeda K., Ohshima K., Tsugu H., Kimura H., Tomonaga M. 1998. Expression and cellular localization of low-density lipoprotein receptor-related protein/alpha 2-macroglobulin receptor in human glioblastoma in vivo. *Brain Tumor Pathol.* **15**:23–30.

92. Yamamoto M., Sawaya R., Mohanam S., Bindal A.K., Bruner J.M., Oka K., et al. 1994. Expression and localization of urokinase-type plasminogen activator in human astrocytomas in vivo. *Cancer Res.* **54**:3656–3661.

93. Yamamoto M., Sawaya R., Mohanam S., Rao V.H., Bruner J.M., Nicolson G.L., Rao J.S. 1994. Expression and localization of urokinase-type plasminogen activator receptor in human gliomas. *Cancer Res.* **54:**5016–5020.

94. Yanamandra N., Konduri S.D., Mohanam S., Dinh D.H., Olivero W.C., Gujrati M., et al. 2000. Downregulation of urokinase-type plasminogen activator receptor (uPAR) induces caspase-mediated cell death in human glioblastoma cells. *Clin. Exp. Metastasis* **18:**611–615.

95. Yang J.L., Seetoo D.Q., Wang Y., Ranson M., Berney C.R., Ham J.M., et al. 2000. Urokinase-type plasminogen activator and its receptor in colorectal cancer: independent prognostic factors of metastasis and cancer-specific survival and potential therapeutic targets. *Int. J. Cancer* **89:**431–439.

96. Yebra M., Goretzki L., Pfeifer M., Mueller B.M. 1999. Urokinase-type plasminogen activator binding to its receptor stimulates tumor cell migration by enhancing integrin-mediated signal transduction. *Exp. Cell Res.* **250:**231–240.

97. Yu W., Kim J., Ossowski L. 1997. Reduction in surface urokinase receptor forces malignant cells into a protracted state of dormancy. *J. Cell Biol.* **137:**767–777.

98. Zhou H.M., Nichols A., Meda P., Vassalli J.D. 2000. Urokinase-type plasminogen activator and its receptor synergize to promote pathogenic proteolysis. *EMBO J.* **19:**4817–4826.

13

Regulation of Cell-Cycle and Apoptosis in Human Brain Tumors

Juan Fueyo, Candelaria Gomez-Manzano, and Timothy J. McDonnell

1. CELL-CYCLE CONTROL IN NORMAL LIFE

Cell division is the result of a series of events involving DNA replication (S phase), and the subsequent production of two daughter cells (M phase). The fundamental task of the cell-cycle is to ensure that DNA is faithfully replicated once during the S phase and that identical chromosomal copies are distributed equally to two daughter cells during the M phase. Cell-cycle progression depends on discrete control points to achieve that end. The control mechanisms that restrain cell-cycle transition or induce apoptotic-signaling pathways after cell stress are known as checkpoints. Ideally, checkpoints retard transition from one stage to another until a specific intrinsic or extrinsic condition has been satisfied. A complex system of positive and negative regulatory mechanisms governs cell-cycle progression, exerting control at various checkpoints. Two key control points in the cell-cycle are at the G1 checkpoint (DNA quality), and at the end of the G2 checkpoint (chromosomal quality) (Fig. 1). Lesions in the checkpoints regulatory pathways occur so frequently in cancer, regardless of patient age or tumor type, that they appear to be part of the life history of most, if not all, cancer cells (26,58, 64,83).

The G1 checkpoint, a coordinated cascade of signals, governs the transition from G1 to the S phase, resulting in normal Retinoblastoma (Rb)-susceptibility protein function. Regulation of Rb protein takes place through the interaction of a series of proteins, including p16, cyclin-dependent kinases 4 and 6 (CDK4/6), cyclin D, and E2F. Under nonreplicating conditions, Rb protein binds to and sequesters key transcriptional factors, including E2F. When it is time for the cell to replicate, cyclin D binds to CDK4 and CDK6, forming active kinases that phosphorylate Rb. The phosphorylated Rb then releases factors that transcriptionally activate S phase genes, permitting transition from G1 to the S phase. The p16 protein is one of the most important regulators of the CDK4-cyclin D complex. It blocks the binding of CDK4 to cyclin D, preventing phosphorylation of Rb, thus arresting the cell in the G1 phase. Inactivation of p16 or Rb, increased cyclin D1, or CDK4/6 activity results in progression to the S phase without regard to genomic integrity (64). In this regard, inactivation of Rb or p16 function, or overexpression of cyclin D or CDK4, are common events in human glioma cells (43).

The end of the G2 checkpoint initiates mitosis. Control of this checkpoint is, however, not as well understood as the factors that regulate the G1 checkpoint (26). In yeast, several genes have been identified as controllers of cell-cycle arrest in G2 after DNA damage (56). In mammalian cells, arrest in the G2 phase is caused by inhibitory phosphorylations of Cdc2. Dephosphorylation of Cdc2 at

From: *Contemporary Cancer Research: Brain Tumors*
Edited by: F. Ali-Osman © Humana Press Inc., Totowa, NJ

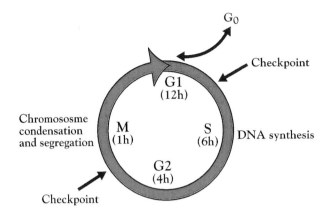

Fig. 1. Cell cycle clock. The active growth cycle of a cell can be divided into four discrete phases. A cell typically spends 6 to 8 h copying its DNA (S phase) and 3 to 4 h preparing for cell division (G2 phase). The formation of two daughter cells in mitosis (M phase) generally requires only about 1 h. After division daughter cells can undergo another division cycle and then will spend 12 h to prepare for the next round of DNA copying (G1). Alternatively, daughter cells can enter in a quiescent, nongrowing state (the G_0 phase). The control of cell-cycle progression occurs at discrete stages of the cell-cycle called checkpoints. Checkpoints are negative controls of cell-cycle progression that play an important role in preventing tumorigenesis. The two main checkpoints, G1 and G2, are located before the S and M phases, respectively.

these sites is catalyzed by the dual-specificity phosphatase Cdc25. Recent evidence suggests that the G2/M checkpoint involves inactivation, and possibly translocation, of Cdc25C into the cytoplasm, similar to that which occurs during the fission of yeast Cdc25 *(11)*. Data from several lines of evidence suggest that ataxia-telangiectasia-mutated (ATM) kinase is an upstream component of the DNA damage-induced cell-cycle checkpoint pathway *(73)*. ATM likely plays an important role in the G2/M checkpoint because, following DNA damage, ATM-deficient cells fail to arrest in the G2 phase of the cell-cycle prior to mitosis. The p53 protein also plays a role at the G2 checkpoint, which is one example of its importance in numerous aspects of cell-cycle control (Fig. 2).

2. ABNORMALITIES IN THE GLIOMA KARYOTYPE INDICATE DEREGULATION OF CELL CYCLE CHECKPOINTS OCCURRING IN GLIOMAS

Malignant gliomas are highly heterogeneous tumors. The number and type of genetic abnormalities that occur are not restricted to deregulation of single genes *(9,32,79)*. Analyses of malignant human glioma tissue obtained from biopsy have shown that more than 50% of tumors demonstrate epithelial growth factor receptor *(EGFR)* amplification *(52)*. The vast majority of tumors (81%) with gene amplification contain double minutes. One study showed that polysomy for chromosome 7 also occurred in more than 50% of tumors *(3)*. Results from another study *(31)* showed loss of constitutional heterozygosity for loci on chromosome 10 in more than 90% of tumors histologically classified as glioblastoma (World Health Organization [WHO], grade IV) but not in gliomas with a lower grade of malignancy. The authors also identified loss of sequences on chromosomes 13, 17, and 22, with at least one instance occurring in each grade of malignancy of adult glioma. The tumors in which loss of constitutional heterozygosity was observed were composed of one or a mixture of glial cell subtypes displaying astrocytic, oligodendrocytic, and/or ependymal differentiation.

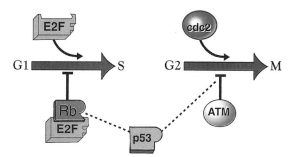

Fig. 2. Schematic representation of the main players in the control of the G1 and G2 checkpoints. The tumor suppressor gene Rb appears to be a critical component of the signaling pathway that arrest cells in G1 by sequestering the positive influence of the transcription factor E2F. After DNA damage, the ATM protein induces arrest of cells before mitosis counteracting the mitogenic stimuli of the cdc2 kinase. The p53 protein is upstream of Rb in controlling the G1 checkpoint. Following DNA damage, p53 is activated and upregulates p21, which in turns inhibits Rb phosphorylation and prevents the release of E2F activity. The p53 protein also participates in the control of the G2 checkpoint.

Taken together, these observations (and many others) suggest that highly malignant gliomas are characterized by the occurrence of multiple and important genetic abnormalities that involve both losses and gains of genetic material. Although some of the targets for amplification (such as *EGFR*) and for losses (such as *p16*) have already been identified, in many other cases (chromosome 6, chromosome 1, chromosome 7, etc.) the target gene and the significance of other abnormalities (such as polysomy of chromosome 7) remain under investigation. However, any conclusions derived from the inactivation, overexpression, or amplification of single genes are best viewed in a larger perspective. Toward that end and whenever possible, single gene abnormalities will be depicted in this chapter in a broad context of networks or pathways that affect or are affected by their abnormal function.

Low-grade gliomas usually express wild-type Rb and p16 proteins. However, inactivation of these two proteins and amplification of cyclin D1 and CDK4, which regulate the phosphorylation of Rb protein, are among the most frequent abnormalities that occur in anaplastic astrocytomas. Several studies have confirmed that inactivation of the *p16* gene by deletion of the *p16* locus in chromosome 9 is a frequent event in high-grade malignant gliomas. Thus, *p16* is deleted in approx 50% of glioblastomas *(33)*. In addition, the *p16* gene is silenced by methylation in a smaller percentage of cases *(13)*. That inactivation of p16 plays a role in the malignant phenotype of gliomas is emphasized by the fact that restoration of p16 activation modifies the unregulated growth of human glioma cells *(2,7,14)*. Immunohistochemical studies showed lack of expression of the *Rb* gene in 30% of glioblastomas *(28)*. Similar to p16, restoration of Rb to human glioma cells repressed their neoplastic phenotype *(15)*. Another important aspect of the inactivation of p16 and Rb is that they appear to be mutually exclusive. Thus, human gliomas expressing a wild-type Rb do not express the p16 protein, and vice versa. For that reason, the actual amount of human malignant gliomas with an abnormal regulation of the p16/Rb pathways exceeds 80% of the cases *(76)*.

The ultimate target of any alteration in the p16/Rb/E2F pathway is deregulation of E2F transcription factors. Among them, the E2F-1 protein transactivates several S-phase genes, and drives cell-cycle progression through the G_1 checkpoint. It has been proved that the activity of "free" E2F-1 is higher in human glioma cells than in human normal cells. E2F-1 fulfills the criteria for being an oncogene and plays probably an important role in the oncogenic properties of gliomas. However, the role of E2F-1, like that of the myc protein, appears to be dual. Indeed, several lines of evidence indicate that E2F-1 may also function as a tumor suppressor gene. In this capacity, E2F-1 protein has been shown to promote apoptosis in several systems, either alone or in association with p53. Furthermore, deletion of the *E2F-1* gene results in spontaneous development of tumors in knockout animals. The transfer of *E2F-1* to gliomas results in apoptosis *(16)*. Additionally, preliminary studies suggest that E2F-1 may be more effective than p53 in eradicating glioma cells, because it is able to induce apoptosis in p53-resistant cells. E2F-1 is also able to override p21 and p16-induced growth arrest, driving the cells to enter the S phase and to undergo apoptosis (two factors that may render cancer cells partially resistant to the apoptotic effect of the p53 protein) *(16)*. The two main disadvantages of the use of this protein as a gene-therapy tool are its potential toxicity and oncogenicity. About the potential role of *E2F-1* as a tumor suppressor in human gliomas it is necessary to remember that there is no report of loss-of-function mutations of the *E2F-1* gene in brain tumors.

In addition to derangement of the *p16* and *Rb* genes, and the deregulation of the E2F-1 protein, other proteins involved in the control of p16/Rb pathway are abnormally expressed in gliomas. Thus, the positive regulators of the cell-cycle, cyclin D1, CDK4, and CDK6 are overexpressed in gliomas *(5,10,63)*. Cyclin D1 is overexpressed in many human cancers as a result of gene amplification or translocations that target the *D1* locus (formally designated *CCND1*) on human chromosome 11q13. The gene encoding its catalytic partner CDK4, located on chromosome 12q13, is similarly amplified in sarcomas and gliomas. These alterations, however, occur less frequently in brain tumor than the inactivation of the tumor suppressor genes *p16* and *Rb*. From a therapeutic point of view, antisense strategies or pharmacological approaches intended to block their function could be designed to counteract the oncogenic effect of these molecules in gliomas.

As mentioned earlier, one alteration that occurs at high frequency in a variety of human tumors is loss of heterozygosity at chromosome 10q23. This change occurs in the vast majority (>70%) of glioblastomas. Independent research teams identified a novel tumor suppressor gene from this region called phosphatase and tensin homolog (*PTEN*) or *MMAC1* (mutated in multiple advanced cancers 1) *(40,70)*. This gene was also described as TEP1 (transforming growth factor [TGF]-β-regulated and epithelial cell-enriched phosphatase) because its expression was rapidly repressed by TGF-β *(67)*. The PTEN gene encodes a protein that functions as a dual-specificity phosphatase in vitro, and it can dephosphorylate the lipid signal transduction molecule PIP3 (phosphatidylinositol 3,4,5-trisphosphate). The N-terminal domain of PTEN also shows extensive homology to the cytoskeletal protein tensin, which plays a role in maintenance of cellular structure and possibly in signal transduction by binding to actin filaments at focal adhesions and to phosphotyrosine-containing proteins through its actin-binding and Src homology-2 (SH2) domains. The majority of the PTEN functions involve the modification of the phosphorylation status of Akt, a master regulator of survival signals and a putative oncogene. Experiments with genetically modified mice have demonstrated that *PTEN* is essential for tumor suppression. Restoration of PTEN activity to glioma cells led to suppression of their neoplastic phenotype, providing evidence that PTEN is a tumor suppressor gene in gliomas *(17,39)*. Although the function of the PTEN protein is not completely understood, data from experiments in knockout mice indicate that PTEN can suppress tumorigenesis through its ability to regulate cellular differentiation and anchorage-independent growth. That PTEN has a role in the control of cell-cycle progression is demonstrated by the fact that transfer of *PTEN* to glioma cells in vitro results in cell-cycle arrest in the G1 phase. Although, PTEN might induce cell-cycle arrest by suppressing or activating several pathways, two cell-cycle regulators are involved in G1-mediated arrest. Transfer of *PTEN* results in upregulation of the cyclin-dependent kinase inhibitor p27 and modification of the function of cyclin D1 *(86)*. The role of PTEN as a tumor suppressor in gliomas is not limited to its ability to negatively regulate cell-cycle progression; PTEN seems to play a critical role in the control of invasion and angiogenesis *(72,85)*. In addition to *PTEN/MMAC1*, at least another potential tumor suppressor gene, *DMBT1* (deleted in multiple malignant brain tumors), is frequently deleted in malignant brain tumors *(49)*.

The p53 gene is the most frequently mutated gene in human cancer and is an archetypal checkpoint regulator *(79)*. Although it is not essential for normal mouse development, one of its roles, for example, is to ensure that in response to genotoxic damage, cells arrest in G1 and attempt to repair their DNA before replication. Although p53 is ordinarily a very short-lived protein, it is stabilized and accumulates in cells following DNA damage or in those responding to certain forms of stress. The precise signal transduction pathway that senses DNA damage and recruits p53 has not been completely elucidated, but after its activation, the wild-type p53 protein suppresses malignant transformation, blocking cell-cycle progression, as well as, inducing apoptosis.

Mutations causing loss of function of the *p53* gene are present in more than 30% of astrocytomas and constitute the earliest detectable genetic alteration in these tumors *(12,54,68)*. Among many other genes, the p53 protein upregulates the expression of the p21 protein, a universal cyclin-dependent kinase inhibitor that negatively regulates progression through the cell-cycle *(79)*. The p53 protein also transcriptionally activates the death gene *BAX*, which is related to the induction of apoptosis *(48)*. Experimental transfer of *p53* to glioma cells first induces expression of p21 protein and growth arrest, and subsequently induces BAX and apoptosis *(19)*. In addition to the direct effects of p53, other molecules may enhance the apoptotic activity of p53. Thus, p14ARF, which is the protein encoded by the alternate reading frame of the *p16* locus in chromosome 9, has recently been implicated in the activation of p53 through its inhibition of the p53-antagonist MDM-2 protein *(6)*.

Because p53 and Rb pathways are both critical in the control of the cell-cycle progression, both proteins are partially inactive in the vast majority of gliomas. This point is supported by one observation based on the geography of the genome. The *p16* locus in chromosome 9 encodes two proteins. One of them, p16, is a key factor in the regulation of Rb. The other, p14ARF, indirectly regulates the function of p53 by inactivating MDM-2. This locus is deleted in 50% of high-grade malignant gliomas. Overexpression of CDK4, with its potential action against the p16 effect on Rb function, and overexpression of MDM-2, with potential inactivation of the p53 function, appear together in gliomas as a result of the proximity of both loci on chromosome 12 (Fig. 3) *(29)*.

Although abnormalities in the control of G2 have not been completely characterized, abnormalities in the germ line of the *ATM* gene result in a syndrome that includes the enhanced frequency of cancer *(50)*. In addition, a recent analyses of chromosome abnormalities of human glioma cells revealed that cell lines with a gain of proximal 5q, where *CCNB1* and *CCNH* reside (genes encoding cyclin B1 and H, respectively), had an increased growth rate. These results suggest that cyclins activating cdc2, the dominant G2/M phase kinase, may play a role in glioma tumorigenesis *(82)*.

3. GENETIC PATHWAYS UNDERLYING THE GENESIS OF PRIMARY AND SECONDARY GLIOBLASTOMA

Carcinogenesis in general and gliomagenesis in particular are multistep processes. The theory of the clonal evolution of tumor cell populations proposes that most neoplasms are of a single-cell origin, and tumor progression results from an acquired genetic variability within the original clone *(55)*. These genetic abnormalities allow sequential selection of the more aggressive subclones. The resultant genetic instability and selection process result in advanced human malignancies. This model fits the malignant progression of astrocytic tumors. Thus, secondary glioblastoma multiforme formation is, not surprisingly, preceded by a series of pathologically recognizable lesions. The timing and order of these changes correlate with the additive presence of abnormalities in different tumor suppressor genes and oncogenes. As mentioned earlier, low-grade astrocytomas may express a mutant-*p53* gene, anaplastic astrocytomas have abnormalities in either *Rb* or *p16* genes, and, in addition, glioblastoma multiforme exhibit alterations of chromosome 10. This stepwise sequence of events might determine the particular biological characteristics of the different grades of malignancy. According to this model, *p53* mutations might be linked to initiation of neoplasia; p16 and Rb abnormalities are associated with malignant progression, and amplification of EGFR and alterations of genes located in chromosome 10 might be related to neovascularization.

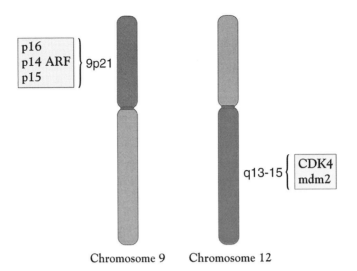

Fig. 3. Gene deletion and gene amplification in malignant gliomas, and the geography of the genome. Deletion of the *p16* locus in chromome 9, a frequent fact in intermediate and high-grade gliomas, produces lack of expression of p16 and p15, and p14ARF. p16 and p15 are key controllers of Rb function. P14ARF indirectly regulates p53 function. Amplification of two locus in chromosome 12 led to overexpression of cdk4 and mdm-2 proteins. Amplification of *cdk4* functionally equals to inactivation of Rb, and amplification of *mdm-2* equals to inactivation of p53. Two simple hits in two different chromosomes are enough to partially inactivate the two main pathways of control of checkpoints in gliomas.

We have described first the model of the stepwise inactivation of genes in the formation of secondary glioblastoma. This multiple-step theory permits a systematic explanation of the functional role that key molecules play in the development of gliomas. There is, however, evidence that different genetic pathways may lead to glioblastoma multiforme as a common endpoint. In fact, it is accepted that there are two major types of human glioblastomas (primary and secondary) that are characterized by different molecular genetic defects *(35)*. Secondary glioblastomas, evolve from low-grade gliomas and often develop over months or years from low-grade or anaplastic astrocytomas. This type of glioblastoma is mainly seen in young adults and before age 50 yr. Primary glioblastomas account for the vast majority of these tumors in older people (> 50 yr), and have a short clinical history, usually less than six months. In these tumors, there is no pre-clinical or histologic evidence of a pre-existing, less malignant, precursor lesion. Characteristically, these tumors show no progression from low, to intermediate and high grades of malignancy. In addition, the molecular abnormalities of primary glioblastomas differ from those observed in secondary glioblastomas. Significantly, *EGFR* amplification occurs most often in elderly patients, without loss of heterozygosity on chromosome 17p or mutations of the *p53* gene. In this group of glioblastomas, amplification of *MDM-2*, a molecule antagonistic of p53 also occurs. The implication is that although p53 is structurally intact, it might be functionally disabled. The dual presence of a mutant *p53* gene and abnormalities in chromosome 10 has been observed in a subset of primary glioblastomas such as the giant cell glioblastoma. The classification of glioblastomas into primary and secondary classes has clinical and therapeutic implications. Thus, single-gene therapy strategies might apply for one class of glioblastoma, but not for the other. However, both classes of glioblastoma display abnormal control of the cell-cycle checkpoints.

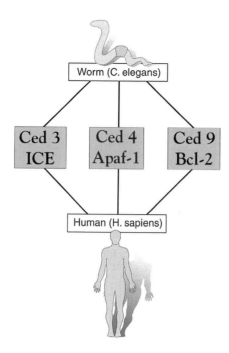

Fig. 4. Control of apoptosis in worm and human. Early work, particularly in the roundworm Caernorhabditis elegans, points out the presence of three key controllers of apoptosis. Interestingly, the three proteins have their homolog in humans. The importance of the control of apoptosis in organism is exemplified by the striking preservation of the major regulators of apoptosis during evolution.

4. CONTROL OF APOPTOSIS IN GLIOMAS

Virtually all human cells are endowed with the capacity to undergo death using an evolutionarily conserved mechanism called apoptosis or programmed cell death (PCD) *(34,87)*. This process typically involves activation of the caspase-family of proteases. Activation of these intracellular proteases is carefully controlled by a delicate balance between anti- and pro-death proteins that precisely regulate the susceptibility of the cell to undergo apoptosis. Unlike accidental cell deaths caused by infarction and trauma, these programmed physiologic deaths culminate in the fragmentation of cells into membrane-encased bodies, which are cleared through phagocytosis by neighboring cells without inciting inflammatory reactions or tissue scarring. Defects in the processes controlling PCD can extend cell longevity, contributing to neoplastic cell expansion independent of cell division. Furthermore, failure in the function of normal apoptotic pathways contributes to carcinogenesis by creating a permissive environment for genetic instability and accumulation of gene mutations. Disruption of normal cell death regulation is associated with resistance to cytotoxic anticancer drugs and radiation.

The critical factors involved in the control of apoptosis have been best defined in the nematode, Caenorhabditis elegans *(47)*. All apoptosis-related events in the developing worm depend upon the normal function of three proteins: Ced-3, Ced-4, and Ced-9 *(27)*. Importantly, Ced-9 is highly homologous to mammalian Bcl-2 and Ced-3 is related to the mammalian interleukin-1b converting enzyme, ICE/caspase 1, and Ced-4 is homologous to mammalian apoptosis protease activation factor-1 (APAF-1) *(88)* (Fig. 4). This model implies the presence of an effective executioner mechanism of apoptosis that is tightly controlled.

5. THE BCL-2 PATHWAY

The worm proteins have turned out to be similar not only in structure but also in function to the mammalian proteins. Thus, Vaux *(78)* showed that the human *Bcl-2* gene, when introduced into the worm, prevents the apoptosis that normally kills cells in the developing worm. Together, the Bcl-2 family of proteins constitutes a critical intracellular checkpoint for apoptosis within a distal common cell death pathway *(21)*. The first known member of this family, *Bcl-2*, was discovered at the interchromosomal breakpoint of t *(14;18)*, the molecular hallmark of follicular B-cell lymphoma. In experimental models using transgenic animals, the *bcl-2*-Ig transgene confers a survival advantage to a population of mature B-cells assessed in vitro. Thus, the *bcl-2*-Ig transgenic mice document a prospective role for the t(14;18) in B-cell growth and the pathogenesis of follicular lymphoma *(45,46)*. The realization that *Bcl-2*, unlike other oncogenes previously studied, functions by preventing PCD instead of promoting proliferation established a new class of oncogenes *(36)*. The identification of multiple Bcl-2 homologs, many of which form homodimers or heterodimers, suggests that these molecules at least partly function through protein-protein interactions. The first pro-apoptotic homolog, BAX, was identified by co-immunoprecipitation with BCL-2 protein. BAX is a 21-kDa protein that shares homology with Bcl-2 and which is clustered in conserved regions, including BH1 and BH2. BAX heterodimerizes with Bcl-2 and also homodimerizes with itself. Following BAX overexpression in cells, apoptotic death is accelerated in response to a cell death signal, earning its designation as a cell death agonist. When BCL-2 is overexpressed, it heterodimerized with BAX and cell death is repressed. Therefore, the ratio of BCL-2 to BAX is important in determining susceptibility to apoptosis *(37)*.

In mammalian cells, a considerable portion of the pro- vs anti-apoptotic BCL-2 members localizes to separate subcellular compartments in the absence of a death signal. Anti-apoptotic members are initially integral membrane proteins found in the mitochondria, endoplasmic reticulum, or nuclear membrane. In contrast, a substantial fraction of the pro-apoptotic members localize to the cytosol or cytoskeleton prior to receiving a death signal. Following a death signal, the pro-apoptotic members that have been examined to date undergo a conformational change that enables them to target and integrate themselves into membranes, especially the mitochondrial outer membrane. The localization of these apoptosis-related molecules indicates that certain cell organellas are directly involved in the control of the apoptosis pathways. In 1996, Wang and colleagues *(42)* reported that cells undergoing apoptosis in vivo showed increased release of cytochrome c (a mitochondrial protein thought related solely to energy production) to their cytosol, suggesting that mitochondria may function in apoptosis by releasing cytochrome c. Subsequent work by Wang's group showed that the activation of caspase 9 requires two other proteins Apaf-1 and cytochrome c, which are released from mitocochondria during apoptosis *(89)*. Importantly, the anti-apoptosis molecule protein BCL-2 can inhibit the release of cytochrome c from the mitochondria (Fig. 5).

There are several hypotheses to explain how the BCL-2-related molecules interact in the course of apoptosis. Although the mechanisms of cytochrome c release from the mitochondria is unclear, one plausible model postulates that it is released via specific channels, such as the voltage-dependent anion-channel, or a channel comprised of BAX alone, or possibly another pro-apoptotic family member acting alone *(62)*. This model proposes that anti-apoptotic BCL-2 molecules are "guarding the mitochondrial gate" from pro-apoptotic BCL-2 members that "gain access" following a death signal. BAX, like BCL-2, has been co-localized to intracellular membranes, including those of mitochondria. That BCL-2 family members may exert their function through direct control of mitochondrial membrane permeability is supported by the finding that the structure of BCL-XL is similar to the structure of members of the colicin family of proteins *(51)*. Colicins are proteins secreted for bacteria that form pores in the surface membranes of other bacterial strains, causing cell death. The veracity of this model is made more convincing by the observation that mitochondria are likely derived from ancient prokaryotes, suggesting that the similarity between BCL-2-related proteins and colicins may be meaningful.

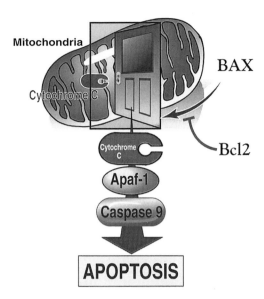

Fig. 5. One of the main pathways of apoptosis works through the mitochondrion. Following a death stimulus, pro-apoptotic members of the BCL-2 family, such as BAX, open new pores or modify existing channels in the mitochondrial membrane, releasing cytochrome c. Release of cytochrome c activates the apaf-1-caspase-9 apoptosome and downstream effector caspases leading to apoptosis. In addition to the mitochondrion, apoptosis can be initiated at multiple sites including plasma membrane, nucleus, and ER.

This theory has prompted a series of electrophysiologic studies, which have revealed the capacity of anti-apoptotic BCL-XL and BCL-2 as well as pro-apoptotic BAX to form distinct ion conductive channels in artificial lipid membranes *(61)*. Although the differences in their selectivity are negligible, BCL-2 and BAX channels display different characteristics. BCL-2 or BAX might regulate an electrochemical gradient or alter critical substrates or protein products residing in the intermembrane space. Because BCL-2 tends to cluster at contact points between the inner and outer membrane, it is a likely candidate for regulating or being a component of the permeability transition pore, which enables the colloidosmotic swelling of mitochondria that sometimes accompanies apoptosis. Alternatively, the BCL-2 family might modify the conductance of ion channels directly or indirectly.

In addition to regulation of apoptosis, Bcl-2 may modulate cell-cycle progression. In this regard, Bcl-2 is a negative regulator of cell-cycle progression *(41,44,57,77)*. Studies with Bcl-2-deficient T-cells showed accelerated cell-cycle progression and increased apoptosis following activation *(41)*. In contrast, thymocytes over-expressing Bcl-2 display an impaired proliferation capability. Furthermore, BCL-2 overexpressing peripheral T-cells exhibit delayed entry to S phase *(41,44,57)*. The anti-apoptotic and cell-cycle regulatory effects seems to be separable functions of the Bcl-2 protein. Thus, a caspase inhibitor that also blocks apoptosis has no substantial effect on cell-cycle progression *(41)*.

In summary, BCL-2 family members reside upstream of irreversible cellular damage. By controlling the flux of ions and molecules, including cytochrome C, between the mitochondria and the cytosol, they play a pivotal role in deciding whether a cell will live or die.

6. THE BCL-2 FAMILY OF PROTEINS IN GLIOMAS

Although the characterization of functional abnormalities of members of the BCL-2 family of proteins in gliomas is still under examination, there is, as mentioned earlier, evidence that BCL-2 protein is overexpressed in malignant gliomas. Louis and colleagues *(1)* examined a series of human gliomas to determine whether BCL-2 is expressed and whether its expression is associated with tumors that express wild-type p53. In this study, gliomas were immunohistochemically stained for BCL-2 and p53. *p53* mutations were identified with single-strand conformation polymorphism and DNA sequencing. 57% of the tumors expressed BCL-2, which was significantly associated with wild-type p53. These findings indicate that p53 and BCL-2 share a common pathway in the control of apoptosis in gliomas. Although Bcl-2 expression is found abnormal in human gliomas, there is not correlation between Bcl-2 expression and prognosis. Thus, Bcl-2 does not constitute a prognosis marker in brain tumors *(23)*.

Although *BAX* maps to the region of chromosome 19 most frequently deleted in gliomas, routine and pulsed-field gel electrophoresis and Southern blotting studies failed to reveal large-scale deletions or rearrangements of the *BAX* gene in gliomas *(8)*. In addition, single-strand conformation polymorphism analysis of all 6 *BAX* exons and flanking intronic sequences did not disclose mutations in 20 gliomas with allelic loss of the second copy of 19q. These data suggest that inactivation of *BAX* does not play a pivotal role in the genesis or malignant progression of gliomas. Despite a lack of structural abnormalities, BAX might be abnormally regulated in gliomas, a theory bolstered by transfer of wild-type *p53* to cell lines in vitro, which induces expression of BAX only in those cell lines that undergo apoptosis *(18,19)*. In addition, transfer of BAX to human glioma cells triggers apoptosis *(24,38,59)*.

7. THE DEATH RECEPTOR SYSTEM

Whereas BCL-2 clearly governs the events that commit a cell to apoptosis upstream of caspase activation, BCL-2-independent pathways for caspase activation and apoptosis induction also exist *(4)*. In mammals, the initiation of PCD can also occur through the interaction of death ligands such as tumor necrosis factor (TNF)-α, Fas (APO-1L/CD95L), or TNF-related apoptosis-inducing ligand (TRAIL/APO-2L), with their respective receptors, followed by aggregation of these receptors *(81)*. Recruitment of adapter proteins, such as Fas-associated death domain (DD) protein, TNF receptor-associated DD protein, and receptor-interacting protein, to a plasma membrane complex ensues through interactions between the DD, present in both the receptor and adapter proteins. The receptor and the C-carboxyterminus of the adapter protein form the death-inducing signaling complex (DISC). The N-terminus of the adapter protein is critical to recruit of the caspases and it is called the death effector domain (DED). Recruitment of the initiator caspase 8 (also called Fas-associated DD-like interleukin 1 β-converting enzyme) through interaction of its DED, results in its subsequent activation, evidently through the mechanism of self-proteolytic cleavage. Activation of caspase 8 triggers the apoptosis executioner mechanisms (Fig. 6) *(4,81)*.

In many types of cells, this "death receptor" pathway for apoptosis is BCL-2-independent and circumvents the participation of mitochondria or other organelles where BCL-2 resides. In some cells, however, apoptosis induced via Fas can be blocked by BCL-2 or BCL-XL overexpression. Recent studies suggest two types of cellular contexts for Fas signaling. In one, Fas ligation leads to processing abundant amounts of pro-caspase-8 (BCL-2-independent). In another, Fas triggers only small amounts of caspase-8 activation (BCL-2-suppressible) *(81)*. The explanation for this phenomenon is currently unknown. However, the basis for this differential sensitivity of BCL-2 might be determined by whether caspase-8 does or does not require a mitochondria-dependent amplification step to achieve sufficient activation of downstream effector caspases. In this regard, the Fas death receptor pathway, which was once thought to require only the activity of caspase 8, has recently been connected to the mitochondrial pathway. In these studies *(22)*, Caspase-8 was directing the signal through the mitochondria by cleaving the BCL-2 family protein, BID. BID is a cytosolic pro-apoptotic protein that, upon cleavage by caspase-8, translocates to mitochondrial membranes, binds to other BCL-2 family proteins, and induces the release of cytochrome C from the mitochondria. Overexpression of BCL-2 or BCL-XL blocks both BID-induced apoptosis and release of cytochrome C from the mitochondria.

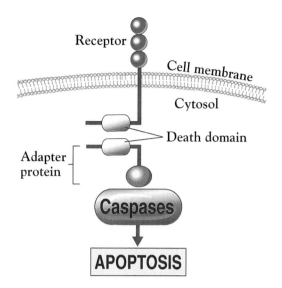

Fig. 6. The death receptor pathway. The pro-apoptotic receptors TNF, Fas, and TRAIL share a related sequence in their C-terminal cytoplasmic domain known as the death domain. Through the death domain, the extracellular signal is connected to cytoplasmic proteins that also contain death receptor domains. These adaptor proteins are able to recruit caspases and therefore activate apoptosis. In the best-known example molecules, such as the so-called Fas ligand, binds to a cell surface protein called Fas. Activation of Fas then triggers caspase-8 activation inside the cell leading to apoptosis.

Even when operating via a BCL-2-independent route, the TNF family death receptor pathway for apoptosis is potentially suppressible by other mechanisms. Most notably, several anti-apoptotic DED-containing proteins have been identified, which compete with DED-containing caspases for recruitment to death receptors, thus functioning as trans-dominant inhibitors of Fas/TNF-signaling. Moreover, some of these anti-apoptotic DED (ADED) family proteins are reportedly overexpressed in cancers. Other mechanisms for tumor cell resistance to apoptosis induction by Fas and related death receptors include downregulation of the receptors; inactivating mutations within the *Fas* gene; and increased expression of soluble or decoy receptors that compete for TNF family ligands.

8. DEATH RECEPTORS IN GLIOMAS

The Fas pathway, CD95 (Fas/APO-1) and its ligand (CD95L), belong to a cytokine and cytokine receptor family that includes nerve growth factor (NGF) and TNF and their corresponding receptors. CD95 expression increases during malignant progression from low-grade to anaplastic astrocytoma. Agonistic antibodies to CD95, or the natural ligand, CD95L, induce apoptosis in human malignant glioma cells in vitro. Glioma cell sensitivity to CD95-mediated apoptosis is regulated by CD95 expression at the cell surface and intracellular apoptosis-regulatory proteins, including BCL-2 family members *(84)*.

TRAIL/APO2L, another TNF-related molecule, is expressed in gliomas. Cultured malignant glioma cells preferentially express agonistic receptors and are susceptible to APO2L-induced apoptosis. The expression of TRAIL has been identified in both human glioma cell lines and primary astrocytic brain tumors, including low-grade astrocytomas and glioblastomas. With the exception of reactive astrocytes, non-neoplastic glia and neurons in the cerebrum lacked immunoreactivity to APO2L *(25)*. The TRAIL pathway has been functionally tested in human gliomas. As mentioned earlier, TRAIL preferentially triggers apoptosis in tumor cells versus normal cells. This mechanism provides a promising therapeutic potential. Hao and colleagues *(25)* analyzed a panel of human malignant glioma cell lines and primary cultures of normal human astrocytes to determine their sensitivity to TRAIL. Although more than 50% of the cell lines tested were sensitive to TRAIL-induced apoptosis, normal astrocytes were resistant. As expected, TRAIL-induced cell death was triggered by activation of caspases 8 and 3. Both sensitive and resistant cell lines expressed TRAIL death receptor (DR5), adapter protein Fas-associated death domain, and caspase-8; but resistant cell lines expressed two-fold higher levels of the apoptosis inhibitor PED/PEA-15 (phosphoprotein enriched in diabetes/phosphoprotein enriched in astrocytes-15 kDa). Transfer of these molecules to sensitive cells resulted in cell resistance, whereas transfection of antisense in resistant cells rendered them sensitive. These results confirm the potential of this pathway to be a promising target for glioma therapies.

9. THE CASPASES

Caspases are cysteine proteases that cleave substrates with an aspartate residue *(25,53,60,71,74, 75)*. Caspase1/ICE is the prototype of this large family of proteins. Caspases are expressed as inactive proenzymes and are activated by proteolytic cleavage following a death stimulus. The first suggestion that proteolysis might be involved in apoptosis came from studies of leukemia cell apoptosis induced by chemotherapeutic drugs. It was shown that the nuclear protein *poly-ADP-ribose-poly*merase (PARP) was cleaved as an early event. Genetic analysis of PCD in the simple nematode, Caenorhabiditis elegans, solidified the significance of this event when it was discovered that the cell death gene *CED-3* encodes a cysteine protease. Because caspases both cleave substrates at Asp residues and are themselves activated by cleavage at Asp residues, the potential for proteolytic cascades exists, with some caspases operating as upstream initiators and others as downstream effectors. All of the upstream initiator caspases contain large N-terminal prodomains, many of which have been shown to bind other proteins involved in triggering the apoptotic cascade. Downstream caspases, which function as the ultimate effectors of apoptosis, uniformly possess small prodomains and are probably predominantly activated by upstream caspases.

The caspases can be divided into three groups, each with distinct substrate specificities. Group I caspases preferentially recognize substrates that are not directly involved in the mechanism(s) of apoptosis. Rather, they have been shown to play an important role in cytokine maturation. Group II caspases are termed "executioner" caspases because they are directly responsible for cleaving and disabling homeostatic and structural proteins during apoptosis. Group III caspases are termed "activator" caspases because their substrate specificity corresponds to the cleavage sites between large and small subunits of most, but not all, group II and group III caspases. Activation of group III activator caspases occurs via an oligomerization-induced autolytic mechanism. Two major cell death pathways have been described: the "extrinsic" pathway and the "intrinsic" pathway. Caspase-8 is the key activator caspase of the extrinsic pathway where it is activated in response to ligand binding to members of the death receptor family. Caspase-9 is the key activator caspase of the intrinsic pathway where it is activated in response to stimuli that cause the release of cytochrome *c* from mitochondria. Cytochrome C induces a conformational change in the adapter molecule Apaf-1, which then recruits caspase-9, resulting in its activation. Although there are few reports of caspase inactivation in human gliomas, inactivation of caspases or caspase co-factors like Apaf-1 have been described in other cancers. Recently, mutations in the *Apaf-1* gene in melanomas have been reported *(69)*.

10. CASPASES AND CASPASE-RELATED PROTEINS IN GLIOMAS

Caspases are a powerful system for destruction so that, under normal circumstances, their function is tightly regulated. Various molecules inhibit caspase function, such as BCL-2, mentioned earlier. BCL-2 inhibits apoptosis by preventing the release of cytochrome C from mitochondria, thus preventing the activation of the caspases. The inhibitor-of-apoptosis (IAP) molecules also have an inhibitory effect on the caspases *(20)*. The IAP proteins are currently being investigated to determine their possible roles in development and cancerogenesis. At least three IAP genes with antiapoptotic properties have been identified: *HIAP-1*, *HIAP-2*, and *XIAP*. These proteins interfere with apoptosis at the level of caspase 3 and 7. HIAP-1, HIAP-2, and XIAP are widely expressed by glioma cell lines *(80)*, suggesting that these proteins may play a role in the striking resistance of gliomas to the induction of apoptosis by radiotherapy and cancer chemotherapy. In contrast, glioma cells did not express NAIP, another member of the IAP family. The lack of NAIP expression in glioma cell lines in vitro is consistent with strictly neuronal NAIP expression in the rat brain in vivo. Survivin, a human gene encoding a new apoptosis inhibitor with structural similarity to IAP, has recently been identified. Survivin is unique in that it is expressed selectively in most commonly occurring human cancers but not in normal adult tissue. Expression of the anti-apoptotic survivin seems to correlate with a histologically more aggressive type of neuroblastoma and its unfavorable prognosis *(30)*. Other investigators have transferred caspases to glioma in order to induce a therapeutic effect. These experiments have shown that transfer of exogenous caspases to glioma cells results in induction of cell death via apoptosis *(65,66)*.

Regulation of caspase activation is one of the key events in apoptosis. Despite rapid progress in the identification of the molecules that are critical for caspase activation, many questions remain unanswered, particularly those related to how apoptosis-inducing stimuli signal the activation of the death machinery inside the cells.

11. APOPTOSIS IN GLIOMAS: CONCLUSIONS

Human malignant glioma cells are paradigmatic for their intrinsic resistance to multiple pro-apoptotic stimuli. The molecular basis for their resistance to apoptosis has not been fully elucidated. A wide variety of stimuli can trigger apoptosis. At least two pathways have been identified, 1. a mitochondria-dependent pathway, which is governed by the BCL-2 family proteins; and 2. a pathway involving activation of upstream initiator caspases, such as, those that contain death effector domains and which are involved in Fas and TNF signaling. Extensive cross-talk probably exists between these two pathways. Members of both pathways are abnormally expressed in gliomas. This fact may be responsible in part for the high resistance of human glioma cells to die after being exposed to high doses of chemotherapeutic drugs and radiotherapy.

The challenge ahead is to map the functions of newly found apoptotic proteins in the biochemical pathways of apoptosis. An equally important task is to study how these pathways are modified in human diseases such as cancer. Finally, it is possible that these basic scientific discoveries on apoptosis may reveal logical strategies for the discovery of new therapeutic drugs for the treatment of cancer in general and gliomas in particular.

ACKNOWLEDGMENTS

We gratefully acknowledge and express deep appreciation to Joann Aaron (Department of Neuro-Oncology, University of Texas M.D. Anderson Cancer Center) for editorial assistance, and Ian Sulk (Department of Scientific Publications, University of Texas M.D. Anderson Cancer Center) for the illustrations

REFERENCES

1. Alderson L.M., Castleberg R.L., Harsh G.R. 4th, Louis D.N., Henson J.W. 1995. Human gliomas with wild-type p53 express bcl-2. *Cancer Res.* **55**:999–1001.
2. Arap W., Nishikawa R., Furnari F.B., Cavenee W.K., Huang H.-S.S. 1995. Replacement of the p16/CDKN2 gene suppresses human glioma cell growth. *Cancer Res.* **55**:1351–1354.
3. Bigner S.H., Schrock E. 1997. Molecular cytogenetics of brain tumors. *J. Neuropathol. Exp. Neurol.* **56**:1173–1181.
4. Budihardjo I., Oliver H., Lutter M., Luo X., Wang X. 1999. Biochemical pathways os caspase activation during apoptosis. *Annu. Rev. Cell Dev. Biol.* **15**:269–290.

5. Buschges R., Weber R.G., Actor B., Lichter P., Collins V.P., Reifenberger G. 1999. Amplification and expression of cyclin D genes (CCND1, CCND2 and CCND3) in human malignant gliomas. *Brain Pathol.* **9:**435–442.

6. Chin L., Pomerantz J., DePinho R.A. 1998. The INK4a/ARF tumor suppressor: one gene—two products—two pathways. *Trends Biochem. Sci.* **23:**291–296.

7. Chintala S.K., Fueyo J., Gomez-Manzano C, et al. 1997. Adenovirus-mediated p16/CDKN2 gene transfer suppresses glioma invasion in vitro. *Oncogene* **15:**2049–2057.

8. Chou D., Miyashita T., Mohrenweiser H.W., Ueki K., Kastury K., Druck T., et al. 1996. The BAX gene maps to the glioma candidate region at 19q13.3, but is not altered in human gliomas. *Cancer Genet. Cytogenet.* **88:**136–140.

9. Collins V.P., James C.D. 1993. Gene and chromosomal alterations associated with the development of human gliomas. *FASEB J.* **7:**926–930.

10. Costello J.F., Plass C., Arap W., Chapman V.M., Held W.A., Berger et al. 1997. Cyclin-dependent kinase 6 (CDK6) amplification in human gliomas identified using two-dimensional separation of genomic DNA. *Cancer Res.* **57:**1250–1254.

11. Ferrell J.E. Jr. 1998. How regulated protein translocation can produce switch-like responses. *Trends Biochem. Sci.* **23:**461–465.

12. Frankel R.H., Bayona W., Koslow M., Newcomb E.W. 1992. p53 mutations in human malignant gliomas: Comparison of loss of heterozygosity with mutation frequency. *Cancer Res.* **52:**1427–1433.

13. Fueyo J., Gomez-Manzano C., Bruner J.M, et al. 1996. Hypermethylation of the CpG island of p16/CDKN2 correlates with gene inactivation in gliomas. *Oncogene* **13:**1615–1619.

14. Fueyo, J., Gomez-Manzano C., Yung W.K.A., et al. 1996. Adenovirus-mediated p16/CDKN2 gene transfer induces growth arrest and modifies the transformed phenotype of glioma cells. *Oncogene* **12:**103–110.

15. Fueyo J., Gomez-Manzano C., Yung W.K.A., et al. 1998. Suppression of human glioma growth by adenovirus-mediated Rb gene transfer. *Neurology* **50:**1307–1315.

16. Fueyo J., Gomez-Manzano C., Yung W.K.A., et al. 1998. Overexpression of E2F-1 in glioma triggers apoptosis and suppresses tumor growth in vitro and in vivo. *Nat. Med.* **4:**685–690.

17. Furnari F.B., Lin H., Huang H.S., Cavenee W.K. 1997. Growth suppression of glioma cells by PTEN requires a functional phosphatase catalytic domain. *Proc. Natl. Acad. Sci. USA* **94:**12,479–12,484.

18. Gomez-Manzano C., Fueyo J., Kyritsis A.P., Steck P.A., Roth J.A., McDonnell, et al. 1996. Adenovirus-mediated transfer of the p53 gene produces rapid and generalized death of human glioma cells via apoptosis. *Cancer Res.* **56:**694–699.

19. Gomez-Manzano C., Fueyo J., Kyritsis A.P., McDonnell T.J., Steck P.A., Levin, V.A. Yung W.K. 1997. Characterization of p53 and p21 functional interactions in glioma cells en route to apoptosis. *J. Natl. Cancer Inst.* **89:**1036–1044.

20. Goyal L. 2001. Cell death inhibition: keeping caspases in check. *Cell* **104:**805–808.

21. Gross A., McDonnell J.M., Korsmeyer S.J. 1999. BCL-2 family members and the mitochondria in apoptosis. *Genes Dev.* **13:**1899–1911.

22. Gross A., Yin X.M., Wang K., Wei M.C., Jockel J., Milliman C. et al. 1999. Caspase cleaved BID targets mitochondria and is required for cytochrome c release, while BCL-XL prevents this release but not tumor necrosis factor-R1/Fas death. *J. Biol. Chem.* **274:**1156–1163.

23. Grzybicki D.M., Moore S.A. 1999. Implications of prognostic markers in brain tumors. *Clin. Lab. Med.* **19:**833–847.

24. Haghighat P., Timiryasova T.M., Chen B., Kajioka E.H., Gridley D.S., Fodor I. 2000. Antitumor effect of IL-2, p53, and bax gene transfer in C6 glioma cells. *Anticancer Res.* **20:**1337–1342.

25. Hao C., Beguinot F., Condorelli G., Trencia A., Van Meir E.G., Yong et al. 2001. Induction and intracellular regulation of tumor necrosis factor-related apoptosis-inducing ligand (TRAIL) mediated apotosis in human malignant glioma cells. *Cancer Res.* **61:**1162–1170.

26. Hartwell L., Kastan M.B. 1994. Cell cycle control and cancer. *Science* **266:**1821–1828.

27. Hengartner M.O., Horvitz H.R. 1994. Programmed cell death in Caenorhabditis elegans. *Curr. Opin. Genet. Dev.* **4:** 581–586.

28. Henson J.W., Schnitker B.L., Correa K.M., et al. 1994. The retinoblastoma gene is involved in malignant progression of astrocytomas. *Ann. Neurol.* **36:** 714–721.

29. Hui A.B., Lo K.W., Yin X.L., Poon W.S., Ng H.K. 2001. Detection of multiple gene amplifications in glioblastoma multiforme using array-based comparative genomic hybridization. *Lab. Invest.* **81:**717–723.

30. Islam A., Kageyama H., Takada N., Kawamoto T., Takayasu H., Isogai E., et al. 2000. High expression of Survivin, mapped to 17q25, is significantly associated with poor prognostic factors and promotes cell survival in human neuroblastoma. *Oncogene* **19:**617–623.

31. James C.D., Carlbom E., Dumanski J.P., Hansen M., Nordenskjold M., Collins V.P., Cavenee W.K. 1988. Clonal genomic alterations in glioma malignancy stages. *Cancer Res.* **48:**5546–5551.

32. James C.D., Collins P.V. 1993. Glial tumors, in *Molecular Genetics of Nervous System Tumors* (Levine A.J., Schmidek H.H., eds.), Wiley-Liss Inc., New York, pp. 241–248.

33. Jen J., Harper J.W., Bigner S.H., et al. 1994. Deletion of p16 and p15 genes in brain tumors. *Cancer Res.* **54:**6353–6358.

34. Kerr J.F., Wyllie A.H., Currie A.R. 1972. Apoptosis: a basic biological phenomenon with wide-ranging implications in tissue kinetics. *Brit. J. Cancer* **26:**239–257.

35. Kleihues P., Ohgaki H. 1997. Genetics of glioma progression and the definition of primary and secondary glioblastoma. *Brain Pathol.* **7:**1131–1136.

36. Korsmeyer S.J. 1995. Regulators of cell death. *Trends Genet.* **11:**101–105.

37. Korsmeyer S.J., Shutter J.R., Veis D.J., Merry D.E., Oltvai Z.N. 1993. Bcl-2/Bax: a rheostat that regulates an antioxidant pathway and cell death. Semin. *Cancer Biol.* **4:**327–332.

38. Lee A., DeJong G., Guo J., Bu X., Jia W.W. 2000. Bax expressed from a herpes viral vector enhances the efficacy of N,N'-bis(2-hydroxyethyl)-N-nitrosourea treatment in a rat glioma model. *Cancer Gene Ther.* **7:**1113.

39. Li D.M., Sun H. 1998. PTEN/MMAC1/TEP1 suppresses the tumorigenicity and induces G1 cell cycle arrest in human glioblastoma cells. *Proc. Natl. Acad. Sci. USA* **95:**15,406–15,411.

40. Li, J., Yen, C., Liaw D., Podsypanina K., Bose S., Wang S.I., et al. 1997. PTEN, a putative protein tyrosine phosphatase gene mutated in human brain, breast, and prostate cancer. *Science* **275:**1943–1947.

41. Linette G.P., Li Y., Roth K.A., Korsmeyer S.J. 1996. Crosstalk between cell death and cell cycle progression: Bcl-2 regulates NFAT-mediated activation. *Proc. Natl. Acad. Sci. USA* **93:**9545–9552.

42. Liu X., Kim C.N., Yang J., Jemmerson R., Wang X. 1996. Induction of apoptotic program in cell-free extracts: requirement for dATP and cytochrome c. *Cell* **86:**147–157.

43. Maher, E.A., Furnari F.B., Bachoo R.M., Rowitch D.H., Louis D.N., Cavenee W.K., DePinho R.A. 2001. Malignant glioma: genetics and biology of a grave matter. *Genes Dev.* **15:**1311–1333.

44. Mazel S., Burrum D., Petrie H.T. 1996. Regulation of cell division cycle progression by bcl-2 expression: a potential mechanism for inhibition of programmed cell death. *J. Exp. Med.* **183:**2219–2226.

45. McDonnell T.J., Deane N., Platt F.M., Nunez G., Jaeger U., McKearn J.P., Korsmeyer S.J. 1989. bcl-2-immunoglobulin transgenic mice demonstrate extended B cell survival and follicular lymphoproliferation. *Cell* **57:**79–88.

46. McDonnell T.J., Korsmeyer S.J. 1991. Progression from lymphoid hyperplasia to high-grade malignant lymphoma in mice transgenic for the t(14; 18). *Nature* **349:**254–256.

47. Metzstein M.M., Stanfield G.M., Horvitz H.R. 1998. Genetics of programmed cell death in C. elegans: past, present and future. *Trends Genet.* **14:**410–416.

48. Miyashita T., Reed J.C. 1995. Tumor suppressor p53 is a direct transcriptional activator of the human bax gene. *Cell* **80:**293–299.

49. Mollenhauer, J., Wiemann S., Scheurlen W., Korn B., Hayashi Y., Wilgenbus K.K., et al. 1997. DMBT1, a new member of the SRCR superfamily, on chromosome 10q25.3-26.1 is deleted in malignant brain tumours. *Nat. Genet.* **17:**32–39.

50. Morrell D., Chase C.L., Swift M. 1990. Cancers in 44 families with ataxia-telangiectasia. *Cancer Genet. Cytogenet.* **50:**119–123.

51. Muchmore S.W., Sattler M., Liang H., Meadows R.P., Harlan J.E., Yoon H.S., et al. 1996. X-ray and NMR structure of human Bcl-xL, an inhibitor of programmed cell death. *Nature* **1381:**335–341.

52. Nagane M., Lin H., Cavenee W.K., Huang H.J. 2001. Aberrant receptor signaling in human malignant gliomas: mechanisms and therapeutic implications. *Cancer Lett.* **162:**17–21.

53. Nicholson D.W., Thornberry N.A. 1997. Caspases: killer proteases. *Trends Biochem. Sci.* **22:**299–306.

54. Nigro J.M., Baker S.J., Preisinger A.C. 1989. Mutations in the p53 gene occur in diverse human tumour types. *Nature* **342:**705–708.

55. Nowell P.C. 1976. The clonal evolution of tumor cell populations. *Science* **194:**23–28.

56. O'Connell M.J., Walworth N.C., Carr A.M. 2000. The G2-phase DNA-damage checkpoint. *Trends Cell Biol.* **10:**296–300.

57. O'Reilly L.A., Huang D.C., Strasser A. 1996. The cell death inhibitor Bcl-2 and its homologues influence control of cell cycle entry. *EMBO J.* **15:**6979–6990.

58. Pardee AB. 1989. G1 events and regulation of cell proliferation. *Science* **246:**603–608.

59. Ruan H., Wang J., Hu L., Lin C.S., Lamborn K.R., Deen D.F. 1999. Killing of brain tumor cells by hypoxia-responsive element mediated expression of BAX. *Neoplasia* **1:**431–437.

60. Salvesen G.S., Dixit V.M. 1997. Caspases: intracellular signaling by proteolysis. *Cell* **91:**443–446.

61. Schendel S.L., Montal M., Reed J.C. 1998. Bcl-2 family proteins as ion-channels. *Cell Death Differ.* **5:**372–580.

62. Shimizu S., Narita M., Tsujimoto Y. 1999. Bcl-2 family proteins regulate the release of apoptogenic cytochrome c by the mitochondrial channel VDAC. *Nature* **399:**483–487.

63. Schmidt E.E., Ichimura K., Reifenberger G., Collins V.P. 1994. CDKN2 (p16/MTS1) gene deletion or CDK4 amplification occurs in the majority of glioblastomas. *Cancer Res.* **54:**6321–6324.

64. Sherr C.J. 2000. The Pezcoller Lecture: Cancer Cell Cycles Revisited. *Cancer Res.* **60:** -3689–3695.

65. Shinoura N., Saito K., Yoshida Y., Hashimoto M., Asai A., Kirino T., Hamada H. 2000. Adenovirus-mediated transfer of bax with caspase-8 controlled by myelin basic protein promoter exerts an enhanced cytotoxic effect in gliomas. *Cancer Gene Ther.* **7:**739–748.

66. Shinoura N., Koike H., Furitu T., Hashimoto M., Asai A., Kirino T., Hamada H. 2000. Adenovirus-mediated transfer of caspase-8 augments cell death in gliomas: implication for gene therapy. *Hum. Gene Ther.* **11:**1123–1137.

67. Simpson L., Parsons R. 2001. PTEN: life as a tumor suppressor. *Exp. Cell Res.* **264:**29–41.

68. Sidransky D., Mikkelsen T., Schwechheimer K., Rosenblum M.L., Cavanee W., Vogelstein B. 1992. Clonal expansion of p53 mutant cells is associated with brain tumour progression. *Nature* **355:**846–847.

69. Soengas M.S., Capodieci P., Polsky D., Mora J., Esteller M., Opitz-Araya X., et al. 2001. Inactivation of the apoptosis effector Apaf-1 in malignant melanoma. *Nature* **409:**207–211.

70. Steck, P.A., Pershouse M.A., Jasser S.A., Yung W.K., Lin H., Ligon A.H., et al. 1997. Identification of a candidate tumour suppressor gene, MMAC1, at chromosome 10q23.3 that is mutated in multiple advanced cancers. *Nat. Genet.* **15:**356–362.

71. Stroh C., Schulze-Osthoff K. 1998. Death by a thousand cuts: an ever increasing list of caspase substrates. *Cell Death Differ.* **5:**997–1000.

72. Tamura M., Gu J., Matsumoto K., Aota S., Parsons R., Yamada K.M. 1998. Inhibition of cell migration, spreading, and focal adhesions by tumor suppressor PTEN. *Science* **280:**1614–1617.

73. Taylor W.R,, Stark G.R. 2001. Regulation of the G2/M transition by p53. *Oncogene* **20:**1803–1815.

74. Thornberry N.A., Lazebnik Y. 1998. Caspases: enemies within. *Science* **281:**1312–1326.

75. Thornberry N.A. 1999. Caspases: a decade of death research. *Cell Death Differ.* **6:**1023–1027.

76. Ueki K., Ono Y., Henson J. W., Efird J. T., von Deimling A., Louis D. N. 1996. CDKN2/p16 or RB alterations occur in the majority of glioblastomas and are inversely correlated. *Cancer Res.* **56:** 150–153.

77. Vairo G., Innes K.M., Adams J.M. 1996. Bcl-2 has a cell cycle inhibitory function separable from its enhancement of cell survival. *Oncogene* **13:**1511–1519.

78. Vaux, D.L., Weissman I.L., Kim S.K. 1992. Prevention of programmed cell death in Caenorhabditis elegans by human bcl-2. *Science* **258:**1955–1957.

79. Vogelstein B., Lane D., Levine A.J. 2000. Surfing the p53 network. Nature **408:**307–310.

80. Wagenknecht B., Glaser T., Naumann U., Kugler S., Isenmann S., Bahr M., et al. 1999. Expression and biological activity of X-linked inhibitor of apoptosis (XIAP) in human malignant glioma. *Cell Death Differ.* **6:**370–376.

81. Walczak H., Krammer P.H. 2000. The CD95 (APO-1/Fas) and the TRAIL (APO-2L) apoptosis systems. *Exp. Cell Res.* **256:**58–66.

82. Weber R.G., Rieger J., Naumann U., Lichter P., Weller M. 2001. Chromosomal imbalances associated with response to chemotherapy and cytotoxic cytokines in human malignant glioma cell lines. *Int. J. Cancer* **91:**213–218

83. Weinberg R.A. 1995. The retinoblastoma protein and cell cycle control. *Cell* **81:**323–330.

84. Weller M., Kleihues P., Dichgans J., Ohgaki H. 1998. CD95 ligand: lethal weapon against malignant glioma? *Brain Pathol.* **8:**285–293.

85. Wen S., Stolarov J., Myers M.P., Su J.D., Wigler M.H., Tonks N.K., Durden D.L. 2001. PTEN controls tumor-induced angiogenesis. *Proc. Natl. Acad. Sci. USA* **98:**4622–4627

86. Weng L.P., Brown J.L., Eng C. 2001. PTEN coordinates G(1) arrest by down-regulating cyclin D1 via its protein phosphatase activity and up-regulating p27 via its lipid phosphatase activity in a breast cancer model. *Hum. Mol. Genet.* **10:**599–604

87. Wyllie A.H. 1980. Glucocorticoid-induced thymocyte apoptosis is associated with endogenous endonuclease activation. *Nature* **284:**555–556.

88. Zou H., Henzel W.J., Liu X., Lutschg A., Wang X. 1997. Apaf-1, a human protein homologous to C. elegans CED-4, participates in cytochrome c-dependent activation of caspase-3. *Cell* **90:**405–413.

89. Zou H., Li Y., Liu X., Wang X. 1999. An APAF-1.cytochrome c multimeric complex is a functional apoptosome that activates procaspase-9. *J. Biol. Chem.* **274:**11,549–11,556.

III Therapeutics

14

Systemic Chemotherapy for Metastatic Tumors of the Central Nervous System

Charles A. Conrad and W. K. Alfred Yung

1. INTRODUCTION

The incidence of brain metastases exceeds 100,000 per year in the United States *(21)*, thus making tumor metastasis to the central nervous system (CNS) a significant challenge in the management of patients with solid tumors. To put this into perspective, brain metastases occur at almost one order of magnitude greater than primary malignant brain tumors. Metastatic tumors to the brain and spine also arise in approx 10 to 15% of patients with systemic cancers. This incidence rises to approx 24% when results from autopsy studies are factored in. Patients with intracranial and intraspinal metastases comprise approx 5% of all cancer patients *(4)*. Despite this preponderance of metastatic tumors to the CNS vs primary malignancies of the nervous system, the amount of research effort directed at the two sources of CNS disease is disparate. This is evidenced by the low number of scientific publications, a little more than 300 on brain metastases published between 1998 and 2000. However, during the same period more than 5000 publications were devoted to primary brain neoplasms. This disparity in attention to metastatic tumors of the CNS may be explained, at least in part, by the clinical complexity inherent in treating metastatic cancer. The diversity of the tumor histologies that metastasize to the brain and spinal cord combined with the absence of good clinical studies of the effectiveness of various forms of therapies, e.g., systemic chemotherapy vs radiation therapy, has hampered progress in developing efficacious therapies. Most clinical trials that have attempted to study the value of systemic chemotherapy for this group of patients have included "all comers" representing patients with multiple histologies. Metastatic tumors to the CNS arise most frequently in patients who have primary lung cancer (35–50%), particularly in patients who have small cell lung cancer (SCLC) *(18)*. Metastases from solid tumors of the breast account for approx 10–30% of metastatic disease, followed by malignant melanoma with a 30–40% frequency of occurrence, and approx 5% for renal and colorectal cancer. The remaining other metastases to the brain (15%) are from systemic neoplasms, including nonsolid tumors, such as leukemia and lymphoma. By the time these diseases are discovered, they have frequently resulted in multiple brain metastases. In contrast to malignant melanoma, lung and breast carcinomas, which frequently have multiple brain metasta-ses, patients who have colorectal and renal cell carcinoma typically have a single brain metastasis at the time of diagnosis *(10,34)*. The challenge of treating patients with tumors metastatic to the CNS is compounded by the fact that these space-occupying lesions are within the closed, confined cranial vault. Patients typically demonstrate a slow decline in their physical, cognitive, and emotional functions as a consequence of the growing metastatic foci. Other patients, however, may have a focus of disease in a relatively silent area of the brain. Few symptoms are obvious in these patients until the brain is overwhelmed and a sudden decompensation and a decreased level of consciousness ensues. Typi-

From: *Contemporary Cancer Research: Brain Tumors*
Edited by: F. Ali-Osman © Humana Press Inc., Totowa, NJ

cally, patients with metastatic tumors to the CNS have symptoms that include headache, change in mental status, somnolence, cranial nerve palsies, dysphasia, visual field defects, hemiparesis, and focal or generalized seizures *(34)*. Because many patients with systemic cancers are living longer, there is an increased likelihood that metastatic disease will occur in the CNS. Furthermore, the incidence of cancers such as malignant melanoma and lung cancer is increasing. The successful management of late-stage metastatic disease has thus become a clinical imperative. Although surgical resection of symptomatic lesions and whole-brain cranial radiotherapy have improved survival, more effective treatments for metastatic disease will ultimately reside in as yet undiscovered treatment strategies *(53)*. These will undoubtedly include innovative, novel chemotherapy regimens.

2. OUTCOME PREDICTION

To properly stratify patients and to develop meaningful study designs, it is important to be familiar with relevant prognostic factors, as elucidated in previous work by Curran et al. *(7)*. Curran and colleagues evaluated 1578 patients with malignant gliomas who were treated in Radiation Therapy Oncology Group (RTOG) trials. Statistical evaluation was accomplished using a recursive partition analysis (RPA) of the data from these trials. A pool of 26 factors was initially culled from the data after RPA was performed. Six distinct prognostic groups were deemed to be of critical importance for determining prognostic outcome. The factors of age (< than 50 vs > than 50 yr of age), tumor histology, Karnofsky Performance Status (KPS), mental status, extent of tumor resection, duration of symptoms prior to diagnosis, neurologic function, and radiotherapy dose appeared to correlate with differences in survival. These data were prospectively validated at a later date.

Patients with metastatic tumors to the CNS have been the subjects of similar analyses. One important study was carried out by Hall et al. *(14)* in a recent retrospective analysis of 740 patients. This study was designed to identify predictors of long-term survival (>2 yr) using a multivariate analysis. Among the 51 long-term survivors, favorable prognostic factors included younger age, single metastasis, extent of surgical resection, having received whole-brain radiotherapy, and treatment with chemotherapy. Because the benefit for long-term survival after treatment with chemotherapy had been previously unknown, these retrospective findings are interesting and pertinent to the present discussion. Previously, there was no known benefit of the addition of chemotherapy and its role in influencing prognostic outcome. Patients with favorable histologies, such as ovarian cancer, were particularly responsive to chemotherapy. Patients with ovarian cancer fared much better (23.9%) than those with SCLC (1.7%).

One of the most useful data sets was analyzed by Gaspar et al. *(11)* using RPA to assess patients with brain metastases enrolled in three separate RTOG trials. The database included 1200 patients who had been assigned to consecutive studies. The characteristics of these patients before treatment are given in Table 1. All statistically significant ($p < 0.5$) variables were used in a RPA approach. Patients were distributed into three distinct prognostic groups on the basis of a small number of pretreatment characteristics, shown in Fig. 1.

Prognosis was defined for patients who had been divided into three classes. Patients in the most favorable class (Class I) had a median survival of 7.1 mo, a KPS of ≥70, were <65 yr of age, and had controlled primary systemic disease with the CNS being the only metastatic site. Class 3 patients had the worst prognosis. Those patients presented with a KPS < 70, and had a median survival of only 2.3 mo. All other patients were assigned to Class 2, and had a median survival of 4.2 mo.

At a later date, Gaspar et al. *(11,12)* prospectively confirmed the previous findings with 445 patients who had solid tumor metastases and who either received accelerated radiotherapy or accelerated hyperfractionated radiotherapy. Although no significant differences were shown between the two treatment arms, RPA based on these three classes revealed a significant difference. Class 1 patients survived 6.2 mo compared to 3.8 mo for class 2 patients. Additional studies *(2,6)* confirmed the usefulness of stratifying patients based on RPA criteria. Thus, it would be prudent in future studies evaluating the effectiveness of systemic chemotherapy regimes to stratify enrolled participants into these classes *(6)*.

Table 1
Demonstrates the Pre-Treatment Characteristics of Patients With Brain Metastasis Used for the Recursive Partitioning Analysis

Characteristic	Classification groups
Brain metastases	Alone or with other metastases
Primary cancer	Controlled or uncontrolled
Primary lesion site	Lung, breast, or other
Histology	Squamous, adenocarcinoma, large cell, small cell, melanoma, or other
Prior brain surgery	Yes or no
Time interval from primary diagnosis to brain metastases	<2 yr or >2 yr
Headache	Absent or present
Seizure	Absent or present
Visual distrubance	Absent or present
Neurologic dysfunction	None, minor, moderate, or major
Midline shift of brain	Yes or no
Mass effect of brain tumors	Yes or no
Location of lesions	Frontal, temporal, parietal, occipital, basal ganglia, cerebellum, or brainstem
Sentinal location of lesions	Frontal, temporal, parietal, occipital, basal ganglia, cerebellum, or brainstem
Sentinal lesion side	Right, left, or midline
Necrotic center in lesion	Yes or no
Number of lesions	Single or multiple
Tumor response to treatment	Complete, partial, stable disease or progression
Karnofsky performance status, 5	30 to 40, 50 to 60, 70 to 80, or 90 to 100
Area of tumor, mm^2	0 to 400, 401 to 900, 901 to 1600, or 1601 +
Age, years	<40, 40 to 44, 45 to 49, 50 to 54, 55 to 59, 60 to 64, 65 to 69, or 70+
Total radiotherapy dose, cGy	2400 to 3499, 3500 to 4000, 4001 to 5279, 5280 to 6079, 6080 to 6719

Adapted from Gilbert (ref. *12a*) and adapted from Gasper (ref. *11*).

3. TREATMENT DIFFICULTIES

Metastatic tumors of the CNS derive from and are discontinuous with the patient's primary systemic neoplasm. The existence of a blood–brain barrier (BBB) creates a privileged anatomical compartment and extension of disease into this compartment is a significant challenge in the overall treatment of the patient. Nationally and internationally, chemotherapy has generally been perceived as being ineffective for treating CNS metastases. The reasons for this are well known, and include 1. impaired delivery of chemotherapy into the CNS; 2. the drug resistance of solid tumor clones that are capable of metastases to the CNS (*9*); 3. CNS metastases occuring in the setting of drug failure of the primary systemic disease; and 4. the small number of patients enrolled in the studies have generally had tumors with mixed histologies. A few larger studies have, however, lent a degree of statistical power to the interpretation of the various treatment protocols undertaken in this complicated field of clinical medicine *(10,13,17,18,29,35,42,43,46)*.

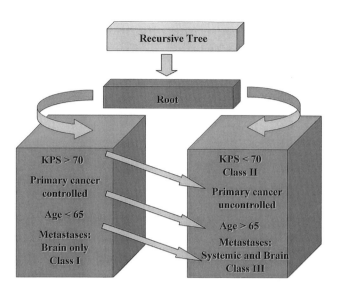

Fig. 1. A recurve partitioning analysis tree which was designed for clinical trials in brain metastases, taken from Gilbert (ref. *12a*) and adapted from Gasper (ref. *11*).

The relative importance to treatment with chemotherapy of an intact BBB has been debated for years. Because it was assumed that an intact BBB was a significant impediment, early chemotherapy trials relied on lipid-soluble drugs such as nitrosoureas. Because nitrosoureas are not typically used to treat the most common histologic sources of brain metastases, it is unclear whether treatment failure was a result of the disparity between histology and the aptness of the chemotherapeutic agent used, or if limitations in delivery of these drugs to the target was a more significant factor. Levin and Landahl *(25)* predicted the effectiveness of chemotherapy for penetrating the BBB on the basis of the molecular weight of the compound used, and the $\log_{10}$ of the ratio of partitioning the compound between an octanol/water interface [log (octanol/water) mol. wt.$^{-1/2}$]. The ability to predict the clearance of drugs from the cerebrospinal fluid (CSF) can be approximated by plotting a constant K_{out} ($K_{out} = Cl_{csf}/Vol_{csf}$) against the octanol /water coefficient (Fig. 2). Table 2 lists drugs detected in the CSF of animals as a percentage of serum concentration. In the setting of a normal BBB, the transport of hydrophilic drugs is limited by tight junctions between the endothelial cells lining capillaries. For strongly hydrophobic drugs, the ability to penetrate normal brain can be predicted by the octanol/ water coefficient. This estimate is often, however, an insufficient predictor, implicating the involvement of carrier systems in transporting drugs out of the CNS in addition to the limitations of the BBB. Many drugs appear to be transported by P-glycoprotein (PGP), which is encoded by the human multidrug resistance-1 (*MDR-1*) gene in humans. The PGP protein is expressed at high levels in brain endothelial cells, which presumably helps maintain the BBB and extrude potential toxic agents *(50)*. Stewart and colleagues *(47,48)* examined drug delivery to tumor and adjacent brain and found that adequate levels of drug were able to reach the center of tumor, with decreasing amounts of drug delivered to the periphery of the tumor and adjacent brain. Additionally, low levels of some drugs were evident in the normal brain interstitium, inferring that micrometastatic foci may be poorly bathed with adequate drug concentrations. Direct measurement of drug concentration within micrometastatic foci have, however, yet to be performed. It has been erroneously thought by some that the drug levels found in the CSF were an adequate surrogate for drug levels attained in brain metastases. In actuality, surgical specimens obtained from symptomatic brain metastasis demonstrated a poor correlation between drug levels in a metastatic focus compared with drug levels in the CSF *(3)*.

Table 2
CSF to Plasma Drug Ratios Following Intravenous
Administration in Rhesus Monkeys or Humans

Drug	CSF-Plamsa ratio	Reference
TEPA	1.0	28
Thiotepa	1.0	52
6-mercaptopurine	0.27	3,38
Zidovudine (Azidothymidine)	0.24	39
5-Fluorouracil	0.155	8
Cytosine arabinoside	0.06–0.25	3
Vincristine	0.05	3
Spiromustine	0.047	5
Cisplatin	0.029	19,48
Etoposide	0.018	37,52
Methotrexate	0.01–0.03	3
INF-α	0.01	1,45
Daunomycin	nd[a]	3

[a]nd, not detectable.

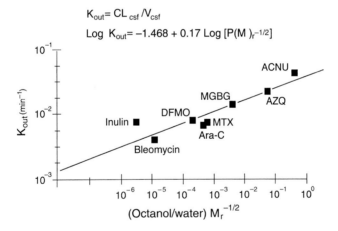

Fig. 2. Relationship between octanol/water coefficient as it relates to molecular weight of the compound of interest and a constant of the particular species able to move out of the CSF (adapted from ref. *25*).

Postmus et al. *(37)* found low levels of etoposide in the CSF after treatment, but found clear evidence of clinical activity in patients with SCLC. Results from animal models have shown that microscopic metastatic foci are required to be at least $1mm^3$ before an intact BBB tends to fail *(9)*. Some researchers have argued that an intact BBB favors the production of an isolated CNS primary relapse, which may in fact be from a predilection for tumors to invade tissues sites on the basis of a favorable growth factor environment *(27,33)*, rather than to a tumor sanctuary created by an intact BBB. Larger metastatic foci significantly or completely abrogate barriers altogether, totally obviating the importance of the BBB. Other clinical data from patients with chemosensitive tumors treated prior to radiation therapy also tend to argue in favor of a minimal role for BBB as a cause of treatment failure. Chemosensitive tumors, such as those from SCLC have been shown by multiple authors to have a high percentage of initial responders with the use of multi-agent chemotherapy *(20)*, including patients with SCLC treated with a combination of cisplatin (CDDP), etopside (VP-16), and vincristine *(20)*. Many of these agents, such as vinca-alkaloids are known to not adequately penetrate normal brain *(47)*. A recent review of pooled data from five previous trials of patients treated for SCLC with different chemotherapy regimens demonstrated a 66% response rate *(33)*. Favorable response data from 97 patients with brain metastases were also demonstrated using a six-drug combination of 6–TG, procarbazine, dibromodulcitol, lomustine (CCNU), 5-FU, and hydroxyurea *(29)*. Overall response rates for non-small cell lung cancer (NSCLC), SCLC, and breast cancer were 52%, 66%, and 60%, respectively. Such responses by patients with SCLC would argue against the limiting role of the BBB. Favorable response rates have also been shown by patients with germ cell tumors that are exclusively sensitive to chemotherapy. Kollmannsberger et al. *(17)*, demonstrated high response rates in patients with germ cell tumors compared with a subset of patients with metastatic CNS disease. High-dose chemotherapy followed by autologous bone marrow transplantation was given and response rates of 91% were seen in the 22 evaluated patients who had metastatic CNS disease. Consistent with these results, Rustin et al. *(42,43)* reported complete responses in 50% of patients with germ cell carcinoma metastatic to the brain who were treated with a combination of CDDP, vincristine, methotrexate, bleomycin, etoposide, dactinomycin, and cyclophosphamide. Similar reports of chemosensitive tumors, such as gestational choriocarcinoma, demonstrated high response rates in approx 75% of patients with CNS metastases *(42,43)*. Because these tumor types respond so well to chemotherapy, the concept that the BBB is of significant importance is arguable. The current consensus is that although the BBB may have some sort of role viz a viz microscopic tumor foci, its overall impediment to treatment failure is questionable at best.

A second commonly stated reason for the ineffectiveness of chemotherapy is that some tumors that metastasize to the CNS have an intrinsic resistance to chemotherapy, which probably accounts for the bulk of CNS treatment failure. Although there are, as discussed, examples of chemosensitive tumors, many of the tumors with a predilection for the brain, such as melanoma, NSCLC, and renal cancer, are relatively insensitive to chemotherapy. Other tumor types such as breast cancer are moderately chemosensitive. There is, in fact, a spectrum of chemotherapy sensitivities. This range exists among different tumor types and among tumors with the same histology. Intrinsic differences such as these are undoubtedly a result of the genetic and biologic characteristics of individual tumors, encompassing both classic and nonclassic (i.e., failure to undergo apoptosis in response to cytotoxic damage) resistance mechanisms. Classic resistance can be broadly understood as cellular strategies used to avoid the toxic effects of chemotherapy. These include drug clearance, bioconversion, and repair pathways *(22–25,50)*. Nonclassic resistance is, on the other hand, described as the ability of malignant cells to resist cell death by inhibiting apoptotic or death pathways via mechanisms linked to cell survival and growth factor signal transduction-mediated pathways *(54)*. Growth factors may produce a selective advantage for clonal cell populations to metastasize, contributing to the resistant phenotype of the tumor *(15,49,54)*. Much attention is presently being directed toward subcellular and genetic mechanisms in which the *p53* tumor suppressor gene has a central role. Invasion promoting genes, such as matrix metalloproteinase (MMP-2) and MMP-9, are known to be regulated in part by p53. Secondary tumors arising from a metastatic-capable primary neoplasm express a higher than normal level of specific genes associated with metastasis *(26)*, such as epidermal growth factor receptor (EGFR), kinase-associated (KA1), MMP-2, and MDR-1, which are regulated in part by p53 protein *(27,49)*. Other mechanisms have been associated with an increased predilection for metastatic spread, including over-expression of CD-44-R1 in choriocarcinoma and c-ERB2 in breast carcinoma *(15,49,54)*. Other investigations have demonstrated characteristic patterns of chromosomal changes in patients with CNS metastases. These perturbations include chromosomal gains on 1q23, 8q24, 17q24, and 20q13, and are present in more than 80% of patients with CNS metastases *(32)*. Those changes that occur in primary tumors to help facilitate metastatic-capable clones may also alter the chemosensitivity of metastatic lesions.

A third consideration while assessing the treatment failure of CNS metastases, is that many patients with brain metastases present after failing chemotherapy for their primary disease, presenting a selection bias as a result of chemotherapy-resistant clones. This concept plays itself out as progressive disease resistance with subsequent treatments and it is quite common. SCLC is a tumor with a high predilection for the CNS and 10% of patients with SCLC have brain metastasis at the time of their original diagnosis *(30,34)*. As patients move through the course of their treatment, and if their disease progresses, an additional 40 to 50% develop CNS metastasis *(22)*. At that point, it becomes more difficult to concomitantly treat the primary disease site and also the CNS disease. This observation of progressive disease resistance with subsequent treatment protocols tends to bias clinical findings. Not many studies have stratified patients according to numbers of previously administered chemotherapy regimens, resulting in an erroneous comparison between response in the CNS and responses by the primary tumor to front-line therapy. A more accurate assessment of response may be provided by observations of CNS tumor chemotherapy responsiveness in patients who have brain metastases at the time of original diagnosis.

4. POTENTIAL SOLUTIONS/STUDY DESIGN

All of these issues, physiologic and methodologic alike, must be addressed in a rational system using intelligently designed studies to obtain the true value for CNS metastases of chemotherapy, biochemotherapy, and perhaps signal transduction inhibitory therapy. Ideally, trials will incorporate the following approaches. Sufficient numbers of patients for any given histology should be enrolled so that the study will be adequately powered to determine if the regimen of interest is superior to current treatment strategies. To do this, estimates of the response for each tumor type must first be obtained to provide a baseline against which to measure outcomes from the clinical trial. These estimates are readily available in the literature for frequently metastatic tumors, such as from SCLC, NSCLC, and breast cancers. Treatment efficacy should initially be demonstrated in patients who have failed whole brain radiation therapy. It would likely be beneficial to stratify study patients into a chemotherapy-naive patient group vs a heavily pretreated patient group. Stratification of patients into RPA classification groups is also essential when initiating a study. Different studies should consistently provide adequate measurements of neurologic versus systemic endpoints. Combination therapies should be tailored to the targeted histology rather than to concerns focused on drug delivery. Postmus and Smit *(35)* suggested that because established brain metastases do not differ significantly in their response to chemotherapy from other metastatic areas in the body, phase II clinical trials for brain metastasis should utilize drug combinations that have shown activity against the specific tumor histology being assessed. These authors contend that the major reason for treatment failure is that the currently used chemotherapy regimens are suboptimal for the specific tumor histology being targeted.

Finally, it is important to obtain relevant tissue after drug(s) treatment to assess biologic endpoints for the specific target of the drug(s) used and to obtain drug levels within the specimen.

5. CHEMOTHERAPY EFFICACY

Specific chemotherapeutic agents exert activity against specific tumor types. This is true of SCLC, NSCLC, and breast carcinoma. Recently, some activity has been reported against melanoma *(15)*. A newly completed phase III study compared early vs delayed whole brain irradiation with concurrent chemotherapy. CDDP and vinorelbine were given to 171 patients with NSCLC, demonstrating a positive chemotherapy effect. The overall objective response rate intracranially was 27% in the chemotherapy-alone arm vs 33% for the chemotherapy arm with early whole brain irradiation. The six-month survival rates for each group were 46% and 40%, respectively, with a median survival duration of 24 and 21 wk, respectively. The results were not significantly different between the two groups and there were no significant differences in observed toxicities between the two groups *(37)*. A smaller study analyzed 30 patients who had brain metastases out of a total enrollment of 121 patients with NSCLC being treated with a combination of CDDP, ifosfamide, and irinotecan. The objective response rate intracranially was an impressive 50% and the patients had no previous radiation therapy to the brain *(10)*. Additionally, in a recently completed phase III trial organized by the European Lung Cancer Cooperative Group *(36)*, patients with SCLC were randomized to receive teniposide with and without whole brain irradiation. A total of 120 patients were randomized. An intracranial response rate was seen in 58% of patients in the combined chemotherapy/radiation arm, compared with a 22% response rate for patients in the chemotherapy arm alone *(17)*. An important finding was that the results from the study showed no differences in the clinical response of intracranial lesions compared with the response of other metastatic sites.

A recent Canadian study *(44)* enrolled 103 patients with NSCLC metastatic to the brain. Patients were randomized to receive docetaxel or best supportive care. Both groups were well-balanced in terms of prognostic factors. The median survival for the two groups was 7.0 mo for the chemotherapy-treated arm vs 4.6 mo for the best supportive care arm ($p = 0.003$). The side effects from chemotherapy fell within acceptable limits, and the conclusion was that the group of patients treated with chemotherapy had a significantly prolonged survival and that the treatment outweighed the risks associated with toxicity.

These larger, better-controlled recent studies are starting to demonstrate a trend toward a positive role for chemotherapy to treat selected tumor histologies. Such success shows the need for a continuing evaluation of chemotherapy combinations that have demonstrated a high degree of activity against particular tumor types. It is of critical importance that adequate numbers of patients with a single histology are enrolled to ensure that the studies are sufficiently powered to meaningfully assess the benefits of these regimens for patients harboring intracranial metastatic disease. Studies currently underway are evaluating a new FDA-approved drug, temozolomide. This drug produces a methyl-alkylating group that exhibits excellent penetration into the CNS. This novel agent may provide benefit for patients who have metastatic melanoma.

An example of the response of metastatic adenocarcinoma originating from the cervix to chemotherapy is demonstrated in Fig. 3. There is a clear response by multiple metastatic lesions to combined protein kinase-C inhibition using cisplatin and ironotecan (CPT-11). Of interest is that this response occurred after whole-brain irradiation and carmustine (BCNU) chemotherapy failure. This demonstration of response is seen with drugs that are typically are not thought of as good penetrators to the CNS, but clearly were more potent to this tumor histology rather than BCNU chemotherapy, which has a good penetration into the CNS.

6. CONCLUSIONS

The management of patients with CNS metastases is tremendously difficult because the patient's physical, cognitive, and emotional functions are slowly eroded as a consequence of growing metastatic foci. Additionally, because many patients are living longer because of better systemic treatment of their primary disease, successful management of late stage metastatic disease becomes more imperative. The treatment of patients with CNS metastases is currently unsatisfactory with current methods. Many obstacles remain in the way of effectively managing patients who have CNS metastases. Of the many factors that appear to limit the effectiveness of chemotherapy, probably least important is the limitation of an intact BBB, which was once thought to be critically important. Intrinsic drug resistance is probably a more relevant issue, which is acquired *de novo* and which emanates from the emergence of drug resistance clones in heavily pretreated patients. Recent large studies have happily begun to demonstrate a positive impact of chemotherapy for selected groups of patients. These limited glimpses of chemotherapy-sensitive tumors that have invaded the CNS impel us to explore novel combinations of drugs. Because of the emergence of targeted signal transduction inhibitors, realistic and rational treatment strategies can now be contemplated with greater hope of relieving patients who endure the burden of metastatic CNS disease.

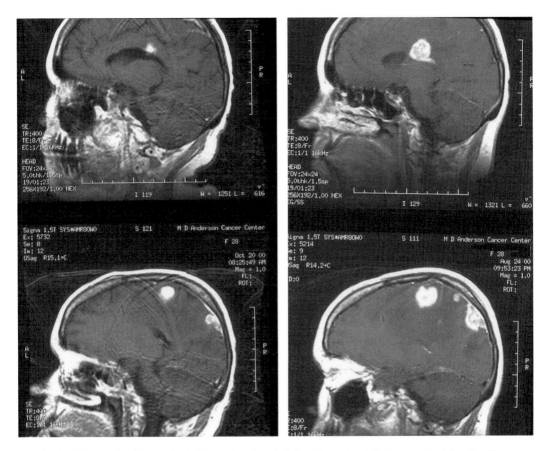

Fig. 3. MRI imaging into sagittal planes after the administration of gadolinium contrast showing the response of multiple metastatic lesions to two courses of chemotherapy.

REFERENCES

1. Adams F., Quesada J.R., Gutterman J.U. 1984. Neuropsychiatric manifestations of human leukocyte interferon therapy in patients with cancer. *JAMA* **252**:938–941.
2. Agoola O., Benoit B., Cross P., et al. 1998. Prognostic factors derived from recursive partition analysis (RPA) of Radiation Therapy Oncology Group (RTOG) brain metastases trials applied to surgically resected and irradiated brain metastatic cases. *Int. J. Radiat. Oncol. Biol. Phys.* **42**:155–159.
3. Balis F.M., Poplack D.G. 1989. Central nervous system pharmacology of antileukemic drugs. *Am. J. Pediatr. Hematol. Oncol.* **11**:74–86.
4. Barron K.D., Hirano A., Araki S., Terry R.D. 1958. Experiences with neoplasm involving the spinal cord. *Neurology* **9**:91–106.
5. Bigler R.E., Zanzonico P.B., Cosma M., Sgouros G. 1988. Adjuvant radioimmunotherapy for micrometastases: a strategy for cancer cure, inRadiolabeled Monoclonal Antibodies for Imaging and Therapy, (Srivastava S.C., ed.), Plenum, New York, pp. 409–429.
6. Chidel M.A., Suh J.H., Reddy C.A., et al. 2000. Application of recursive partitioning analysis and evaluation of the use of whole brain radiation among patients treated with sterotactic radiosurgery for newly diagnosed brain metastases. *Int. J. Radiat. Oncol. Biol. Phys.* **47**:993–999.
7. Curran W.J., Scott C.B., Horton J., et al. 1993. Recursive partitioning analysis of prognostic factors in three radiation therapy oncology group malignant glioma trials. *J. Natl. Cancer Inst.* **85**:704–710.
8. Doge H., Hliscs R. 1984. Intrathecal therapy with [198]Au-colloid formeningosis prophylaxis. *Eur. J. Nucl. Med.* **9**:125–128.

9. Donelli, M.G., Zucchetti M., D'Incalco M. 1992. Do anticancer agents reach the tumor target in the human brain? *Cancer Chemother. Pharmacol.* **30:**251–260.

10. Fujita A., Fukuoka S., Takabatake H., Tagaki S., Sekine K. 2000. Combination chemotherapy of cisplatin, ifosfamide, and irinotecan with rhG-CSF support in patients with brain metastases from non-small cell lung cancer. *Oncology* **59:** 291–295.

11. Gaspar L., Scott C., Rotman M., et al. 1997. Recursive partitioning analysis (RPA) of prognostic factors in three radiation therapy oncology group (RTOG) brain metastases trials. *Int. J. Radiation Oncology Biol. Phys.* **37:**745–751.

12. Gaspar L.E., Scott C., Murray K., et al. 2000. Validation of the RTOG recursive partitioning analysis (RPA) classification for brain metastases. *Int. J. Radiat. Oncol. Biol. Phys.* **47:**1001–1006.

12a. Gilbert M.R. 2001. Brain metastatses: still on "orphan" disease? *Curr. Oncol. Rep.* **3:**463–466.

13. Grossi F., Scolaro T., Tixi L., Loprevite M., Ardizzoni A. 2001. The role of systemic chemotherapy in the treatment of brain metastases from small-cell lung cancer. *Crit.l Rev. Oncology-Hematology* **37:**61–67.

14. Hall W.A., Djalilian H.R., Nussbaum E.S., Cho K.H. 2000. Long-term survival with metastatic cancer to the brain. *Med. Oncol.* **17:**279–286.

15. Hwu W.J. 2000. New approaches in the treatment of metastatic melanoma: thalidomide and temozolomide. *Oncology* **14:**25–28.

16. Kaba S.E., Kyritsis A.P., Hess K., et al. 1997. TPDC-FuHu chemotherapy for the treatment of recurrent metastatic brain tumors. *J. Clin. Oncol.* **15:**1063–1070.

17. Kollmannsberger C., Nichol C., Bamberg M., Hartmann J.T., Schleucher N., Beyer J., et al. 2000. First-line high-dose chemotherapy +/– radiation therapy in patients with metastatic germ-cell cancer and brain metastases. *Ann. Oncol.* **11:** 553–559.

18. Komaki R, Cox J.D., Stark R. 1983. Frequency of brain metastasis in adenocarcinoma and large-cell carcinoma of the lung: Correlation with survival. *Int. J. Rad. Oncol. Biol. Phys.* **9:**1467–1470.

19. Kovacs E.J., Beckner S.K., Longo D.L., Varesio L., Young H.A. 1989. Cytokine gene expression during the generation of human lymphokine-activated killer cells: early induction of interleukin 1 beta by interleukin 2. *Cancer Res.* **49:**940–944.

20. Krisjansen, PE.G., Sorenson P.S., Hansen, M.S., et al. 1993. Prospective evaluation of the effect on initial brain metastases from small-cell lung cancer of platinum-etoposide based induction chemotherapy followed by an alternating drug regimen. *Ann. Oncol.* **4:**579–583.

21. Landis S.H., Murray T., Bolden S., et al. 1998. Cancer Statistics. *CA Cancer J.* **48:**6–29

22. Lesser G.J. 1996. Chemotherapy of cerebral metastases from solid tumors. *Neurosurgery Clin. North Am.* **7:**527–536.

23. Levin V.A. 1980. Relationship of octanol/water partition coefficient and molecular weight to rat brain capillary permeability. *J. Med. Chem.* **23:**682–684.

24. Levin V.A., Patlak C.S., Landahl H.D. 1980. Heuristic modeling of drug delivery to malignant brain tumors. *Pharmacokinet. Biopharm.* **8:**257–296.

25. Levin V.A., Landahl H.D. 1985. Pharmacokinetic approaches to drug distribution in the cerebrospinal fluid based on ventricular administration in beagle dogs. *J. Pharmacokinet. Biopharm.* **13:**387–403.

26. Lloyd B.H., Platt-Higgins A., Rudland P.S., Barraclough R. 1998. Human S100A4 (p9ka) induces the metastatic phenotype upon benign tumour cells. *Oncogene* **17:**465–473.

27. Mashimo T., Watabe M., Hirota S., Hosobe S., Miura K., Tegtmeyer P.J., et al. 1998. The expression of the KA11 gene, a tumor metastasis suppressor, is directly activated by p53. *Proc. Natl. Acad. Sci. USA* **95:**11,307–11,311.

28. Mencel P.J., L.M.DeAngelis, R.J. Motzer. 1994. Hormonal ablation as effective therapy for carcinomatous meningitis from prostatic carcinoma. *Cancer* **73:**1892–1894.

29. Murray N., Livingston R.B., Shepherd F.A., James K., Zee B., Langleben A., et al. 1999. Randomized study of CODE versus alternating CAV/EP for extensive-stage small-cell lung cancer: an Intergroup Study of the National Cancer Institute of Canada Clinical Trials Group and the Southwest Oncology Group. *J. Clin. Oncol.* **17:**2300–2308.

30. Nugent, J.K., Bunn P.A., Matthews M.J., et al. 1979. CNS metastases in small cell bronchogenic carcinoma: Increasing frequency and changing pattern with lengthening survival. *Cancer* **44:**1885–1893.

31. Opp M.R., Obal F.R., Krueger J.M. 1988. Effects of alpha-MSH on sleep, behavior and brain temperature: interactions with IL 1. *Am. J. Physiol.* **255:**R914–R922.

32. Petersen I., Hildalgo A., Petersen S., Schluens K., Schewe C., Pacyna-Gengelbach M, et al. 2000. Chromosomal imbalances in brain metastases of solid tumors. *Brain Pathol.* **10:**395–401.

33. Ponta H., Sleeman J., Herrlich P. 1994. Tumor metastasis formation, cell-surface proteins confer metastasis-promoting or suppressing properties. *Biochim. Biophys. Acta.* **1198:**1–10.

34. Posner J.B., Chernik N.L. 1978. Intracranial metastases from systemic cancer. *Adv. Neurol.* **19:**579–592.

35. Postmus P.E., Smit E.F. 1999. Chemotherapy for brain metastases of lung cancer: A review. *Ann. Oncol.* **10:**753–759.

36. Postmus P.E., Haaxma-Reiche H., Smit E.F., Groen H.J., Karnicka H., Lewinski T., et al. 2000. Treatment of brain metastases of small-cell lung cancer: comparing teniposide and teniposide with whole-brain radiotherapy—a phase III study of the European Organization for the Research and Treatment of Cancer Lung Cancer Cooperative Group. *J.Clin. Oncol.* **18:**3400–3408.

37. Postmus P.E., Holthuis J.J.M., Haaxma-Reiche H., et al. 1984. Penetration of VP 16-213 into cerebrospinal fluid after high-dose administration. *J. Clin. Oncol.* **2**:215–220.

38. Reddeman H., Bartelt G., Blau H-J. 1986. Intrathekale radiogoldprohylaxe un liquorbefunde bei kindern mit akuter lymphoblastischer leukose. *Folia Haematol.* **113**:466–473.

39. Rigon A., Sotti G., Zanesco L., et al. Profilassi meningea con radiocolloidi nell leucemia e nel linoofa non-Hodgkin dell'infanzia. *Radiol. Med.* **71**:517–520.

40. Robinet G, Thomas P., Breton P.J.L., Lena H., Gouva S., Dabouis G., et al. 2001. Results of a phase III study of early versus delayed whole brain radiotherapy with concurrent cisplatin and vinorelbine combination in inoperable brain metastasis of non-small-cell lung cancer. *Ann. Oncol* **12**:59–67.

41. Roetger A., Merschjann A., Dittmar T., Jackisch C., Barnekow A., Brandt B. 1998. Selection of potentially metastatic subpopulations expressing c-erB-2 from breast cancer tissue by use of an extravasation model. *Am. J. Pathol.* **153**:1797–1806.

42. Rustin G.J.S., Newlands E.S., Bagshaew K.D., Begent R.H.J., Crawford S.M. 1986. Successful management of metastatic and primary germ cell tumors in the brain. *Cancer* **57**:2108–2113.

43. Rustin G.J.S., Newlands E.S., Begent R.H.J., Dent J., Bagshawe K.D. 1989. Weekly alternating etoposide, methotrexate, and actinomycin/vincristine and cyclophosphamide chemotherapy for the treatment of CNS metastases of choriocarcinoma. *J. Clin. Oncol.* **7**:900–903.

44. Shepherd F.A., Dancey J., Ramlau R., Mattson K., Gralla R., O'Rourke M., et al. 2000. Prospective randomized trial of docetaxel versus best supportive care in patients with non-small-cell lung cancer previously treated with platinum-based chemotherapy. *J. Clin. Oncol.* **18**:2095–2103.

45. Smedley H., Katrak M., Sikora K., Wheeler T. 1983. Neurological effects of recombinant human interferon. *Br. Med. J.* **286**:262–264.

46. Sorensen J.B., Stenbygaard L.E., Dombernowsky P., Hansen H.H. 1999. Paclitaxel, gemcitabine, and cisplatin in non-resectable non-small-cell lung cancer. *Ann. Oncol.* **10**:1043–1049.

47. Stewart D.J., Lu K., Benjamin R.S., et al. 1983. Concentrations of vinblastine in human intracerebral tumor and other tissues. *J. Neuro-oncol.* **1**:139–144.

48. Stewart D.J., Leavens M., Maor M., et al. 1982. Human central nervous system distribution of cis-diaminedichloroplatinum and use as radiosensitizer in malignant brain tumors. *Cancer Res.* **42**:2472–2479.

49. Sun Y., Wicha M., Leopold W.R. 1999. Regulation of metastasis-related gene expression by p53: a potential clinical implication. *Mol. Carcinog.* **24**:25–28.

50. Thiebaut F., Tsuoro T., Hamada H., et al. 1987. Cellular localization of the multidrug resistance gene product in normal human tissues. *Proc. Natl. Acad. Sci. USA* **84**:7735–7738.

51. Twelves C.J., Souhami R.L., Harper P.G., Ash C.M., Spiro S.G., Earl H.M., et al. 1990. The response of cerebral metastases in small cell lung cancer to systemic chemotherapy. *Br. J. Cancer* **61**:147–150.

52. Va der Gaast A., Sonneveld P., Mans D.R., Splinter I.A. 1992. Intrathecal administration of etoposide in the treatment of malignant meningitis: feasibility and pharmacokinetic data. *Cancer Chemother. Pharmacol.* **29**:335–337.

53. Wheldon T.E., O'Donoghue J.A., Hilditch T.E., Barrett A. 1988. Strategies for systemic radiotherapy of micrometastases using antibody-targeted [131]. I. *Radiother. Oncol.* **11**:133–142.

54. Wu C.S., El-Deiry W.S. 1996. Apoptotic death of tumor cells correlates with chemosensitivity, independent of p53 or Bcl-2. *Clin. Cancer Res.* **2**:623–633.

15

Radiation Biology and Therapy of Tumors of the Central Nervous System

Nalin Gupta, John R. Fike, Penny K. Sneed,
Philip J. Tofilon, and Dennis F. Deen

1. RADIATION BIOLOGY

1.1. Radiation-Induced Deoxyribonucleic Acid Damage and Repair

Interaction of ionizing radiation with any biological material results in uneven energy deposition, which results in a variety of chemical modifications. This is the *direct* action of radiation that predominates for particulate radiation (protons, neutrons, or α-particles). Another mechanism is the interaction of a photon with orbital electrons of the absorbing intracellular medium, of which water molecules are the most common. This interaction ejects fast electrons from outer shells that create multiple ionizations along their tracks. This mechanism, the *indirect* action of radiation, is the predominant one for X-rays and γ-rays. The initial ionization occurs in 10^{-15} seconds while ion radicals and free radicals exist for only 10^{-10} to 10^{-5} s. The consequences of radiation-induced chemical alterations may not be expressed for hours or days, if the parameter is cell killing; and potentially years if genetic changes are not manifest until following generations *(56)*.

Whereas radiation produces ionizations randomly throughout the cell, it has been assumed that deoxyribonucleic acid (DNA) damage determines cell survival *(72,115)*. Damage to other cellular components, such as proteins, messenger ribonucleic acid (mRNA), and lipids, are not believed to be significant because many copies of these components exist and damaged molecules are presumably replaced by normal turnover. The major types of DNA lesions caused by X-rays and γ-rays are base damage, DNA–DNA or DNA–protein crosslinks, and scissions of the phosphodiester backbone leading to single-strand breaks (SSBs) or double-strand breaks (DSBs). Lesions are characterized as being *simple*, i.e., with no damage to neighboring groups, or *complex*, where combinations of lesions or multiple lesions exist. These represent only broad categories of lesions because the exact chemical changes are extremely diverse. It is unlikely that these different types of damage are repaired with equal efficiency or fidelity. The majority of data acquired so far support the theory that DNA DSBs are the significant lesions that cause cell killing following ionizing radiation.

Physiologic DSBs are created in order to initiate homologous recombination during meiosis and during immunologic development, particularly V(D)J recombination. Therefore, eukaryotic cells have evolved two distinct molecular mechanisms to repair DNA DSBs: homologous recombination (HR) and nonhomologous end-joining (NHEJ) *(54,77)*. HR requires an undamaged DNA double strand template that is used to fill in homologous areas that have been lost on the damaged DNA helix. NHEJ does not require a template and this results in repair being error-prone with small regions of DNA being deleted. The activation of these repair processes by DNA DSBs not only leads to struc-

From: *Contemporary Cancer Research: Brain Tumors*
Edited by: F. Ali-Osman © Humana Press Inc., Totowa, NJ

tural repair of DNA, but also triggers a variety of cellular signaling pathways that in turn produce many other cellular effects.

In yeast, HR is performed by proteins encoded by the *RAD52* epistasis group of genes, of which there are corresponding proteins in mammalian cells. One of these proteins, Rad51, appears to be required as a component of the replication fork during normal DNA replication and damage repair *(173)*. Rad51 localizes to discrete foci within the nucleus after ionizing radiation and during S phase in undamaged cells. Transgenic mice knocked out for *Rad51* are nonviable and die early during embryogenesis *(176)*. In addition to being essential, the mammalian Rad51 protein interacts with a number of other proteins that are involved in the response to cell injury, including p53, Brca1, and Brca2 (the latter two are products of tumor suppressor genes implicated in hereditary breast cancer). Brca2, in particular, appears crucial for this interaction because Rad 51 foci do not accumulate in nuclei of Brca2 deficient cells *(193)*. Brca1 and Brca2 interact with components of the chromatin scaffolding and appear to participate with other repair complexes; possibly preparing or priming the DNA helix prior to repair. Similar to the role that mismatch repair gene mutation plays in the onco-genesis of colon cancer, the interaction between Rad51 and the products of the *BRCA1* and *BRCA2* genes suggests a role for defective DNA DSB repair in oncogenesis *(77)*.

Other components of the cellular DNA repair machinery have been discovered by identifying the genes responsible for a number of related human genetic syndromes such as Nijmegen breakage syndrome, Bloom syndrome, Werner syndrome *(47)*, and ataxia telangiectasia (AT). AT is character-ized by radiosensitivity, predisposition to cancer, and neurodegeneration (particularly in the cerebel-lum) *(76)*. Cells derived from AT patients show increased genetic instability with increased rates of chromosomal breakage, translocations, and recombination. The ataxia telangiectasia mutated (ATM) protein appears to be involved in the activation of HR following ionizing radiation. A host of proteins involved in DNA damage such as c-Abl, p53, and Brca1, directly or indirectly, interact with ATM.

Not surprisingly, a distinct set of proteins are involved in NHEJ, even though functional overlap exists between HR and NHEJ. It is believed that NHEJ is the preferred method of DSB repair in mammalian cells, despite its inaccuracy. The crucial participant is DNA-dependent protein kinase (DNA-PK), which consists of a heterodimer of the Ku protein (which directs the complex to DNA damaged ends) and, the catalytic domain which is related to the family of phosphatidyl-inositol 3-kinases (PI3-K) *(163)*. DNA-PK recognizes DBSs in vitro and is believed to subsequently recruit other proteins involved in NHEJ. One of these components, DNA ligase IV, when lost in transgenic mice, results in widespread neuronal loss.

1.2. Cell-Cycle Alterations Following Radiation Treatment

Early experiments noted that eukaryotic cells do not arrest randomly in the cell-cycle in response to ionizing radiation *(117,121–123)*. Cells tended to arrest in late G_1 (just prior to S phase), during S phase, and at the late G_2/M phase boundary. The molecular basis of these observations remained obscure until genetic experiments in yeast revealed a complex series of biochemical pathways that regulate the progress of cells through the cell-cycle. Normal yeast cells (*S. cerevisiae*) arrest in G_2 following irradiation. A large number of yeast mutants, identified by the designation *rad*, were known to be radiation sensitive. Weinert and Hartwell *(186)* screened several of these mutants for failure to delay in G_2 following irradiation. They reasoned that the function of the G_2 delay was to allow repair to occur before progression into M phase, so cells defective for a G_2 delay should be more sensitive to DNA damage. Using this strategy, one mutant, *rad9*, was identified that failed to arrest in G_2. Weinert and Hartwell coined the term "checkpoint" to indicate a decision point in the cell-cycle where specific gene products that monitor cell-cycle progression respond to cell damage by delaying the cell-cycle thereby increasing the chances for repair. This concept was expanded by Murray *(118)* when he postulated that components of such a monitoring system consisted of (a) a sensor to detect damage, (b) a signaling pathway that communicates this information, and (c) a component of the cell-cycle machinery that mediates the actual arrest at a precise point, i.e., the checkpoint. The mamma-

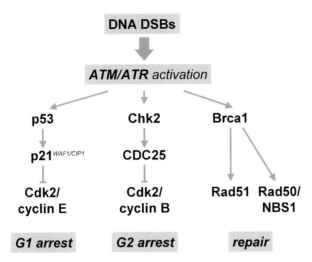

Fig. 1. A simplified schematic description of ATM/ATR dependent events following the formation of DNA DSBs. Multiple interactions between these pathways are known to exist. Some of these individual proteins (i.e., p53) are also capable of activating apoptotic pathways.

lian G_2/M checkpoint is controlled by a specific enzyme, CDC2, which belongs to a group of cyclin dependent kinases (CDK). The activity of CDC2 is modulated, in turn, by other kinases that are members of the upstream signaling pathway that Murray referred to earlier *(111)*.

Similar to yeast, mammalian cells also demonstrate a G_1 and G_2/M block following radiation, with varying degrees of an S phase delay *(99)*. However, the regulation of mammalian cell-cycle checkpoints is considerably more complex. ATM (along with a related gene named ATR) is believed to be relatively high in the hierarchy of signaling following DNA damage (Fig. 1). The activation of ATM and/or ATM- and Rad3-related (ATR) following ionizing radiation leads to the activation of downstream targets such as p53, Mdm2, Brca 1 & 2. Through these secondary genes, specific cell-cycle checkpoints such as those in late G_1, and at the G_2/M boundary are triggered. p53 appears crucial for activation of the G_1 checkpoint whereas Chk1, another intermediary protein is responsible for progression through late G_2 *(19)*. Additional functional interactions occur between members of the G_1 and G_2 checkpoints. Although there is some evidence that the length of the G_2 delay correlates with increased survival *(106,169)*, the functional link between cell-cycle alterations and DNA repair remains unclear. It is possible that these two events occur in parallel following DNA damage.

1.3. Radiation-Induced Apoptosis

In past studies, irradiated cells were reported to a "reproductive" or mitotically-linked death. This was usually measured by a standard clonogenic assay, although this assay does not formally determine the mechanism of cell death. Through the production of DNA DSBs, cells cannot execute mitosis faithfully and experience either a permanent mitotic arrest eventually leading to loss of viability, or progress through several cycles of cell division with grossly abnormal chromosomal structure leading to growth arrest *(7,131)*. Cellular damage created by radiation also can activate apoptosis, a process of cellular death that is characterized by specific morphological and biochemical features including cellular shrinkage, chromatin condensation, nuclear blebbing, and nonrandom DNA fragmentation. This differs from acute necrosis, which is distinguished by cell swelling and lysis and often produces an inflammatory response *(132,133)*. Apoptosis also requires specific gene products and can be attenuated by inhibitors of protein synthesis. The precise relationship between radiation-induced cell damage and execution of apoptosis remains unclear.

There appears to be a substantial degree of cell type specificity with respect to the exact mechanism of cell death. Cells that display an acute post-radiation apoptotic response are those derived from lymphoid and myeloid lineages. p53 can play an important role in postirradiation apoptosis. Although wild-type p53 is known to have antiproliferative effects when introduced into most cells in culture *(38,107)*, introduction of the wild-type gene into leukemia or colon cancer cell lines causes apoptosis *(153,191)*. More convincing evidence for the role of p53 in apoptosis comes from studies using cells derived from knockout mice. Using mice homozygous for a *p53* deletion, two groups of investigators demonstrated that the absence of p53 protects thymocytes against apoptosis following ionizing radiation but not in response to stimuli that mimic T-cell receptor engagement (such as phorbol esters) or glucocorticoids *(27,95)*. This effect was dramatic because 50% of wild-type thymocytes lost viability after 2.5 Gy, whereas only 20% of cells null for p53 lost viability after 20 Gy of radiation.

The intermediate components of the apoptotic response have been identified during the past several years *(59)*. Two major pathways appear to lead to apoptosis. The first pathway, receptor mediated apoptosis, begins with the activation by a specific extracellular ligand such as tumor necrosis factor-α (TNF-α) or CD95-L. Downstream signaling pathways eventually trigger activation of a number caspases (a specific class of proteases); with activation of the effector caspases resulting in irreversible initiation of apoptosis *(41)*. The second pathway is mitochondria-dependent and involves the activation of intracellular signaling molecules (such as p53) that modulate the balance of proapoptotic and anti-apoptotic factors, eventually leading to the release of pro-apoptotic factors, such as cytochrome c from the mitochondria *(90)*.

In the nervous system, apoptosis is essential during development and is regulated by similar molecules (Bcl-2, Apaf-1) identified in other cell types *(192)*. In the immature nervous system, the presence of neurotrophic factors (e.g., nerve growth factor [NGF]) is responsible for maintaining viability of neurons, whereas the absence of these factors triggers apoptosis. Stem cells in particular appear to be exquisitely sensitive to injury caused by radiation (see below). Adult neuronal populations, being post-mitotic in nature, have traditionally been thought to be relatively resistant to radiation but indirect evidence suggests that apoptosis plays a significant role in the response to cell injury. Increased expression of injury-associated transcription factors has been identified in the rodent cerebral cortex *(135)*. Apoptosis has been identified following cellular ischemia, in Alzheimer's disease, and Huntington's disease. In addition, caspase-independent cell death has been observed in cultured hippocampal cells following ionizing radiation *(71)*. Finally, *ATM* null mice demonstrate increased resistance to radiation induced apoptosis in specific areas of the hippocampus and external granule layer of the cerebellum in rodent brain and in the retina *(60)*.

2. NORMAL TISSUE EFFECTS

2.1. Timing of Radiation-Induced Central Nervous System Injury

Radiotherapy remains a major treatment modality for primary and metastatic neoplasms located in the central nervous system (CNS). In addition, exposure of the brain and spinal cord is often unavoidable in the radiotherapeutic management of tumors located in close proximity to the CNS such as head and neck cancers. In each cancer treatment situation, the radiation dose that can be safely administered is limited by the potential for injury to the normal CNS tissue. Whereas any type of normal tissue damage is undesirable, the CNS injury that can occur after radiotherapy is associated with a high rate of morbidity and mortality and is especially devastating. Classically, based on time of expression, radiation-induced CNS injury has been divided into three reactions: acute, early delayed and late delayed *(64,145,154,178)*. Acute injury (acute radiation encephalopathy) is expressed in days to weeks after irradiation and is fairly uncommon under current radiotherapy protocols. Early delayed injury typically occurs from 1 to 6 mo and can involve transient demyelination with somno-lence and L'Hermitte's syndrome after brain and spinal cord irradiation, respectively. Although acute and early delayed injuries can result in severe symptoms, they are normally reversible and resolve spontaneously. In contrast, late-delayed effects, which occur at times greater than 6 mo, are usually irreversible and progressive and have been causally associated with the morbidity and mor-tality of radiation-induced CNS injury. Late delayed injury is characterized by demyelination, vascu-lar abnormalities and ultimately necrosis (both focal and diffuse), which is generally restricted to the white matter. It is this late delayed injury that is generally assumed to be responsible for the morbid-ity and mortality associated with radiation-induced CNS injury.

2.2. Cellular Targets

Although the CNS damage occurring after radiotherapy has been well described in terms of histological and functional criteria, the specific cellular and biochemical processes responsible for its pathogenesis remain poorly defined. Because vascular abnormalities and demyelination domi-nate the histological presentation, considerable effort has been focused on the radioresponse of the vasculature and the oligodendrocyte lineage. The apparent aim of such studies has been to identify the primary cell population or "target" within the CNS, whose death or inactivation after irradia-tion results in white matter necrosis. In the vascular damage scenario, white matter necrosis is considered to be a secondary response to ischemia. Substantial data are available describing radia-tion-induced vascular abnormalities including vessel wall thickening, vessel dilation, and endothelial cell nuclear enlargement, which are presumed to be the result of endothelial cell dam-age *(16,137,145,161)*. Time and dose-related reductions in blood vessel density and a slight loss of endothelial cells, which is extremely variable between individual vessels, have been reported prior to the development of necrosis in white matter *(16,137)*, whereas Siegal et al. *(161)* have reported transient increases in vascular permeability in the rat spinal cord at 1 d after irradiation, the vascu-lar abnormalities considered to be responsible for white matter necrosis are slowly developing and, although preceding necrosis, still require greater than 20 wk to evolve. Thus, although after stan-dard irradiation procedures the appearance of vascular abnormalities is well correlated with necro-sis, whether they are the result of endothelial cell death or other pathophysiological changes remain to be determined. Delineating the specific etiology of the vascular damage would be of consider-able value in understanding the processes responsible for the precipitation of late delayed injury in the irradiated CNS.

Radiation-induced necrosis also has been reported in the absence of vascular changes *(103,145)*, which argues against the absolute dependence on vascular damage for its expression. Furthermore, as mentioned, the vascular basis for radiation-induced injury assumes that ischemia is ultimately respon-sible for the precipitation of the necrosis. However, the CNS phenotype that is by far the most sensitive to oxygen deprivation is the neuron *(98)*, which is located in the gray matter, a relatively radioresis-tant region. Consequently, although the differences in blood flow between gray and white matter may be involved *(98)*, the predilection of radiation-induced necrosis for white matter is inconsistent with a solely vascular basis. On the other hand, recent boron neutron capture therapy (BNCT) studies have clearly indicated that delivery of a high radiation dose almost entirely to the vasculature can result in necrosis *(112)*. Thus, although it seems unlikely that radiation injury can be attributed to a singular target, there is little doubt that vascular damage and, presumably, endothelial cell loss play a signifi-cant role in the expression of white matter necrosis.

In addition to vascular abnormalities, the histological presentation of radiation-induced CNS injury is typically dominated by demyelination, which implicates oligodendrocytes as a target cell population. The glial hypothesis for radiation-induced CNS injury is focused on oligodendrocytes. These terminally differentiated cells provide the myelin sheath for neurons and their loss is an obvi-ous source of demyelination. The glial hypothesis gained strength in the 1980s with the identifica-tion of the O-2A progenitor cell, which serves as a precursor and source of new oligodendrocytes

(134). With the development of an in vivo/in vitro excision assay, van der Kogel and colleagues demonstrated that irradiation results in the loss of reproductive capacity of the O-2A progenitor cells in both the brain and spinal cord of adult rats *(179–181).* Identification of the O-2A progenitor allowed for the application of the classical stem cell model of radiation-induced tissue injury to the CNS. That is, radiation induces the loss of O-2A progenitors, which then results in the failure to replace normally turned-over oligodendrocytes with the eventual consequence being demyelination. The strength of the glial hypothesis is that it accounts for the white matter selectivity of radiation-induced CNS injury and is consistent with the established concept of using stem cells (in this case progenitor or precursor cells) as a continual source of functional, terminally differentiated cells (oligodendrocytes). Furthermore, in contrast to endothelial cells and the vascular hypothesis, an acute loss of O-2A progenitor cells can be detected after irradiation with their recovery being time and dose dependent.

However, as for the vascular hypothesis, there are inconsistencies that argue against the oligodendrocyte lineage as being the sole source of radiation-induced white matter necrosis. In other demyelinating conditions (e.g., multiple sclerosis) the degeneration of denuded axons is not a general finding *(18),* strongly suggesting that oligodendrocyte loss is not sufficient for necrosis. In addition, whereas oligodendrocyte kinetics may be consistent with the relatively early transient demyelination detected after irradiation, they are not consistent with the late onset of necrosis *(65,103).* Furthermore, glial cell depletion has been detected in rat, dog and human brain after relatively low radiation doses, which are not associated with a significant risk of necrosis *(3,44,178).* Thus, although there is the detectable loss of O-2A cells and eventually oligodendroglia after irradiation, there appears to be additional factors required to result in white matter necrosis and late delayed injury.

In summary, there is evidence both for and against the vasculature and oligodendrocyte lineage as being the primary targets for radiation-induced CNS injury. It has been suggested that both are involved with their relative contributions dependent on dose and time of evaluation *(145,178).* Although probably correct, this conclusion continues to leave critical questions unanswered regarding the pathogenesis of radiation-induced CNS injury. In retrospect, a disadvantage to the approach of focusing solely on a single cell type is that the CNS is comprised of a number of different cell types organized in a highly integrated system. Following standard radiation protocols, not only the vasculature and O-2A progenitors will be irradiated but also astrocytes, microglia, neurons and the recently identified neural stem cells. Each will be expected to have some type of response to radiation, which may involve death, compromised function and/or changes in gene expression and it would appear that these responses need to be taken into account when attempting to understand the radioresponse of the CNS.

2.3. Cell–Cell Interactions

Because of the highly integrated nature of the CNS and its reliance on cell–cell interactions, an understanding of the radioresponse of the other neural phenotypes assumes further significance. Cells of the CNS, as in most normal tissue, do not operate as independent entities; their function is contingent on the appropriate interactions with neighboring and in some cases distant cells. For example, appropriate propagation of neuronal impulses requires axonal myelination; neurons provide both growth factors *(18,190)* and electrical cues *(4)* that regulate the proliferation of the oliogodendrocyte lineage. The maintenance of the blood–brain barrier is another illustration of a critical intercellular interaction, in this case it is between endothelial cells and astrocytes. Many other examples exist and it is clearly evident that under both normal and pathological conditions, the CNS is highly dependent on cellular interactions occurring via a variety of endocrine, paracrine, juxtacrine and contact mediated processes. The implication of this cell interaction dependence is that, whereas the vasculature and oligodendrocyte lineage may be the primary radiation targets within the CNS, their radioresponse will be influenced by the radioresponse of other cell types.

Thus, given the number of phenotypes in the CNS and its almost total reliance on cell–cell interactions, the radioresponse of this critical normal tissue should be viewed as an integrated system and not as a collection of functionally autonomous parts. In 1993, Chiang et al. *(26)* noted the necessity of accounting for the interdependence of glial, vascular, and neuronal components in the radioresponse of the CNS. Thus, delineating the pathogenesis of radiation-induced CNS injury will require an understanding not only of the radioresponse of the vasculature and oligodendrocyte lineage, but also of the other phenotypes as well as critical cell–cell interactions.

In addition to considering the various neural cell types, insights into the pathogenesis of radiation injury in the CNS may also be gained through analogies with its response to other types of damage. This perspective is based on the assumption that the CNS, as for most normal tissue, has a limited repertoire of responses to injury. Histologically, CNS lesions induced after radiation are not unique and are actually quite similar to those that occur after other types of injury. This lack of a defining lesion for radiation-induced CNS injury led Schultheiss and Stephens *(145)* to speculate that the radioresponse of the CNS and its reaction to other forms of damage may have similar components. After other types of injury (traumatic, ischemic, and excitotoxic) it is now recognized that in addition to the incipient cell death a significant proportion of the resulting tissue damage is from secondary reactive processes that take place in hours to days after the initial injury *(146)*. Many of these events like membrane breakdown and phospholipid hydrolysis, cationic fluxes, excitatory amino acid release and the induction of specific genes lead to or result from the production of reactive oxygen species (ROS). Along with these deleterious events, however, there is also the activation of competing processes, which involve changes in gene expression and the induction of cytokines. Cytokines, such as basic fibroblast growth factor (bFGF), TNF-α, and assorted neurotrophins have been shown to limit the spread of brain infarction or injury *(13,109,114)*. The induction of these cytokines appears to comprise an intrinsic mechanism of recovery and/or repair.

Thus, although there is indeed some specificity in its reaction to traumatic, ischemic and excitotoxic types of insult, the general injury response of the CNS involves acute cell death, initiation of secondary reactive (oxidative) processes and enhanced cytokine gene expression. It is well established in other systems that ionizing radiation can induce cell death, initiate oxidative events and modify gene expression. One working model of the radioresponse of the CNS involves these three cellular reactions to irradiation and incorporates many of the same elements that have been described for the CNS response to other types of insults. Radiation directly induces a certain level of acute cell death. This has been demonstrated after in vivo irradiation for O-2A progenitors, subependymal neural stem cells and oligodendrocytes *(91,172,179,181)*. In addition, we propose that radiation also activates molecular and biochemical cascades resulting in secondary reactive processes that generate a persistent oxidative stress, which ultimately contributes to tissue injury. Furthermore, at the same time a competing process is initiated involving the induction of genes coding for protective cytokines. Irradiation of rodent brain has been shown to increase the expression of bFGF *(135)* and TNF-α *(61,135)*. Moreover, Daigle et al. *(35)* have shown that p75 TNF receptor (TNFR) knockout mice are more susceptible to radiation induced brain injury.

The level of tissue injury expressed after CNS irradiation then reflects the balance between these three reactions. After higher doses that result in functional and morphological deficits, the induction of acute cell death and/or the activation of secondary reactive processes dominate. In contrast, after lower doses (e.g., 15 Gy) that do not produce detectable injury, the induction of recovery/repair related cytokines will dictate the outcome. Viewed from this perspective, radiation-induced CNS injury is not the result of a single, instantaneous event, but of a dynamic, multi-faceted process operating over time. The portion of the process corresponding to the direct cell death or initial loss of clonogenicity induced by radiation is unlikely to be susceptible to modulation, especially in a tumor treatment setting. However, an understanding of the secondary events involved in the precipitation of tissue injury as well as the intrinsic protection mechanisms may identify processes or molecules that are susceptible to manipulation and thus provide the basis for developing interventional therapies for radiation induced CNS toxicity.

2.4. Neural Stem Cells

For decades it was assumed that the mature brain does not have the innate ability to replenish neurons in response to injury or neurodegenerative conditions *(96)*. It is now recognized that neurogenesis occurs in the mammalian brain throughout life *(48,174)*. There are two major regions of neurogenesis in the mammalian forebrain, the subventricular zone (SVZ) and the subgranular zone (SGZ) of the dentate gyrus, and both areas have been shown to contain stem cells with multipotential character *(39,70,152)*. The precise role of neurogenesis under normal and pathologic conditions has not yet been fully elucidated, but it has been suggested that SVZ cells may act as a reserve population of undifferentiated cells that can be recruited after tissue injury *(40,97,113)*. Because irradiation can induce normal tissue injury as a sequelae to therapeutic treatment, it is possible that neurogenesis plays a role in subsequent cell/tissue response. Given that proliferation, migration and differentiation, the hallmarks of neurogenesis, are apparently under the control of specific growth factors *(31,84)*, it may be possible to use such factors to modulate neurogenesis and perhaps affect the development or severity of tissue injury.

The radiation response of the SVZ was first reported over 25 yr ago by Hopewell and colleagues *(22,62,63,68)*. Based on counts of mitotic and total cells, those studies noted that after irradiation there was a dose-dependent loss of cellularity within the SVZ, or as they called it, the subependymal plate. It was suggested that after irradiation with high doses, cell depletion within the SVZ was a result of the loss of a glial precursor. However, after small doses of X-rays, the repair capacity of the SVZ cells allowed for a gradual restoration of the supply of neuroglia *(68)*. Hopewell et al. suggested that the depletion of the cells of the SVZ could play a role in radiation-induced late effects, contending that if the restorative response observed in the SVZ should fail, a gradual decline in number of glial cells in the brain would ultimately lead to necrosis *(68)*. Despite interesting correlative data, a cause and effect relationship between the radiation response of the SVZ and later effects has not yet been established.

The SVZ is a highly mitotic area with a growth factor of almost 40% *(172)*. Cells produced in the SVZ are able to migrate long distances, primarily into the olfactory bulb where they differentiate into neurons *(92,94)*. Recent studies have revealed that the cells of the SVZ are extremely sensitive to irradiation, undergoing apoptosis after doses as low as 1 Gy *(157)*; 24 h after exposure there is a 96–98% reduction in cell proliferation *(172)*. Although in the first week following irradiation there is a subsequent increase in the number of proliferating cells, the repopulation of the SVZ, in terms of total cell number, number of proliferating cells and number of immature neurons remains impaired in a dose-dependent fashion up to 180 d after treatment *(172)*. Based on these observations and because of the potential for SVZ stem cells to migrate and also to differentiate into cells known to play a role in radiation injury (astrocytes, oligodendrocytes), SVZ cells may play a role in radioresponse of the CNS. The ability to manipulate these multipotential stem cells in situ using exogenous factors or transplant them at a site of injury would not only provide a means of investigating the intrinsic repair/recovery processes that occur after CNS irradiation, but also could provide the basis for the design of new therapeutic strategies.

Although measurable tissue destruction is generally considered to be the most significant adverse effect of ionizing irradiation on the CNS, less severe morphologic injury can also occur after radiotherapy, which may lead to cognitive dysfunction, particularly in children *(1,15,36,42,81)*. Much of the available clinical literature suggests that the cognitive effects of ionizing irradiation reflect impaired attention and memory more than low intellectual performance *(32,69,139)*. Based on such data it has been suggested that the hippocampus, a critical component of the medial temporal lobe memory system *(166)*, may be involved in the cognitive changes observed after irradiation *(1)*. Indirect evidence of the role of hippocampal damage in this cognitive dysfunction comes from clinical studies of head and neck cancer in which patients received high radiation doses to the inferomedial portion of the temporal lobes. Those patients reported subjective memory impairment, and relative to nonirradiated controls, showed poorer performance on measures of nonverbal recent memory *(89)*.

Within the hippocampus, memory functions are associated with the principal cells of the hippocampal formation, i.e., the pyramidal cells and the granule cells of the dentate gyrus *(29)*. Studies of the radiation response of the brain in late gestational or neonatal mice have shown that damage to the granule cell layer of the hippocampus or substantial reductions in dentate granule cell number are associated with cognitive impairments *(33,108,110,162,184)*. In the SGZ of rodents, new neurons are continuously generated *(6,17,49,50,74)*, migrate into the granule cell layer *(83)*, develop granule cell morphology and neuronal markers *(17)*, and connect with their target area, CA3 of the hippocampus *(167)*. Recent data also show that neurogenesis occurs in the adult human hippocampus beyond age 70 *(43)*. Although many new neurons are produced in the SGZ each day *(49)*, their significance has not been fully understood *(83)*. However, a direct association between hippocampus-dependent learning and survival of neurons generated in the mature hippocampal formation has been suggested *(49)*. Recently, investigators used a toxin to reduce the number of newly formed neurons and found that a hippocampal-dependent form of associated memory formation was impaired *(158)*. Given that SGZ neurogenesis may play some role in cognitive function, radiation-induced alterations in cognition may thus be mediated through changes in SGZ stem cells and/or their progeny.

Neuronal precursor cells in the rat SGZ are quite sensitive to irradiation, undergoing apoptosis 3–6 h after exposure *(124,126,171)* (Fig. 2). Recent work by Tada et al. *(171)*, showed that 24 h after irradiation cell proliferation was significantly reduced relative to sham-irradiated controls. Further, the number of apoptotic nuclei increased rapidly with radiation dose, reaching a plateau at about 3 Gy. The maximum number of apoptotic nuclei was substantially higher than the number of proliferating cells, suggesting that non-proliferating as well as proliferating cells in the subgranular zone were sensitive to irradiation. In addition, measures of SGZ proliferation obtained up to 120 d after X-irradiation showed significant reductions in the numbers of proliferating cells, suggesting a prolonged radiation-induced reduction in neurogenesis in the dentate gyrus *(171)*. Although the use of proliferation alone to define neurogenesis is less precise in adult than in developing tissue *(75)*, it has previously been shown that low dose x-irradiation reduces turned-on-after-division protein, 64 kDa (TOAD-64) and polysialylated-neural cell adhesion molecule (PSA-NCAM) labeling, proteins which are expressed specifically in immature neurons in the dentate gyrus and are used as measures of neurogenesis *(124)*. Thus, significant effects on SGZ neurogenesis occur after radiation doses that do not result in gross tissue changes or necrosis *(16)*.

Clearly neural stem cells are sensitive to the effects of ionizing irradiation. Similar X-ray sensitivity and long-term depression of proliferative activity in the SVZ *(172)* and the SGZ *(171)* suggest a common responsiveness to ionizing irradiation among stem/precursor cells of the mammalian forebrain. Whether that responsiveness is causally related or contributory to the late developing morphologic or functional sequelae associated with therapeutic irradiation needs to be determined.

3. NEW AND RECENT CLINICAL TECHNOLOGIES

Radiation therapy has proven efficacy against many types of brain tumors. There is a dose-response relationship for high grade gliomas, with higher radiation doses up to 60–70 Gy resulting in longer survival times *(8,142,183)*. But radiation also damages normal tissue, causing white matter demyelination and malacia and vascular damage characterized by endothelial alterations, telangiectasia, hyalinosis, and fibrinoid necrosis *(2)*. Neurocognitive changes may occur after exposure to doses at or above 18 Gy in 10 fractions *(2)* and there is a significant risk of symptomatic brain necrosis with doses at or above 60 Gy in 30–33 fractions *(102,154)*.

The key issue in the radiation therapy of these tumors is clearly a matter of therapeutic ratio; doses of radiation that are tolerable to the patient may be insufficient to control the tumor at its primary site. By definition, the therapeutic ratio can be increased by therapies that 1, increase damage to tumor cells; 2, decrease damage to irradiated normal brain cells; or 3, do both. A variety of ways to achieve an improved therapeutic ratio have been or are being studied.

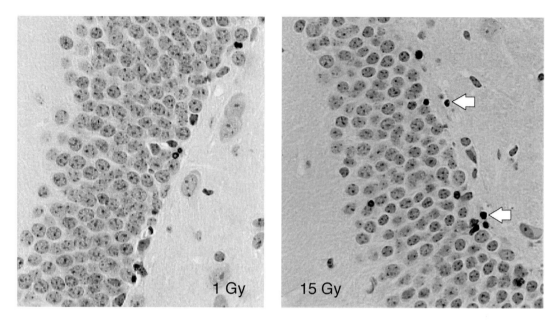

Fig. 2. The subgranular zone of the dentate gyrus in a rodent demonstrating apoptosis of neural stem cells following irradiation with 15 Gy.

3.1. Three-Dimensional Conformal Radiotherapy and Intensity-Modulated Radiotherapy

Improved targeting of radiation therapy has been made possible by advances in imaging of brain tumors and through advances in radiation treatment planning and delivery techniques. More precise targeting of radiation may decrease late toxicity by minimizing the volume of normal brain tissue that is irradiated and by limiting the radiation dose to critical structures. Tumor control may be improved by allowing dose escalation to the tumor because of better sparing of normal tissue and by helping to ensure that portions of tumor are not missed as a result of crude localization methods.

Several decades ago, radiation therapy for brain tumors was routinely accomplished using whole or partial brain lateral opposed radiation fields. The radiation oncologist estimated tumor extent manually based on hard copies of axial computed tomography (CT) imaging or other available imaging. Many centers now routinely immobilize brain tumor patients using a mask and/or bite-block device and perform CT-based treatment planning (sometimes merging the treatment planning CT scan with diagnostic magnetic resonance imaging) in order to concentrate radiation dose in the target region. In the past, it was possible to combine two or more beams to localize dose predominantly on one side of the brain, but available planning systems required all of the beams to lay in a single plane. With three-dimensional conformal radiotherapy, computerized treatment planning systems allow multiple noncoplanar intersecting radiation beams, each of which is individually shaped to conform to the tumor from its particular angle. Beam directions can be chosen to give excellent tumor coverage, whereas limiting dose to critical structures and limiting the volume of normal brain tissue receiving significant doses of radiation. Three-dimensional conformal technique produces a fairly uniform dose to the target region (generally 5–10% dose variation) and moderate dose fall-off outside the target. An example of a three-dimensional conformal plan for a glioblastoma is shown in Fig. 3.

In its most advanced form, intensity-modulated radiotherapy (IMRT) is an extremely sophisticated computer-driven technique that delivers a more heterogeneous dose within the target region

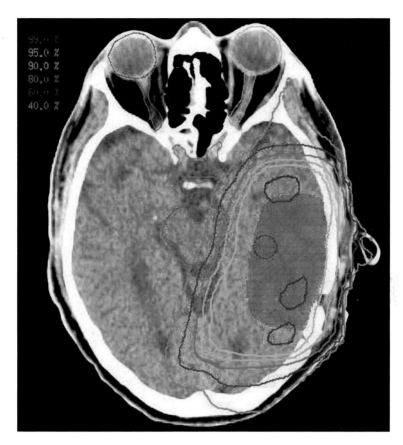

Fig. 3. An axial CT image from a three-dimensional conformal treatment plan for a left temporal lobe glioblastoma multiforme treating the tumor plus margin with 2.0 Gy per daily fraction at the 95% isodose contour. There is good dose fall-off in the brainstem and low dose to the optic chiasm and optic nerves. The 99% hot spots are shown, as well as the 90%, 80%, 60%, and 40% isodose contours.

(generally 15–25% dose variation) but also has a much more rapid dose fall-off of dose outside the target region. Hundreds or thousands of small beams with different intensities are combined together as fixed fields or using an arc technique. Inverse treatment planning is generally used, with operator entry of the desired tumor dose and normal tissue constraints and iterative calculation of a solution by the treatment planning software. An example of an IMRT plan for a glioblastoma is shown in Fig. 4. In a study comparing three-dimensional conformal radiotherapy to IMRT for seven challenging intracranial targets and two paraspinal targets, IMRT increased target coverage by an average of 36% and conformity by an average of 10% *(127)*. Dose-escalation using IMRT in the treatment of high-grade gliomas is currently under investigation. It is hypothesized that IMRT will result in significantly improved tumor control, but this remains to be proven. IMRT may also reduce normal tissue toxicity. In a retrospective study of pediatric medulloblastoma patients receiving conventional radiotherapy (11 patients) vs IMRT (15 patients), IMRT reduced the median radiation dose to the auditory apparatus to 35.2 Gy from 53.2 Gy and resulted in lower ototoxicity. Thirteen percent of the IMRT patients had grade 3 or 4 hearing loss compared with 64% of the conventionally irradiated patients ($p < 0.014$) *(66)*.

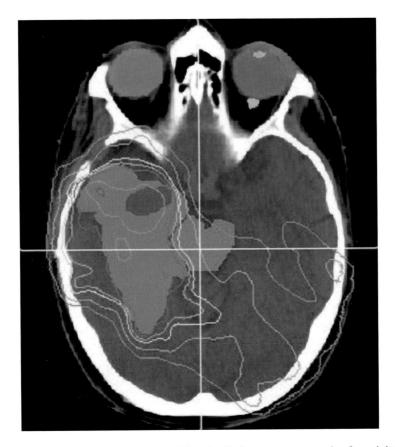

Fig. 4. An axial CT image from an intensity modulated radiotherapy treatment plan for a right temporal lobe glioblastoma multiforme treating the gross tumor at the 85% isodose contour and the presumed region of microscopic tumor at the 70% isodose contour, with some underdosing near the chiasm (because this patient had received previous radiation to the sella and chiasm). The 95% hot spot is shown as well as the 65%, 60%, 45%, and 30% isodose contours.

3.2. Proton Beam Therapy

Protons are radiobiologically only slightly more effective than conventional radiation but physically different in that beams can be controlled much more precisely, allowing for very rapid fall-off of dose outside the target volume, especially deep to the target. Proton therapy has accepted superiority over standard radiotherapy in the treatment of skull base chondrosarcomas and chordomas, producing 5-yr actuarial local control rates of 97% and 67%, respectively (116). Dose escalation trials were undertaken between 1992 and 1996 at Massachusetts General Hospital/Harvard Cyclotron Laboratory giving 68.2 Gy equivalent (GyE), 79.7 GyE, and 90 GyE to Grade II, III, and IV gliomas, respectively (45,46). There was no suggestion of a survival benefit in 20 patients with grade II or III tumors, and radiation necrosis (with or without tumor) was documented in 18 of 22 postradiation surgeries (45). There was a suggestion of benefit in 23 glioblastoma patients who underwent an accelerated proton boost to 90 GyE after 55–65 Gy of conventional radiation; the median survival time was 20 mo with 34% and 18% actuarial survival at 2 and 3 yr. This is longer than expected by Radiation Therapy Oncology Group (RTOG) prognostic criteria. Recurrences were generally seen in the volumes that received 60–70 GyE and not in regions that received 90 GyE, but treatment of larger volumes to 90 GyE was not felt to be advisable owing to the risk of radiation necrosis *(46)*.

3.3. Temporary and Permanent Brachytherapy

Interstitial brachytherapy is another technique allowing delivery of a high focal dose of radiation to a tumor region using radiation sources placed directly in tissue or within catheters. Dose falls off with the square of the distance away from point sources of radiation and is also attenuated by tissue, resulting in excellent sparing of surrounding normal brain tissue. There may also be radiobiological advantages of continuous low dose-rate radiation from the accumulation of cells in late G_2, a radio-sensitive phase of the cell-cycle, and elimination of repopulation as a result of inhibition of mitosis.

Major series of temporarily implanted high-activity iodine-125 sources delivering approx 50–65 Gy over 5–7 d have resulted in median survival times of 18–19 mo from the date of diagnosis when used as a boost in conjunction with external beam radiotherapy in 56 and 159 patients with newly diagnosed glioblastoma *(164,187)*, 12 and 11.5 mo from the date of brachytherapy in 66 and 32 patients with recurrent glioblastomas *(160,164)*, and 12 mo from brachytherapy in 45 patients with recurrent Grade III gliomas *(164)*. A major drawback of temporary brachytherapy is the significant risk of symptomatic radiation necrosis using this technique; in the series referenced above, 44–64% of patients underwent reoperation showing tumor and/or necrosis *(160,164,187)*. Furthermore, two prospective, randomized trials in 140 and 299 patients with newly diagnosed malignant gliomas comparing external beam radiotherapy (plus BCNU in one trial) with or without a 60 Gy temporary brachytherapy boost failed to show a significant survival benefit for the brachytherapy arm *(85,149)*.

An alternative approach is the permanent implantation of low-activity iodine-125 sources directly into gross tumor or lining a resection cavity. Low-dose-rate radiation gives a much lower risk of radiation necrosis than high-dose-rate radiation. A large number of low-grade glioma patients have been treated in Germany using permanently implanted low-activity iodine-125 sources beginning in 1979 and 20–30 d temporary implants of iodine-125 since 1985. Among patients treated from 1979–1991, the 5- and 10-yr survival probabilities were 85% and 83%, respectively, for 97 patients with pilocytic astrocytomas, and 61% and 51% for 250 patients with Grade II astrocytomas *(82)*. Only 2.6% of patients experienced progressive, symptomatic radiation necrosis. However, there is no evidence to date that these results are superior to those achieved with conventional therapy.

Permanently implanted low-activity iodine-125 sources have also been used successfully to line resection cavities at the time of reoperation for recurrent skull base tumors, malignant meningiomas, brain metastases, or malignant gliomas *(53,57,105,125)*. The median survival times after re-operation with brachytherapy were 47 wk in 47 patients with recurrent glioblastoma in one series without any cases of symptomatic radiation necrosis *(125)* and 64 weeks in 18 patients with recurrent glioblastoma in another series with only one case of symptomatic radiation necrosis *(57)*. The median survival time was 14.7 mo after temporary brachytherapy in 30 patients with recurrent brain metastases *(105)*.

3.4. Intra-Operative Radiotherapy

Intra-operative radiotherapy involves the delivery of a single dose of radiation at the time of open surgery, usually given to a resection cavity using electrons and a dose of 15–25 Gy. The depth of penetration is controlled by the choice of electron energy and dose falls off fairly rapidly beyond the effective treatment range. One series from Japan reported a median survival time of 119 wk in 30 patients with glioblastoma who underwent IORT to a mean dose of 18.3 Gy prior to external beam radiotherapy to a mean dose of 58.5 Gy *(104)*.

3.5. Radiosurgery

Radiosurgery involves the delivery of a single high-dose fraction of carefully focused radiation to a small intracranial target, often using a Gamma Knife with 201 collimated beams of cobalt-60 radiation or a specially adapted linear accelerator. Very rapid fall-off of radiation dose outside the target is required to limit normal tissue toxicity to an acceptable level (Fig. 5). No prospective, randomized trials evaluating the role of radiosurgery in the treatment of brain tumors have been reported to date except for one small trial showing significantly improved control of brain metastases treated with whole brain radiotherapy plus radiosurgery boost vs whole brain radiotherapy alone *(80)*. There are numerous retrospective reviews demonstrating the efficacy of radiosurgery in the treatment of a wide variety of benign and malignant brain tumors such as meningiomas, acoustic neuromas, pituitary adenomas, brain metastases, and glial tumors *(79)*. Benign tumors tend to shrink slowly over years after radiosurgery and brain metastases tend to shrink over months; most tumors do not disappear completely, except for metastases less than 1 cm in diameter. Representative 5-yr actuarial freedom-from-progression rates after radiosurgical treatment are 89–95% for benign meningiomas, 94–98% for acoustic neuromas, and 90–94% for brain metastases with about a 5% incidence of radiosurgery-related complications in patients with meningioma or brain metastases *(79)*. At an institution with a large experience, median survival times were 10.2 mo after radiosurgery for 86 patients with recurrent glioblastoma *(160)* and 19.9 mo after diagnosis in 78 patients treated with radiosurgery boost in conjunction with radiotherapy for newly diagnosed glioblastoma *(159)*, similar to results of temporary brachytherapy.

3.6. Heavy Particle Therapy

Heavy particles such as helium or neon deposit DNA-damaging energy densely, allow excellent dose precision and conformity, and are not subject to hypoxic cell radioresistance. A total of 37 patients with previously unirradiated glioblastoma underwent heavy charged particle radiotherapy or treatment with a combination of photons and particles (helium, carbon, and/or neon) at Lawrence Berkeley Laboratory from 1976 to 1992, including 22 patients treated with photons and < 20 Gy particle boost and 15 patients treated on a randomized trial comparing 20 vs 25 Gy of neon irradiation given over 4 wk *(20)*. The median survival times were 11 mo for the first 22 patients and 13 vs 14 mo for patients randomized to 20 vs 25 Gy neon irradiation. Results did not appear to be better than those achieved with standard therapy, although there was one case of autopsy-proven absence of tumor in a patient who died of pneumonia and gastrointestinal hemorrhage 19 mo post-treatment *(20)*.

3.7. Neutron Beam Therapy

Neutrons differ radically from conventional photon (X-ray) radiation in that DNA-damaging energy is deposited much more densely, resulting in greater cell kill and a much higher relative biological effect. Also, there is less resistance of hypoxic cells to neutron radiation than to conventional photon radiation. Interestingly, clinical trials utilizing neutrons to treat malignant gliomas have resulted in a much higher control rate than for photons, but no improvement in survival, presumably from necrosis *(5,21,52,88)*. Of fifteen patients autopsied in one trial, only one had tumor and the other 14 patients had coagulative necrosis of the tumor site and surrounding white matter *(87)*. No beneficial combination was found in a randomized study searching for the optimal dose of neutrons for a limited volume neutron boost combined with photon whole brain radiotherapy to 45 Gy *(86)*.

3.8. Boron Neutron Capture Therapy

Boron neutron capture therapy (BNCT) was first proposed in 1936, just 4 yr after discovery of the neutron *(93)*. Although clinical trials of BNCT began in this country in the 1950s and have continued in Japan up to the present, BNCT is still in its infancy in terms of effective implementation. Numerous papers and reviews have been written on this topic (e.g., *see* ref. *28* for a more detailed description of BNCT and its history). BNCT requires the accumulation of a stable isotope of boron, ^{10}B, in tumor cells prior to broad-beam low-energy thermal or epithermal neutron irradiation of both tumor and normal tissue, with one or a small number of neutron radiation treatments.

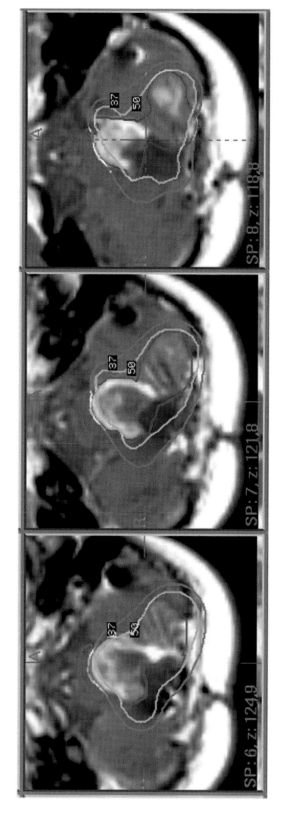

Fig. 5. An axial MR image from a Gamma Knife radiosurgery treatment plan for a recurrent posterior fossa ependymoma. A dose of 16 Gy in one fraction was delivered at the 50% isodose contour. Plugging allowed the anterior isodose contour adjacent to the brain stem to be reduced to 12 Gy.

293

The ^{10}B nuclei have a high probability of thermal neutron capture which results in nuclear fission creating high linear energy transfer (LET) particles with a range of only one cell diameter, killing only the cells in the immediate vicinity of the boron compound. The success of BNCT depends heavily upon the availability of a ^{10}B-containing compound with highly selective concentration in tumor cells as opposed to blood, scalp, and normal brain tissue. The major compound used in clinical trials to date, *p*-boronophenylalanine (BPA), yields ^{10}B concentrations 3.5-fold higher in tumor and 1.5-fold higher in scalp than in blood *(23)*.

In a recent Phase I/II dose-escalation clinical study at Brookhaven National Laboratory, patients with glioblastoma (GBM) were infused intravenously with BPA-fructose and then irradiated with neutrons. These patients had all undergone resection of their tumor 3–5 wk prior to BNCT and they received BNCT in place of standard radiation therapy. An interim report on the outcome for 38 of these patients indicates that the median time to tumor progression was 31.6 wk, whereas the median survival time was 13.0 mo *(24)*. These times are very similar to those resulting from standard radiation therapy *(185)*. Thus, BNCT using systemic administration of a compound that does not exhibit ideal tumor-localizing properties and a low energy neutron beam that is contaminated with higher energy neutron beams and gamma rays produced patient outcomes essentially equal to standard therapy.

Clearly, improvements to this specific BNCT protocol seem possible. First, better boronated compounds could be made that selectively target tumor cells over normal cells, second these compounds could be administered locally to the brain tumor—thereby increasing their concentration in tumor cells, and third purer sources of low energy neutrons could be used.

The concept of neutron capture therapy (NCT) is not limited solely to using boron, although NCT and BNCT have often been used interchangeably. Other transition metals also can capture neutrons and undergo nuclear fission. For example, gadolinium also undergoes fission upon bombardment with neutrons and produces short-lived radioactive atoms. Therefore, the search for a better compound should not be limited to boron, and irrespective of the metal chosen, attempts should be made to specifically target these compounds to the tumor cell. For example, targets might be ligands that are found on the brain tumor cell membrane and not on normal brain cells, such as epidermal growth factor receptor (EGFR), its mutant EGFRvIII, interleukin-13 receptor (IL-13R), and low-density lipoprotein receptor (LDLR) *(100)*.

3.9. Radiation Modifiers

Another general approach is to combine photon irradiation with hypoxic cell sensitizers (such as misonidazole or etanidazole) or radiation sensitizers (such as bromo-deoxyuridine [BudR], or iodo-deoxyuridine [IudR]). No benefit was suggested for hypoxic cell sensitization in any of four randomized studies using misonidazole *(9,51,119,177)* or in a Phase I trial of etanidazole for malignant gliomas *(25)*. Halogenated pyrimidines such as BUdR and IUdR are incorporated into the DNA of cycling cells in place of thymidine, rendering the DNA more susceptible to radiation damage. Results appeared to be promising for patients with Grade III gliomas in a Phase II Northern California Oncology Group trial of conventional radiotherapy to 59.4 Gy at 1.8 Gy daily with weekly 96-h intravenous infusions of BUdR followed by six cycles of chemotherapy with procarbazine, CCNU, and vincristine (PCV). This trial became a Phase III randomized intergroup study in 1994 comparing radiation/BUdR/PCV with radiation/PCV. Preliminary analysis of the randomized trial did not suggest any benefit of BUdR *(129)*. Other radiation modifiers under investigation include hemoglobin substitutes and hemoglobin modifiers to try to overcome the problem of radioresistance as a result of tumor hypoxia as well as Tirapazamine, a hypoxic cell toxin.

3.10. Altered Fractionation

There is a limit to the amount of radiation that can be given safely owing to the significant risk of brain necrosis above doses of 60–70 Gy using standard fractionation doses of 1.8–2.0 Gy per d

(102,154). Two different altered fractionation schemes have been studied fairly extensively for malignant gliomas and other tumor types and appeared to be promising in early trials *(168)*. Hyperfractionation involves more than one radiation fraction daily using smaller than conventional fraction size (often 1.0-1.2 Gy twice daily) separated in time by at least 4–6 h, keeping the overall treatment time similar to conventional once-daily radiotherapy. The use of smaller size fractions increases the radiation tolerance of late-responding tissues such as normal brain, allowing a higher total dose to be given without increasing normal tissue toxicity. Accelerated hyperfractionation involves more than one radiation fraction daily (often 1.6 Gy twice daily), with a total daily dose significantly larger than for conventional fractionation, resulting in significantly shortened overall time for the radiotherapy course. This approach should decrease the opportunity for tumor cell repopulation during the treatment course. Unfortunately, recent prospective randomized trials have not confirmed a benefit of altered fractionation in the treatment of malignant gliomas. A Phase III study, RTOG 90–06, randomized 712 patients from 1990–1994 to 60 Gy at 2.0 Gy per daily fraction vs 72 Gy at 1.2 Gy twice daily and found no survival difference between the two arms after adjusting for known prognostic factors *(147)*. Similarly, hyperfractionation failed to improve time to progression or survival in a Pediatric Oncology Group Phase III trial for children with brainstem gliomas comparing 54 Gy at 1.8 Gy per daily fraction to 70.2 Gy at 1.17 Gy twice daily *(101)*. Another prospective, randomized trial, Northern California Cancer Center protocol 6G-90-1, compared conventional radiotherapy (59.4 Gy at 1.8 Gy daily) to accelerated hyperfractionated radiotherapy (70.4 Gy at 1.6 Gy twice daily), with or without difluoromethylornithine (DFMO) as a radiosensitizer for glioblastoma multiforme. No survival differences were seen among the four arms *(130)*.

3.11. Hyperthermia

Hyperthermia inhibits repair of sublethal radiation damage and is particularly effective against S phase cells and low-pH hypoxic cells that tend to be resistant to radiation *(37)*. In addition, hyperthermia may cause tumor reoxygenation, thereby helping to overcome hypoxia-associated radioresistance *(120)*. Numerous investigators have performed Phase I and Phase I/II trials using various forms of external or interstitial hyperthermia for brain tumors *(148)*. One randomized Phase II/III trial was performed at the University of California San Francisco in patients with GBM, suggesting a survival benefit for hyperthermia *(165)*. From 1990 to 1995, patients with KPS $\geq$70 and technically implantable GBM $\leq$5 cm in diameter were enrolled postoperatively, treated with partial brain radiotherapy to 59.4 Gy at 1.8 Gy per daily fraction, and then patients who were still eligible for brachytherapy were randomized to brachytherapy alone (60 Gy over 5–6 d using high-activity iodine-125 sources) vs brachytherapy with hyperthermia (with a goal of heating the tumor to at least 42.5°C for 30 minutes before and after brachytherapy using interstitial microwave antennas). Of the 112 eligible patients enrolled, 68 actually underwent brachytherapy $\pm$ hyperthermia. The median freedom from progression time was 49 wk for "heat" vs 33 wk for "no heat" (one-tailed $p = 0.045$) and the median survival times were 85 vs 76 wk with 18-mo survival probabilities of 59% vs 38% for "heat" vs "no heat" (one-tailed $p = 0.02$) *(165)*. Interstitial hyperthermia is technically difficult to perform and only a subset of patients are candidates.

4. NEW THERAPEUTIC STRATEGIES

4.1. Hypoxic Cell Toxins

Whereas solid tumors are heterogeneous and are composed of physiologically distinct subpopulations of cells, from a radiobiologic perspective, hypoxic cells are the most important subpopulation because of their well-documented resistance to radiation. Radiation kills cells and induces damage by producing free radicals that attack DNA and make it a free radical. If oxygen is present, the damaged DNA becomes irreparable, whereas if oxygen is absent much of the damage can be repaired *(55)*.

Historically, the radiobiologically important hypoxic cells have been thought to be those that arise in tumors whenever tumor growth produces cells that are > 150 μm from a blood vessel *(175)*. This is the approximate distance that O_2 can diffuse in solid tissue and beyond this point, necrosis occurs. Cells at this distance from blood vessels have a partial oxygen pressure (pO_2) < 0.5 mmHg, and their destruction typically requires ~3 times the radiation dose that is required to kill well-oxygenated cells (pO_2 > 20 mmHg) *(55)*. Hypoxic cells can also develop through intermittent blood flow, a phenomenon that is known to occur in a variety of disease states including tumors *(182)*. In addition to containing extremely hypoxic cells, tumors contain cells with pO_2 between 0.5 and 20 mmHg. The radiation dose required to kill hypoxic cells divided by the radiation dose required to kill the same fraction of oxic cells defines the oxygen enhancement ratio (OER), and cells at intermediate pO_2 have an OER between 1 and 3 *(55)*. Because of the many cells in solid tumors that are intermediately hypoxic, it is important to devise therapies that kill cells under all degrees of hypoxia *(189)*.

In addition to hindering attempts to cure brain tumors with radiation, hypoxia can produce other unwanted effects. Recent clinical studies of patients with solid tumors elsewhere in the body show a correlation between tumor hypoxia and metastases *(10)* and between hypoxia and tumor progression *(170)*. These observations provide addition rationale for developing therapies that target hypoxic cells.

Several studies show that human brain tumors contain regions of hypoxia. Kayama et al. *(73)* used a Clark electrode to make single pO_2 measurements in 16 malignant brain tumors whose pO_2 ranged from 5 to 38 mmHg with an average pO_2 of 15.3 + 2.3 mmHg. The numbers of patients in each group were too small to permit comparisons of pO_2 among groups, but there was no significant difference between the mean values measured in primary brain tumors (14.9 + 3.2 mmHg) and metastatic tumors (16.5 + 2.0 mmHg). All tumor pO_2 levels were considerably lower than in surrounding normal brain, which ranged from 40 to 114 mmHg (mean of 59.8 + 6.5 mmHg). A more recent study by Rampling et al. *(136)* employed an Eppendorf polarographic microelectrode to take multiple measurements of pO_2 at various locations in primary and metastatic brain tumors. The mean pO_2 in GBM ranged from 0.1 to 24.3 mmHg, and the percentage of measurements that were < 2.5 mmHg (OER > 1.5) in each of these tumors ranged from 9.5 to 68.5%. Collingridge et al. *(30)* also used the Eppendorf apparatus in their study of low and high grade gliomas. The average percentage of measurements < 2.5 mmHg was 40.6% for low-grade tumors and 49.4% for high-grade tumors.

Because normal tissues do not contain regions of hypoxia, hypoxic cells provide a means for selectively targeting tumor tissue to the exclusion of normal tissue *(12)*. Recent studies suggest that it may be possible to develop a hypoxic cell-targeted gene therapy that can be administered during radiation therapy and improve the therapeutic ratio. The DNA construct to be delivered to the tumor cells would contain hypoxia-responsive elements (HREs) in the enhancer region of the promoter and a suicide gene. Under hypoxic conditions, the transcriptional complex hypoxia inducible factor-1 (HIF-1) builds up in cells and binds to HREs. This, in turn, activates the adjacent promoter and causes expression of the downstream suicide gene that kills the cell. The groundwork for such a proposal has been provided by the innovative studies of several scientists. HIF-1 was initially discovered during a search for factors that regulate erythropoietin (Epo) expression. It was quickly discovered that HIF-1 activity can be found in nearly every cell type studied, making it a prime candidate for a master regulator of the transcriptional response to hypoxia. HIF-1 activity is initiated upon heterodimerization of the two bHLH-PAS proteins, HIF-1*a* and the arylhydrocarbon receptor nuclear translocator (ARNT), leading to the formation of a functional transcription factor complex. ARNT is also responsible for mediating responses to environmental pollutants such as dioxin via heterodimerization with the arylhydrocarbon receptor *(144)*. HIF-1 is a novel member of the rapidly growing bHLH-PAS family of transcription factors. DNA-binding sites, or HREs, for this complex have been localized to the promoters or enhancers of most of the previously identified hypoxia responsive genes, including Epo, phosphoglycerate kinase (PGK), and vascular endothelial growth factor (VEGF) *(150,151,188)*. HIF-1α normally has a very short half-life. Hypoxia stabilizes this protein such that its half-life is increased, allowing for the build-up of HIF-1 levels within the hypoxic cells *(67,143)*, which in turn can bind to HRE and turn on the adjacent genes.

Several investigators have shown that this system actually works. Dachs *(34)* constructed plasmids in which HREs from the PGK promoter region were used to regulate both the CD2 marker gene and cytosine deaminase, which activates the prodrug 5-fluorocytosine (5-FC) to 5-fluorouracil (5-FU). These investigators showed that CD2 was expressed in vitro only when oxygen concentrations were ≤2%; normoxic concentrations in cell culture are approx 5%. They also showed that expression of cytosine deaminase under hypoxia activates the prodrug resulting in cell growth inhibition in vitro. Lastly, they showed that CD2 was expressed in tumor xenografts and that its expression was localized near areas of pyknosis and necrosis, which are presumed to indicate regions of hypoxia.

Shibata et al. *(155)* prepared reporter plasmids by inserting HIF-1 binding regions from human VEGF and/or Epo genes into the pGL3 promoter vector, which contains luciferase as the reporter gene. These constructs were transiently transfected into two mouse tumor cell lines (SCCVII and EMT-6/KU) and two human tumor cell lines (HT1080 and Hep G2). The pGL3/Epo construct did not increase gene expression in hypoxic mouse cells, but it did increase gene expression in hypoxic human cells two- to five-fold over that seen in oxic human cells. pGL3/VEGF and pGL3/VEGF/ Epo constructs increased gene expression in hypoxic cells compared to oxic cells by ratios of 3 to 12 in all four cell lines. The investigators then prepared and studied constructs that contained five copies of HRE, pGL3, VEGF and/or the E1b minimal promoter sequence. Gene expression ratios for hypoxic to oxic cells were approx 5 (pGL3/VEGF), approx 20 (5xHRE/pGL3/VEGF), and approx 45 (5xHRE/pGL3/VEGF/E1b). Shibata et al. *(156)* also found that five copies of HRE derived from the 5'-UTR of the human VEGF gene with an E1b minimal promoter showed 50- and 110-fold increases in reporter gene expression for 6 h and 18 h incubation periods, respectively, under hypoxic conditions.

Brown's group *(156)* at Stanford University has recently reported the use of *E. coli* nitroreductase (NTR) for killing hypoxic cells. NTR works by converting a nontoxic prodrug (CB1954) into a potent cross-linking agent. They placed the NTR suicide gene under the control of five copies of HRE and the cytomegalovirus (CMV) minimal promoter (Pcmv) and generated stably transfected clones from the HT1080 cell line. These clones were approx 20-fold more sensitive to CB1954 as compared to parent cells under anoxic conditions, whereas the sensitivities of both cell lines to CB1954 under oxic conditions were the same.

The Deen laboratory at University of California at San Francisco has also begun investigating the use of HRE to control gene expression in hypoxic cells. Plasmids containing up to nine copies of HRE have been tested to see whether expression of the LacZ reporter gene was induced in U-251 MG and U-87 MG brain tumor cells during hypoxia *(140)*. Under anoxic conditions (95% N_2/5% CO_2), no increased gene expression was observed for two copies of HRE, whereas a 5- to 15-fold increase was noted for three and six copies of HRE, and nine copies of HRE yielded 27 to 37-fold increases in both cell lines. Less severe hypoxia (0.3 and 1% O_2) produced a 10- to 40-fold increase in gene expression, depending upon cell line and the HRE copy number. Moreover, when the plasmid was delivered to cells via a recombinant adeno-associated virus (AAV), gene expression was increased approx 100-fold under anoxic conditions. This laboratory has transfected cells with the *Bax* gene under control of HRE and showed that anoxic brain tumor cells were preferentially killed through apoptosis; thus *Bax* is a potential suicide gene for this type of therapy.

Based on the findings of these laboratory studies, development of a hypoxia-targeted gene therapy appears to be feasible. There are, however, a number of issues to be resolved before this approach is likely to be successful in human studies *(140)*. First, suitable constructs must be developed, which kill slowly and nonproliferating hypoxic tumor cells and exhibit minimal toxicity to surrounding normal cells. Elements of these constructs include the copy number of HRE, the promoter and the suicide gene. Then it will be necessary to efficiently deliver this construct to the hypoxic cells of interest by viruses, lipoproteins or other delivery agents. Once it has been shown that the construct can indeed target and selectively kill hypoxic cells, it will be necessary to evaluate the construct in combination with radiation. Some early studies of combined therapy have been done using cell cultures. Sakakura et al. *(141)* have shown that overexpression of *Bax* in human breast cancer cells enhances their sensitivity to radiation, and 5-FU is a known radiation sensitizer *(138)*. Thus, cells that escape direct killing by certain suicide genes may be more vulnerable to radiation, further supporting the rationale for developing this type of hypoxia-targeted gene therapy for use in combination with radiation therapy. Last, animal studies will be necessary to provide convincing evidence of this.

4.2. Anti-Angiogenesis and XRT/Metronomic Therapy

Chemotherapy given alone or in combination with another agent is typically given at a maximum tolerated dose (MTD), and because of its toxicity, regimens of chemotherapy are usually separated by relatively long periods of time (i.e., weeks). Thus, during the course of a standard 6-wk radiation therapy protocol, attempts to enhance the therapeutic ratio by MTD drug treatment are limited to very few doses, and the overall effect of adding drug to the radiation protocol will mostly likely be minute. This rather bleak prediction has in fact been the case for brain tumor therapy in that none of the drugs tested in combination with radiation have dramatically improved the therapeutic outcome.

Recent advances in anti-angiogenic research have opened up a novel approach for enhancing radiation therapy. Browder et al. *(11)* at the Folkman laboratory, have shown that low doses of chemotherapy administered repeatedly for long periods of time can markedly improve the efficacy of the treatment, as compared to a more standard cytotoxic therapy. They also showed that combining prolonged, low dose chemotherapy with an anti-angiogenic drug could cure these normally drug-resistant tumors. The notion behind this is that endothelial cells in blood vessels are refractory to normal high dose chemotherapy, which normally targets more rapidly dividing cells such as tumor cells. Whereas, the prolonged low dose chemotherapy can eventually kill the endothelial cells comprising blood vessels. In one type of experiment, they used both a drug-resistant Lewis lung carcinoma model to show that 16 doses of 170 mg/kg cyclophosphamide spaced 6 days apart was more effective than a "conventional" protocol in which three courses of drug treatment were begun every 20 d; each course consisted of 150 mg/kg every other day for three doses.

Others have confirmed that this strategy of targeting the blood vessels in tumors can be efficacious in producing tumor regression. Klement et al. *(78)* used neuroblastoma xenografts to investigate low doses of vinblastine in combination with the DC101 antibody, which inhibits a VEGF receptor and thereby inhibits angiogenesis. They also found that prolonged treatment of tumors with low dose vinblastine slower tumor growth, and that combination of this treatment with DC101 could cure these normally drug-resistant tumors.

Commentaries by others *(58)* point out the importance of these findings and encourage the rethinking of dosing for chemotherapy alone and in combination with other agents. Brain tumor patients are allowed a recovery period following surgery, which typically delays radiation therapy for approx 2 wk. Because it is nontoxic, a low dose anti-angiogenic therapy could be initiated immediately after surgery and continue through radiation therapy. This could potentially inhibit angiogenesis during this period and, at the least, keep the tumor burden low before the onset of radiation therapy.

5. SUMMARY

Radiation is rightfully one of the primary modalities used in the treatment of brain tumors. Nonetheless, efforts to increase the efficacy of radiation using high-LET particles, BNCT, radiation modifiers, and altered fractionation have been largely unsuccessful in improving outcomes to date. Further investigations in one or more of these areas may be fruitful in the future. A variety of techniques are available to increase radiation dose to the tumor whereas limiting normal tissue dose, but improved efficacy of these approaches remains to be proven. Dose escalation may be more successful after incorporation of three-dimensional tumor mapping using a technique such as magnetic resonance spectroscopy *(128)*. Last, because tumor cells can be found at far distances from the primary site

(14), for cures to become common, it will be necessary to combine radiation therapy with targeted therapies that seek out and selectively destroy outlying tumor cells. Both of the new therapeutic strategies mentioned above could potentially meet this requirement.

ACKNOWLEDGMENTS

Dennis Deen is supported by NIH P01 NS42927 and NIH R01 CA85356. John Fike is supported by R01 CA 76141, R21 NS40088, DAMD17-01-1-0820.

REFERENCES

1. Abayomi O.K. 1996.Pathogenesis of irradiation-induced cognitive dysfunction. *Acta. Oncol.* **35**:659–663.
2. Ang K.K. 2000. Radiobiology of the central nervous system, in *Neuro-Oncology: The Essentials* (Bernstein M., Berger M.S. eds.),Thieme Medical Publishers, Inc., New York, pp. 160–168.
3. Asai A., Matsutani M., Kohno T., Nakamura O., Tanaka H., Fujimaki T., et al. 1989. Subacute brain atrophy after radiation therapy for malignant brain tumor. *Cancer* **63**:1962–1974.
4. Barres B.A., Raff M.C. 1993. Proliferation of oligodendrocyte precursor cells depends on electrical activity in axons. *Nature* **361**:258–260.
5. Battermann J.J. 1980.Fast neutron therapy for advanced tumors. *Intl. J. Rad. Oncol. Bio. Phys.* **6**:333–335.
6. Bayer S.A. 1982. Changes in the total number of dentate granule cells in juvenile and adult rats: a correlated volumetric and 3H-thymidine autoradiographic study. *Exp. Brain Res.* **46**:315–323.
7. Bedford J.S., Mitchell J.B., Griggs H.G., Bender M.A. 1978. Radiation-induced cellular reproductive death and chromosome aberrations. *Radiat. Res.* **76**:573–586.
8. Bleehen N.M., Stenning S.P. 1991. A Medical Research Council trial of two radiotherapy doses in the treatment of grades 3 and 4 astrocytoma. *Br. J. Cancer* **64**:769–774.
9. Bleehen N.M., Wiltshire D.R., Plowman P.N., Watson J.V., Gleave J.R.W., Holmes A.E., et al. 1981. A randomized study of misonidazole and radiotherapy for grade 3 and 4 cerebral astrocytoma. *Br. J. Cancer* **43**:436–441.
10. Brizel D.M., Scully S.P., Harrelson J.M., Layfield L.J., Bean J.M., Prosnitz L.R., Dewhirst M.W. 1996. Tumor oxygenation predicts for the likelihood of distant metastases in human soft tissue sarcoma. *Cancer Res.* **56**:941–943.
11. Browder T., Butterfield C.E., Kraling B.M., Shi B., Marshall B., O'Reilly M.S., Folkman J. 2000. Antiangiogenic scheduling of chemotherapy improves efficacy against experimental drug-resistant cancer. *Cancer Res.* **60**:1878–1886.
12. Brown J.M., Giaccia A.J. 1998. The unique physiology of solid tumors: opportunities (and problems) for cancer therapy. *Cancer Res.* **58**:1408–1416.
13. Bruce A.J., Boling W., Kindy M.S., Peschon J., Kraemer P.J., Carpenter M.K., et al. Altered neuronal and microglial responses to excitotoxic and ischemic brain injury in mice lacking TNF receptors. *Nat. Med.* **2**:788–794.
14. Burger P.C., Dubois P.J., Schold S.C., Jr., Smith K.R., Jr., Odom G.L., Crafts D.C., Giangaspero F. 1983. Computerized tomographic and pathologic studies of the untreated, quiescent, and recurrent glioblastoma multiforme. *J. Neurosurg.* **58**:159–169.
15. Butler R.W., Hill J.M., Steinherz P.G., Meyers P.A., Finlay J.L. 1994. Neuropsychologic effects of cranial irradiation, intrathecal methotrexate, and systemic methotrexate in childhood cancer. *J. Clin. Oncol.* **12**:2621–2629.
16. Calvo W., Hopewell J.W., Reinhold H.S., Yeung T.K. 1988. Time- and dose-related changes in the white matter of the rat brain after single doses of X rays. *Brit. J. Radiol.* **61**:1043–1052.
17. Cameron H.A., Woolley C.S., McEwen B.S., Gould E. 1993. Differentiation of newly born neurons and glia in the dentate gyrus of the adult rat. *Neuroscience* **56**:337–344.
18. Cannella B., Hoban C.J., Gao Y.L.,Garcia-Arenas R., Lawson D., Marchionni M., et al. 1998. The neuregulin, glial growth factor 2, diminishes autoimmune demyelination and enhances remyelination in a chronic relapsing model for multiple sclerosis. *Proc. Natl. Acad. Sci. USA* **95**:10,100–10,105.
19. Caspari T. 2000. How to activate p53. *Curr. Biol.* **10**:R315–317.
20. Castro J.R., Phillips T.L., Prados M., Gutin P., Larson D.A., Petti P.L., et al. 1997. Neon heavy charged particle radiotherapy of glioblastoma of the brain. *Int. J. Radiat. Oncol. Biol. Phys.* **38**:257–261.
21. Catteral M., Bloom H.J.G., Ash D.V., Walsh L., Richardson A., Uttley D., et al. 1980. Fast neutrons compared with megavoltage X-rays in the treatment of patients with supratentorial glioblastoma: a controlled pilot study. *Int. J. Radiat. Oncol. Biol. Phys.* **6**:261–266.
22. Cavanagh J.B., Hopewell J.W. 1972. Mitotic activity in the subependymal plate of rats and the long-term consequences of X-irradiation. *J. Neurol. Sci.* **15**:471–482.
23. Chadha M., Capala J., Coderre J.A., Elowitz E.H., Iwai J.-I., Joel D.D., et al. 1998. Boron neutron-capture therapy (BNCT) for glioblastoma multiforme (GBM) using the epithermal neutron beam at the Brookhaven National Laboratory. *Int. J. Radiat. Oncol. Biol. Phys.* **40**:829–834.

24. Chanana A.D.Capala J., Chadha M., Coderre J.A., Diaz A.Z., Elowitz E.H., et al. 1999. Boron neutron capture therapy for glioblastoma multiforme: interim results from the phase I/II dose-escalation studies. *Neurosurgery* **44:**1182–1192.

25. Chang E.L., Loeffler J.S., Riese N.E., Wen P.Y., Alexander E., III, Black P.M., Coleman C.N. 1998. Survival results from a phase I study of etanidazole (SR2508) and radiotherapy in patients with malignant glioma. *Int. J. Radiat. Oncol. Biol. Phys.* **40:**65–70.

26. Chiang C.S., McBride W.H., Withers H.R. 1993. Radiation-induced astrocytic and microglial responses in mouse brain. *Radiother. Oncol.* **29:**60–68.

27. Clarke A.R., Purdie C.A., Harrison D.J., Morris R.G., Bird C.C., et al. 1993. Thymocyte apoptosis induced by p53-dependent and independent pathways. *Nature* **362:**849–852.

28. Coderre J.A., Morris G.M. 1999. The radiation biology of boron neutron capture therapy. *Radiat. Res.* **151:**1–18.

29. Collier T.J., Quirk G.J., Routtenberg A. 1987. Separable roles of hippocampal granule cells in forgetting and pyramidal cells in remembering spatial information. *Brain Res.* **409:**316–328.

30. Collingridge D.R., Piepmeier J.M., Knisely J.P., Rockwell S. 1998. Polarographic measurement of oxygen tension in human brain glioma. *Int. J. Radiat. Oncol. Biol. Phys.* **42:**267.

31. Craig C.G., Tropepe V., Morshead C.M., Reynolds B.A., Weiss S., van der Kooy D. 1996. In vivo growth factor expansion of endogenous subependymal neural precursor cell populations in the adult mouse brain. *J. Neurosci.* **16:** 2649–2658.

32. Crossen J.R., Garwood D., Glatstein E., Neuwelt E.A. 1994. Neurobehavioral sequelae of cranial irradiation in adults: A review of radiation-induced encephalopathy. *J. Clin. Oncol.* **12:**627–642.

33. Czurko A., Czeh B., Seress L., Nadel L., Bures J. 1997. Severe spatial navigation deficit in the Morris water maze after single high dose of neonatal X-ray irradiation in the rat. *Proc. Natl. Acad. Sci. U S A* **94:**2766–2771.

34. Dachs G.U., Patterson A.V., Firth J.D., Ratcliffe P.J., Townsend K.M.S., Stratford I.J., Harris A.L. 1997. Targeting gene expression to hypoxic tumor cells. *Nature Med.* **3:**515–520.

35. Daigle J.L., Hong J.H., Chiang C.S., McBride W.H. 2001. The role of tumor necrosis factor signaling pathways in the response of murine brain to irradiation. *Cancer Res.* **61:**8859–8865.

36. Dennis M., Spiegler B.J., Obonsawin M.C., Maria B.L., Cowell C., Hoffman H.J., et al. 1992. Brain tumors in children and adolescents–III. Effects of radiation and hormone status on intelligence and on working, associative and serial-order memory. *Neuropsychologia* **30:**257–275.

37. Dewey W.C., Freeman M.L., Raaphorst G.P., Clark E.P., Wong R.S.L., Highfield D.P., et al. 1980. Cell biology of hyperthermia and radiation, in *Radiation Biology in Cancer Research* (Meyn, R.E., Withers, H.R., eds.), Raven Press, New York, pp. 589–621.

38. Diller L., Kassel J., Nelson C.E., Gryka M.A., Litwak G., Gebhardt M., et al. 1990. p53 functions as a cell cycle control protein in osteosarcomas. *Mo. Cellular Biol.* **10:**5772–5781.

39. Doetsch F., Caille I., Lim D.A., Garcia-Verdugo J.M., Alvarez-Buylla A. 1999. Subventricular zone astrocytes are neural stem cells in the adult mammalian brain. *Cell* **97:**703–716.

40. Doetsch F., Garcia-Verdugo J.M., Alvarez-Buylla A. 1997. Cellular composition and three-dimensional organization of the subventricular germinal zone in the adult mammalian brain. *J. Neurosci.* **17:**5046–5061.

41. Earnshaw W.C., Martins L.M., Kaufmann S.H. 1999. Mammalian caspases: structure, activation, substrates, and functions during apoptosis. *Ann. Rev. Biochem.* **68:**383–424.

42. Ellenberg L., McComb J.G., Siegel S.E., Stowe S. 1987. Factors affecting intellectual outcome in pediatric brain tumor patients. *Neurosurgery* **21:**638–644.

43. Eriksson P.S., Perfilieva E., Bjork-Eriksson T., Alborn A.M., Nordborg C., Peterson D.A., Gage F.H. 1998. Neurogenesis in the adult human hippocampus. *Nat. Med.* **4:**1313–1317.

44. Fike J.R., Cann C.E., Turowski K., Higgins R.J., Chan A.S., Phillips T.L., Davis R.L. 1988. Radiation dose response of normal brain. *Int. J. Radiat. Oncol. Biol. Phys.* **14:**63–70.

45. Fitzek M.M., Thornton A.F., Harsh G., IV, Rabinov J.D., Menzenrider J.E., Lev M., et al. 2001. Dose-escalation with proton/photon irradiation for Daumas-Duport lower-grade glioma: results of an institutional phase I/II trial. *Int. J. Radiat. Oncol. Biol. Phys.* **51:**131–137.

46. Fitzek M.M., Thornton A.F., Rabinov J.D., Lev M.H., Pardo F.S., Menzenrider J.E., et al. 1999. Accelerated fractionated proton/photon irradiation to 90 cobalt gray equivalent for glioblastoma multiforme: results of a phase II prospective trial. *J. Neurosurgery* **91:**251–260.

47. Futaki M., Liu J.M. 2001. Chromosomal breakage syndromes and the BRCA1 genome surveillance complex. *Trends Mol. Med.* **7:**560–565.

48. Gage F.H. 2000. Mammalian neural stem cells. *Science* **287:**1433–1438.

49. Gould E., Beylin A., Tanapat P., Reeves A., Shors T.J. 1999. Learning enhances adult neurogenesis in the hippocampal formation. *Nat. Neurosci.* **2:**260–265.

50. Gould E., McEwen B.S., Tanapat P., Galea L.A., Fuchs E. 1997. Neurogenesis in the dentate gyrus of the adult tree shrew is regulated by psychosocial stress and NMDA receptor activation. *J. Neurosci.* **17:**2492–2498.

51. Green S.B., Byar D.P., Strike T.A., Alexander E., Brooks W.H., Burger P.C., et al. Randomized comparisons of BCNU, streptozotocin, radiosensitizer, and fractionation of radiotherapy in the postoperative treatment of malignant glioma (study 7702) (abstr.). *Proc. Am. Soc. Clin. Oncol.* **3:**260, 1984.

52. Griffin T.W., Davis R. Laramore G. 1983. Fast neutron radiation therapy for glioblastoma multiforme—results of an RTOG study. *Am. J. Clin.l Oncol.* **6:**661–667.

53. Gutin P.H., Leibel S.A., Hosobuchi Y., Crumley R.L., Edwards M.S., Wilson C.B., et al. 1987. Brachytherapy of recurrent tumors of the skull base and spine with iodine-125 sources. *Neurosurgery* **20:**938–945.

54. Haber J.E. 2000. Partners and pathwaysrepairing a double-strand break. *Trends Genet.* **16:**259–264.

55. Hall E.J. 1988. *Radiobiology for the Radiologist.* J. B. Lippincott Co., Philadelphia, PA.

56. Hall E.J. 1994. *Radiobiology for the Radiologist.* J. B. Lippincott Co., Philadelphia, PA.

57. Halligan J.B., Stelzer K.J. Rostomily R.C., Spence A.M., Griffin T.W., Berger M.S. 1996. Operation and permanent low activity ^{125}I brachytherapy for recurrent high-grade astrocytomas. *Int. J. Radiat. Oncol. Biol. Phys.* **35:**541–547.

58. Hanahan D., Bergers G., Bergsland E. 2000. Less is more, regularly: metronomic dosing of cytotoxic drugs can target tumor angiogenesis in mice. *J. Clin. Invest.* **105:**1045–1047.

59. Hengartner M.O. 2000. The biochemistry of apoptosis. *Nature* **407:**770–776.

60. Herzog K.H., Chong M.J., Kapsetaki M., Morgan J.I., McKinnon P.J. 1998. Requirement for Atm in ionizing radiation-induced cell death in the developing central nervous system. *Science* **280:**1089–1091.

61. Hong J.H., Chiang C.S., Campbell I.L., Sun J.R., Withers H.R., McBride W.H. 1995. Induction of acute phase gene expression by brain irradiation. *Int. J. Radiat. Oncol. Biol. Phys.* **33:**619–626.

62. Hopewell J.W. 1971. A quantitative study on the mitotic activity in the subependymal plate of adult rats. *Cell Tissue Kinet.* **4:**273–278.

63. Hopewell J.W., Cavanagh J.B. 1972. Effects of X irradiation on the mitotic activity of the subependymal plate of rats. *Br.. J. Radiol.* **45:**461–465.

64. Hopewell J.W., Wright E.A. 1970. The nature of latent cerebral irradiation damage and its modification by hypertension. *Br. J. Radiol.* **43:**161–167.

65. Hornsey S., Myers R., Coultas P.G., Rogers M.A., White A. 1981. Turnover of proliferating cells in the spinal cord after X irradiation and its relation to time-dependent repair of radiation damage. *Br. J. Radiol.* **54:**1081–1085.

66. Huang E., Teh B.S., Strother D.R., Davis Q.G., Chiu J.K., Lu H.H., Carpenter L.S., et al. 2002. Intensity-modulated radiation therapy for pediatric medulloblastoma: early report on the reduction of ototoxicity. *Int J Radiat Oncol Biol Phys* **52:**599–605.

67. Huang L.E., Gu J. Schau M., Bunn H.F. 1998. Regulation of hypoxia-inducible factor 1alpha is mediated by an O2- dependent degradation domain via the ubiquitin-proteasome pathway. *Proc. Natl. Acad. Sci. USA* **95:**7987–7992.

68. Hubbard B.M., Hopewell J.W. 1980. Quantitative changes in cellularity of the rat subependymal plate after x-irradiation. *Cell Tissue Kinet.* **13:**403–413.

69. Imperato J.P., Paleologos N.A., Vick N.A. 1990. Effects of treatment on long-term survivors with malignant astrocytomas. *Ann. Neurol.* **28:**818–822.

70. Johansson C.B., Momma S., Clarke D.L., Risling M., Lendahl U., Frisen J. 1999. Identification of a neural stem cell in the adult mammalian central nervous system. *Cell* **96:**25–34.

71. Johnson M.D., Xiang H., London S., Kinoshita Y., Knudson M., Mayberg M, et al. 1998. Evidence for involvement of Bax and p53, but not caspases, in radiation-induced cell death of cultured postnatal hippocampal neurons. *J. Neurosci. Res.* **54:**721–733.

72. Kaplan M.I., Morgan W.F. 1998. The nucleus is the target for radiation-induced chromosomal instability. *Radiat. Res.* **150:**382–390.

73. Kayama T., Yoshimoto T., Fujimoto S., Sakurai Y. 1991. Intratumoral oxygen pressure in malignant brain tumor. *J. Neurosurg.* **74:**55–59.

74. Kempermann G., Kuhn H.G., Gage F.H. 1997. More hippocampal neurons in adult mice living in an enriched environment. *Nature* **386:**493–495.

75. Kempermann G. Kuhn H.G., Gage F.H. 1998. Experience-induced neurogenesis in the senescent dentate gyrus. *J. Neurosci.* **18:**3206–3212.

76. Khanna K.K. 2000. Cancer risk and the ATM gene: a continuing debate. *J. Natl. Cancer Inst.* **92:**795–802.

77. Khanna K.K., Jackson S.P. 2001. DNA double-strand breaks: signaling, repair and the cancer connection. *Nat. Genet.* **27:**247–254.

78. Klement G., Baruchel S., Rak J., Man S., Clark K., Hicklin D.J., et al. 2000. Continuous low-dose therapy with vinblastine and VEGF receptor-2 antibody induces sustained tumor regression without overt toxicity. *J. Clin. Invest.* **105:**15–24.

79. Kondziolka D., Flickinger J.C., Lunsford L.D. 2000. Stereotactic radiosurgery and radiation therapy, in *Neuro-Oncology: The Essentials* (Berstein M., Berger M.S., eds.) Thieme Medical Publishers, Inc., New York, pp. 183–197.

80. Kondziolka D., Patel A., Lunsford L.D., Kassam A., Flickinger J.C. 1999. Stereotactic radiosurgery plus whole brain radiotherapy versus radiotherapy alone for patients with multiple brain metastases. *Inl. J. Rad. Oncol. Biol. Phys* **45:** 427–434.

81. Kramer J.H., Crittenden M.R., Halberg F.E., Wara W.M., Cowan M.J. 1992. A prospective study of cognitive functioning following low-dose cranial radiation for bone marrow transplantation. *Pediatrics* **90:**447–450.

82. Kreth F.W., Faist M., Warnke P.C., Roßner R., Volk B., Ostertag C.B. 1995. Interstitial radiosurgery of low-grade gliomas. *J. Neurosurgery* **82:**418–429.

83. Kuhn H.G., Dickinson-Anson H., Gage F.H. 1996. Neurogenesis in the dentate gyrus of the adult rat: age-related decrease of neuronal progenitor proliferation. *J. Neurosci.* **16:**2027–2033.

84. Kuhn H.G., Winkler J., Kempermann G., Thal L.J., Gage F.H. 1997. Epidermal growth factor and fibroblast growth factor-2 have different effects on neural progenitors in the adult rat brain. *J. Neurosci.* **17:**5820–5829.

85. Laperriere N.J., Leung P.M.K., McKenzie S., Milosevic M., Wong S., Glen J., Pintilie M., Bernstein M. 1998. Randomized study of brachytherapy in the initial management of patients with malignant astrocytoma. *Int. J. Radiat. Oncol. Biol. Phys.* **41:**1005–1011.

86. Laramore G.E., Diener-West M., Griffin T.W., Nelson J.S., Griem M.L., Thomas F.J., et al. 1988. Randomized neutron dose searching study for malignant gliomas of the brain: results of an RTOG study. *Int. J. Radiat. Oncol. Biol. Phys.* **14:**1093–1102.

87. Laramore G.E., Griffin T.W., Gerdes A.J., Parker R.G. 1978. Fast neutron and mixed (neutron/photon) beam teletherapy for grades III and IV astrocytomas. *Cancer* **42:**96–103.

88. Laramore G.E., Martz K.L., Nelson J.S., Nelson D.F., Griffin T.W., Chang C.H., Horton J. 1988. RTOG survival data on anaplastic astrocytoma of the brain: does a more aggressive form of treatment adversely impact survival? (abstr.). *Int. J. Radiat. Oncol. Biol. Phys.* **15(Suppl. 1):**195.

89. Lee P.W., Hung B.K., Woo E.K., Tai P.T., Choi D.T. 1989. Effects of radiation therapy on neuropsychological functioning in patients with nasopharyngeal carcinoma. *J. Neurol. Neurosurg. Psychiatry* **52:**488–492.

90. Li P. Nijhawan D., Budihardjo I., Srinivasula S.M., Ahmad M., Alnemri E.S., Wang X. 1997. Cytochrome c and dATP-dependent formation of Apaf-1/caspase-9 complex initiates an apoptotic protease cascade. *Cell* **91:**479–489.

91. Li Y.Q.Jay V., Wong C.S. 1996. Oligodendrocytes in the adult rat spinal cord undergo radiation-induced apoptosis. *Cancer Res* **56:**5417–5422.

92. Lim D.A., Fishell G.J., Alvarez-Buylla A. 1997. Postnatal mouse subventricular zone neuronal precursors can migrate and differentiate within multiple levels of the developing neuraxis. *Proc. Natl. Acad. Sci. USA* **94:**14,832–14,836.

93. Locher G.L. 1936. Biological effects and therapeutic possibilities of neutrons. *Am. J Roentgenol.* **36:**1–13.

94. Lois C., Alvarez-Buylla A. 1994. Long-distance neuronal migration in the adult mammalian brain. *Science* **264:**1145–1148.

95. Lowe S.W., Schmitt E.M., Smith S.W., Osborne B.A., Jacks T. 1993. p53 is required for radiation-induced apoptosis in mouse thymocytes. *Nature* **362:**847–849.

96. Lowenstein D.H., Parent J.M.. 1999. Brain, heal thyself. *Science* **283:**1126–1127.

97. Luskin M.B., McDermott K. 1994. Divergent lineages for oligodendrocytes and astrocytes originating in the neonatal forebrain subventricular zone. *Glia* **11:**211–226.

98. Lutz P.L. 1992. Mechanisms for anoxic survival in the vertebrate brain. *Ann. Rev. Physiol.* **54:**601–618.

99. Maity A., McKenna W.G., Muschel R.J. 1994. The molecular basis for cell cycle delays following ionizing radiation: a review. *Radiother. Oncol.* **31:**1–13.

100. Maletinska L.E., Blakely E.A., Bjornstad K.A., Deen D.F., Knoff L.J., Forte T.M. 2000. Human glioblastoma cell lines: levels of low-density lipoprotein receptor and low-density lipoprotein receptor-related protein. *Cancer Res.* **60:**2300–2303.

101. Mandell L.R., Kadota R., Freeman C., Douglass E.C., Fontanesi J., Cohen M.E., et al. 1999. There is no role for hyperfractionated radiotherapy in the management of children with newly diagnosed diffuse intrinsic brainstem tumors: results of a Pediatric Oncology Group Phase III trial comparing conventional vs. hyperfractionated radiotherapy. *Int. J. Radiat. Oncol. Biol. Phys.* **43:**959–964.

102. Marks J.E., Baglan R.J., Prassad S.C., Blank W.F. 1981. Cerebral radionecrosis: incidence and risk in relation to dose, time, fractionation and volume. *Int. J. Radiat. Oncol. Biol. Phys.* **7:**243–252.

103. Mastaglia F.L., McDonald W.I., Watson J.V., Yogendran K. 1976. Effects of x-radiation on the spinal cord: an experimental study of the morphological changes in central nerve fibres. *Brain* **99:**101–122.

104. Matsutani M., Nakamura O., Nagashima T., Asai A., Fujimaki T., Tanaka H., et al. 1994. Intra-operative radiation therapy for malignant brain tumors: rationale, method, and treatment results of cerebral glioblastomas. *Acta. Neurochirurgica (Wien)* **131:**80–90.

105. McDermott M.W., Cosgrove G.R., Larson D.A., Sneed P.K., Gutin P.H. 1996. Interstitial brachytherapy for intracranial metastases. *Neurosurgery Clinics of North America* **7:**485–495.

106. McKenna W.G., Iliakis G., Weiss M.C., Bernhard E.J., Muschel R.J. 1991. Increased G2 delay in radiation-resistant cells obtained by transformation of primary rat embryo cells with the oncogenes H-*ras* and V-*myc*. *Radiat. Res.* **125:**283–287.

107. Mercer W.E., Shields M.T., Amin M., Sauve G.J., Appella E., Romano J.W., Ullrich S.J. 1990. Negative growth regulation in a glioblastoma tumor cell line that conditionally expresses human wild-type p53. *Proc. Nat. Acad. Sci. USA* **87:**6166–6170.

108. Mickley G.A., Ferguson J.L., Mulvihill M.A., Nemeth T.J. 1989. Progressive behavioral changes during the maturation of rats with early radiation-induced hypoplasia of fascia dentata granule cells. *Neurotoxicol. Teratol.* **11**:385–393.

109. Mocchetti I., Wrathall J.R. 1995. Neurotrophic factors in central nervous system trauma. *J. Neurotrauma* **12**:853–870.

110. Moreira R.C.M., Moreira M.V., Bueno J.L.O., Xavier G.F. 1997. Hippocampal lesions induced by ionizing radiation: a parametric study. *J. Neurosci. Meth.* **75**:41–47.

111. Morgan D.O. 1995. Principles of CDK regulation. *Nature* **374**:131–134.

112. Morris G.M., Coderre J.A., Bywaters A., Whitehouse E., Hopewell J.W. 1996. Boron neutron capture irradiation of the rat spinal cord: histopathological evidence of a vascular-mediated pathogenesis. *Radiat. Res.* **146**:313–320.

113. Morshead C.M., van der Kooy D. 1992. Postmitotic death is the fate of constitutively proliferating cells in the subependymal layer of the adult mouse brain. *J. Neurosci.* **12**:249–256.

114. Moyer J.A., Wood A., Ay I., Finklestein S.P., Protter A.A. Basic fibroblast growth factor: a potential therapeutic agent for the treatment of acute neurodegenerative disorders and vascular insufficiency. *Exp. Opin. Ther. Pat.* **8**:1425–1445.

115. Munro T.R. 1970. The relative radiosensitivity of the nucleus and cytoplasm of Chinese hamster fibroblasts. *Radiat. Res.* **42**:451–470.

116. Munzenrider J.E., Crowell C. 1994. Charged particles, in *Radiation Oncology Technology and Biology* (Mauch P.M., Loeffler J.S., eds.), W. B. Saunders, Philadelphia, PA, pp. 34–55.

117. Murnane J.P. 1995. Cell cycle regulation in response to DNA damage in mammalian cells: A historical perspective. *Cancer and Metastasis Reviews* **14**:17–29.

118. Murray A.W. 1992. Creative blocks: cell cycle checkpoints and feedback controls. *Nature* **359**:599–604.

119. Nelson D.F., Schoenfeld D., Weinstein A.S., Nelson J.S., Wasserman T., Goodman R.L., Carabell S. 1983. A randomized comparison of misonidazole sensitized radiotherapy plus BCNU and radiotherapy plus BCNU for treatment of malignant glioma after surgery: preliminary results of an RTOG study. *Int. J. Radiat. Oncol. Biol. Phys.* **9**:1143–1151.

120. Oleson J.R. 1995. Hyperthermia from the clinic to the laboratory: a hypothesis. *Int. J. Hyperthermia* **11**:315–322.

121. Painter R.B. 1962. The direct effect of X-irradiation on HeLa S3 deoxyribonucleic acid synthesis. *Radiat. Res.* **16**:846–859.

122. Painter R.B., Robertson J.S. 1959. Effect of irradiation and theory of role of mitotic delay on the time course of labeling of HeLa S3 cells with tritiated thymidine. *Radiat. Res.* **11**:206–217.

123. Painter R.B., Young B.R. 1975. X-ray-induced inhibition of DNA synthesis in Chinese hamster ovary, human HeLa, and mouse L cells. *Radiat. Res.* **64**:648–656.

124. Parent J.M., Tada E., Fike J.R., Lowenstein D.H. 1999. Inhibition of dentate granule cell neurogenesis with brain irradiation does not prevent seizure-induced mossy fiber synaptic reorganization in the rat. *J. Neurosci.* **19**:4508–4519.

125. Patel S., Breneman J.C., Warnick R.E., Albright R.E., Jr., Tobler W.D., van Loveren H.R., Tew J.M., Jr.. 2000. Permanent iodine-125 interstitial implants for the treatment of recurrent glioblastoma multiforme. *Neurosurgery* **46**:1123–1128.

126. Peissner W., Kocher M., Treuer H., Gillardon F. 1999. Ionizing radiation-induced apoptosis of proliferating stem cells in the dentate gyrus of the adult rat hippocampus. *Brain Res. Mol. Brain Res.* **71**:61–68.

127. Pirzkall A., Carol M., Lohr F., Hoss A., Wannenmacher M., Debus J. 2000. Comparison of intensity-modulated radiotherapy with conventional conformal radiotherapy for complex-shaped tumors *Int. J. Radiat. Oncol. Biol. Phys.* **48**:1371–1380.

128. Pirzkall A., McKnight T.R., Graves E.E., Carol M.P., Sneed P.K., Wara W.M., et al. 2001. MR-spectroscopy guided target delineation for high-grade gliomas. *Int. J. Radiat. Oncol. Biol. Phys.* **50**:915–928.

129. Prados MD, Scott C, Sandler H, Buckner JC, Phillips T, Schultz C, et al. 1999. A phase 3 randomized study of radiotherapy plus procarbazine, CCNU, and vincristine (PCV) with or without BUdR for the treatment of anaplastic astrocytoma: a preliminary report of RTOG 9404. *Int. J. Radiat. Oncol. Biol. Phys.* **45**:1109–1115.

130. Prados M.D., Wara W.M., Sneed P.K., McDermott M., Chang S.M., Rabbit J., et al. Phase III trial of accelerated hyperfractionation with or without difluoromethylornithine (DFMO) versus standard fractionated radiotherapy with or without DFMO for newly diagnosed patients with glioblastoma multiforme. *Int. J. Radiat. Oncol. Biol. Phys.* **49**:71–77.

131. Puck T.T. 1958. Action of radiation on mammalian cells. III. Relationship between reproductive death and induction of chromosome anomalies by X-irradiation of euploid human cells *in vitro. Proc. Nat. Acad. Sci. USA* **44**:772–780.

132. Raff M.C. Social controls on cell survival and cell death. *Nature* **356**:397–400.

133. Raff M.C., Barres B.A., Burne J.F., Coles H.S., Ishizaki Y., Jacobson M.D. 1993. Programmed cell death and control of cell survival: Lessons from the nervous system. *Science* **262**:695–700.

134. Raff M.C., Miller R.H., Noble M. 1983. A glial progenitor cell that develops in vitro into an astrocyte or an oligodendrocyte depending on culture medium. *Nature* **303**:390–396.

135. Raju U., Gumin G.J., Tofilon P.J. 2000. Radiation-induced transcription factor activation in the rat cerebral cortex. *Int. J. Radiat. Biol.* **76**:1045–1053.

136. Rampling R., Cruickshank G., Lewis A.D., Fitzsimmons S.A., Workman P. 1994. Direct measurement of pO2 distribution and bioreductive enzymes in human malignant brain tumors. *Int. J. Radiat. Oncol. Biol. Phys.* **29**:427–431.

137. Reinhold H.S., Calvo W., Hopewell J.W., van der Berg A.P. 1990. Development of blood vessel-related radiation damage in the fimbria of the central nervous system. *Int. J. Radiat. Oncol. Biol. Phys.* **18**:37–42.

138. Rogulski K.R., Kim J.H., Kim S.H., Freytag S.O. 1997. Glioma cells transduced with an Escherichia coli CD/HSV-1 TK fusion gene exhibit enhanced metabolic suicide and radiosensitivity. *Hum. Gene. Ther.* **8**:73–85.

139. Roman D.D., Sperduto P.W. 1995. Neuropsychological effects of cranial radiation: current knowledge and future directions. *Int. J. Radiat. Oncol. Biol. Phys.* **31**:983–998.

140. Ruan H. Su H., Hu L., Lamborn K.R., Kan Y.W., Deen D.F. 2001. A hypoxia-regulated adeno-associated virus vector for cancer-specific gene therapy. *Neoplasia* **3**:255–263.

141. Sakakura C., Sweeney E.A., Shirahama T., Igarashi Y., Hakomori S., Tsujimoto H., et al. Overexpression of bax enhances the radiation sensitivity in human breast cancer cells. *Surg. Today* **27**:90–93.

142. Salazar O.M., Rubin P., Feldstein M.L., Pizzutiello R. 1979. High dose radiation therapy in the treatment of malignant gliomas: final report. *Int. J. Radiat. Oncol. Biol. Phys.* **5**:1733–1740.

143. Salceda S., Caro J. 1997. Hypoxia-inducible factor 1alpha (HIF-1alpha) protein is rapidly degraded by the ubiquitin-proteasome system under normoxic conditions. Its stabilization by hypoxia depends on redox-induced changes. *J. Biol. Chem.* **272**:22,642–22,647.

144. Schmidt J.V. Bradfield C.A. 1996. Ah receptor signaling pathways. *Ann. Rev. Cell. Dev. Biol.* **12**:55–89.

145. Schultheiss T.E., Stephens L.C. 1992. Invited review: permanent radiation myelopathy. *Br. J. Radiol.* **65**:737–753.

146. Schwab M.E., Bartholdi D. 1996. Degeneration and regeneration of axons in the lesioned spinal cord. *Physiol. Rev.* **76**:319–370.

147. Scott C.B., Scarantino C., Urtasun R., Movsas B., Jones C.U., Simpson J.R., Fischbach A.J., Curran W.J., Jr. 1998. Validation and predictive power of Radiation Therapy Oncology Group (RTOG) recursive partitioning analysis classes for malignant glioma patients: a report using RTOG 90-06. *Int. J. Radiat. Oncol. Biol. Phys.* **40**:51–55.

148. Seegenschmiedt M.H., Klautke G., Grabenbauer G.G., Sauer R. 1995. Thermoradiotherapy for malignant brain tumors: review of biological and clinical studies. *Endocurietherapy/Hyperthermia Oncology* **11**:201–221.

149. Selker R.G., Shapiro W.R., Green S., Burger P., Van Gilder J., Saris S., et al. 1995. A randomized trial of interstitial radiotherapy (IRT) boost for the treatment of newly diagnosed malignant glioma (glioblastoma multiforme, anaplastic astrocytoma, anaplastic oligodendroglioma, malignant mixed glioma): BTCG study 87-01 (abstract). Presented at Program of the Congress of Neurological Surgeons 45th Annual Meeting, San Francisco, CA.

150. Semenza G.L. 1998. Hypoxia-inducible factor 1 and the molecular physiology of oxygen homeostasis. *J. Lab. Clin. Med.* **131**:207–214.

151. Semenza G.L., Wang G.L. 1992. A nuclear factor induced by hypoxia via de novo protein synthesis binds to the human erythropoietin gene enhancer at a site required for transcriptional activation. *Mol. Cell Biol.* **12**:5447–5454.

152. Seri B., Garcia-Verdugo J.M., McEwen B.S., Alvarez-Buylla A. 2001. Astrocytes give rise to new neurons in the adult mammalian hippocampus. *J. Neurosci.* **21**:7153–7160.

153. Shaw P. Bovey R., Tardy S., Sahli R., Sordat B., Costa J. 1992. Induction of apoptosis by wild-type p53 in a human colon tumor-derived cell line. *Proc. Nat. Acad. Sci. USA* **89**:4495–4499.

154. Sheline G.E., Wara W.M., Smith V. 1980. Therapeutic irradiation and brain injury. *Int. J. Radiat. Oncol. Biol. Phys.* **6**:1215–1228.

155. Shibata T., Akiyama N., Noda M., Sasai K., Hiraoka M. 1998. Enhancement of gene expression under hypoxic conditions using fragments of the human vascular endothelial growth factor and the erythropoietin genes. *Int. J. Radiat. Oncol. Biol. Phys.* **42**:913–916.

156. Shibata T., Giaccia A.J., Laderoute K.R., Brown J.M. 1999. Tumor-specific gene therapy using hypoxia-responsive gene expression. *AACR Proc.* **40**:632.

157. Shinohara C., Gobbel G.T., Lamborn K.R., Tada E., Fike J.R. 1997. Apoptosis in the subependyma of young adult rats after single and fractionated doses of X-rays. *Cancer Res.* **57**:2694–2702.

158. Shors T.J., Miesegaes G., Beylin A., Zhao M., Rydel T., Gould E. 2001. Neurogenesis in the adult is involved in the formation of trace memories. *Nature* **410**:372–376.

159. Shrieve D.C., Alexander E., 3rd, Black P.M., Wen P.Y., Fine H.A., Kooy H.M., Loeffler J.S. 1999. Treatment of patients with primary glioblastoma multiforme with standard postoperative radiotherapy and radiosurgical boost: prognostic factors and long-term outcome. *J. Neurosurgery* **90**:72–77.

160. Shrieve D.C., Alexander E., 3rd, Wen P.Y., Fine H.A., Kooy H.M., Black P.M., Loeffler J.S. 1995. Comparison of stereotactic radiosurgery and brachytherapy in the treatment of recurrent glioblastoma multiforme. *Neurosurgery* **36**:275–284.

161. Siegal T., Pfeffer M.R. 1995. Radiation-induced changes in the profile of spinal cord serotonin, prostaglandin synthesis, and vascular permeability. *Int. J. Radiat. Oncol. Biol. Phys.* **31**:57–64.

162. Sienkiewicz Z.J., Saunders R.D., Butland B.K. 1992. Prenatal irradiation and spatial memory in mice: investigation of critical period. *Int. J. Radiat. Biol.* **62**:211–219.

163. Smith GC, Jackson SP. 1999. The DNA-dependent protein kinase. *Genes Dev.* **13**:916–934.

164. Sneed P.K., McDermott M.W., Gutin P.H. 1997. Interstitial brachytherapy procedures for brain tumors. *Sem. Surg. Oncol.* **13**:157–166.

165. Sneed P.K., Stauffer P.R., McDermott M.W., Diederich C.J., Lamborn K.R., Prados M.D., et al. 1998. Survival benefit of hyperthermia in a prospective, randomized trial of brachytherapy boost ± hyperthermia for glioblastoma multiforme. *Int. J. Radiat. Oncol. Biol. Phys.* **40**:287–295.

166. Squire L.R., Zola-Morgan S. 1991. The medial temporal lobe memory system. *Science* **253**:1380–1386.

167. Stanfield B.B., Trice J.E. 1988. Evidence that granule cells generated in the dentate gyrus of adult rats extend axonal projections. *Exp. Brain Res.* **73**:399–406.

168. Stuschke M., Thames H.D. 1997. Hyperfractionated radiotherapy of human tumors: overview of the randomized clinical trials. *Int. J. Radiat. Oncol. Biol. Phys.* **37**:259–267.

169. Su L.N., Little J.B. 1993. Prolonged cell cycle delay in radioresistant human cell lines transfected with activated *ras* oncogene and/or Simian Virus 40 T-antigen. *Rad. Res.* **133**:73–79.

170. Sutherland R.M. 1998. Tumor hypoxia and gene expression - implications for malignant progression and therapy. *Acta. Oncologica* **37**:567–574.

171. Tada E., Parent J.M., Lowenstein D.H., Fike J.R. 2000. X-irradiation causes a prolonged reduction in cell proliferation in the dentate gyrus of adult rats. *Neuroscience* **99**:33–41.

172. Tada E., Yang C., Gobbel G.T., Lamborn K.R., Fike J.R. 1999. Long term impairment of subependymal repopulation following damage by ionizing irradiation. *Exptl. Neurol.* **160**:66–77.

173. Tashiro S., Walter J., Shinohara A., Kamada N., Cremer T. 2000. Rad51 accumulation at sites of DNA damage and in postreplicative chromatin. *J. Cell Biol.* **150**:283–291.

174. Temple S., Alvarez-Buylla A. 1999. Stem cells in the adult mammalian central nervous system. *Curr. Opin. Neurobiol.* **9**:135–141.

175. Thomlinson R.H., Gray L.H. 1955. The histological structure of some human lung cancers and the possible implications for radiotherapy. *Br. J. Cancer* **9**:539–549.

176. Tsuzuki T., Fujii Y., Sakumi K., Tominaga Y., Nakao K., Sekiguchi M., et al. 1996. Targeted disruption of the Rad51 gene leads to lethality in embryonic mice. *Proc. Natl. Acad. Sci. USA* **93**:6236–6240.

177. Urtasun R., Felstein M.L., Partington J., Tanasichuk H., Miller J.D.R., Russell D.B., et al. 1982. Radiation and nitroimidazoles in supratentorial high grade gliomas: a second clinical trial. *Br. J Cancer* **46**:101–108.

178. van der Kogel AJ. 1991. Central nervous system injury in small animal models, in *Radiation Injury to the Nervous System* (Gutin R.H., Leibel S.A., Sheline G.E. eds), Raven Press, Ltd., New York, pp. 91–111.

179. van der Maazen R.W., Kleiboer B.J., Verhagen I., van der Kogel A.J. 1991. Irradiation in vitro discriminates between different O-2A progenitor cell subpopulations in the perinatal central nervous system of rats. *Radiat. Res.* **128**:64–72.

180. van der Maazen R.W., Kleiboer B.J., Verhagen I., van der Kogel A.J. 1993. Repair capacity of adult rat glial progenitor cells determined by an in vitro clonogenic assay after in vitro or in vivo fractionated irradiation. *Int. J. Radiat. Biol.* **63**:661–666.

181. van der Maazen R.W., Verhagen I., Kleiboer B.J., van der Kogel A.J. 1991. Radiosensitivity of glial progenitor cells of the perinatal and adult rat optic nerve studied by an in vitro clonogenic assay. *Radiother. Oncol.* **20**:258–264, 1991.

182. Vaupel P.W. 1993.Oxygenation of solid tumors, in *Drug Resistance in Oncology* (Teicher B.A. ed.),Marcel Dekker, New York, pp. 53–85.

183. Walker M.D. Strike T.A., Sheline G.E. 1979. An analysis of dose-effect relationship in the radiotherapy of malignant gliomas. *Int. J. Radiat. Oncol. Biol. Phys.* **5**:1725–1731.

184. Wallace R.B., Graziadei R., Werboff J. 1981. Behavioral correlates of focal hippocampal x-irradiation in rats II. Behavior related to adaptive function in a natural setting. *Exp. Brain Res.* **43**:207–212.

185. Wallner K.E., Galicich J.H., Krol G., Arbit E., Malkin M.G. 1989. Patterns of failure following treatment for glioblastoma multiforme and anaplastic astrocytoma. *Int. J. Rad.Oncol. Biol. Phys.* **16**:1405–1409.

186. Weinert T.A., Hartwell L.H. 1988. The *RAD9* gene controls the cell cycle response to DNA damage in *Saccharomyces cerevisiae*. *Science* **241**:317–322.

187. Wen P.Y., Alexander E., 3rd, Black P.M., Fine H.A., Riese N., Levin J.M., Coleman C.N., Loeffler J.S. 1994. Long term results of stereotactic brachytherapy used in the initial treatment of patients with glioblastomas. *Cancer* **73**:3029–3036.

188. Wenger R.H., Gassman M. 1997. Oxygen(es) and the hypoxia-inducible factor-1. *J. Biol. Chem.* **378**:609–616.

189. Wouters B.G., Brown J.M. 1997. Cells at intermediate oxygen levels can be more important than the "hypoxic fraction" in determining tumor response to fractionated radiotherapy. *Radiat. Res.* **147** :541–550.

190. Yeh H.J., Ruit K.G., Wang Y.X., Parks W.C., Snider W.D., Deuel T.F. 1991. PDGF A-chain gene is expressed by mammalian neurons during development and in maturity. *Cell* **64**:209–216.

191. Yonish-Rouach E., Resnitzky D., Lotem J., Sachs L., Kimchi A., Oren M. 1991. Wild-type p53 induces apoptosis of myeloid leukaemic cells that is inhibited by interleukin-6. *Nature* **352**:345–347.

192. Yuan J., Yankner B.A. 2000. Apoptosis in the nervous system. *Nature* **407**:802-809.

193. Yuan S.S., Lee S.Y., Chen G., Song M., Tomlinson G.E., Lee E.Y. 1999. BRCA2 is required for ionizing radiation-induced assembly of Rad51 complex in vivo. *Cancer Res.* **59**:3547–3551.

16

Advances in the Management of Cerebral Metastases

Fadi Hanbali and Raymond Sawaya

1. INTRODUCTION

Brain metastases are the most common intracranial tumors in adults *(23,48,62)*. Their incidence is thought to be increasing as a result of several factors, namely, early detection secondary to advances in diagnostic technology and prolonged survival from improved systemic chemotherapy.

A single brain metastasis refers to the presence of a single lesion in the brain with no reference to the systemic status of the primary cancer; a solitary brain metastasis, on the other hand, refers to the presence of a single cerebral lesion with no evidence of metastatic spread elsewhere in the body. The management of cerebral metastasis has been complex and controversial over the years. Steroids and whole-brain radiation therapy (WBRT) have been the mainstay of treatment of brain metastasis since the 1950s *(82)*. In the early 1990s, two prospective randomized trials demonstrated that surgery followed by WBRT is superior to radiation alone in patients with a single metastasis *(75,100)*. Since its introduction, radiosurgery has become an important alternative to surgery *(2,5,41,58,90)*.

2. EPIDEMIOLOGY

Cerebral metastases are encountered in 15 to 40% of all patients with systemic malignancies, depending on whether autopsy, surgical, or radiological data are reviewed *(13,27,55,60,68,73,88)*. Autopsy studies indicate that about two-thirds of patients with brain metastases have multiple lesions *(4,20)*. Metastases may develop in any part of the brain; approx 80 to 85% of lesions are located supratentorially, whereas 15 to 20% arise infratentorially *(27,60,87)*.

The most common malignancies to metastasize to the brain in order of decreasing frequency are lung carcinoma (40–60%), breast carcinoma (15–20%), melanoma (10–20%), renal cell carcinoma (5–10%) and colorectal carcinoma (5–10%) *(56)*. Melanoma, choriocarcinoma, and small cell lung carcinoma metastases tend to be multiple, whereas adenocarcinoma of the lung, thyroid, breast, kidney, and colorectal carcinoma usually occur as single metastases *(27,60,87)*. Melanoma has the highest propensity to metastasize to the brain. Among lung primaries, adenocarcinoma and small cell carcinoma metastasize to the brain quite frequently, although squamous cell carcinoma does so less commonly. Small cell lung cancers tend to be particularly radiosensitive, thereby representing only a minority of cases in most surgical series *(60)*.

The mode of extension to the brain is almost always hematogenous through the arterial circulation. Venous dissemination via Batson's plexus of veins in the spinal epidural space has been proposed as an alternative mechanism of metastasis *(8,89)*. The distribution of cerebral metastases usually correlates with the cerebral blood flow and the brain weight; this would explain why most metastatic tumors arise near the temporoparieto-occipital junction. Delattre and Posner *(79)* reported

From: *Contemporary Cancer Research: Brain Tumors*
Edited by: F. Ali-Osman © Humana Press Inc., Totowa, NJ

that gastrointestinal and genitourinary malignancies frequently metastasize to the posterior fossa (53%) via Batson's plexus of veins. However, Graf *(46)* demonstrated site-specific localization of metastases within the brain. According to Graf *(46),* large cell lung carcinomas had a predilection for the occipital lobe, and squamous cell lung carcinoma was more common in the cerebellum. Breast carcinoma metastases were most frequently identified in the cerebellum and the basal ganglia. Melanoma metastasized most commonly to the frontal and temporal lobes. The reason for this site-specific localization is unknown.

3. DIAGNOSIS

Cerebral metastases tend to have characteristic features on radiological images. Lesions that appear on computed tomography (CT) and/or magnetic resonance (MR) imaging that are well circumscribed, enhancing after contrast administration, multiple, and located at the gray-white junction, with significant surrounding vasogenic edema favor the diagnosis of brain metastases. The differential diagnosis of cerebral metastases includes primary brain tumors, abscesses, encephalitis, resolving hematoma, cerebral infarcts, demyelinating lesions, and radiation necrosis.

Around 20 to 40% of patients with symptomatic cerebral metastasis present with previously undiagnosed primaries *(67,85).* Franzini *(42)* showed that only 15% of patients with multiple cerebral lesions with no previous history of systemic malignancy had evidence of brain metastasis based on stereotactic biopsy. Therefore, one should try to determine the histology of the lesion early in the course of the disease prior to the initiation of treatment *(99)*

In general, newly diagnosed brain lesions in patients known to have systemic cancer are most likely to be metastases. However, the diagnosis of a single brain metastasis in patients with known systemic cancer based on MR imaging findings was found to be erroneous in 11 to 15% of cases following resection or stereotactic biopsy *(75,103).* Consequently, all patients with systemic cancer and single brain metastases, except possibly those with end-stage systemic disease, should have histologic confirmation of the newly diagnosed brain lesions by either open or stereotactic biopsy prior to initiation of treatment *(60).*

4. PATHOPHYSIOLOGY

Several authors have tried to explain the pathogenesis of brain metastasis. In 1889, Paget analyzed the autopsy records of more than 1000 women with breast cancer. He described a nonrandom pattern of metastasis and introduced the theory of "seed" and "soil." He suggested that certain tumor cells had a specific affinity for the milieu of certain organs. Metastases result only when the "seed" and the "soil" are compatible *(72).* Several series have shown that certain tumors metastasize to specific organs independently of vascular anatomy, rate of blood flow, and number of tumor cells delivered to that organ *(37,97).*

Ewing *(30),* on the other hand, hypothesized that metastatic dissemination occurs by purely mechanical factors as a result of the anatomical structure of the vascular system. These theories have been adopted either separately or in conjunction to explain the metastatic site preferences of different neoplastic diseases. Regional metastatic spread can be ascribed to anatomical factors, such as efferent venous circulation or lymphatic drainage to regional lymph nodes, whereas distant organ metastasis can be attributed to the "seed" and "soil" concept *(97).*

In general, primary tumors are biologically heterogenous. The metastatic process consists of a series of sequential steps that must be completed by tumor cells for the metastasis to develop. This phenomenon is highly selective for a pre-existing subpopulation of cells that possess the biological prerequisites for favorable interactions with host microenvironment and homeostatic mechanisms, which allow these cells to segregate from the parent tumor and migrate to distant sites where they can evolve into new growths. Therefore, metastases can have a clonal origin, and different metastases may originate from the proliferation of different single cells *(1,35,39,40,53,72,98).*

The first step in this process would be proper vascularization of the tumor mass through the secretion of several proangiogenic factors by tumor and host cells and the absence of antiangiogenic factors. The next step would be local invasion of the host vascular or lymphatic channels through the expression of a series of enzymes (collagenases). Tumorous cells may then grow in these channels and shower tumor emboli into the circulatory system. These emboli must survive a variety of obstacles (immune defenses, turbulence in the vascular system) before arresting in the capillary beds of receptive organs. These cells must then extravasate into the organ parenchyma, proliferate, and establish a micrometastasis. When these metastases develop, they will shed, in turn, tumor cells into the circulation, resulting in metastasis of metastases. This represents the metastatic cascade *(31–34,36)*.

This process represents an alteration of normal homeostatic processes that are routinely active during growth of the human embryo, tissue renewal, and injury repair. Fidler noted that fewer than 0.1% of tumor cells survive to potentially evolve into a metastatic lesion 24 hr after entry into the circulation; failure to complete any one of the above steps eliminates most of the neoplastic cells *(7,38,72)*.

5. MANAGEMENT STRATEGIES

The development of brain metastases denotes a poor prognosis. The median survival time is about 1 mo without treatment *(65)* and is prolonged to 2 mo with corticosteroids *(82)*. The survival may be boosted up to 3 to 6 mo with a combination of steroids and whole-brain radiation therapy (WBRT) *(19,59,75,86)*. Surgical resection followed by WBRT has prolonged survival up to 11 mo *(74,75,100)*.

In 1926, Grant *(47)* first reviewed the controversial surgical treatment of metastatic brain tumors. Patchell et al. *(75)* and Vecht *(100)* have indicated that surgical resection followed by WBRT is superior to treatment with WBRT alone in patients with single brain metastasis in good clinical condition with no progression of the extracranial tumor during the previous 3 mo *(75,100)*. These two prospective randomized trials have established surgery as the gold standard treatment for single brain metastasis.

The current principal options for the treatment of cerebral metastases include surgery, WBRT, and radiosurgery. To follow is a discussion of each of these modalities.

5.1. Role of Surgery

In general, resection of the metastatic brain tumor does not impact systemic progression of cancer, which is the cause of death in the majority of this group of patients *(11,45,69,70)*. In patients with "absent" or "limited" systemic cancer, controlled neurologic disease is translated into a longer and more functional survival.

Not all patients with brain metastases are candidates for surgical resection. A major consideration in the decision-making process should be the immediate risk of surgical intervention compared to the potential long-term benefits of quality survival. The patient's clinical status, histology of the primary tumor, and the location and number of tumors in the brain must all be considered during patient selection *(60,61)*.

5.1.1. Clinical Criteria

Several studies have shown that the status of the primary cancer may be the most significant predictor of overall survival in patients undergoing resection of cerebral metastases *(13,61,75)*. Surgery is best offered for patients whose systemic cancer is "absent," "limited," or "controlled." One indication of the status of the systemic cancer is the expected survival time of the patients, excluding the presence of cerebral metastases. At M. D. Anderson Cancer Center (Houston, TX), patients whose expected overall survival time is beyond 3 to 4 mo are considered to be good candidates for surgical resection.

The general medical condition of the patient is another important factor in deciding about surgical resection. Cardiac or respiratory conditions that increase the anesthesia risk and may be life threatening to the patient may call for nonsurgical management, even in patients who might survive longer than 4 mo *(60,61)*.

The patient's preoperative neurological status is also a major determinant in patient selection. The potential for neurologic recovery after surgical intervention is closely related to the preoperative neurologic status. Several studies have shown that patients with Karnofsky Performance Scale (KPS) scores of less than 70 have shorter postoperative survival times than patients with a score more than of 70 or more *(60,61)*. Surgical intervention, sometimes, may be indicated despite a low KPS score. Elevated intracranial pressure, mass effect on eloquent (functionally critical) cerebral cortex, and decreased cerebral blood flow may all contribute to a poor neurologic status. Surgery can significantly improve function by reversing the deleterious effect of the intraparenchymal lesion. One way to assess the potential for recovery is to monitor the effect of preoperative steroids. Patients whose function improves with high dose steroids have a higher probability of recovery after surgery *(60,61)*.

Several authors have demonstrated a direct relationship between survival and the interval between diagnosis of the primary cancer and the brain metastasis *(18,61,74,78)*. In one study, patients who presented with cerebral metastasis 1 yr or more after diagnosis of their primary cancer had a significantly longer survival time than those in whom the metastasis was detected within 1 yr *(44)*. Patients of advanced age and male sex also have a worse prognosis for cerebral metastasis *(12,75,104,105)*.

5.1.2. Histological Criteria

The histology of the primary tumor plays an important factor in patient selection. Some metastases are especially radiosensitive or responsive to chemotherapy, and may be optimally treated using these modalities instead of surgery *(61)*. Metastases from small cell lung cancer, primary lymphomas, and germ cell tumors are particularly sensitive to chemotherapy and radiation. Other metastatic tumors like non-small cell lung cancer and breast cancer show intermediate sensitivity to radiation, and surgery should be considered as one arm of the multi-disciplinary treatment. In contrast, metastatic renal cell carcinoma, melanoma, and most sarcomas tend to be radioresistant, and surgery provides a better option for treatment of these lesions (Table 1).

5.1.3. Location of Lesions

The location of the metastatic lesion in the brain plays an important role in the decision-making process. Metastases that are deep within the brain parenchyma or adjacent to eloquent cortex carry a higher surgical risk than those located on the surface of the brain or within noneloquent regions. Several new technologies have emerged in the last decade or so that improve the surgeon's ability to perform a safer and more complete surgical resection for many tumors previously deemed unresectable (Fig. 1). Such advances include intraoperative ultrasound, intraoperative cortical mapping, image-guided, computer-assisted frameless surgical navigation systems, and intraoperative MR imaging. The potential surgical morbidity and consequent recovery time must always be taken into consideration when deciding about surgery for a patient with systemic cancer and a limited survival expectation *(60,61)*.

5.1.4. Number of Lesions

At this time, surgery should be considered the gold standard for treating single brain metastases. This fact has been proven by several retrospective studies but was well documented by two prospective randomized trials in the early 1990s *(75,100)*. Patchell et al. *(75)* and Vecht et al. *(100)* showed that surgical resection of the metastatic brain tumor followed by WBRT resulted in a longer survival, fewer recurrences, and a better quality of life than treatment with WBRT alone in this patient population with single cerebral metastases.

Table 1
Sensitivity of Brain Metastases to Radiation Therapy

Highly sensitive	Intermediately sensitive	Poorly sensitive
Choriocarcinoma	Non-small cell lung cancer	Renal cell carcinoma
Germinoma	Colon	Sarcoma
Lymphoma	Breast	Melanoma
Small-cell lung Cancer		

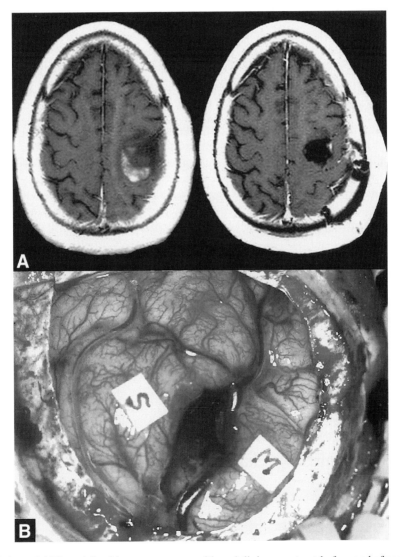

Fig. 1. (A) An axial T1-weighted image sequence with gadolinium contrast before and after resection of a metastatic tumor in the sensorimotor cortex. **(B)** The corresponding intraoperative picture of the brain depicting the area of resection of the tumor (S, sensory cortex; M, motor cortex).

Regardless of the site of origin, 50 to 75% of brain metastases are multiple *(101)*. Surgery for multiple cerebral metastases has always been a controversial issue. The presence of multiple metastases has been considered by many centers a contraindication to surgery, even when the tumors are surgically accessible *(50,80)*. Bindal et al. *(13)*, based on the experience at M. D. Anderson Cancer Center, retrospectively reviewed 56 patients who underwent resection for multiple brain metastases (a maximum of three lesions) between 1984 and 1992. Of these, 30 had one or more lesions left unresected (Group A), and 26 underwent resection of all lesions (Group B). The latter were matched to a control group of 26 patients with single surgically resected metastases (Group C). There was no difference in surgical mortality (3%, 4%, and 0% for groups A, B, and C, respectively) or morbidity (8%, 9%, and 8% for groups A, B, and C, respectively) regardless of treatment group. Patients who had all their lesions resected (Group B, median, 14 mo) had a longer survival period than those who had lesions left unresected (Group A, median, 6 mo). The survival time was very similar between patients who had all their multiple metastases resected and patients who had resected single metastases *(13)*. It is imperative, however, for all lesions to be surgically accessible and not to exceed four. A common guideline followed at M. D. Anderson is that all patients with multiple brain metastases with limited systemic disease and in whom all lesions are surgically accessible should have all their lesions (not to exceed 4) removed, even if multiple craniotomies are required (Fig. 2). We have found that this practice can significantly improve the length and quality of life for this group of patients.

5.1.5. Surgical Adjuncts

Many technological advances in the last decade have enabled us to perform a safer surgical intervention and provide a better outcome for patients with brain metastases. These neurosurgical adjuncts have allowed for better localization of the tumor, whether within an eloquent cortex region or deep within the brain parenchyma, and more accurate delineation of the surgical route for a safer resection of the metastasis. Optimum tumor resection can be achieved when the tumor is specifically localized, the borders are clearly elucidated, the residual tumor is readily identified, and the adjacent functional brain is safely preserved.

5.1.5.1. Ultrasound

The intraoperative ultrasound (IOUS) has been shown to be especially efficacious during resection of metastatic tumors (Fig. 3). Most metastatic lesions are typically echogenic relative to the surrounding brain, and can be readily differentiated from surrounding edema *(51)*. The IOUS can also well define the extent of resection and can readily, in real time, detect residual tumor after complete excision was attempted. The IOUS can also show the relationship of the tumor to surrounding structures, such as the ventricles or adjacent sulci.

5.1.5.2. Cortical Mapping

Although the medial and lateral aspects of the rolandic cortex can often be appreciated on preoperative MR images, their anatomy may be so perturbed by a tumor growing in that area that intraoperative cortical mapping should be performed to identify those sites. Identification of the precentral gyrus provides the surgeon with the opportunity to identify the adjacent central sulcus, the postcentral gyrus, and the sylvian fissure relative to the lesion in question. Evoked responses record electrical activity from the cortical surface. An average of these is then taken to reduce background activity in order to identify a phase shift across the Rolandic sulcus *(9,102)*. Proximity of the lesion to the functionally identified motor cortex can then be determined (Fig. 4). Cortical mapping can also be performed by direct brain stimulation in an awake patient. This technique may provide more information than phase shift as it can further subdivide and classify functional and nonfunctional areas within the motor cortex itself. Another major advantage of direct cortical stimulation is that it is an excellent tool for mapping the language cortex in the awake patient. This information can then be used to direct the placement of the cortical incision for resection of the metastatic tumor.

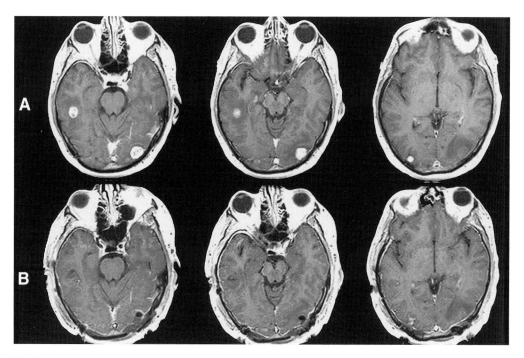

Fig. 2. Gadolinium-enhanced magnetic resonance imaging of the brain. **(A)** Preoperative imaging showing three metastatic melanoma lesions in the right temporal, right occipital, and left occipital lobes. **(B)** Postoperative imaging of the same patient after resection of the previously described three lesions during the same operative procedure.

5.1.5.3. Image-Guided, Computer-Assisted Frameless Surgical Navigation Systems

Another intraoperative adjunct is the image-guided, computer-assisted frameless surgical navigation systems. This technology allows pre-operative planning as well as real-time intraoperative guidance, localization, and orientation. In addition to showing cortical anatomy and displaying the trajectory on underlying anatomy, the navigation system also allows visualization of major vessels such as principal arteries and major surface-draining veins. It also permits less exposure of the normal brain because the cranial and dural openings are smaller. However, loss of cerebrospinal fluid, insinuation of air into the subdural space, changes in the anatomic position of a lesion with decompression, and surgically induced edema or hemorrhage are all contributing factors to the inaccuracies that can occur with the surgical navigation systems that rely on preoperatively acquired images. More recently, these systems have incorporated an ultrasound technology that would correct for all these inaccuracies.

5.1.5.4. Intraoperative MR Imaging

Operating under interactive MR imaging guidance offers the surgeon several advantages over the aforementioned navigation systems. With intraoperative MR imaging, there is no need for fiducials and registration. Intraoperative MR imaging provides superior localization of a lesion and allows dynamic updating of this information as changes in the fluid and tissue compartments of the brain occur. In addition, intraoperative MR imaging allows precise pre-operative delineation of the optimal trajectory of a surgical approach as well as dynamic guidance and verification of the execution of the chosen approach. Finally, intraoperative MR imaging allows tissue characterization, which helps the surgeon identify any residual tumor and rule out intraoperative complications such as hemorrhage *(14,108)*.

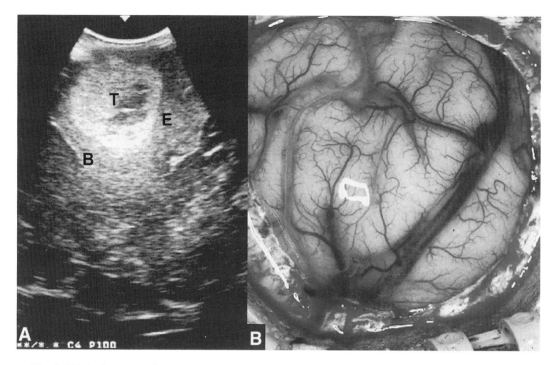

Fig. 3. (A) An intraoperative ultrasound image of a high-grade glioma depicting the hyperechogenic tumor (T), the edema (E) surrounding the brain metastasis, and the normal brain (B). **(B)** The corresponding intraoperative picture of the brain showing widened gyri overlying the brain tumor.

5.1.6. Surgical Outcome

Major advances in diagnostic measures and therapeutic interventions have significantly improved the outcome of patients after surgery for brain metastases. Craniotomy for cerebral metastases carries a 1-yr survival of 44% (range, 22–68%) and a median survival of 10 mo (range, 6–16 mo) *(60,61)*. Death as a result of neurological progression accounts for 30 to 40% of the cases, with the rest being secondary to systemic disease progression. The age of the patient, his functional status, and systemic status at the time of diagnosis of the brain metastasis are the most important prognostic variables *(11,45,68,69,75,100)*. Tumor histology may also be a determinant of survival. Melanomas are usually associated with the shortest survival (median, 7 mo), whereas lung, breast, or renal cell carcinomas carry a longer survival internal (median, 12, 12, and 10 mo, respectively) *(61)*.

Morbidity from craniotomy for metastasis consists of both neurologic deficits (speech dysfunction, hemiparesis) and nonneurologic complications (pulmonary embolus, deep vein thrombosis, wound infection). Neurologic complications can be expected to occur in 6% (range, 0–13%), and nonneurologic complications in 8% (range, 0–21%) of patients. Surgical mortality ranges from 0 to 10% WBRT *(61)*.

5.2. Role of WBRT

5.2.1. Indications for WBRT

External beam WBRT has been considered the mainstay of treatment for the majority of patients with brain metastases since its value was first documented in 1954 *(94)*. Historically, WBRT has been shown to improve or stabilize neurologic status in 50 to 75% of patients with cerebral metastases *(16,71,94,101)*.

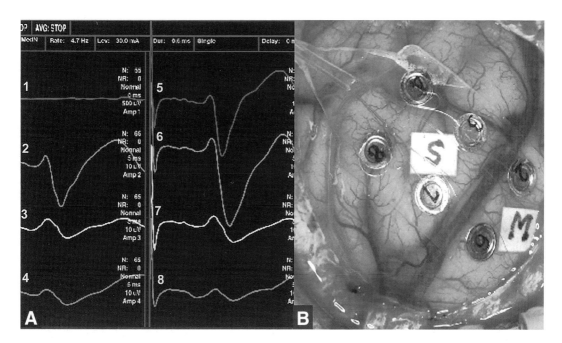

Fig. 4. (A) Cortical mapping. A phase reversal can be appreciated between electrodes 2, 5, and 6 (M, motor) and electrodes 3 and 7 (S, sensory). **(B)** The corresponding intraoperative picture showing the electrode plate and the mapped sensorimotor cortex.

The first two randomized trials that provided a detailed analysis of symptomatic improvement in 1812 patients treated by different radiation dose schedules were conducted by the Radiation Therapy Oncology Group (RTOG). Trials I and II reviewed different radiation fractionation schemes to compare the rate and the duration of response, time to disease progression, survival, and ultimate cause of death *(16)*. The median survival time in Trial I was 18 wk and that in Trial II was 15 wk. Survival time was independent of the radiation fraction size or total dose. In both studies, brain metastases were a cause of death in 40% of patients on average. Because of these patients' limited life expectancy, an improved or stable neurologic function was maintained throughout the patient's life in 75 to 80% of those treated.

However, the local control rate may be inadequate, especially in patients who live longer than a few months. In the randomized study reported by Patchell et al. *(75)*, the median time to local disease progression was only 21 wk for patients treated with WBRT-only compared to 59 wk for surgery plus WBRT. Recurrence at the site of the original metastasis was more frequent in the WBRT group compared with the surgery plus WBRT group. The overall length of survival was significantly shorter in the WBRT group (Table 2), and the patients treated with surgery plus WBRT remained functionally independent longer (median, 38 wk vs 8 wk in the WBRT only group).

Another randomized study by Vecht et al. *(100)* confirmed that patients presenting with single cerebral metastases had prolonged overall survival when treated with surgery followed by WBRT (Table 2). They also maintained a longer functional independent survival (median, 9 mo in the surgery plus WBRT group vs 4 mo in the WBRT-only group, $p = 0.06$).

Postoperative adjuvant WBRT theoretically destroys residual cancer cells at the site of the resection. It is also intended to inactivate tumor emboli at other sites in the brain that may not yet be detected by MR imaging, thereby preventing new tumors from subsequently developing. Many retrospective reviews have demonstrated enhanced local control and survival in select individuals with a

Table 2
Different Series Comparing the Incidence of Intracranial Tumor Progression (%)
and the Median Patient Survival (mo) With Different Modalities of Treatment
for Metastatic Brain Tumors

Reference	N	Type of treatment	Intracranial recurrence (%)	p	Survival (mo)	p
75	23	WBRT	52		15	
	25	Surgery + WBRT	20	0.02	40	0.01
100	31	WBRT	NA		6	
	32	Surgery + WBRT	NA		10	0.04
28	21	Surgery	52		10	
	12	Surgery + RT	50	NS	8	NS
26	19	Surgery	65		14.4	
	79	Surgery + WBRT	45	0.03	20.6	NS
74	46	Surgery	70		43	
	49	Surgery + WBRT	18	<0.01	48	0.39
43	6	Radiosurgery	100		70	
	10	Radiosurgery + WBRT	20	<0.01	72	0.37
10	62	Surgery ± WBRT	33.9		16.4	
	31	Radiosurgery ± WBRT	48.4	0.05	7.5	<0.01
88	66	Surgery + WBRT	31.8		9	
	67	Radiosurgery + WBRT	14.9	0.05	12	0.55
93	62	Radiosurgery	58		11.3	
	43	Radiosurgery + WBRT	37	0.01	11.1	0.80

NS, not significant; NA, not available; WBRT, whole-brain radiation therapy.

solitary brain metastasis receiving WBRT following surgical resection *(26,91,92)* (Table 2). A randomized trial by Patchell et al. showed that adjuvant WBRT after resection for a single metastasis had a local control rate of 90% (compared to 54% in the observation group, $p < 0.001$) as well as a distant control rate of 86% (compared to 63% in the observation group, $p < 0.01$). Patients in the adjuvant WBRT group were less likely to die of neurologic causes than patients in the observation group (14 vs 44%, respectively; $p = 0.003$). However, there was no difference in overall survival between the two groups *(74)* (Table 2).

In contrast, other authors have questioned the value of postoperative WBRT in the treatment of patients with cerebral metastases. The length of survival, as reported by Dosoretz et al. *(28)*, was similar in patients with single cerebral metastases treated with surgery alone compared to those managed by surgery followed by WBRT (Table 2). Wronski et al. *(106)* showed, in a retrospective study of 236 patients with brain metastases from nonsmall cell lung cancer, no statistically significant difference in overall survival between patients treated with surgery alone compared to those treated with surgery followed by WBRT.

Several authors advocate the administration of prophylactic WBRT in the management of patients with small cell lung cancer based on the findings that this practice would reduce the incidence of brain metastases *(22,52,54)*. Others have shown major concerns regarding potential detrimental neurologic sequelae from WBRT in patients surviving for longer than 1 yr *(29,49,83)*. Auperin et al. showed a small but statistically significant survival benefit of 5.4% at 3 yr and a reduction in the incidence of brain metastases by around 25% in patients in complete remission *(6)*. The authors recommended prophylactic WBRT as a standard treatment for patients with small cell lung cancer who are in complete remission following the initial treatment. There was no support for this practice in patients who were not in complete remission.

5.2.2. Complications of WBRT

Patients who have a potential for long-term survival are at risk for complications from WBRT. Acute sequelae of WBRT include mild fatigue, epilation, and mild to moderate skin erythema and hyperpigmentation. Early delayed radiation reactions may develop 3 to 10 wk after treatment and can result in the somnolence syndrome (somnolence, anorexia, and irritability) or transient neurologic deterioration that resolves within 6 wk *(15,63,94)*. Radiation-induced progressive mental disturbances and neurologic abnormalities including dementia, ataxia, and death in the absence of tumor recurrence have all been described *(24,25)*. These late side effects, however, are seldom noted because most patients with brain metastases have a short life expectancy as a result of progressing systemic disease *(101)*. DeAngelis et al. *(25)*, estimated a 19% risk of radiation-induced dementia developing within a median time interval of 14 mo when radiation fraction sizes of 3 Gy or higher were administered as WBRT. In order to minimize the risk of serious late sequelae of WBRT, patients with a life expectancy greater than 6 m who require WBRT should be treated with 1.8 Gy to 2.0 Gy per daily fraction to a total whole-brain dose of 40 Gy to 45 Gy.

At M. D. Anderson Cancer Center, the administration of WBRT as an adjuvant in the treatment of single brain metastases is individualized for each patient. WBRT is usually deferred after resection for a single cerebral metastasis in patients with radiosensitive tumors, those with a postoperative MR imaging scan showing no residual tumor, or primary tumors, such as renal cell carcinoma that are associated with a higher survival potential following surgery. For patients with multiple metastases, treatment with postoperative WBRT remains standard practice *(60,61)*. A retrospective review of 120 patients with single cerebral metastases is currently underway at M. D. Anderson Cancer Center to assess the benefits of WBRT after surgical resection in this group of patients.

5.3. Role of Radiosurgery

5.3.1. Indications for Radiosurgery

The relatively small size of brain metastases, their well-demarcated shape, and their relative lack of invasion into surrounding brain parenchyma make them ideal radiosurgical targets.

Several retrospective nonrandomized studies have provided similar local control rates of brain metastases treated with radiosurgery when compared to surgical series at a reduced cost *(84,95)*, with decreased morbidity and mortality and a shorter hospital stay *(21,43,66,69,75,86)*. A local tumor control rate of 84 to 96% was demonstrated in the literature *(2,3,5,17,41,43,66,90,107)*. Another advantage of this technique is that, unlike surgery, few lesions may be considered inaccessible to radiosurgical treatment as a result of their location in the brain. Yet, radiosurgery is limited to treatment of small lesions, usually not exceeding 3 cm in maximal diameter (10–12 cm^3). The dose of radiation delivered to the surrounding brain increases rapidly, and the risk of complications increases accordingly, as the size of the lesion goes beyond 3.5 cm *(96,107)*. The number of individual metastatic lesions is not in itself a contraindication to radiosurgical treatment unless combined with a low performance score (KPS < 70) and/or the presence of uncontrolled systemic cancer. Another relative contraindication would be posterior fossa metastases associated with cerebrospinal fluid flow obstruction and hydrocephalus *(107)*.

To date, no prospective randomized trial has been performed to compare the results of surgery to those of radiosurgery in the treatment of brain metastasis. Several retrospective series, though, have tried to resolve this issue without much success. Bindal et al. *(10)* followed 31 patients treated by radiosurgery and 62 well-matched patients from a pool of over 500 patients who underwent surgery (Table 2). They noted a shorter median survival time and a poorer local control rate in the radiosurgi-

cal group. The local control rate was 38.7% for the radiosurgery group vs 8.1% for the surgical group
(p = 0.05). The neurological survival in patients treated with radiosurgery was significantly shorter
than those managed with surgery (1-yr freedom from neurologically-caused death, 40% in the radiosurgery group vs 83% in the surgery group, p = 0.05). Schöggl et al. *(88)*, matched 67 patients treated
with radiosurgery to 66 patients managed by surgical resection (Table 2). All patients received WBRT
as adjuvant treatment. Statistical analysis of their data showed no difference in survival between the
two groups; however, the local control rate was significantly better with radiosurgery (95 vs 83% in
the surgery group). This difference was attributed to a lower local control rate for radioresistant
metastases to fractionated WBRT in the surgical group. The median interval time to local control
failure was 3.9 mo in the surgical group compared with 4.9 mo in the radiosurgical group. Currently,
a prospective randomized trial is being conducted at M. D. Anderson Cancer Center to objectively
analyze the results of surgery and radiosurgery in the management of brain metastasis.

The fact that adjuvant WBRT after surgical resection has been proved to prolong survival and
lower the recurrence rate would argue in favor of giving adjuvant WBRT in patients treated with
radiosurgery in place of surgery. Retrospective studies have suggested a benefit of WBRT after radiosurgery for solitary brain metastases *(5,41,43,66)*; no prospective randomized trial, however, has
confirmed these results. Fuller et al. reported an 80% regional intracranial tumor control for patients
receiving WBRT in addition to radiosurgery as compared to 0% regional intracranial control rate for
those treated with radiosurgery alone *(43)* (Table 2). Auchter et al., in addition, showed an overall
local control rate of 86%, with a median survival of 56 wk in a group of patients with single brain
metastases treated with radiosurgery and WBRT who met Patchell's eligibility criteria for surgical
resection *(5)*.

In contrast, many authors consider the benefit achieved from WBRT after a surgical resection does
not hold true in the case of radiosurgery. Sneed et al. *(93)* mentioned that complete tumor coverage is
achieved by the computerized radiosurgery treatment planning, and that the prescribed isodose contour, although steep, may also help to ensure adequate treatment of the tumor or tumor bed. Her series
included 62 patients treated by radiosurgery alone and another 43 managed by radiosurgery and
WBRT (Table 2). Survival time and local control were the same for both the radiosurgery and radiosurgery plus WBRT groups (median survival 11.3 vs 11.1 mo, respectively; p = 0.80; local freedom
from progression by patient 71% vs 79%, respectively; p = 0.30). The intracranial control rate, however, was significantly worse for patients in the radiosurgery group than those with adjuvant WBRT
(1-yr intracranial freedom from progression, 28 vs 69%, respectively; p = 0.008). The authors concluded that the omission of WBRT in the initial management of patients treated with radiosurgery for
up to 4 metastases does not appear to compromise survival. Kihlstrom et al. *(57)* confirmed the
failure of WBRT to have an impact on survival in patients treated with stereotactic radiosurgery. This
lack of survival difference between these two groups is most likely from the fact that most patients
die of systemic complications of cancer once the intracranial disease is stabilized by radiosurgery.

5.3.2. Complications of Radiosurgery

The complication rate of radiosurgery treatment varies among different studies. Acute radiation-
induced toxicity occurs from the first day up to the 90th day after treatment. After this period the
toxicity is called late toxicity *(76,81)*. Acute toxicities are reported to be between 4.7% and 10%,
whereas late toxicities vary between 2.3% and 6% *(17,64,77,90,93)*. Common complications included
nausea and vomiting, transient worsening of neurological symptoms, seizures, tumoral hemorrhage,
deep vein thrombosis, and symptomatic radiation necrosis (Table 3). 11% of patients treated by
Loeffler et al. *(64,77)* complained of nausea and vomiting, whereas 12.1% of those reviewed by
Bindal et al. *(10)* developed deep vein thrombosis within 30 d of treatment. The 30-d mortality of this
procedure varied between 0% and 3.2% *(5,10, 17,90,93)*. Failure of radiosurgery, as denoted by the
need of a surgical intervention after radiosurgical treatment, was reported to be in the range of 1.9 to
9.7% of cases *(10,41,93)*.

Table 3
Mortality and Morbidity After Radiosurgery Treatment for Metastastic Brain Tumors

Reference	N	Mortality (%)	Radiation necrosis (%)	Neurologic deterioration (%)	Seizures (%)	Tumoral hemorrhage (%)
90	237	0	2.5	1.7	1.3	0
41	116	0	0.8	3.4	0	2.5
10	31	3.2	12.9	NA	0	9.7
17	84	0	2.4	5.9	3.6	0
93	105	0.9	5.7	0.9	0	0
43	27	0	11.1	0	0	0

NA, not available.

6. CONCLUSION

Surgery has been recognized by several prospective series as the gold standard in the treatment of single cerebral metastasis. Surgery has also been proven helpful in the management of multiple metastases as well as recurrent metastases. Radiosurgery, more recently, has provided local control rates that are similar to those of surgery, at a reduced cost and with decreased morbidity and mortality, for lesions smaller than 3 cm in maximal diameter. The use of adjuvant WBRT with surgery or radiosurgery is still a controversial issue. Therefore, to better understand the role of these multiple disciplinary approaches in the management of cerebral metastases, additional prospective randomized trials should be conducted.

REFERENCES

1. Akslen L.A., Heuch I., Hartveit F. 1988. Metastatic patterns in autopsy cases of cutaneous melanoma. *Invasion Metastasis* **8**:193–204.
2. Alexander E. 3rd, Moriarty T.M., Davis R.B., Wen P.Y., Fine H.A., Black P.M., et al. 1995. Stereotactic radiosurgery for the definitive, noninvasive treatment of brain metastases. *J. Natl. Cancer Inst.* **87**:34–40.
3. Alexander E. 3rd, Moriarty T.M., Loeffler J.S. 1996. Radiosurgery for metastases. *J. Neurooncol.* **27**:279–285.
4. Amer M.H., Al-Sarraf M., Baker L.H., Vaitkevicius V.K. 1978. Malignant melanoma and central nervous system metastases: incidence, diagnosis, treatment and survival. *Cancer* **42**:660–668.
5. Auchter R.M., Lamond J.P., Alexander E., Buatti J.M., Chappell R., Friedman W.A., et al. 1996. A multiinstitutional outcome and prognostic factor analysis of radiosurgery for resectable single brain metastasis. *Int. J. Radiat. Oncol. Biol. Phys.* **35**:27–35.
6. Auperin A., Arriagada R., Pignon J.P., Le Pechoux C., Gregor A., Stephens R.J., et al. 1999. Prophylactic cranial irradiation for patients with small-cell lung cancer in complete remission. Prophylactic Cranial Irradiation Overview Collaborative Group. *N. Engl. J. Med.* **341**:476–484.
7. Aznavoorian S., Murphy A.N., Stetler-Stevenson W.G., Liotta L.A. 1993. Molecular aspects of tumor cell invasion and metastasis. *Cancer* **71**:1368–1383.
8. Batson O. 1941. The role of the vertebral veins in metastatic processes. *Ann. Int. Med.* **16**:38–45.
9. Berger M.S., Rostomily R.C. 1997. Low grade gliomas: functional mapping resection strategies, extent of resection, and outcome. *J. Neurooncol.* **34**:85–101.
10. Bindal A.K., Bindal R.K., Hess K.R., Shiu A., Hassenbusch S.J., Shi W.M., Sawaya R. 1996. Surgery versus radiosurgery in the treatment of brain metastasis. *J. Neurosurg.* **84**:748–754.
11. Bindal R.K., Bindal A.K., Sawaya R. 1997. Outcome of surgical therapy for metastatic cancer to the brain. *Advances in Surgery* **31**:351–373.
12. Bindal R.K., Sawaya R., Leavens M.E., Hess K.R., Taylor S.H. 1995. Reoperation for recurrent metastatic brain tumors. *J. Neurosurg.* **83**:600–604.
13. Bindal R.K., Sawaya R., Leavens M.E., Lee J.J. 1993. Surgical treatment of multiple brain metastases. *J. Neurosurg.* **79**:210–216.
14. Black P.M., Moriarty T., Alexander E., Stieg P., Woodard E.J., Gleason P.L., et al. 1997. Development and implementation of intraoperative magnetic resonance imaging and its neurosurgical applications. *Neurosurgery* **41**:831–842; discussion 842–845.

15. Boldrey E., Sheline G. 1966. Delayed transitory clinical manifestations after radiation treatment of intracranial tumors. *Acta. Radiol. Ther. Phys. Biol.* **5:**5–10.

16. Borgelt B., Gelber R., Kramer S., Brady L.W., Chang C.H., Davis L.W., et al. 1980. The palliation of brain metastases: final results with the first two studies by the Radiation Therapy Oncology Group. *Int. J. Radiat. Oncol. Biol. Phys.* **6:**1–9.

17. Breneman J.C., Warnick R.E., Albright R.E. Jr., Kukiatinant N., Shaw J., Armin D., Tew J. Jr. 1997. Stereotactic radiosurgery for the treatment of brain metastases. Results of a single institution series. *Cancer* **79:**551–557.

18. Burt M., Wronski M., Arbit E., Galicich J.H. 1992. Resection of brain metastases from non-small-cell lung carcinoma. Results of therapy. Memorial Sloan-Kettering Cancer Center Thoracic Surgical Staff. *J. Thorac. Cardiovasc. Surg.* **103:**399–410; discussion 410–411.

19. Cairncross J.G., Kim J.H., Posner J.B. 1980. Radiation therapy for brain metastases. *Ann. Neurol.* **7:**529–541.

20. Chason J., Walker F., Landers J. 1963. Metastatic carcinoma in the central nervous system and dorsal root ganglia. A prospective autopsy study. *Cancer* **16:**781–787.

21. Coffey R.J., Flickinger J.C., Bissonette D.J., Lunsford L.D. 1991. Radiosurgery for solitary brain metastases using the cobalt-60 gamma unit: methods and results in 24 patients. *Int. J. Radiat. Oncol. Biol. Phys.* **20:**1287–1295.

22. Cox J.D., Stanley K., Petrovich Z., Paig C., Yesner R. 1981. Cranial irradiation in cancer of the lung of all cell types. *Jama* **245:**469–472.

23. Crowley M.J., O'Brien D.F. 1993. Epidemiology of tumours of the central nervous system in Ireland. *Ir. Med. J.* **86:** 87–88.

24. DeAngelis LM. 1994. Management of brain metastases. *Cancer Invest.* **12:**156–165.

25. DeAngelis L.M., Delattre J.Y., Posner J.B. 1989. Radiation-induced dementia in patients cured of brain metastases. *Neurology* **39:**789–796.

26. DeAngelis L.M., Mandell L.R., Thaler H.T., Kimmel D.W., Galicich J.H., Fuks Z., Posner J.B. 1989. The role of postoperative radiotherapy after resection of single brain metastases. *Neurosurgery* **24:**798–805.

27. Delattre J.Y., Krol G., Thaler H.T., Posner J.B. 1988. Distribution of brain metastases. *Arch. Neurol.* **45:**741–744.

28. Dosoretz D.E., Blitzer P.H., Russell A.H., Wang C.C. 1980. Management of solitary metastasis to the brain: the role of elective brain irradiation following complete surgical resection. *Int. J. Radiat. Oncol. Biol. Phys.* **6:**1727–1730.

29. Einhorn L.H., 3rd. 1995. The case against prophylactic cranial irradiation in limited small cell lung cancer. *Semin. Radiat. Oncol.* **5:**57–60.

30. Ewing E. 1928. *Neoplastic Diseases*, 6th ed. W.B. Saunders Co, Philadelphia, PA.

31. Fidler I.J. 2000. Angiogenesis and cancer metastasis. *Cancer J. Sci. Am.* **6(Suppl 2):**S134–S141.

32. Fidler I.J. 1991. Cancer metastasis. *Br. Med. Bull.* **47:**157–177.

33. Fidler I.J. 1990. Critical factors in the biology of human cancer metastasis: twenty-eighth G.H.A. Clowes memorial award lecture. *Cancer Res.* **50:**6130–6138.

34. Fidler I.J. 1990. Host and tumour factors in cancer metastasis. *Eur. J. Clin. Invest.* **20:**481–486.

35. Fidler I.J. 1995. Modulation of the organ microenvironment for treatment of cancer metastasis. *J. Natl. Cancer Inst.* **87:** 1588–1592.

36. Fidler I.J. 1997. Molecular biology of cancer: invasion and metastasis, in *Cancer: Principles and Practice of Oncology* (DeVita V.T, Hellman S., Rosenberg S.A., eds.), Lippincott-Raven, Philadelphia, PA, pp. 135-152.

37. Fidler I.J. 1991. Orthotopic implantation of human colon carcinomas into nude mice provides a valuable model for the biology and therapy of metastasis. *Cancer Metastasis Rev.* **10:**229–243.

38. Fidler I.J., Hart I.R. 1982. Biological diversity in metastatic neoplasms: origins and implications. *Science* **217:**998–1003.

39. Fidler I.J., Kripke M.L. 1977. Metastasis results from preexisting variant cells within a malignant tumor. *Science* **197:** 893–895.

40. Fidler I.J., Talmadge J.E. 1986. Evidence that intravenously derived murine pulmonary melanoma metastases can originate from the expansion of a single tumor cell. *Cancer Res.* **46:**5167–5171.

41. Flickinger J.C., Kondziolka D., Lunsford L.D., Coffey R.J., Goodman M.L., Shaw E.G., et al. 1994. A multi-institutional experience with stereotactic radiosurgery for solitary brain metastasis. *Int. J. Radiat. Oncol. Biol. Phys.* **28:**797–802.

42. Franzini A., Leocata F., Giorgi C., Allegranza A., Servello D., Broggi G. 1994. Role of stereotactic biopsy in multifocal brain lesions: considerations on 100 consecutive cases. *J. Neurol. Neurosurg. Psychiatry* **57:**957–960.

43. Fuller B.G., Kaplan I.D., Adler J., Cox R.S., Bagshaw M.A. 1992. Stereotaxic radiosurgery for brain metastases: the importance of adjuvant whole brain irradiation. *Int. J. Radiat. Oncol. Biol. Phys.* **23:**413–418.

44. Galicich J.H., Sundaresan N., Arbit E., Passe S. 1980. Surgical treatment of single brain metastasis: factors associated with survival. *Cancer* **45:**381–386.

45. Gaspar, L., C. Scott, M. Rotman, S. Asbell, T. Phillips, T. Wasserman, et al. 1997. Recursive partitioning analysis (RPA) of prognostic factors in three Radiation Therapy Oncology Group (RTOG) brain metastases trials. *Int. J. Radiat. Oncol. Biol. Phys.* **37:**745–751.

46. Graf A.H., Buchberger W., Langmayr H., Schmid K.W. 1988. Site preference of metastatic tumours of the brain. *Virchows Arch. A. Pathol. Anat. Histopathol.* **412:**493–498.

47. Grant F. 1926. Concerning intracranial malignant metastases. Their frequency and the value of surgery in their treatment. *Ann. Surg.* **84:**635.

48. Grant R., Whittle I.R., Collie D.A., Gregor A., Ironside J.W. 1996. Referral pattern and management of patients with malignant brain tumours in south east Scotland. *Health Bull. (Edinb)* **54:**212–222.

49. Gregor A., Cull A., Stephens R.J., Kirkpatrick J.A., Yarnold J.R., Girling D.J., et al. 1997. Prophylactic cranial irradiation is indicated following complete response to induction therapy in small cell lung cancer: results of a multicentre randomised trial. United Kingdom Coordinating Committee for Cancer Research (UKCCCR) and the European Organization for Research and Treatment of Cancer (EORTC). *Eur. J. Cancer* **33:**1752–1758.

50. Haar F., Patterson R.H. Jr. 1972. Surgical for metastatic intracranial neoplasm. *Cancer* **30:**1241–1245.

51. Hammoud M.A., Ligon B.L., elSouki R., Shi W.M., Schomer D.F., Sawaya R. 1996. Use of intraoperative ultrasound for localizing tumors and determining the extent of resection: a comparative study with magnetic resonance imaging. *J. Neurosurg.* **84:**737–741.

52. Hansen H.H., Dombernowsky P., Hirsch F.R., Hansen M., Rygard J. 1980. Prophylactic irradiation in bronchogenic small cell anaplastic carcinoma. A comparative trial of localized versus extensive radiotherapy including prophylactic brain irradiation in patients receiving combination chemotherapy. *Cancer* **46:**279–284.

53. Hu F.N., Wang R.Y., Hsu T.C. 1987. Clonal origin of metastasis in B16 murine melanoma: a cytogenetic study. *J. Natl. Cancer Inst.* **78:**155–163.

54. Jackson D.V. Jr., Richards F. 2nd, Cooper M.R., Ferree C., Muss H.B., White D.R., Spurr C.L. 1977. Prophylactic cranial irradiation in small cell carcinoma of the lung. A randomized study. *Jama* **237:**2730–2733.

55. Johnson J.D., Young B. 1996. Demographics of brain metastasis. *Neurosurg. Clin. N. Am.* **7:**337–344.

56. Kehrli P. 1999. Epidemiology of brain metastases. *Neurochirurgie* **45:**357–363.

57. Kihlstrom L., Karlsson B., Lindquist C. 1993. Gamma Knife surgery for cerebral metastases. Implications for survival based on 16 years experience. *Stereotact. Funct. Neurosurg.* **61:**45–50.

58. Kondziolka D., Patel A., Lunsford L.D., Kassam A., Flickinger J.C. 1999. Stereotactic radiosurgery plus whole brain radiotherapy versus radiotherapy alone for patients with multiple brain metastases. *Int. J. Radiat. Oncol. Biol. Phys.* **45:**427–434.

59. Kurtz J.M., Gelber R., Brady L.W., Carella R.J., Cooper J.S.. 1981. The palliation of brain metastases in a favorable patient population: a randomized clinical trial by the Radiation Therapy Oncology Group. *Int. J. Radiat. Oncol. Biol. Phys.* **7:**891–895.

60. Lang F.F., Sawaya R. 1996. Surgical management of cerebral metastases. *Neurosurg. Clin. N. Am.* **7:**459–484.

61. Lang F.F., Sawaya R. 1998. Surgical treatment of metastatic brain tumors. *Semin. Surg. Oncol.* **14:**53–63.

62. Lassouw G.M., Twijnstra S., Schouten L.J., van de Pol M. 1992. The Neuro-Oncology Register. *Neuroepidemiology* **11:**261–266.

63. Littman P., Rosenstock J., Gale G., Krisch R.E., Meadows A., Sather H., et al. 1984. The somnolence syndrome in leukemic children following reduced daily dose fractions of cranial radiation. *Int. J. Radiat. Oncol. Biol. Phys.* **10:**1851–1853.

64. Loeffler J.S., Alexander E. 1993. Radiosurgery for the treatment of intracranial metastases, in *Stereotactic Radiosurgery* (Alexander E., Loeffler J.S., Lunsford L.D., eds.), McGraw-Hill, New York, pp. 197–206.

65. Markesbery W.R., Brooks W.H., Gupta G.D., Young A.B. 1978. Treatment for patients with cerebral metastases. *Arch. Neurol.* **35:**754–756.

66. Mehta M.P., Rozental J.M., Levin A.B., Mackie T.R., Kubsad S.S., Gehring M.A., Kinsella T.J. 1992. Defining the role of radiosurgery in the management of brain metastases. *Int. J. Radiat. Oncol. Biol. Phys.* **24:**619–625.

67. Merchut M.P. 1989. Brain metastases from undiagnosed systemic neoplasms. *Arch. Intern. Med.* **149:**1076–1080.

68. Mintz A.H., Kestle J., Rathbone M.P., Gaspar L., Hugenholtz H., Fisher B., et al. 1996. A randomized trial to assess the efficacy of surgery in addition to radiotherapy in patients with a single cerebral metastasis. *Cancer* **78:**1470–1476.

69. Noordijk E.M., Vecht C.J., Haaxma-Reiche H., Padberg G.W., Voormolen J.H., Hoekstra F.H., et al. 1994. The choice of treatment of single brain metastasis should be based on extracranial tumor activity and age. *Int. J. Radiat. Oncol. Biol. Phys.* **29:**711–717.

70. Oneschuk D., Bruera E. 1998. Palliative management of brain metastases. *Support Care Cancer* **6:**365–372.

71. Order S.E., Hellman S., Von Essen C.F., Kligerman M.M. 1968. Improvement in quality of survival following whole-brain irradiation for brain metastasis. *Radiology* **91:**149–153.

72. Paget S. 1989. The distribution of secondary growths in cancer of the breast. 1889. *Cancer Metastasis Rev.* **8:**98–101.

73. Patchell R. A. 1991. Brain metastases. *Neurol. Clin.* **9:**817–824.

74. Patchell R.A., Tibbs P.A., Regine W.F., Dempsey R.J., Mohiuddin M., Kryscio R.J., et al. 1998. Postoperative radiotherapy in the treatment of single metastases to the brain: a randomized trial. *Jama* **280:**1485–1489.

75. Patchell R.A., Tibbs P.A., Walsh J.W., Dempsey R.J., Maruyama Y., Kryscio R.J., et al. 1990. A randomized trial of surgery in the treatment of single metastases to the brain. *N. Engl. J. Med.* **322:**494–500.

76. Pavy J.J., Denekamp J., Letschert J., Littbrand B., Mornex F., Bernier J., et al. 1995. EORTC Late Effects Working Group. Late effects toxicity scoring: the SOMA scale. *Radiother. Oncol.* **35:**11–15.

77. Petrovich Z., Luxton G., Formenti S., Jozsef G., Zee C.S., Apuzzo M.L. 1996. Stereotactic radiosurgery for primary and metastatic brain tumors. *Cancer Invest* **14:**445–454.

78. Posner J.B. 1977. Management of central nervous system metastases. *Semin. Oncol.* **4:**81–91.

79. Posner J.B., Chernik N.L. 1978. Intracranial metastases from systemic cancer. *Adv. Neurol.* **19:**579–592.

80. Ransohoff J. 1975. Surgical management of metastatic tumors. *Semin. Oncol.* **2:**21–27.
81. Rubin P., Constine L.S. 3rd, Fajardo L.F., Phillips T.L., Wasserman T.H. 1995. EORTC Late Effects Working Group. Overview of late effects normal tissues (LENT) scoring system. *Radiother. Oncol.* **35:**9–10.
82. Ruderman N., Hall T. 1965. Use of glucocorticoids in the palliative treatment of metastatic brain tumors. *Cancer* **18:** 298–306.
83. Russell A.H., Pajak T.E., Selim H.M., Paradelo J.C., Murray K., Bansal P., et al. 1991. Prophylactic cranial irradiation for lung cancer patients at high risk for development of cerebral metastasis: results of a prospective randomized trial conducted by the Radiation Therapy Oncology Group. *Int. J. Radiat. Oncol. Biol. Phys.* **21:**637–643.
84. Rutigliano M.J., Lunsford L.D., Kondziolka D., Strauss M.J., Khanna V., Green M. 1995. The cost effectiveness of stereotactic radiosurgery versus surgical resection in the treatment of solitary metastatic brain tumors. *Neurosurgery* **37:**445–453; discussion 453–455.
85. Salvati M., Cervoni L., Raco A. 1995. Single brain metastases from unknown primary malignancies in CT-era. *J. Neurooncol.* **23:**75–80.
86. Sause W.T., Crowley J.J., Morantz R., Rotman M., Mowry P.A., Bouzaglou A., et al. 1990. Solitary brain metastasis: results of an RTOG/SWOG protocol evaluation surgery + RT versus RT alone. *Am. J. Clin. Oncol.* **13:**427–432.
87. Schaefer P.W., Budzik R.F. Jr., Gonzalez R.G. 1996. Imaging of cerebral metastases. *Neurosurg. Clin. N. Am.* **7:**393–423.
88. Schöggl A., Kitz K., Reddy M., Wolfsberger S., Schneider B., Dieckmann K., Ungersbock K. 2000. Defining the role of stereotactic radiosurgery versus microsurgery in the treatment of single brain metastases. *Acta. Neurochir.* **142:**621–626.
89. Shah S.H., Soomro I.N., Hussainy A.S., Hassan S.H. 1999. Clinico-morphological pattern of intracranial tumors in children. *J. Pak. Med. Assoc.* **49:**63–65.
90. Simonova G., Liscak R., Novotny J. Jr., Novotny J. 2000. Solitary brain metastases treated with the Leksell gamma knife: prognostic factors for patients. *Radiother. Oncol.* **57:**207–213.
91. Skibber J.M., Soong S.J., Austin L., Balch C.M., Sawaya R.E. 1996. Cranial irradiation after surgical excision of brain metastases in melanoma patients. *Ann. Surg. Oncol.* **3:**118–123.
92. Smalley S.R., Schray M.F., Laws E.R., O'Fallon J.R. 1987. Adjuvant radiation therapy after surgical resection of solitary brain metastasis: association with pattern of failure and survival. *Int. J. Radiat. Oncol. Biol. Phys.* **13:**1611–1616.
93. Sneed P.K., Lamborn K.R., Forstner J.M., McDermott M.W., Chang S., Park E., et al. 1999. Radiosurgery for brain metastases: is whole brain radiotherapy necessary? *Int. J. Radiat. Oncol. Biol. Phys.* **43:**549–558.
94. Sneed P.K., Larson D.A., Wara W.M. 1996. Radiotherapy for cerebral metastases. *Neurosurg. Clin. N. Am.* **7:**505–515.
95. Sperduto P.W., Hall W.A. 1996. Radiosurgery, cost-effectiveness, gold standards, the scientific method, cavalier cowboys, and the cost of hope. *Int. J. Radiat. Oncol. Biol. Phys.* **36:**511–513.
96. Sturm V., Kimmig B., Engenhardt R., Schlegel W., Pastyr O., Treuer H., et al. 1991. Radiosurgical treatment of cerebral metastases. Method, indications and results. *Stereotact. Funct. Neurosurg.* **57:**7–10.
97. Sugarbaker E.V. 1979. Cancer Metastasis: a product of tumor-host interactions. *Curr. Prob. Cancer* **3:**1–59.
98. Talmadge J.E., Wolman S.R., Fidler I.J. 1982. Evidence for the clonal origin of spontaneous metastases. *Science* **217:** 361–363.
99. Vecht C.J. 1998. Clinical management of brain metastasis. *J. Neurol.* **245:**127–131.
100. Vecht C.J., Haaxma-Reiche H., Noordijk E.M., Padberg G.W., Voormolen J.H., Hoekstra F.H., et al. 1993. Treatment of single brain metastasis: radiotherapy alone or combined with neurosurgery? *Ann. Neurol.* **33:**583–590.
101. Vermeulen S.S. 1998. Whole brain radiotherapy in the treatment of metastatic brain tumors. *Sem. Surg. Oncol.* **14:**64–69.
102. Vives K.P., Piepmeier J.M. 1999. Complications and expected outcome of glioma surgery. *J. Neurooncol.* **42:**289–302.
103. Voorhies R.M., Sundaresan N., Thaler H.T. 1980. The single supratentorial lesion. An evaluation of preoperative diagnostic tests. *J. Neurosurg.* **53:**364–368.
104. White K.T., Fleming T.R., Laws E.R. 1981. Single metastasis to the brain. Surgical treatment in 122 consecutive patients. *Mayo Clin. Proc.* **56:**424–428.
105. Winston K.R., Walsh J.W., Fischer E.G. 1980. Results of operative treatment of intracranial metastatic tumors. *Cancer* **45:**2639–2645.
106. Wronski M., Arbit E., Burt M., Galicich J.H. 1995. Survival after surgical treatment of brain metastases from lung cancer: a follow-up study of 231 patients treated between 1976 and 1991. *J. Neurosurg.* **83:**605–616.
107. Young R.F. 1998. Radiosurgery for the treatment of brain metastases. *Semin. Surg. Oncol.* **14:**70–78.
108. Zakhary R., Keles G.E., Berger M.S. 1999. Intraoperative imaging techniques in the treatment of brain tumors. *Curr. Opin. Oncol.* **11:**152–156.

17

Immunotherapy of Central Nervous System Tumors

Contemporary Cancer Research

**Amy B. Heimberger, David A. Reardon,
Darell D. Bigner, and John H. Sampson**

1. INTRODUCTION

The overall objective of this chapter is to evaluate significant progress and research advances within the field of immunotherapy and to delineate the challenges associated with the utilization of immunotherapies that are unique to central nervous system (CNS) tumors. Immunotherapy of CNS tumors is complicated by multiple factors, such as, tumor heterogeneity, immunosuppression, and immunologic privilege. The study of immunotherapies requires a thorough knowledge of immunological response within the CNS and its potential consequences, including the induction of autoimmune disorders, is mandatory.

2. GLIOMA BIOLOGY

2.1. Heterogeneity

Gliomas are characterized by diverse karotypes *(8,115)*, at the genetic level, and at the protein antigenic level, a marked heterogeneity. The use of antibodies of various specificities has allowed elucidation of such complex antigenic diversity, both in animal tumor models *(38,84,94)* and in human glial tumors *(2,18,73)*. Even among clones derived from a single established cell line, reactivity with a panel of monoclonal antibodies (MAbs) of varied specificity demonstrated an individualized pattern of antigenicity *(133,134)*. This diversification renders tumor cells differentially susceptible to various therapeutic modalities, which offers one explanation for therapeutic resistance.

2.2. Immunosuppression

Immunosuppression in patients with primary intracranial tumors has been well documented. Although not all patients with glioblastoma have subnormal systemic immune competence, many have been found to have low peripheral lymphocyte counts and reduced delayed hypersensitivity reactions, indicating a degree of anergy that is proportional to the degree of anaplasia of the neoplasm *(75)*. The lymphocyte deficit involves both B-cells with diminished induction of Ig synthesis *(107)* and T-helper (CD4+) subsets with decreased T-helper activity *(39,83,106)*. Diminished lymphocyte activation has been attributed to diminished interleukin (IL)-2 production *(30,31)*. Recent data also suggest that diminished responsiveness of peripheral T-cells is associated with impaired early transmembrane signaling through the T-cell receptor-CD3 complex *(86)*.

Numerous reports of decreased or defective systemic cell-mediated immunity in patients with brain tumors are counterbalanced by the demonstration of a seemingly exuberant, but probably inef-

From: *Contemporary Cancer Research: Brain Tumors*
Edited by: F. Ali-Osman © Humana Press Inc., Totowa, NJ

fective local immune response within the CNS tumors *(37)*. Mononuclear cell infiltrates are common within the parenchyma of human gliomas, and several studies have attempted to correlate the intensity of lymphocytic infiltration with survival *(16,91,128)*. However, the lymphocytes isolated from gliomas are dysfunctional. For example, these lymphocytes do not express IL-2 or interferon (IFN)-γ, but rather IL-4 and granulocyte-macrophage-colony stimulating factor (GM-CSF), which suggests a predominant type 2 (TH-2) intratumoral immune response that does not promote cell-mediated activity *(108)*. These findings suggest an intrinsic defect in the TH-1 cytokine response that results in diminished cell-mediated immunity.

This impairment or alteration of immune activation may be mediated by immunosuppressive cytokines produced by tumor cells in vivo *(83)*. Human malignant glioma cell culture supernatants have been shown to suppress immune responses in vitro *(11,39,61)*, specifically, IL-2 synthesis and IL-2R expression *(29,106)*. Production of IL-10 *(53,55)*, prostaglandin PGE_2 *(3,111)*, and transforming growth factor-β (TGF-β) *(11,26,39,136)* has been implicated. TGF-β has many systemic immunosuppressive properties including the reduction of IL-1, IL-2, and IFN-γ; down-regulation of major histocompatibility complex (MHC) II; and depression of cytotoxicity by natural killer (NK) cells. Furthermore, TGF-β has a suppressive effect on glioma-infiltrating lymphocyte proliferation and cytotoxic activity *(60)*.

Inhibition of immunosuppressive factors, such as TGF-β, may render glioma cells more immunogenic and is a potential immunotherapy. In animal studies, after a highly immunogenic and easily rejected subcutaneous fibrosarcoma cell line was transfected with TGF-β, the cell line completely escaped immune rejection *(120)*. In a reciprocal experiment, rodents bearing intracranial 9L were subcutaneously immunized with 9L cells genetically modified with an antisense plasmid vector to inhibit TGF-β expression, which resulted in 100% survival and increased lytic activity of tumor cells *(36)*. Clinical trials evaluating the efficacy of antisense TGF-β transformed autologous tumor cells are ongoing.

2.3. Immunological Privilege

The brain has been characterized as "immunologically privileged," largely based on evidence of a protective environment provided to allografts and xenografts by the brain. Most of the early studies demonstrated, through attempts to transplant MHC-mismatched tissues into various organs, that the brain was a more permissive host than other organs *(89)*. Data from this paradigm indicated that sensitization to antigens present within the brain was relatively diminished. In animals that had previously been sensitized to foreign tissue, subsequent rechallenge demonstrated that the immune responses were often delayed or incomplete *(81)*. Additionally, a number of vaccination strategies in experimental animals were quite effective against tumors outside the CNS, but completely failed to have impact on tumors grown within the CNS *(59,112)*. In a clinical study, patients successfully treated with biomodulators had tumor relapses within the brain despite remissions extracranially *(85)*. Taken together, the data indicates that the relationship between the brain and the immune system is not the same as that between the immune system and other organs. Possible explanations for the "immunological privilege" of the brain include the absence of conventional lymphatics, the presence of the blood–brain barrier (BBB), and the paucity of antigen-presenting cells within the neural parenchyma.

The absence of lymphatic drainage within the brain was thought to block the afferent limb of the immune response, thus also partially explaining immunological privilege. However, cerebrospinal fluid is drained either into dural sinuses or along the subarachnoid space to the spleen or deep cervical lymph nodes, respectively *(24)*. Following injection of radiolabeled albumin into brain parenchyma, albumin begins to appear in lymph in about 1 h. Maximal concentrations are achieved in 15–20 h and drainage persists for several days *(137)*, indicating that there is in fact lymphatic exposure of antigens from the brain. The "immunological privilege" of the CNS is therefore a relative term.

3. IMMUNOLOGICAL RESPONSES
WITHIN THE CENTRAL NERVOUS SYSTEM

3.1. Antigen Presentation Within the Central Nervous System

The ability of cells within the CNS to initiate an immunological response and present antigens has been the subject of controversy. The presence of MHC is a fundamental requirement for the participation in antigen presentation and the induction of immune responses. MHC class I expression in the normal CNS is concentrated on the endothelial cells, and no definitive class I staining is associated with normal neurons or glial cells *(63,117,121)*. Weak or occasional class I staining is identified on microglia *(1,77,125)*. ependymal cells *(125)*, and stromal cells. Class II MHC molecule expression in the normal CNS is limited to select microglial cells, especially in the white matter *(78,125)*. There is general agreement that neurons and oligodendrocytes do not express class II MHC molecules under normal conditions. Disagreement does occur as to whether endothelial cells and astrocytes express these molecules, especially under pathologic conditions such as multiple sclerosis (MS) and experimental autoimmune encephalomyelitis (EAE) *(52,65,77,121,126)*.

Candidates for intrinsic antigen presentation within the CNS include microglia, macrophages, and dendritic cells (DCs). Microglia, in addition to expressing MHC and co-stimulatory molecules *(80,135)*, have phenotypic and functional characteristics of both macrophages and DCs *(5,71,119,124,135,138)* and are capable of antigen presentation to helper T-cells *(50,124)*.

Initially, DCs were thought to have a minimal role within the CNS. This conclusion was based on immunohistochemical investigations of class II expression in conventional tissue preparations in a variety of species in which only rare isolated cells were reported *(48)*. Recent observations indicate that the choroid plexus does contain an extensive population of MHC class II positive cells with the immunofluorescence and morphological appearance of DCs *(114)*. Additionally, cells consistent with the DCs have been identified in whole mounts of rat dura *(80)*. Responses elicited by placement of inflammatory stimuli into the neural parenchyma are minimal compared with responses elicited similarly in the ventricles or subarachnoid space, and McMenamin and Forrester *(80)* have proposed that this may be due to the paucity of DCs within the parenchyma. The paraventricular, leptomeningeal, and perivascular sites are often involved in the initial stages of autoimmune disorders, which may be a consequence of the extensive antigen-presenting cells present at these sites.

3.2. T-Cell Responses Within the Central Nervous System

Lymphocytes are a rare finding in the CNS of healthy humans or rodents *(44,51)*. During neuro-inflammatory illnesses, such as MS, lymphocytes are abundant within the CNS *(51,93)*. Activated lymphocytes have been shown to infiltrate into the CNS *(49,51)* and can be directed against a tumor target *(110)*. For example, when mice were vaccinated systemically with an irradiated, syngeneic murine melanoma line transfected with cytokines and then challenged intracranially with melanoma there was a significant increase in survival. By performing depletion studies, CD8+ T-cells were shown to be essential for the rejection of intracranial melanoma. Interestingly, CD4+ T-cells seemed to play a limited role in the effector arm of the immune response against tumors within the brain since efficacious responses were seen even after apparent depletion of CD4+ cells *(110)*. This data suggested that the CNS might pose a barrier that preferentially discriminates against certain CD4+ T-cell subsets in the absence of activated CD8+ T-cells. Overall, however, there is solid evidence that at least some subsets of lymphocytes can mediate an immune response within the CNS.

3.3. Humoral Responses Within the Central Nervous System

Humoral responses may also contribute to the immune response within the CNS. Although most studies examine humoral responses within the CNS based on pathological states (32–34), systemic antibodies have been shown to penetrate into gliomas within the CNS. Specifically, MAbs specific to tumor antigens, such as epidermal growth factor receptor (EGFR) or tenascin delivered intravenously, can penetrate into CNS tumors, but only 0.001 to 0.01% of the total injected dose *(113,143,144)*. Nonetheless, in some cases this may be sufficient to bind the majority of the cell surface antigens *(35)*. Recently, antibodies within the CNS have been shown to induce autonomous, complement-mediated, and antibody-dependent cell-mediated cytotoxicity *(109)*.

3.4. Induction of Autoimmunity

Induction of EAE, an autoimmune, inflammatory demyelinating process, is a potential risk when using various forms of immunotherapy. EAE can be induced by immunization with myelin basic protein (MBP), myelin proteolipid protein *(123,130)*, myelin oligodendrocyte glycoprotein *(69)*, glial fibrillary acidic protein, β-crystalloid, and the astroglial calcium-binding protein S-100β *(131)*. Since there is the ability to induce autoimmune encephalitis not only with myelin proteins but also with many of the CNS components, a preparation containing these components, as well as other undiscovered components, has the potential to induce EAE. EAE can be readily induced in nonhuman primates after a single injection of complete Freund's adjuvant and either autologous or heterologous CNS tumor homogenate *(9)*.

Given the ranges of protocols that routinely use vaccination with CNS tissue for the production of lethal EAE in nonhuman primates *(9)* and the documented susceptibility of humans to post-vaccination encephalitis, the induction of such autoimmune responses is of particular concern. Because of previous immunotherapy trials of humans with brain tumors in which there were two possible cases of EAE *(10,122)*, a potential autoimmune response remains a consideration—although in most studies involving active immunization with human glioma tissue there were no cases of EAE *(74)*. In the scenario of an immunotherapy with the potential to induce EAE, several strategies have been reported to inhibit EAE development; however, it is this concern for induction of fatal autoimmunity that has directed tumor-specific approaches.

4. CELLULAR VACCINES

4.1. Nonspecific

Since the 1960s, immunotherapy of patients with brain tumors has been ongoing and has included systemic vaccination of patient's glioma cell lines and gliomas both with and without adjuvants. Starting in the 1970s, localized therapy was introduced and delivered via intratumoral injection. These first studies were based on the in vitro observation of lymphocyte cytotoxicity to glioblastoma cells. In glioma patients receiving autologous leukocytes delivered into the tumor, 50% of the patients (9/18) had a clinical improvement; however, overall mean survival was only 64 wk *(139)*. This is in comparison to the median survival for patients with newly diagnosed glioblastoma multiforme (GBM), which is between 40 and 72 wk.

To increase the potency of the immune cells, lymphokine-activated killer (LAK) cells were activated in vitro with cytokines, such as IL-2. However, treatment in mice with metastatic CNS sarcoma with LAK cells, plus IL-2 administered systemically was not effective against intracranial disease. These cells were functional in vitro and significantly reduced the number of pulmonary metastases in vivo, which indicated that the LAK cells were a viable treatment systemically *(79)*. The differences in these results may be secondary to the differential trafficking of LAK cells, the inability to bypass the BBB, or the inability to fully activate the immune system.

To bypass the potential problem of delivery of LAK cells into the brain from the systemic circulation, patients with malignant gliomas were treated with intracavitary LAK cells, but this resulted in only a modest increase in the disease-free interval *(82)* or partial tumor responses radiographically *(56)*. However, when patients were treated with intracavitary LAK cells plus a bispecific antibody (an anti-CD3 antibody conjugated to an antiglioma antibody—NE150), 4/10 showed regression of tumor, and in another 4/10 patients, computed tomography or histology suggested eradication of the glioma cells left behind after surgery. This was in contrast to the group of patients who received LAK cells alone whose survival rate was similar to that of patients receiving conventional treatment *(90)*.

Alternative sources of T-cells that have been sensitized to tumor-specific antigens are tumor-draining lymph nodes. In treatment experiments, mice with intracranial gliomas were treated systemically with cells harvested from draining lymph nodes and activated with anti-CD3 and IL-2, which resulted in a significant increase in median survival *(96)*. However, in a human clinical trial, only 2/6 GBM patients treated systemically with T-cells obtained from systemic draining lymph nodes showed a partial radiographic response *(95)*.

Another source of lymphocytes that have been "exposed" to tumor antigens is the harvesting of T-cells directly from the tumor, and these are referred to as tumor-infiltrating lymphocytes (TILs). In a study of patients with malignant gliomas, TILs were isolated and expanded in vitro with IL-2. The patients were then treated by injecting the TILs directly into the surgical bed. Cell phenotyping demonstrated that 95% of these cells were T-cells, with 66% demonstrating the CD8 phenotype (cytotoxic) and 33% expressing the CD4 phenotype (helper). No significant toxicity was observed; however, all patients developed transient and asymptomatic cerebral swelling, noted on the immediate post-treatment imaging studies. Conclusions regarding efficacy could not be made secondary to the limited numbers of patients enrolled within the trial *(97)*. The wider application of treating patients with TILs is limited by the difficulty in obtaining sufficient tumor samples to derive the TILs in vitro.

More recently, immunotherapy has been directed to activating the immune system with DCs, which are specialized antigen-presenting cells that play a pivotal role in the induction of T- and B-cell immunity. These cells have the exceptional ability to activate naive CD4+ and CD8+T-cells in vitro and in vivo. Furthermore, these cells seem to be sufficiently "potent" to activate the immune system systemically with efficacy against intracranial tumors. This was first demonstrated by treating mice with intracranial melanoma systemically with DCs pulsed with either melanoma extract or melanoma RNA. Vaccination resulted in the induction of specific cytotoxic T-cells as well as a >280% increase in median survival *(4)*. These studies were extended by our group in a syngeneic murine glioma model created to closely recapitulate astrocytomas in human gliomas in which DCs were pulsed with tumor homogenate derived from the astrocytoma. Not only was there a significant increase in median survival in animals but immunological memory was also demonstrated. In vitro studies confirmed that both humoral and cell-mediated immunity was induced without the induction of autoimmunity *(47)*. Acid-eluted peptides derived from autologous tumors yielded similar results in a gliosarcoma treatment tumor model *(68)*.

Recently, DC immunotherapy has been evaluated in a phase I clinical trial in patients with malignant gliomas. These patients received biweekly intradermal injections of peripheral-blood-derived DCs pulsed with acid-eluted peptides from the surface of autologous glioma cells. After vaccination, 4/7 patients developed systemic cytotoxicity directed toward autologous glioma cells, and both cytotoxic and memory T-cells infiltrated the tumors of patients who underwent reoperation after vaccination *(140)*. Although toxicity was minimal and included only mild fever and lymphadenopathy, the use of nonantigen-specific approaches is worrisome for the possible induction of potentially fatal autoimmunity *(9)*. In the case of acid-eluted tumor antigens, contaminating antigens such as MBP could induce autoimmunity.

4.2. Specific

Recently, DC immunotherapy has been shown to be capable of initiating significant autoimmunity *(28,40,72)*. Although autoimmunity could be a desirable outcome for nonessential tissues, such as the prostate, when infiltrated with tumor, autoimmune encephalomyelitis would be a lethal consequence of using this approach against primary brain tumors. Targeting the DCs to a tumor-specific antigen such as the EGFR variant III (EGFRvIII), which is found on a high percentage of malignant primary tumors of the brain, could eliminate the risk of inducing autoimmunity. The mutation is characterized by a consistent in-frame deletion of 801 base pairs from the extracellular domain that splits a codon and produces a novel glycine amino acid at the fusion junction (Fig. 1). This fusion junction encodes a tumor-specific protein sequence expressed on the surface of tumor cells that is not

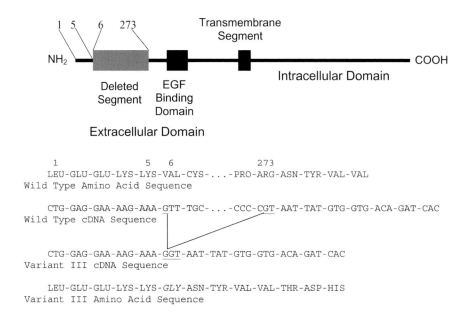

Fig. 1. Amino acid and cDNA sequence of the wild type and mutation epidermal growth factor receptor. An 801-base-pair *EGFR* gene deletion (upper) results in the fusion of normally distant *EGFR* gene and protein sequences (lower). A glycine amino acid is inserted at the fusion point as a result of the in-frame mutation that splits a codon.

present in normal tissues, making it an ideal target for anti-tumor immunotherapy. Additionally, because this molecule confers enhanced tumorigenicity, and is clonally expressed in the more malignant tumors, targeting it would direct therapy to a large proportion of the most malignant cells.

Systemic vaccination with DCs mixed with a peptide designated PEP-3, specific only to the mutated splice site of EGFRvIII, generated antigen-specific immunity. In mice challenged with intracerebral tumors, this resulted in a > 600% increase in median survival, which compared favorably with the survival of mice vaccinated with an equivalent amount of PEP-3 alone or saline (Fig. 2). Sixty-three percent of mice treated with DCs mixed with the tumor-specific peptide survived long-term, and 100% survived rechallenge with tumor, which indicated that anti-tumor immunological memory was also induced *(46)*. Whether this approach will result in significant immunological or clinical responses is currently being investigated in a phase I/II clinical trial at Duke University Medical Center and M.D. Anderson Cancer Center.

Although tumor specificity has obvious advantages, significant potential problems are recognizable with an agent that selectively targets a single tumor-specific mutation: the intrinsic heterogeneity of cells that constitute malignant tumors, the propensity for the development of antigen-loss variants within malignant tumors, and the limited number of sites available for immune recognition within such mutations. Although EGFRvIII seems to represent a nearly terminal branch of malignant progression for brain tumors, neoplastic cells not expressing this epitope may have a selective growth advantage under the conditions of therapy with such a vaccination protocol. This traditional limitation of a narrowly specific immunotherapeutic agent may be overcome by identifying other tumor-specific antigens that could be utilized with the DCs as adjuvant or in combination with other therapeutic approaches. Although the identification of tumor antigens in the past has been difficult for many types of cancer, the data generated by techniques such as serial analysis of gene expression (SAGE) from the Cancer Genome Anatomy project has already revealed many new potential targets within public gene expression databases *(62)*.

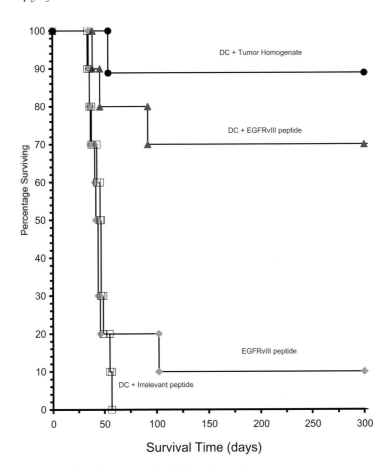

Fig. 2. Vaccination with DCs mixed with EGFRvIII peptide protects against intracerebral challenge with K1735EGFRvIII melanoma cells in C3H mice. C3H mice received three i.p. vaccinations, spaced 1 wk apart of phosphate-buffered serum (PBS, negative control), DCs mixed with an irrelevant 13-mer peptide (negative control), EGFRvIII 13-mer peptide spanning the splice junction alone, DCs mixed with the EGFRvIII 13-mer peptide, or DCs mixed with K1735EGFRvIII tumor homogenate. C3H mice were subsequently challenged intracerebrally one week later with the lethal dose of 2×10^3 viable K1735EGFRvIII cells. Median days of survival, number of mice, and significance compared with data for PBS-immunized mice based on log-rank analysis for each group are as follows: open square, DCs mixed with irrelevant peptide: 47, n = 10, $p > 0.05$; closed diamond, EGFRvIII peptide: 43, n = 9, $p > 0.05$; closed triangle, DCs mixed with PEP-3-keyhole limpet hemocyanin: >300, n = 8, $p < 0.001$; closed circle, DCs mixed with tumor homogenate: >300, n = 9, $p < 0.001$. A > 552% increase in median survival compared with that for PBS controls was observed for mice vaccinated with either DCs mixed with tumor homogenate or with DCs mixed with EGFRvIII peptide.

5. ANTIBODY-MEDIATED IMMUNOTHERAPY

5.1. Conjugated Antibodies

Although localization of polyvalent antibodies to human gliomas was demonstrated in the 1960s, the promise of passive immunotherapy for CNS neoplasms was not recognized until the identification of tumor-associated or tumor-specific antigens, production of homogenous, high-affinity MAbs to such antigens, and the use of compartmental administration (intracavitary, intratumoral, or intrathecal). MAbs can be deployed as biological response modifiers to induce apoptosis or mediate immune responses, or as a delivery system for chemotherapeutic agents, toxins, or radionucleotides.

The most widely exploited treatment modality in clinical trials has been the use of MAbs conjugated to radionucleotides. An early example of such an approach involved the administration of ^{125}I-labeled 425, a MAb directed against wild-type EGFR, to 25 patients with newly diagnosed GBM or anaplastic astrocytoma. In this phase II trial, patients received 40–224 mCi of ^{125}I-labeled 425 via either intravenous or intra-arterial infusion following surgical resection and radiation therapy. The median survival achieved was 62 wk, with no significant associated toxicity (15).

Subsequent clinical trials have utilized a compartmental approach to optimize delivered dose. One of the first adaptations of compartmental delivery was the intrathecal administration of radiolabeled MAbs for patients with neoplastic meningitis. Neoplastic meningitis, a devastating late-stage complication affecting 3–8% of all cancer patients, has a median survival of only 8–24 wk with conventional chemotherapy and/or radiotherapy (43). Administration of the ^{131}I-labeled F(ab')$_2$ fragment of Me1-14, a murine IgG$_{2a}$ developed to react with a proteoglycan chondroitin sulfate expressed by many types of cancer cells including melanoma and gliomas (19), induced encouraging responses among 11 patients with neoplastic meningitis (7). Three patients had complete CSF responses (two consecutive negative CSF cytology results after an initial positive cytology), two others had partial radiographic response, and the other six patients remained alive for six months or longer including one patient who achieved an apparent cure (20). The intrathecal administration of radiolabeled MAbs has been used in a similar fashion to improve the outcome of patients who have been diagnosed with a wide variety of other types of neoplastic meningitis including malignant glioma, ependymoma, pineoblastoma, lymphoma, medulloblastoma, and ovarian, bladder, breast and lung carcinoma (17,87).

The compartmental approach has also been successfully exploited in the treatment of patients who have intracerebral malignant gliomas. Tenascin, an extracellular matrix hexabrachion glycoprotein, is expressed ubiquitously in malignant gliomas and in breast, lung, and squamous cell carcinomas, but not in normal brain. MAb 81C6 is a murine IgG$_{2b}$ that binds to an epitope within the alternatively spliced fibronectin Type III region of tenascin (12,14). This tenascin isoform is abundantly expressed in gliomas (127,144). Preclinical studies have confirmed the specificity of 81C6 for tenascin-expressing tumors in cell culture and xenograft model systems. Bourdon et al. (13) first demonstrated preferential localization of radioiodinated anti-tenascin 81C6 MAb in subcutaneous and intracranial human xenografts in athymic mice and rats using paired-label analysis. Additional preclinical studies with ^{131}I-labeled 81C6 demonstrated significant tumor growth delay and regression in athymic mice bearing subcutaneous D-54/MG human glioma xenografts and prolongation of median survival for athymic rats bearing intracranial tumors (22,66,67). These promising results in preclinical animal studies led to a paired-label study in humans with recurrent malignant glioma. In this study, biopsy specimens obtained after intravenous injection of ^{123}I-labeled 81C6 demonstrated tumor-to-normal brain ratios up to 25:1, and single photon emission computed tomography (SPECT) localization indices showed an up to five-fold higher tumor accumulation of 81C6 compared with control IgG$_{2b}$ murine immunoglobulin (113).

We have performed a series of phase I clinical trials to establish the maximum tolerated dose (MTD) of ^{131}I-labeled murine 81C6 (mu81C6) MAb injected directly into a patient's surgically created resection cavity (SCRC). The MTD for three subgroups of patients with CNS tumors was established by these studies: (a) 80 mCi for adult patients with leptomeningeal neoplasms or brain tumor resection cavities that communicate with the subarachnoid space (7), (b) 100 mCi for patients with recurrent malignant gliomas who received prior radiation therapy with or without chemotherapy (6), and (c) 120 mCi for newly diagnosed and previously untreated adult patients with malignant gliomas (21). In the latter group, delayed neurological toxicity was dose-limiting, and the median survival for all patients and those with GBM was 79 and 69 wk, respectively.

In a recently completed phase II clinical trial, 33 patients with newly diagnosed and previously untreated malignant glioma, including 27 with GBM, received 120 mCi of ^{131}I-labeled mu81C6 directly into the SCRC, followed by conventional external beam radiotherapy and a year of alkylator-based chemotherapy. Median survival for all patients and those with GBM treated on this study was

86.7 and 79.4 wk, respectively (Fig. 3). Of note, only one patient (3%) required reoperation for radionecrosis. Figure 4 depicts serial MRI and *F*-fluoro-deoxy-ᴅ-glucose positron emission tomography ([18]FDG PET) images of a representative patient treated on this study *(98)*. The median survival achieved with ^{131}I-labeled 81C6 in this study significantly surpassed that of historical controls treated with conventional radiotherapy and chemotherapy, even after accounting for established prognostic factors including age and Karnofsky performance status *(25)*. In addition, the median survival associated with ^{131}I-labeled 81C6 exceeded that achieved with the administration of interstitial chemotherapy using carmustine-loaded polymers placed in the surgical resection cavity *(132)*. Finally, the rate of re-operation for radionecrosis associated with the administration of ^{131}I-labeled 81C6 was substantially lower than that observed with other methods aimed at delivering a local radiotherapeutic boost to the tumor bed including ^{125}I-interstitial brachytherapy and stereotactic radiosurgery *(70,76,116)*. Other investigators have confirmed that the compartmental administration of radiolabeled MAbs directed against tumor-associated antigens improves survival for patients with malignant glioma. Riva et al. demonstrated that the injection of ^{131}I-labeled antitenascin MAbs BC-2 and BC-4 significantly improved outcome for patients with newly diagnosed and recurrent malignant glioma without significant toxicity *(102–104)*. Similarly encouraging responses among patients with malignant gliomas have been observed using a MAb directed against eryrthropoietin-induced c-DNA-1 (ERIC-1) radiolabeled with either ^{131}I or ^{90}Y and administered to the primary tumor site *(54,92)*.

Two major ongoing efforts are directed at further improving the outcome associated with the compartmental administration of radiolabeled 81C6 for patients with malignant glioma. In the first of these efforts, genomic cloning has been used to generate a chimeric MAb consisting of the variable-region genes of murine 81C6 and the human constant-region domains of human IgG_2 (ch81C6). The reactivity pattern of ch81C6 with recombinant tenascin fragments and the affinity constant for binding of radioiodinated ch81C6 were virtually identical to those for mu81C6 *(45)*. In addition, preclinical studies have demonstrated a superior uptake of ^{131}I-ch81C6 compared to mu81C6 in human glioma xenografts which is most likely related to an increased stability of ch81C6 *(141)*. Phase I clinical trials have established the MTD of ^{131}I-labeled ch81C6 to be 80 mCi when administered into the SCRC of patients with newly diagnosed malignant glioma. Dose-limiting toxicity (DLT) was hematologic and most likely reflects the enhanced stability of ch81C6 in the systemic circulation relative to mu81C6. To date, 57 patients with newly diagnosed malignant glioma have received ^{131}I-ch81C6 in an ongoing combined phase I/II study. No episodes of DLT have been encountered among 30 patients treated at the MTD, and the median survival for the 44 patients with newly diagnosed GBM treated on this study is a highly encouraging 89 wk, while that for the entire treated cohort has yet to be established *(99)*.

The second ongoing effort to further improve the efficacy of compartmental 81C6 administration for patients with malignant glioma is the use of alternative radioisotopes. Astatine 211 is an alpha-particle emitting radioisotope produced at the Duke University Medical Center cyclotron by using a novel internal target system via the ^{209}Bi(alpha,2n)^{211}At nuclear reaction *(64)*. We have developed a method for labeling MAbs and antibody fragments with [211]At using the acylation agent *N*-succinimidyl 3-[[211]At]astatobenzoate (SAB) *(101)*. Monoclonal antibodies labeled with alpha particle-emitting radionuclides may be valuable for the treatment of CNS malignancies for several reasons. The range of [211]At alpha particles in tissue is only 55–70 μm, so their toxic effects are confined to a region equivalent to only a few cell diameters. Their high energy and short range combine to generate radiation of high linear energy transfer (LET). The mean LET of [211]At alpha particles is 97 keV/μm, about 500 times higher than the LET for the beta particles of [131]I. The LET of [211]At alpha-emissions is nearly ideal for maximizing biological effectiveness because the distance between ionizing events approximates that between DNA strands. Thus, the probability of double DNA strand breaks is high. These lesions are generally nonrepairable, enhancing cytotoxicity. In addition, since their effectiveness is nearly independent of dose rate, oxygen presence, and cell-cycle position, high LET radiation is particularly attractive for applications such as radioimmunotherapy

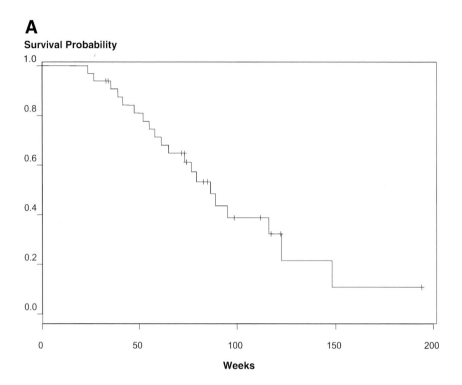

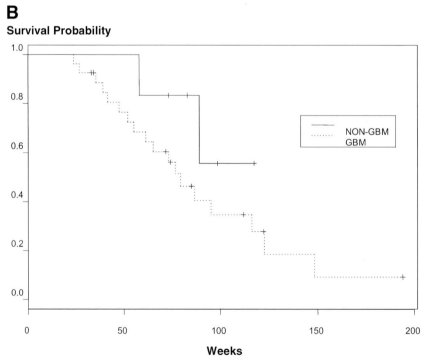

Fig. 3. Kaplan-Meier overall survival estimates for patients with newly diagnosed malignant glioma treated on a phase II study with 120 mCi of ^{131}I-labeled 81C6. (**A**) Median survival for all patients (A) was 86.7 wk and for those with GBM was 79.4 wk (**B**). (Reprinted with permission from ref. *98.*)

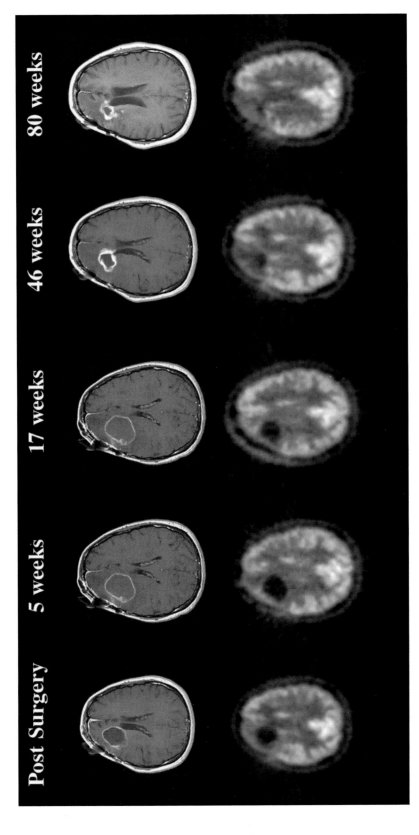

Fig. 4. Serial MRI and [18]FDG PET scan results of a representative patient following injection of 120 mCi of ^{131}I-labeled 81C6 into the surgically created resection cavity. The cavity gradually collapses over time as the rim develops more prominent enhancement with limited metabolic activity. (Reprinted with permission from ref. 98.)

Post Surgery 5 weeks 17 weeks 46 weeks 80 weeks

(142). Dosimetry calculations suggest that it might be possible to treat cystic brain tumors with cyst fluid activity concentrations less than 1/10 of those required with beta-emitting radionuclides such as ^{131}I and ^{90}Y *(105).* To date, 17 patients with recurrent malignant glioma have been treated on a phase I study with ^{211}At-labeled ch81C6. Accrual is ongoing at the 6.7-mCi dose level, and median survival for patients with recurrent GBM is an encouraging 53 wk and includes two patients who remained alive for 152 and 153 wk after ^{211}At-labeled ch81C6 administration *(100).*

In conclusion, studies to date confirm that the local administration of monoclonal antibodies against tumor-specific antigens conjugated to radioisotopes is feasible, well-tolerated and associated with a significantly improved survival for patients with malignant gliomas.

5.2. Unconjugated Antibodies

Naked antibodies may have direct effects without conjugation to immunotoxins or radioactive isotopes. In glioma cell lines that are dependent on autocrine growth factors, inhibition of the receptor with a neutralizing MAb may lead to apoptosis. Treatment of human glioma cell lines with a MAb to fibroblast growth factor inhibited in vitro and in vivo tumor growth secondary to DNA fragmentation and presumably deprivation of the autocrine dependent growth factor *(88).* In a phase I/II trial, a MAb directed against EGFR was administered intravenously at the time of malignant glioma recurrence to 16 patients that had failed surgery, radiotherapy and chemotherapy. Infusion of the antibody was well tolerated, but no therapeutic benefit was demonstrated in the patients, whose median survival was 39 wk *(118);* however, it should be noted that tumor debulking was not performed prior to initiation of therapy. Alternatively, insufficient amounts of the antibody may have reached or penetrated the tumor at the administered dose. A way to ensure adequate delivery of MAbs is by the local administration directly into the tumor. For example, when the MAb Herceptin (Genentech, Inc., San Francisco, CA) is delivered directly into intracranial breast carcinoma expressing HER-2/neu in athymic mice, there is a 57% increase in median survival compared with survival in a saline-treated group *(42).*

Antibodies also mediate immune responses directly within the CNS. Y10, an IgG$_{2a}$ antibody that recognizes the EGFRvIII mutation, was found *in vitro* to inhibit DNA synthesis and cellular proliferation and to induce autonomous, complement-mediated, and antibody-dependent cell-mediated cytotoxicity *(109).* Systemic treatment with Y10 of subcutaneous B16 melanomas that were transfected to maintain stabile expression of the murine EGFRvIII led to long-term survival in all mice. Similar therapy with systemic Y10 failed to increase median survival of mice with EGFRvIII-expressing B16 melanomas in the brain; however, treatment with a single intracerebral injection of Y10 increased median survival by an average 286%, with 26% long-term survivors. The mechanism of action of Y10 in vivo was shown to be independent of complement, granulocytes, NK cells, and T-cells through in vivo complement and cell subset depletions. Treatment with Y10 in Fc receptor knockout mice demonstrated the mechanism of Y10 to be Fc receptor-dependent (Fig. 5). This data indicates that an unarmed, tumor-specific MAb may be an effective immunotherapy against intracerebral tumors delivered locally.

6. CYTOKINE THERAPY

6.1. Local Therapy

A variety of cytokines have been used to modulate the immune system or for their direct effects on tumor cell proliferation or invasion. The development of recombinant human IL-2 generated the initial interest in cytokine immunotherapy. Presumably, IL-2 does not have a direct toxic effect on cancer cells but is required for the growth of CD8+ cells and stimulates these cells to engage in cytotoxic activity, and it enhances the activity of NK cells. The use of IL-2 as an immunotherapy initially held promise for patients with malignant gliomas, who have decreased IL-2 production and down-regulated IL-2R expression. Many of the first attempts to modulate the immune system by

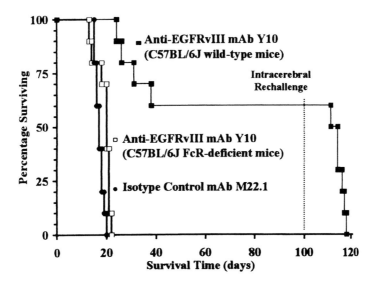

Fig. 5. Survival of C57BL6/J mice with intracerebral B16EGFRvIII tumors treated with anti-EGFRvIII monoclonal antibody (MAb) Y10. B16 EGFRvIII cells are B16 murine melanoma cells stably transfected to express a murine homologue of the human tumor-specific EGFR mutation EGFRvIII. Y10 is a murine IgG_{2a} MAb that specifically recognizes EGFRvIII. M22.1 is an isotype-matched control murine MAb. Mice were challenged with 500 B16EGFRvIII cells intracerebrally and treated 24 h later with a single bolus of 10 μg of MAb injected directly into the tumor. In wild-type mice, intratumoral injection of Y10 significantly increased median survival by >488% relative to treatment with M22.1, and 60% of mice treated with Y10 survived for >90 days without evidence of tumor ($p < 0.001$). Mice that were rechallenged with intracerebral tumor at this point all succumbed to tumor. In mice with deletions of both FcRγ and FcγRII genes, treatment with Y10 failed to increase median survival ($p > 0.4$). (Reprinted with permission from ref. *109*.)

employing cytokines were with local intralesional administration in which the cytokine was delivered with nonspecific activators of the immune system such as *Corynebacterium parvum (23)* or with activated killer cells *(57)*. Many of the initial local immunotherapy cytokine clinical trials failed to demonstrate efficacy, however.

Secondary to its potent immune stimulatory effects such as the induction of γ-IFN and enhancement of cytolytic function of T-cells, IL-12 has also been delivered locally with modest efficacy. After systemic delivery to rats of IL-12 with irradiated 9L gliosarcoma cells, the rats rejected challenge with both flank and intracerebral tumors *(58)*. To provide a constant supply of IL-12, the 9L gliosarcoma cell line was genetically engineered to express IL-12. Rats challenged intracranially with malignant glioma after local delivery of IL-12 had a 70% increase in median survival times *(27)*.

6.2. Transduced Cells

Comprehensive evaluations of the efficacy of subcutaneous vaccines consisting of transfected melanoma cells producing cytokines such as IL-1α, IL-2, IL-3, IL-4, IL-6, IL-12 γ-IFN, TNF-α, granulocyte colony-stimulating factor, leukemia inhibitory factor, macrophage migration inhibitory factor, or GM-CSF could in some cases increase the median survival of mice. In one study, cells producing IL-3, IL-6 or GM-CSF increased the survival of mice challenged with viable B16 cells in the brain. Vaccination with B16 cells producing IL-4 or γ-IFN had no effect, and vaccination with B16 cells producing IL-2 decreased survival time. GM-CSF-producing vaccines increased survival in mice with pre-established tumors *(110)*. Similar results were obtained in another study but the combination of GM-CSF and IL-4 or TNF-α induced the most potent antitumor activity *(129)*.

The application of cytokine secreting tumor cells in human clinical trials, however, has been limited by the constraints of the in vitro protocols. Viable tumor cells are not readily available for all patients and the transfection of these cells is heterogenous. A potential way to overcome this limitation is by genetically engineering allogeneic fibroblasts to secrete these cytokines *(41)*.

7. CONCLUSION

Although the conventional teaching has been that tumors within the CNS are "immunologically privileged," this statement must be qualified by evidence that systemically induced immune responses are quite capable of eradicating tumors within this compartment – at least in animal models. A risk of utilizing nonspecific immunotherapies is the induction of autoimmune disease. Antigen-specific vaccines may circumvent this potential risk; however, they may prove to be less efficacious secondary to antigen-negative escape variants. Currently, immunotherapeutic modalities for the treatment of CNS tumors are derivative of systemic immunotherapy protocols. An interesting future direction of study that has not yet been exploited, in part because of the difficulties of isolation and characterization of these cells, is the intrinsic activation of localized immune cells within the CNS. Whether these cells are capable of initiating an immune response is unclear, but further areas of investigation include evaluating the potency of these cells in initiating an immune response, as well as the type of immune responses that can be intrinsically generated.

ACKNOWLEDGMENTS

Supported by NIH Grants NS20023 and CA11898 and by NIH Grant MO1 RR 30, GCRC Program, NCRR.

REFERENCES

1. Akiyama H., Itagaki S., McGeer P.L. 1988. Major histocompatibility complex antigen expression on rat microglia following epidural kainic acid lesions. *J. Neurosci. Res.* **20:**147–157.
2. Albino A.P., Lloyd K.O., Houghton A.N., Oettgen H.F., Old L.J. 1981. Heterogeneity in surface antigen and glycoprotein expression of cell lines derived from different melanoma metastases of the same patient. Implications for the study of tumor antigens. *J. Exp. Med.* **154:**1764–1778.
3. Alleva D.G., Burger C.J., Elgert K.D. 1994. Tumor-induced regulation of suppressor macrophage nitric oxide and TNF-α production. Role of tumor-derived IL-10, TGF-β, and prostaglandin E$_2$. *J. Immunol.* **153:**1674–1686.
4. Ashley D.M., Faiola B., Nair S., Hale L.P., Bigner D.D., Gilboa E. 1997. Bone marrow-generated dendritic cells pulsed with tumor extracts or tumor RNA induce antitumor immunity against central nervous system tumors. *J. Exp. Med.* **186:**1177–1182.
5. Banati R.B., Graeber M.B. 1994. Surveillance, intervention and cytotoxicity: Is there a protective role of microglia? *Dev. Neurosci.* **16:**114–127.
6. Bigner D.D., Brown M.T., Friedman A.H., Coleman R.E., Akabani G., Friedman H.S., et al. 1998. Iodine-131-labeled antitenascin monoclonal antibody 81C6 treatment of patients with recurrent malignant gliomas: phase I trial results. *J. Clin. Oncol.* **16:**2202–2212.
7. Bigner D.D., Brown M., Coleman R.E., Friedman A.H., Friedman H.S., McLendon R.E, et al. 1995. Phase I studies of treatment of malignant gliomas and neoplastic meningitis with ^{131}I-radiolabeled monoclonal antibodies anti-tenascin 81C6 and anti-chondroitin proteoglycan sulfate Me1-14 F(ab')$_2$ – a preliminary report. *J. Neurooncol.* **24:**109–122.
8. Bigner D.D., Bigner S.H., Ponten J., Westermark B., Mahaley M.S., Ruoslahti E., et al. 1981. Heterogeneity of genotypic and phenotypic characteristics of fifteen permanent cell lines derived from human gliomas. *J. Neuropathol. Exp. Neurol.* **40:**201–229.
9. Bigner D.D., Pitts O.M., Wikstrand C.J. 1981. Induction of lethal experimental allergic encephalomyelitis in nonhuman primates and guinea pigs with human glioblastoma multiforme tissue. *J. Neurosurg.* **55:**32–42.
10. Bloom H.J.G., Peckham M.J., Richardson A.E., Alexander P.A., Payne P.M. 1973. Glioblastoma multiforme: a controlled trial to assess the value of specific active immunotherapy in patients treated by radical surgery and radiotherapy. *Br. J. Cancer* **27:**253–267.
11. Bodmer S., Strommer K., Frei K., Siepl C., de Tribolet N., Heid I., Fontana A. 1989. Immunosuppression and transforming growth factor-β in glioblastoma. Preferential production of transforming growth factor-β2. *J. Immunol.* **143:** 3222–3229.

12. Bourdon M.A., Matthews T.J., Pizzo S.V., Bigner D.D. 1985. Immunochemical and biochemical characterization of a glioma-associated extracellular matrix glycoprotein. *J. Cell Biochem.* **28:**183–95.

13. Bourdon M.A., Coleman R.E., Blasberg R.G., Groothuis D.R., Bigner D.D. 1984. Monoclonal antibody localization in subcutaneous and intracranial human glioma xenografts: paired-label and imaging analysis. *Anticancer Res.* **4:**133–140.

14. Bourdon M.A., Wikstrand C.J., Furthmayr H., Matthews T.J., Bigner D.D. 1983. Human glioma-mesenchymal extracellular matrix antigen defined by monoclonal antibody. *Cancer Res* **43:**2796–805.

15. Brady L.W., Miyamoto C., Woo D.V., Rackover M., Emrich J., Bender H., et al. 1992. Malignant astrocytomas treated with iodine-125 labeled monoclonal antibody 425 against epidermal growth factor receptor: A phase II trial. *Int. J. Radiat. Oncol. Biol. Phys.* **22:**225–230.

16. Brooks W.H., Markesbery W.R., Gupta G.D., Roszman T.L.. 1978. Relationship of lymphocyte invasion and survival of brain tumor patients. *Ann. Neurol.* **4:**219–224.

17. Brown M.T., Coleman R.E., Friedman A.H., Friedman H.S., McLendon R.E., Reiman R., et al. 1996. Intrathecal ^{131}I-labeled antitenascin monoclonal antibody 81C6 treatment of patients with leptomeningeal neoplasms or primary brain tumor resection cavities with subarachnoid communication: phase I trial results. *Clin. Cancer. Res.* **2:** 963–972.

18. Byers V.S., Johnston J.O.. 1977. Antigenic differences among osteogenic sarcoma tumor cells taken from different locations in human tumors. *Cancer Res.* **37:**3173–3182.

19. Carrel S., Accola R.S., Carmagnola A.L., Mach J.P. 1980. Common human melanoma-associated antigen(s) detected by monoclonal antibodies. *Cancer Res.* **40:**2523–2528.

20. Cokgor I., Akabani G., Friedman H.S., Friedman A.H., Zalutsky M.R., Zehngebot L.M., et al. 2001. Long term response in a patient with neoplastic meningitis secondary to melanoma treated with ^{131}I-radiolabeled anti-chondroitin proteoglycan sulfate Me1-14 F(ab')₂: a case study. *Cancer* **91(9):**1809–1813.

21. Cokgor I., Akabani G., Kuan C-T, Friedman H.S., Friedman A.H., Coleman R.E., et al. 2000. Phase I trial results of iodine-131-labeled antitenascin monoclonal antibody 81C6 treatment of patients with newly diagnosed malignant gliomas. *J. Clin. Oncol.* **18:**3862–3872.

22. Colapinto E.V., Lee Y.S., Humphrey P.A., Zalutsky M.R., Friedman H.S., Bullard D.E., Bigner D.D. 1988. The localisation of radiolabelled murine monoclonal antibody 81C6 and its Fab fragment in human glioma xenografts in athymic mice [published erratum appears in Br J Neurosurg;2(4):548]. *Br. J. Neurosurg.* **2:**179–191.

23. Conley F.K., Adler J.R., Duncan J.A., Kennedy J.D., Sutton R.C. 1990. Intralesional immunotherapy of brain tumors with combined *Corynebacterium parvum* and recombinant interleukin-2 in mice. *J. Natl. Cancer Inst.* **82:**1340–1344.

24. Cserr H.F., Knopf P.M. 1997. Cervical lymphatics, the blood-brain barrier, and immunoreactivity of the brain, in *Immunology of the Nervous System* (Keane, R.W., Hickey, W.F., eds.), Oxford University Press, New York, pp. 195–202.

25. Curran W.J., Scott C.B., Horton J., Nelson J.S., Weinstein A.S., Fischbach A.J., et al. 1993. Recursive partitioning analysis of prognostic factors in three Radiation Therapy Oncology Group malignant glioma trials. *J. Natl. Cancer Inst.* **85:**704–710.

26. De Martin R., Haendler B., Hofer-Warbinek R., Gaugitsch H., Wrann M., Schlusener H., et al. 1987. Complementary DNA for human glioblastoma-derived T cell suppressor factor, a novel member of the transforming growth factor-β gene family. *EMBO J.* **6:**3673–3677.

27. DiMeco F., Rhines L.D., Hanes J., Tyler B.M., Brat D., Torchiana E., et al. 2000. Paracrine delivery of IL-12 against intracranial 9L gliosarcoma in rats. *J. Neurosurg.* **92:**419–427.

28. Dittel, B.N., Visintin I., Merchant R.M., Janeway C.A. 1999. Presentation of the self antigen myelin basic protein by dendritic cells leads to experimental autoimmune encephalomyelitis. *J. Immunol.* **163:**32–39.

29. Elliott L.H., Brooks W.H., Roszman T.L. 1992. Suppression of high affinity IL-2 receptors on mitogen activated lymphocytes by glioma-derived suppressor factor. *J. Neurooncol.* **14:**1–7.

30. Elliott L., Brooks W., Roszman T. 1987. Role of interleukin-2 (IL-2) and IL-2 receptor expression in the proliferative defect observed in mitogen-stimulated lymphocytes from patients with gliomas. *J. Natl. Cancer Inst.* **78:**919–922.

31. Elliott L.H., Brooks W.H., Roszman T.L. 1984. Cytokinetic basis for the impaired activation of lymphocytes from patients with primary intracranial tumors. *J. Immunol.* **132:**1208–1215.

32. Esiri M.M., Oppenheimer D.R., Brownell B., Haire M. 1982. Distribution of measles antigen and immunoglobulin-containing cells in the CNS in subacute sclerosing panencephalitis (SSPE) and atypical measles encephalitis. *J. Neurol. Sci.* **53:**29–43.

33. Esiri M.M. 1980. Multiple sclerosis: A quantitative and qualitative study of immunoglobulin-containing cells in the central nervous system. *Neuropathol. Appl. Neurobiol.* **6:**9–21.

34. Esiri M.M. 1980. Poliomyelitis: immunoglobulin-containing cells in the central nervous system in acute and convalescent phases of the human disease. *Clin. Exp. Immunol.* **40:**42–48.

35. Faillot T., Magdelenat H., Mady E., Stasiecki P., Fohanno D., Gropp P., et al. 1996. A phase I study of an anti-epidermal growth factor receptor monoclonal antibody for the treatment of malignant gliomas. *Neurosurgery* **39:**478–483.

36. Fakhrai H., Dorigo O., Shawler D.L., H. Lin H., Mercola D., Black K.L., et al. 1996. Eradication of established intracranial rat gliomas by transforming growth factor β antisense gene therapy. *Proc. Natl. Acad. Sci. U. S. A.* **93:**2909–2914.

37. Farmer J-P., Antel J.P., Freedman M., Cashman N.R., Rode H., Villemure J-G. 1989. Characterization of lymphoid cells isolated from human gliomas. *J. Neurosurg.* **71:**528–533.

38. Fogel M., Gorelik E., Segal S., Feldman M. 1979. Differences in cell surface antigens of tumor metastases and those of the local tumor. *J. Natl. Cancer Inst.* **62:**585–588.

39. Fontana A., Hengartner H., de Tribolet N., Weber E. 1984. Glioblastoma cells release interleukin 1 and factors inhibiting interleukin 2-mediated effects. *J. Immunol.* **132:**1837–1844.

40. Gautam A.M., Glynn P. 1989. Lewis rat lymphoid dendritic cells can efficiently present homologous myelin basic protein to encephalitogenic lymphocytes. *J. Neuroimmunol.* **22:**113–121.

41. Glick R.P., Lichtor T., de Zoeten E., Deshmukh P., Cohen E.P. 1999. Prolongation of survival of mice with glioma treated with semiallogeneic fibroblasts secreting interleukin-2. *Neurosurgery* **45:**867–874.

42. Grossi P.M., Ocahai H., Archer G.E., Chewning T., McLendon R.E., Friedman A.H., et al. 2002. Intracerebral microinfusion of Herceptin in an athymic rat model of intracranial metastatic breast cancer. Unpublished results.

43. Grossman S.A., Krabak M.J. 1999. Leptomeningeal carcinomatosis. *Cancer Treatment Rev.* **25:**103–19.

44. Hauser S.L., Bhan A.K., Gilles F.H., Hoban C.J., Reinherz E.L., Schlossman S.F., Weiner H.L. 1983. Immunohistochemical staining of human brain with monoclonal antibodies that identify lymphocytes, monocytes and the Ia antigen. *J. Neuroimmunol.* **5:**197–205.

45. He X., Archer G.E., Wikstrand C.J., Morrison S.L., Zalutsky M.R., Bigner D.D., Batra S.K. 1994. Generation and characterization of a mouse/human chimeric antibody directed against extracellular matrix protein tenascin. *J. Neuroimmunol.* **52:**127–137.

46. Heimberger A.B., Archer G.E., Crotty L.E., McLendon R.E., Friedman A.H., Friedman H.S., et al. 2002. Dendritic cells pulsed with a tumor-specific peptide induce long-lasting immunity and are effective against murine intracerebral melanoma. *Neurosurgery* **50:**158–166.

47. Heimberger A.B., Crotty L.E., Archer G.E., McLendon R.E., Friedman A., Dranoff G., et al. 2000. Bone marrow-derived dendritic cells pulsed with tumor homogenate induce immunity against syngeneic intracerebral glioma. *J. Neuroimmunol.* **103:**16–25.

48. Hickey W.F., Vass K., Lassmann H. 1992. Bone marrow-derived elements in the central nervous system: An immunohistochemical and ultrastructural survey of rat chimeras. *J. Neuropathol. Exp. Neurol.* **51:**246–256.

49. Hickey W.F., Hsu B.L., Kimura H. 1991. T-lymphocyte entry into the central nervous system. *J. Neurosci. Res.* **28:**254–260.

50. Hickey W.F., Kimura H. 1988. Perivascular microglial cells of the CNS are bone marrow-derived and present antigen *in vivo. Science* **239:**290–292.

51. Hickey W.F., Kimura H.. 1987. Graft-vs.-host disease elicits expression of class I and class II histocompatibility antigens and the presence of scattered T lymphocytes in rat central nervous system. *Proc. Natl. Acad. Sci. USA* **84:**2082–2086.

52. Hickey W.F., Osborn J.P., Kirby W.M. 1985. Expression of Ia molecules by astrocytes during acute experimental allergic encephalomyelitis in the Lewis rat. *Cell. Immunol.* **91:**528–535.

53. Hishii M., Nitta T., Ishida H., Ebato M., Kurosu A., Yagita H., et al. 1995. Human glioma-derived interleukin-10 inhibits antitumor immune responses *in vitro. Neurosurgery* **37:**1160–1166.

54. Hopkins K., Chandler C., Bullimore J., Sandeman D., Coakham H., Kemshead J.T. 1995. A pilot study of the treatment of patients with recurrent malignant gliomas with intratumoral yttrium-90 radioimmunoconjugates. *Radiother. Oncol.* **34:**121–31, 1995.

55. Huettner C., Paulus W., Roggendorf W. 1995. Messenger RNA expression of the immunosuppressive cytokine IL-10 in human gliomas. *Am. J. Pathol.* **146:**317–322.

56. Ibayashi Y., Yamaki T., Kawahara T., Daibo M., Kubota T., Uede T., et al. 1993. Effect of local administration of lymphokine-activated killer cells and interleukin-2 on malignant brain tumor patients. *Neurol. Med. Chir.* **33:**448–457.

57. Jacobs S.K., Wilson D.J., Kornblith P.L., Grimm E.A. 1986. Interleukin-2 or autologous lymphokine-activated killer cell treatment of malignant glioma: Phase I trial. *Cancer Res.* **46:**2101–2104.

58. Jean W.C., Spellman S.R., Wallenfriedman M.A., Hall W.A., Low W.C. 1998. Interleukin-12-based immunotherapy against rat 9L glioma. *Neurosurgery* **42:**850–857.

59. Kida Y., Cravioto H., Hochwald G.M., Hochgeschwender U., Ransohoff J. 1983. Immunity to transplantable nitrosourea-induced neurogenic tumors. II. Immunoprophylaxis of tumors of the brain. *J. Neuropathol. Exp. Neurol.* **42:**122–135.

60. Kuppner M.C., Hamou M-F., Sawamura Y., Bodmer S., de Tribolet N. 1989. Inhibition of lymphocyte function by glioblastoma-derived transforming growth factor β2. *J. Neurosurg.* **71:**211–217.

61. Kuppner M.C., Hamou M-F., Bodmer S., Fontana A., de Tribolet N. 1988. The glioblastoma-derived T-cell suppressor factor/transforming growth factor beta 2 inhibits the generation of lymphokine-activated killer (LAK) cells. *Int. J. Cancer* **42:**562–567.

62. Lal A., Lash A.E., Altschul S.F., Velculescu V., Zhang L., McLendon R.E., et al. 1999. A public database for gene expression in human cancers. *Cancer Res.* **59:**5403–5407.

63. Lampson L.A., Hickey W.F. 1986. Monoclonal antibody analysis of MHC expression in human brain biopsies: Tissue ranging from "histologically normal" to that showing different levels of glial tumor involvement. *J. Immunol.* **136:**4054–4062.

64. Larsen R.H., Akabani G., Welsh P., Zalutsky M.R. 1998. The cytotoxicity and microdosimetry of astatine-211-labeled chimeric monoclonal antibodies in human glioma and melanoma cells *in vitro. Radiat. Res.* **149:**155–162.

65. Lee S.C., Moore G.R.W., Golenwsky G., Raine C.S. 1990. Multiple sclerosis: A role for astroglia in active demyelination suggested by class II MHC expression and ultrastructural study. *J. Neuropathol. Exp. Neurol.* **49:**122–136.

66. Lee Y.S., Bullard D.E., Zalutsky M.R., Coleman R.E., Wikstrand C.J., Friedman H.S., et al. 1988. Therapeutic efficacy of antiglioma mesenchymal extracellular matrix 131I-radiolabeled murine monoclonal antibody in a human glioma xenograft model. *Cancer Res.* **48:**559–566.

67. Lee Y.S., Bullard D.E., Wikstrand C.J., Zalutsky M.R., Muhlbaier L.H., Bigner D.D. 1987. Comparison of monoclonal antibody delivery to intracranial glioma xenografts by intravenous and intracarotid administration. *Cancer Res.* **47:** 1941–1946.

68. Liau L.M., Black K.L., Prins R.M., Sykes S.N., DiPatre P.L., Cloughesy T.F., et al. 1999. Treatment of intracranial gliomas with bone marrow-derived dendritic cells pulsed with tumor antigens. *J. Neurosurg.* **90:**1115–1124.

69. Linington C., Berger T., Perry L., Weerth S., Hinze-Selch D., Zhang Y., et al. 1993. T cells specific for the myelin oligodendrocyte glycoprotein mediate an unusual autoimmune inflammatory response in the central nervous system. *Eur. J. Immunol.* **23:**1364–1372.

70. Loeffler J.S., Alexander E.I., Wen P.Y., Shea W.M., Coleman N., Kooy H.M.,et al. 1990. Results of stereotactic brachytherapy used in initial management of patients with glioblastoma. *J. Natl. Cancer Inst.* **82:**1918–1921.

71. Lowe J., Maclennan K.A., Powe D.G., Pound J.D., Palmer J.B. 1989. Microglial cells in human brain have phenotypic characteristics related to possible function as dendritic antigen presenting cells. *J. Pathol.* **159:**143–149.

72. Ludewig B., Ochsenbein A.F., Odermatt B., Paulin D., Hengartner H., Zinkernagel R.M. 2000. Immunotherapy with dendritic cells directed against tumor antigens shared with normal host cells results in severe autoimmune disease. *J. Exp. Med.* **191:**795–803.

73. MacLean G.D., Seehafer J., Shaw A.R.E., Kieran M.W., Longenecker B.M. 1982. Antigenic heterogeneity of human colorectal cancer cell lines analyzed by a panel of monoclonal antibodies. I. Heterogeneous expression of Ia-like and HLA-like antigenic determinants. *J. Natl. Cancer Inst.* **69:**357–364.

74. Mahaley M.S. Jr., Bigner D.D., Dudka L.F., Wilds P.R., Williams D.H., Bouldin T.W., et al. 1983. Immunobiology of primary intracranial tumors. Part 7: Active immunization of patients with anaplastic human glioma cells: a pilot study. *J. Neurosurg.* **59:**201–207.

75. Mahaley M.S. Jr., Brooks W.H., Roszman T.L., Bigner D.D., Dudka L., Richardson S. 1977. Immunobiology of primary intracranial tumors. Part I: Studies of the cellular and humoral general immune competence of brain-tumor patients. *J. Neurosurg.* **46:**467–476.

76. Masciopinto J.E., Levin A.B., Mehta M.P., Rhode B.S. 1995. Stereotactic radiosurgery for glioblastoma: a final report of 31 patients. *J. Neurosurg.* **82:**530–535.

77. Matsumoto Y., Kawai K., Fujiwara M. 1989. *In situ* Ia expression on brain cells in the rat: autoimmune encephalomyelitis-resistant strain (BN) and susceptible strain (Lewis) compared. *Immunology* **66:**621–627.

78. Mattiace L.A., Davies P., Dickson D.W. 1990. Detection of HLA-DR on microglia in the human brain is a function of both clinical and technical factors. *Am. J. Pathol.* **136:**1101–1114.

79. McCutcheon I.E., Baranco R.A., Katz D.A., Saris S.C. 1990. Adoptive immunotherapy of intracerebral metastases in mice. *J. Neurosurg.* **72:**102–109.

80. McMenamin P.G., Forrester J.V. 1999. Dendritic cells in the central nervous system and eye and their associated supporting tissues, in *Dendritic Cells: Biology and Clinical Applications* (Loetze, M.T., Thomson, A.W., eds.),. Academic, New York, pp. 205–248.

81. Medawar P.B. 1948. Immunity to homologous grafted skin. III. The fate of skin homografts transplanted to the brain, to subcutaneous tissue, and to the anterior chamber of the eye. *Br. J. Exp. Pathol.* **29:**58–69.

82. Merchant R.E., Merchant L.H., Cook S.H.S., McVicar D.W., Young H.F. 1988. Intralesional infusion of lymphokine-activated killer (LAK) cells and recombinant interleukin-2 (rIL-2) for the treatment of patients with malignant brain tumor. *Neurosurgery* **23:**725–732.

83. Miescher S., Whiteside T.L., de Tribolet N., von Fliedner V. 1988. *In situ* characterization, clonogenic potential, and antitumor cytolytic activity of T lymphocytes infiltrating human brain cancers. *J. Neurosurg.* **68:**438–448.

84. Miller F.R., Heppner G.H. 1979. Immunologic heterogeneity of tumor cell subpopulations from a single mouse mammary tumor. *J. Natl. Cancer Inst.* **63:**1457–1463.

85. Mitchell M.S. 1989. Relapse in the central nervous system in melanoma patients successfully treated with biomodulators. *J. Clin. Oncol.* **7:**1701–1709.

86. Morford L.A., Elliott L.H., Carlson S.L., Brooks W.H., Roszman T.L. 1997. T-cell receptor-mediated signaling is defective in T cells obtained from patients with primary intracranial tumors. *J. Immunol.* **159:**4415–4425.

87. Moseley R.P., Davies A.G., Richardson R.B., Zalutsky M., Carrell S., Fabre J., et al. 1990. Intrathecal administration of ¹³¹I radiolabeled monoclonal antibody as a treatment for neoplastic meningitis. *Br. J. Cancer* **62:**637–642.

88. Murai N., Ueba T., Takahashi J.A., Yang H-Q, Kikuchi H., Hiai H., et al. 1996. Apoptosis of human glioma cells *in vitro* and *in vivo* induced by a neutralizing antibody against human basic fibroblast growth factor. *J. Neurosurg.* **85:** 1072–1077.

89. Murphy J.B., Sturm E. 1923. Conditions determining the transplantability of tissues in the brain. *J. Exp. Med.* **38:** 183–196.

90. Nitta T., Sato K., Yagita H., Okumura K., Ishii S. 1990. Preliminary trial of specific targeting therapy against malignant glioma. *Lancet* **335:**368–371.

91. Palma L., Di Lorenzo N., Guidetti B. 1978. Lymphocytic infiltrates in primary glioblastomas and recidivous gliomas. *J. Neurosurg.* **49:**854–861.

92. Papanastassiou V., Pizer B.L., Coakham H.B., Bullimore J., Zananiri T., Kemshead J.T. 1993. Treatment of recurrent and cystic malignant gliomas by a single intracavity injection of 131I monoclonal antibody: feasibility, pharmacokinetics and dosimetry. *Br. J. Cancer* **67:**144–151.

93. Paterson P.Y., Day E.D. 1981–1982. Current perspectives of neuroimmunologic disease: multiple sclerosis and experimental allergic encephalomyelitis. *Clin. Immunol. Rev.* **1:**581–697.

94. Pimm M.V., Baldwin R.W. 1977. Antigenic differences between primary methylcholanthrene-induced rat sarcomas and post-surgical recurrences. *Int. J. Cancer* **20:**37–43.

95. Plautz G.E., Miller D.W., Barnett G.H., Stevens G.H.J., Maffett S., Kim J., et al. 2000. T cell adoptive immunotherapy of newly diagnosed gliomas. *Clin. Cancer Res.* **6:**2209–2218.

96. Plautz G.E., Touhalisky J.E., Shu S. 1997. Treatment of murine gliomas by adoptive transfer of *ex vivo* activated tumor-draining lymph node cells. *Cell. Immunol.* **178:**101–107.

97. Quattrocchi K.B., Miller C.H., Cush S., Bernard S.A., Dull S.T., Smith M., et al. 1999. Pilot study of local autologous tumor infiltrating lymphocytes for the treatment of recurrent malignant glioma. *J. Neurooncol.* **45:**141–157.

98. Reardon D.A., Akabani G., Coleman R.E., Friedman A.H., Friedman H.S., Herndon J.E., et al. 2002a. Phase II trial of murine ^{131}I-labeled anti-tenascin monoclonal antibody 81C6 administered into surgically created resection cavities of patients with newly diagnosed malignant gliomas. *J. Clin. Oncol.* **20:**1389–1397.

99. Reardon D.A., Akabani G., Friedman A., Friedman H., Herndon J., McLendon R., et al. 2002b. Phase I Trial Results: Treatment of Patients With Newly Diagnosed Malignant Gliomas using 131-Iodine Labeled Human/Murine Chimeric Antitenascin Monoclonal Antibody 81C6 Via Surgically Created Resection Cavities. Abstract 2440. Presented at Minisymposium Clinical Research 9. American Association for Cancer Research, 93rd Annual Meeting, April 6–10. *Proc. Am. Assoc. Cancer Res.* **43:**491.

100. Reardon D.A., Akabani G., Friedman A., Friedman H., Herndon J., McLendon R., et al. 2001. A phase I study of astatine-211 labeled human/murine chimeric antitenascin monoclonal antibody 81C6 via surgically created resection cavities for patients with high grade gliomas. Abstract 390. Presented at World Federation of Neuro-Oncology First Quadrennial Meeting and Society for Neuro-Oncology Sixth Annual Meeting, November 15–18. *Neuro-Oncol.* **3:**365.

101. Reist C.J., Garg P.K., Alston K.L., Bigner D.D., Zalutsky M.R. 1996. Radioiodination of internalizing monoclonal antibodies using N-succinimidyl 5-iodo-3-pyridinecarboxylate. *Cancer Res.* **56:**4970–4977.

102. Riva P., Franceschi G., Frattarelli M. 1999. Loco-regional radioimmunotherapy of high-grade malignant gliomas using specific monoclonal antibodies labeled with 90Y: a phase I study. *Clin. Cancer Res.* **5:**3275s–3280s.

103. Riva P., Franceschi G., Arista A., Frattarelli M., Riva N., Cremonini A.M., et al. 1997. Local application of radiolabeled monoclonal antibodies in the treatment of high grade malignant glioma. A six-year clinical experience. *Cancer* **80:**2733–2742.

104. Riva P., Arista A., Tison V., Sturiale C., Franceschi G., Spinelli A., et al. 1994. Intralesional radioimmunotherapy of malignant gliomas. An effective treatment in recurrent tumors. *Cancer* **73:**1076–1082.

105. Roeske J.C., Chen G.T.Y. 1991. Dosimetry model for intracavitary radioimmunotherapy of cystic brain tumors, antibody immunoconjugates. *Radiopharmaceuticals* **4:**637–647.

106. Roszman T.L., Brooks W.H., Elliott L.H. 1987. Inhibition of lymphocyte responsiveness by a glial tumor cell-derived suppressive factor. *J. Neurosurg.* **67:**874–879.

107. Roszman T.L., Brooks W.H., Steele C., Elliott L.H. 1985. Pokeweed mitogen-induced immunoglobulin secretion by peripheral blood lymphocytes from patients with primary intracranial tumors. Characterization of T helper and B cell function. *J. Immunol.* **134:**1545–1550.

108. Roussel E., Gingrass M.C., Grimm E.A., Bruner J.M., Moser R.P. 1996. Predominance of type 2 intratumoural immune response in fresh tumour-infiltrating lymphocytes from human gliomas. *Clin. Exp. Immunol.* **105:**344–352.

109. Sampson J.H., Crotty L.E., Lee S., Archer G.E., Ashley D.M., Wikstrand C.J, et al. 2000. Unarmed, tumor-specific monoclonal antibody effectively treats brain tumors. *Proc. Natl. Acad. Sci. USA* **97:**7503–7508.

110. Sampson J.H., Archer G.E., Ashley D.M., Fuchs H.E., Hale L.P., Dranoff G., Bigner D.D. 1996. Subcutaneous vaccination with irradiated, cytokine-producing tumor cells stimulates CD8+ cell-mediated immunity against tumors located in the "immunologically privileged" central nervous system. *Proc. Natl. Acad. Sci. USA* **93:**10,399–10,404.

111. Sawamura Y., Diserens A-C., de Tribolet N. 1990. *In vitro* prostaglandin E$_2$ production by glioblastoma cells and its effect on interleukin-2 activation of oncolytic lymphocytes. *J. Neurooncol.* **9:**125–130.

112. Schackert H.K., Itaya T., Schackert G., Fearon E., Vogelstein B., Frost P. 1989. Systemic immunity against a murine colon tumor (CT-26) produced by immunization with syngeneic cells expressing a transfected viral gene product. *Int. J. Cancer* **43:**823–827.

113. Schold S.C., Zalutsky M.R., Coleman R.E., Glantz M.J., Friedman A.H., Jaszczak R.J., et al. 1993. Distribution and dosimetry of I-123–labeled monoclonal antibody 81C6 in patients with anaplastic glioma. *Invest. Radiol.* **28:**488–496.

114. Serot J-M., Foliguet B., Bene M-C., Faure G-C. 1997. Ultrastructural and immunohistological evidence for dendritic-like cells within human choroid plexus epithelium. *Neuroreport* **8:**1995–1998.

115. Shapiro J.R., Yung W.K.A., Shapiro W.R. 1981. Isolation, karyotype, and clonal growth of heterogeneous subpopulations of human malignant gliomas. *Cancer Res.* **41:**2349–2359.

116. Shrieve D.C., Alexander E. 3rd, Wen P.Y., Fine H.A., Kooy H.M., Black P.M., Loeffler J.S. 1995. Comparison of stereotactic radiosurgery and brachytherapy in the treatment of recurrent glioblastoma multiforme. *Neurosurgery* **36:** 275–282; discussion 282–284.

117. Sobel R.A., Ames M.B. 1988. Major histocompatibility complex molecule expression in the human central nervous system: Immunohistochemical analysis of 40 patients. *J. Neuropathol. Exp. Neurol.* **47:**19–28.

118. Stragliotto G., Vega F., Stasiecki P., Gropp P., Poisson M., Delattre J-Y. 1996. Multiple infusions of anti-epidermal growth factor receptor (EGFR) monoclonal antibody (EMD 55 900) in patients with recurrent malignant gliomas. *Eur. J. Cancer* **32A:** 636–640.

119. Thomas W.E. 1992. Brain macrophages: evaluation of microglia and their functions. *Brain Res. Brain Res. Rev.* **17:**61–74.

120. Torre-Amione G., Beauchamp R.D., Koeppen H., Park B.H., Schreiber H., Moses H.L., Rowley D.A. 1990. A highly immunogenic tumor transfected with a murine transforming growth factor type β_1 cDNA escapes immune surveillance. *Proc. Natl. Acad. Sci. USA* **87:**1486–1490.

121. Traugott U. 1987. Multiple sclerosis: relevance of class I and class II MHC-expressing cells to lesion development. *J. Neuroimmunol.* **16:**283–302.

122. Trouillas P. 1973. Immunologie et immunotherapie des tumeurs cerebrals. Etat actuel. *Rev. Neurol.* **128:**23–38.

123. Tuohy V.K., Lu Z.J., Sobel R.A., Laursen R.A., Lees M.B. 1988. A synthetic peptide from myelin proteolipid protein induces experimental allergic encephalomyelitis. *J. Immunol.* **141:**1126–1130.

124. Ulvestad E., Williams K., Bjerkvig R., Tiekotter K., Antel J., Matre R. 1994. Human microglial cells have phenotypic and functional characteristics in common with both macrophages and dendritic antigen-presenting cells. *J. Leukocyte Biol.* **56:**732–740.

125. Vass K., Lassmann H. 1990. Intrathecal application of interferon gamma. Progressive appearance of MHC antigens within the rat nervous system. *Am. J. Pathol.* **137:**789–800.

126. Vass K., Lassmann H., Wekerle H., Wisniewski H.M. 1986. The distribution of Ia antigen in the lesions of rate acute experimental allergic encephalomyelitis. *Acta Neuropathol.* **70:**149–160.

127. Ventimiglia J.B., Wikstrand C.J., Ostrowski L.E., Bourdon M.A., Lightner V.A., Bigner D.D. 1992. Tenascin expression in human glioma cell lines and normal tissues. *J. Neuroimmunol.* 36:41–55.

128. Von Hanwehr R.I., Hofman F.M., Taylor C.R., Apuzzo M.L.J. 1984. Mononuclear lymphoid populations infiltrating the microenvironment of primary CNS tumors. Characterization of cell subsets with monoclonal antibodies. *J. Neurosurg.* **60:**1138–1147.

129. Wakimoto H., Abe J., Tsunoda R., Aoyagi M., Hirakawa K., Hamada H. 1996. Intensified antitumor immunity by a cancer vaccine that produces granulocyte-macrophage colony-stimulating factor plus interleukin 4. *Cancer Res.* **56:**1828–1833.

130. Waksman B.H., Porter H., Lees M.B., Adams R.D., Folch J. 1954. A study of the chemical nature of components of bovine white matter effective in producing allergic encephalomyelitis in the rabbit. *J. Exp. Med.* **100:**451–471.

131. Wekerle H., Kojima K., Lannes-Vieira J., Lassmann H., Linington C. 1994. Animal models. *Ann. Neurol.* **36**S47–S53.

132. Westphal M., Delavault P., Hilt D., Olivares R., Belin V., Daumas-Duport C. 2000. Placebo controlled multicenter double-blind randomized prospective phase III trial of carmustine implants (Gliadel™) in 240 patients with malignant gliomas: Final results. Abstract 230. Presented at Fifth Annual Meeting of the Society for Neuro-Oncology. November 9–12, Chicago. *Neuro-Oncology* **2:**301.

133. Wikstrand C.J., Grahmann F.C., McComb R.D., Bigner D.D. 1985. Antigenic heterogeneity of human anaplastic gliomas and glioma-derived cell lines defined by monoclonal antibodies. *J. Neuropathol. Exp. Neurol.* **44:**229–241.

134. Wikstrand C.J., Bigner S.H., Bigner D.D. 1983. Demonstration of complex antigenic heterogeneity in a human glioma cell line and eight derived clones by specific monoclonal antibodies. *Cancer Res.* **43:**3327–3334.

135. Williams K. Jr., Ulvestad E., Cragg L., Blain M., Antel J.P. 1993. Induction of primary T cell responses by human glial cells. *J. Neurosci. Res.* **36:**382–390.

136. Wrann M., Bodmer S., de Martin R., Siepl C., Hofer-Warbinek R., Frei K., et al. 1987. T cell suppressor factor from human glioblastoma cells is a 12.5-kd protein closely related to transforming growth factor-β. *EMBO J.* **6:**1633–1636.

137. Yamada S., DePasquale M., Patlak C.S., Cserr H.F. 1991. Albumin outflow into deep cervical lymph from different regions of rabbit brain. *Am. J. Physiol.* **261:**H1197–H1204.

138. Yao J., Harvath L., Gilbert D.L., Colton C.A. 1990. Chemotaxis by a CNS macrophage, the microglia. *J. Neurosci. Res.* **27:**36–42.

139. Young H., Kaplan A., Regelson W. 1977. Immunotherapy with autologous white cell infusions ("lymphocytes") in the treatment of recurrent glioblastoma multiforme: a preliminary report. *Cancer* **40:**1037–1044.

140. Yu J.S., Wheeler C.J., Zeltzer P.M., Ying H., Finger D.N., Lee P.K., et al. 2001. Vaccination of malignant glioma patients with peptide-pulsed dendritic cells elicits systemic cytotoxicity and intracranial T-cell infiltration. *Cancer Res.* **61:**842–847.

141. Zalutsky M.R., Archer G.E., Garg P.K., Batra S.K., Bigner D.D. 1996. Chimeric anti-tenascin antibody 81C6: increased tumor localization compared with its murine parent. *Nucl. Med. Biol.* **23:**449–458.

142. Zalutsky M.R., Bigner D.D. 1996. Radioimmunotherapy with alpha-emitting radioimmunoconjugates. *Acta Oncol* **35:**373–379.

143. Zalutsky M.R., Moseley R.P., Benjamin J.C., Colapinto E.V., Fuller G.N., Coakham H.P., Bigner D.D. 1990. Monoclonal antibody and F(ab')$_2$ fragment delivery to tumor in patients with glioma: Comparison of intracarotid and intravenous administration. *Cancer Res.* **50:**4105–4110.

144. Zalutsky M.R., Moseley R.P., Coakham H.B., Coleman R.E., Bigner D.D. 1989. Pharmacokinetics and tumor localization of ^{131}I-labeled anti-tenascin monoclonal antibody 81C6 in patients with gliomas and other intracranial malignancies. *Cancer Res.* **49:**2807–2813.

18

Targeting Drugs to Tumors of the Central Nervous System

Maciej S. Lesniak, James Frazier, and Henry Brem

1. INTRODUCTION

Central nervous system (CNS) tumors represent one of the most devastating forms of human illness. In the United States, approx 16,800 people are diagnosed with primary brain tumors each year *(33)*. Of these, half are glial cell neoplasms and more than three quarters of all gliomas are astrocytomas. Astrocytomas represent a heterogeneous group of tumors that can vary from low-grade to the most aggressive-glioblastoma multiforme-based on histopathological classification. Conventional therapy for glioblastomas consists primarily of surgical debulking followed by radiation therapy. Unfortunately, the median survival after surgical intervention alone is 6 mo with only 7.5% of patients surviving for 2 yr. While systemic chemotherapy has been minimally effective, the addition of radiation therapy has extended the median survival to 9 mo *(2,44)*. In spite of these efforts, little progress has been made in extending long-term patient survival, and new therapies and novel approaches are urgently needed to treat this disease.

2. RATIONALE FOR LOCAL DELIVERY

To date, one of the most significant challenges encountered in treating malignant brain tumors has been the unique environment of the CNS. With few exceptions, all of the neurons and supportive glial cells within the CNS are protected from the outside environment by two important barriers. The first of these is the blood–brain barrier (BBB). Tight junctions between endothelial cells of the capillaries form a physiological and pharmacological barrier that prevents the influx of molecules from the bloodstream into the brain. In general, only small, electrically neutral, lipid-soluble molecules can penetrate this capillary endothelium and many chemotherapeutic agents do not fall in this category (Fig. 1). The second important feature of the CNS is the presence of the blood–cerebrospinal fluid barrier (BCB). This barrier is formed by the tightly bound choroid epithelial cells that are responsible for the production of cerebrospinal fluid (CSF). Because the BCB closely regulates the exchange of molecules between the blood and CSF, it can control the penetration of molecules within the interstitial fluid of the brain parenchyma. Furthermore, because the BCB is fortified by an active organic acid transport system, it can actively remove from the CSF a number of agents, such as methotrexate, and therefore actively prevent the diffusion of chemotherapeutic agents directly into the brain parenchyma.

Several approaches have been attempted to overcome the natural boundaries of the CNS and to increase the delivery of chemotherapeutic agents to the tumor bed. The first of these builds upon the physical properties of the BBB and seeks through pharmacological manipulation to create a more

From: *Contemporary Cancer Research: Brain Tumors*
Edited by: F. Ali-Osman © Humana Press Inc., Totowa, NJ

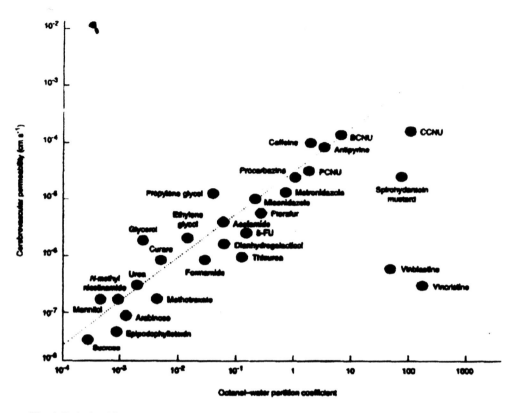

Fig. 1. Relationship between the cerebrovascular permeability and the octanol-water partition coefficient of selected chemicals and drugs. (Reprinted with permission from ref. *1*.)

lipophilic, and thus more BBB-traversable, agents. Both lomustine (CCNU) and semustine (methyl-CCNU) are two lipophilic variants of a known chemotherapeutic agent carmustine (BCNU) that has been shown to modestly improve the survival in patients with malignant brain tumors. However, clinical trials utilizing systemic administration of lomustine or semustine have not shown efficacy of these drugs over BCNU in treating glial tumors *(29)*. A different approach involves increasing the permeability of a hydrophilic agent by linking the drug to a carrier capable of traversing the BBB. For example, the lipophilic dihydropyridine carrier readily crosses the BBB and has been shown to increase intracranial concentrations of a variety of drugs, including neurotransmitters, antibiotics, and antineoplastic agents *(48)*. Likewise, new transport vectors such as a modified protein or receptor-specific monoclonal antibody, have also led to a successful delivery of a number of drugs across the BBB *(47)*.

Another strategy involves disrupting the BBB by means of either an intra-arterial infusion of hyperosmolar mannitol or a novel bradykinin agonist, RMP-7. The rationale for the use of a hyperosmolar solution is that it can cause an acute dehydration of endothelial cells resulting in cell shrinkage, which in turn widens the tight junctions connecting adjacent membranes. In a recent clinical study, Williams et al. *(72)* examined the efficacy of the co-administration of the antineoplastic agents carboplatin and etoposide in conjunction with mannitol in 34 patients with intracranial tumors. While four out of four patients with primitive neuroectodermal tumors (PNETs) and two out of four patients with CNS lymphomas had some degree of response, no benefit was seen in patients with oligodendrogliomas, glioblastomas multiforme, or metastatic carcinomas. These results were further supported by another study in which the survival of patients treated with intra-arterial BCNU was unchanged or worse than those for patients treated with conventional intravenous therapy *(55)*. In contrast to mannitol, the bradykinin agonist RMP-7 directly disrupts the BBB *(53)*. Furthermore, intravenous administration of RMP-7 has been shown to selectively increase the uptake of carboplatin in experimental brain tumors, suggesting a potential use for this agent as adjunctive therapy for selective delivery of chemotherapeutic drugs to the brain *(18)*.

An attractive approach that does not depend on the penetration or disruption of any physiological barrier involves the direct delivery of an antineoplastic agent to the tumor. This may be accomplished by implanting one end of a catheter within the tumor bed and leaving the opposite end easily accessible for injection. One such system, the Ommaya reservoir, has been in clinical use for a number of years and is used to deliver intermittent bolus injections of chemotherapy to the tumor. Most recently, the advent of implantable pumps has permitted a constant infusion of drugs over an extended period of time. The prototype for this model is the Infusaid pump (Infusaid Corp., Norwood, MA) that depends on compressed vapor pressure to deliver a solution at a constant rate *(11)*. Other systems include the MiniMed PIMS system (MiniMed, Sylmar, CA) that delivers drugs by a solenoid pumping mechanism *(40)*, and the Medtronic SynchroMed system (Medtronic, Minneapolis, MN) which uses a peristaltic mechanism to deliver the infused agent *(26)*. All of these devices are limited by mechanical failure, obstruction by tissue debris, and varying rates of infection. None has proven superior over another in the treatment of patients with malignant gliomas.

3. POLYMER-MEDIATED DRUG DELIVERY

Implantable polymers that release chemotherapeutic agents directly into the CNS provide a novel approach to brain tumor therapy. In 1976, Langer and Folkman *(31)* first described these polymers and reported the sustained and predictable release of macromolecules from a non-biodegradable ethylene vinyl acetate (EVAc) copolymer. A drug incorporated into this type of polymer is released by means of diffusion through the micropores of its matrix. The rate of diffusion depends on the chemical properties of the drug itself, including molecular weight, charge, and water solubility. In general, the smaller the molecule, the faster it is released from the polymer. Once released, the drug retains its biological activity. The EVAc polymer has found application in various clinical settings, including glaucoma, asthma, and contraceptive therapy. It has also been experimentally used to deliver drugs intratumorally for glioma therapy *(60)*. The primary limitation of these nonbiodegradable, controlled release polymers is that once the drug has been released, they are inert. Consequently, they remain in place permanently as foreign bodies.

In contrast to EVAc, a new generation of biodegradable polymer systems release drugs by a combination of polymer degradation and drug diffusion (Fig. 2A,B). The polyanhydride poly[*bis*(p-carboxyphenoxy)propane-sebacic acid] (PCPP-SA) matrix is an example of a biodegradable polymer that breaks down to dicarboxylic acids by spontaneous reaction with water *(34)*. There are several advantages of these polymers over EVAc. First, the polyanhydrides can be made to release the active drug at a nearly constant rate. Thus, any drug can be theoretically incorporated into the polymer as long as it does not react with the matrix. Second, by modifying the ratio of carboxyphenoxypropane (CPP) to sebacic acid (SA), one can adjust the polymer breakdown rate from one day to several years. For example, a 1-mm thick polymer composed of pure CPP would require 3 yr to completely degrade, compared to 3 wk when SA is added to reach 80% *(12)*. Third, the PCPP:SA polymer can be manufactured in an endless variety of shapes, such as sheets, rods, or wafers, thereby facilitating its clinical application and method of surgical delivery. Finally, because the matrix itself is completely degraded, there is no foreign body that needs to be surgically removed after the drug is released. The degradation products are noncytotoxic, nonmutagenic, and nonteratogenic *(35)*.

Recently, the spectrum of drugs that can be optimally released from the polyanhydride matrix has been broadened with the introduction of second generation of biodegradable polymers. One such matrix is the fatty acid dimer-sebacic acid (FAD-SA) copolymer. This polymer was developed in light of the finding that PCPP-SA does not release a high percentage of many hydrophilic agents or

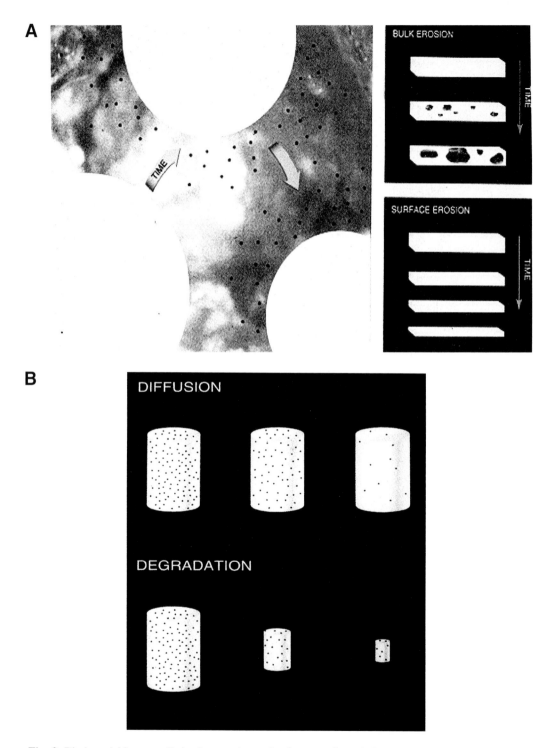

Fig. 2. Biodegradable controlled release polymer implants are intended to release their drug content at a nearly constant rate as they dissolve in a body of water, as depicted in the large illustration **(A)**. Their desirable properties therefore include surface erosion rather than bulk erosion and release of drug by degredation rather than by diffusion. These properties are shown schematically in the smaller diagrams **(A,B)** and depend on the nature of the chemical bonds in the polymer. (Reprinted with permission from ref. *8*.)

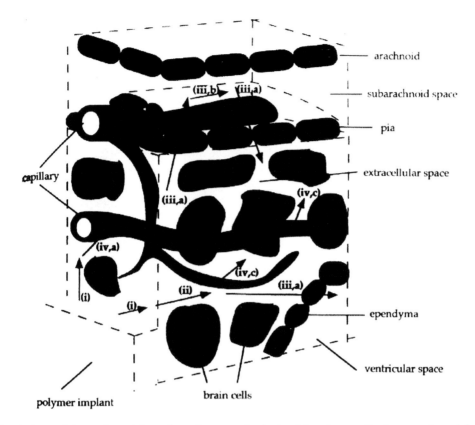

Fig. 3. Fate of drug released from the polymer to the brain. After drug molecules are released from the polymer matrix, they enter the extracellular space of the brain; they can be transported by diffusion due to drug concentration gradients (i); convection due to fluid pressure gradients (ii); drug migration into ventricular space via pial or ependymal surface (iii,a); circulation in the subarachnoid or ventricular spaces (iii,b); subsequent diffusion back into the brain interstitium (iii,c); permeation through the endothelium (iv,a); circulation in the cerebral blood vessels (iv,b); and reentry by permeation back into the brain interstitium (iv,c). (Reprinted with permission from ref. *19*.)

hydrolytically unstable compounds such as methotrexate or carboplatin *(17)*. In another development, Menei et al. *(42)*, introduced a poly(lactide-co-glycolide) polymer that can be formed into microspheres and stereotactically injected into the brain. When covalently linked to polyethylene glycol coating, this polymer matrix has also been shown to reduce opsonization and elimination by the immune system *(23)*. Other new discoveries include polyethyleneglycol-coated liposomes that encapsulate anthracyclines *(20)*, and gelatin-chondroitin sulfate coated microspheres that have been shown to reproducibly release cytokines in vivo *(21)*. The fate of these drug molecules, once released from the polymer, is illustrated in Fig. 3.

3.1. Development of Gliadel®

The choice of carmustine, or BCNU, as the prodrug in the development of polymer-based chemotherapy stems from the well known activity of nitrosoureas against malignant brain tumors. In general, nitrosoureas are low molecular weight alkylating agents that are relatively lipid soluble, and therefore capable of crossing the BBB and achieving potentially tumoricidal concentrations *(39)*.

These pharmacologic considerations have been exploited in a number of clinical trials where systemic administration of BCNU has been shown to modestly prolong the survival of patients with brain tumors *(22,65)*. On the other hand, the relatively short half-life (about 15 min) when given intravenously combined with severe toxicity, such as myelosuppression and pulmonary fibrosis, have precluded the widespread use of systemic BCNU. In an effort to improve its effectiveness and limit the dose-related side effects, BCNU was incorporated into polymers and tested for efficacy against intracranial tumors.

The preclinical studies of BCNU-polymer preparations were performed in several stages. First, it was important to establish the distribution and pharmacokinetics of active drug release in vitro and in vivo. This was done through several experiments, all of which demonstrated that a prolonged, controlled, and sustained release of intact BCNU can be achieved with the polymer system *(24,73–74)*. Next, the efficacy of BCNU-polymers was tested against a rat intracranial glioma. The results clearly showed that local delivery of BCNU by polymer was superior to systemic administration, and led to significant prolongation of survival in animals with malignant glioma *(60)*. Finally, toxicity studies performed in primates showed that BCNU-polymers were well tolerated and that concomitant external beam radiotherapy did not increase toxicity *(4)*. Cumulatively, these studies proved the safety and efficacy of the polymer technology and set the stage for clinical trials.

In a phase I-II clinical trial, 21 patients were treated with three different doses of BCNU loaded in PCPP-SA polymers (1.93%, 3.85%, and 6.35% BCNU by polymer weight) *(5)*. Enrollment criteria included patients with a diagnosis of recurrent malignant glioma who had previously undergone a craniotomy for debulking and in whom standard therapy had failed. All of the patients required an indication for reoperation, such as a unilateral single focus of tumor in the cerebral cortex with an enhancing volume of at least $1.0 \, cm^3$ on computed tomography (CT) or magnetic resonance imaging (MRI) scans, a Karnofsky performance scale score of at least 60 (indicating that the patient is able to function independently), completion of external-beam radiotherapy, and no nitrosoureas for up to 6 wk prior to enrollment. At the time of re-operation, up to eight BCNU-loaded polymer wafers were implanted within the tumor cavity (Fig. 4). The treatment was well tolerated and no patient experienced any signs of local or systemic toxicity. The overall median survival times were 46 wk after implant and 87 wk after initial diagnosis, with 86% of the patients alive more than 1 yr after diagnosis. On the basis of this work, the 3.85% BCNU-loaded polymers were chosen for further clinical study.

A phase III prospective, randomized, double-blind, placebo-controlled clinical trial of PCPP-SA polymer containing 3.8% BCNU by weight was conducted in 222 patients with recurrent malignant gliomas at 27 medical centers in the United States and Canada *(6)*. Patients with recurrent malignant gliomas were randomized to receive either the BCNU-polymer or an empty placebo implanted within the tumor cavity. Selection criteria were the same as for phase I–II study, namely the diagnosis of a recurrent malignant glioma, failure of standard therapy, and the need for reoperation. All of the patients previously underwent external beam radiotherapy, and 52.7% of the BCNU-polymer group and 48.2% of the control group had undergone previous chemotherapy. Whereas the BCNU-polymer treatment group had a median survival of 31 wk, the median survival of the control group was 23 wk (hazard ratio = 0.69, $p = 0.005$) (Fig. 5). The results were even more striking in the glioblastoma multiforme group, with 50% greater survival at 6 mo in patients treated with BCNU-polymers than with placebo alone ($p = 0.02$). There were no significant toxicities attributable to the treatment observed in the BCNU-polymer group. Consequently, this study established that BCNU-polymers are safe and effective in the treatment of recurrent malignant gliomas. In 1996, the FDA approved Gliadel® as the first new treatment against malignant brain tumors in 23 yr. To date, Gliadel® has received regulatory approval in 21 countries.

In general, any treatment for cancers that has been found effective at recurrence has been subsequently shown to be even more effective as initial therapy. Having established Gliadel® as a useful agent in recurrent brain tumors, we naturally turned our attention to further elucidating its role in

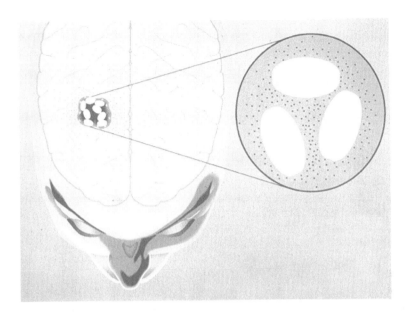

Fig. 4. Up to eight polymer implants line the tumor resection cavity, where the loaded drug is gradually released as it dissolves. The inset shows conceptually how drug molecules diffuse away from these implants. (Reprinted with permission from ref. *8*.)

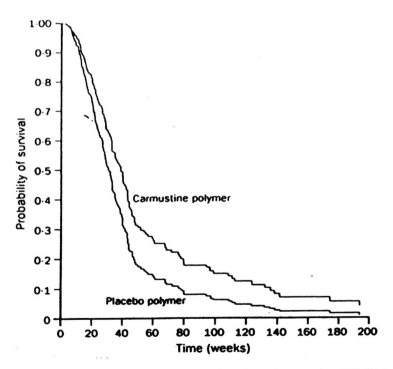

Fig. 5. Overall survival for patients receiving implantation of carmustine (BCNU)-loaded polymers or placebo controls at the time of operation for a recurrent brain tumor after adjustment for prognostic factors. (Reprinted with permission from ref. *6*.)

initial therapy. First, a phase I study involving 22 patients with newly diagnosed malignant gliomas was conducted to evaluate the overall safety of the BCNU-polymer combination *(7)*. None of the 22 patients experienced any local or systemic side effects attributable to Gliadel®. Valtonen et al. *(64)*, conducted a prospective, randomized, double-blind clinical trial in Europe involving 32 patients with newly diagnosed malignant gliomas. Half the patients received 3.85% BCNU wafers with the other half receiving placebo wafers at the time of the initial resection. The median survival was 58 wk for the BCNU treatment group and 40 wk for the placebo group ($p = 0.001$) (Fig. 6). At 1 yr, 63% of the patients treated with BCNU-polymers were alive vs 19% for the control group; at two years, the differences remained highly significant with 31% of the Gliadel® group surviving vs 6% of the control group. Moreover, even after 3 yr, 25% of patients treated with Gliadel® were alive vs 6% of the control group. Based on these highly promising results, a larger phase III study involving 240 patients was carried out to fully assess the role of Gliadel® in initial therapy. This study by Westphal et al. *(70a)*, confirmed the previous findings and showed a statistically significant improvement in survival when patients were treated with Gliadel® initially. This benefit was maintained over a 3 yr follow-up period.

3.2. Potential Drug–Polymer Combinations

3.2.1. Taxol

Taxol, a microtubule-binding agent, has been shown to have tumoricidal activity against several human neoplasms, including ovarian, breast, and nonsmall cell lung cancer. While this chemotherapeutic agent does not cross an intact BBB, it has been shown to exhibit tumoricidal activity against rat and human glioma cells in vitro *(9,51)*. Incorporation of taxol into a biodegradable polymer allowed the BBB to be bypassed, and resulted in a threefold increase in the survival time of rats challenged with intracranial 9L glioma *(66)*. In addition, the implant maintained tumoricidal taxol concentrations within the brain for more than 1 mo after implantation *(66)*. Currently, clinical trials utilizing taxol-loaded polymers are in progress for ovarian cancer, and trials involving brain tumor patients are being planned in the nearby future.

3.2.2. Cyclophosphamide and 4-HC

The chemotherapeutic agent cyclophosphamide has been widely used for the treatment of systemic malignancies. Local delivery of cytoxan is not feasible because it requires enzymatic activation by the hepatic p450 cytochrome oxidase system. The active metabolite of cytoxan, 4-hydroperoxycyclophosphamide (4-HC), poorly crosses the BBB, which necessitates high doses of the parent compound. However, high doses of cytoxan result in severe systemic toxicity. Two reports have demonstrated the use of 4-HC against intracranial F98 gliomas in rat models *(17,28)*. In these studies, 4-HC was incorporated into a polymer matrix consisting of FAD-SA, extending the median survival of treated rats to 77 vs 14 d for the controls.

Recently, it was demonstrated that L-buthionine sulfoximine (BSO) potentiates the antitumor effect of 4-HC in the rat 9L glioma model *(59)*. BSO inhibits glutathione synthesis and modulates tumor resistance to some akylating agents. The glutathione *S*-transferase (GST) enzyme system seems to play an important role in the inactivation of alkylating agents by catalyzing their reaction with glutathione to produce stable, nontoxic conjugates. Increased cellular GST activity or glutathione content has been shown to be associated with resistance to alkylating agents in a variety of human and animal malignancies. Rats challenged with intracranial 9L gliosarcoma and treated with 20% 4-HC and 10% BSO co-loaded in the same FAD-SA polymer had a median survival time 4.6 times greater than that of rats treated with empty polymers (61.5 d vs 13 d). In contrast, the median survival of rats treated with polymers containing only 4-HC was 2.3 times greater than that of controls, and systemic BSO therapy did not improve this survival time. Furthermore, this method of treatment may be safer than systemic administration of BSO, because the study demonstrated that local delivery of BSO within the brain did not deplete glutathione levels systemically.

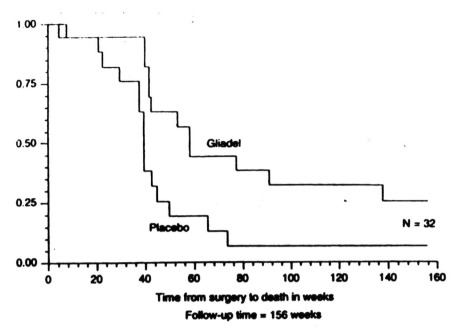

Fig. 6. Kaplan–Meier survival curve for patients with initial therapy for grade III and grade IV gliomas treated with BCNU-loaded polymer implants or placebo polymer. (Reprinted with permission from ref. *64*.)

3.2.3. 5-Fluorouracil

5-Fluorouracil (5-FU), a pyrimidine analog, interferes with the conversion of deoxyuridylic acid to thymidylic acid, thus depriving the cell of one of the essential precursors for DNA synthesis. One of the earlier polymeric delivery systems for intratumoral 5-FU chemotherapy involved the incorporation of 5-FU, adriamycin, or mitomycin C into a matrix consisting of "glassified monomers" with 10% polymetacrylic methyl acid *(30)*. These agents were implanted into 55 patients and achieved a 47% 1-yr survival rate in patients with malignant gliomas. A later study utilized 5-FU-loaded poly(lactic acid-co-glycolic acid) (PLAGA) microspheres in a rat C6 glioma model *(43)*. Intratumoral implantation of these microspheres decreased the mortality of C6 tumor-bearing rats. This effect was attributed to the local and sustained delivery of 5-FU, because systemic administration is ineffective against brain tumors.

Furthermore, Choti et al. *(13)* demonstrated that fluorodeoxyuridine, a related compound, can be successfully delivered from FAD-SA polymers in vitro and in vivo. This study was based on the results of another work in which the continuous infusion of fluorodeoxyuridine from a Medtronic SynchroMed pump was used to treat a single patient with an intracranial metastases from renal cell carcinoma *(14)*. A complete response was achieved in 3 mo and maintained for 22 mo.

3.2.4. Adriamycin

Adriamycin is an anthracycline antibiotic that has tumoricidal activity. The antineoplastic activity is based on its ability to intercalate with DNA, resulting in strand scission and double-stranded cross breaks *(10)*. In one study, an Ommaya reservoir was used after surgical resection to deliver adriamycin to the tumor bed in 22 patients with malignant gliomas *(27)*. A total dose of 5.0 mg in 0.5-mg aliquots was intermittently injected into the Ommaya reservoir. This treatment was combined with cobalt-60 irradiation and immunotherapy. The patients achieved a 1-yr survival rate of 41% and a 2-yr survival rate of 13%. In comparison to the intravenous injection, local delivery increased the concentration of adriamycin up to 38 times. The drug also penetrated within 3 cm into the brain parenchyma.

EVAc needles have been utilized in the development of a polymer-based delivery system for adriamycin *(37)*. This polymer formulation delivered adriamycin with zero-order kinetic release in vitro and significantly inhibited growth of brain tumor xenografts in nude mice. Further animal studies are currently underway, incorporating adriamycin into pCPP-SA.

3.2.5. Methotrexate

The first large-scale trials of intratumoral methotrexate (MTX) were reported in 1987, in which 269 patients were divided into five groups to receive treatment as follows: 1. surgical resection; 2. resection and radiotherapy; 3. resection, radiotherapy; 4. resection and systemic and local chemotherapy; and 5. resection, radiotherapy, and systemic and local chemotherapy *(16)*. The implantation of a Spongostan matrix soaked with MTX was the mode of local delivery. The longest median survivals were achieved when resection, radiotherapy, and systemic chemotherapy were combined. The median survivals for Groups 3 and 5 were 83 and 75 wk, respectively. Median survivals for Groups 1, 2, and 4 were 10.2, 34.8, and 36.8 wk, respectively. These results suggest that local MTX had little effect on overall survival, but there were more long-term survivors in the group receiving local MTX than in the other groups.

Data from clinical trials have shown that intratumoral MTX is minimally toxic *(52,70)*, but there are case reports of toxicity associated with this drug. One patient developed an abulic-hypokinetic syndrome and left hemiparesis after receiving intraventricular MTX for meningeal carcinoma *(63)*. Two patients have also been reported to have formation of enlarged cysts at the site of intracavitary therapy with MTX administered from an Ommaya reservoir *(56)*.

The use of polymeric drug delivery devices to administer MTX has been described in two experimental reports. In one study, rats harboring intracranial ethylnitrosurea-induced tumors were treated with MTX delivered from a polymethylmethacrylate pellet *(49)*. The survival of the treated rats improved 69% compared with that of the controls. In the second study, a polylactide-MTX formulation significantly inhibited glioma growth in the rat flank *(75)*.

MTX has been modified by covalent linkage to dextran via an amide bond. This modification confers biological stability upon the compound and resistance to degradation. The MTX conjugate should have a slower elimination rate in the brain than unmodified MTX and have the ability to diffuse farther into the extracellular matrix. Intratumoral delivery of the MTX-dextran amide conjugate to rats with intracranial glial tumors improved the survival of rats with tumors compared with that of controls *(15)*.

3.2.6. Other Agents

Several other drugs have been incorporated into polymers for the treatment of intracranial neoplasms. Carboplatin, a second-generation platinum analog that is less neurotoxic than its parent compound, cisplatin, has been incorporated into a biodegradable polyanhydride matrix consisting of a FAD-SA. The carboplatin FAD-SA matrix improved median survival 3.3-fold in rats with intracranial F98 gliomas when implanted intracranially *(46)*. Camptothecin, an inhibitor of DNA-replicating enzyme topoisomerase I, significantly prolonged survival in rats challenged with intracranial 9L gliosarcoma; 59% of treated rats remained long-term survivors *(68)*. Systemically administered camptothecin had no effect on survival in this study.

Minocycline is a broad-spectrum antibiotic with known antiangiogenic properties. When incorporated into EVAc polymers, minocycline inhibited neovascularization in the rabbit cornea stimulated by a VX2 carcinoma implant *(62)*. The intracranial implantation of these controlled-release polymers in rats challenged with 9L gliosarcoma tumors prolonged survival and showed a synergistic effect with systemically administered BCNU *(69)*.

Vasogenic edema is induced by malignant gliomas secondary to breakdown of the blood-brain barrier. High-dose corticosteroid therapy usually alleviates the cerebral edema but is associated with major side effects, such as osteoporosis, diabetes, weight gain, and myopathies. It has been demonstrated that dexamethasone can be released from a controlled-release polymer for up to 21 d when intracranially implanted in a rat *(50,57)*. This implant was as effective as systemic dexamethasone in ameliorating cerebral edema in a rat model of tumor-induced edema.

Finally, cytokines, such as IL-2, when delivered locally via microspheres, have been shown to be highly effective in protecting animals challenged with fatal tumor doses *(21,25)*.

An up to date summary of the preclinical studies with various polymer-drug formulations for the treatment of brain tumors is presented in Table 1.

4. FUTURE DIRECTIONS

4.1. Convection-Enhanced Delivery Systems

Fluid convection is currently an area of active investigation for drug delivery to the CNS. Whereas diffusion of a compound in a tissue depends solely on the free concentration gradient and the diffusivity of that compound in that tissue, convection results from a simple pressure gradient and is independent of molecular weight. Convection can be used to supplement diffusion for distribution of certain compounds to treat much larger volumes of brain than can be achieved by diffusion alone and with a greater pharmacokinetic advantage over systemic administration. Several studies have shown that interstitial infusion of a drug into the cerebral white matter creates a pressure gradient that increases convection and can be used to deliver high concentrations of drugs to large regions of the brain without functional or structural damage *(3,32,36)*. Convection-enhanced drug delivery (CEDD) of excitotoxic agents has been used in the treatment of Parkinsonian symptoms in nonhuman primates *(38)*. Recently, a study has demonstrated the utilization of diffusion-weighted MRI (DWMRI) to monitor the effects of intratumoral convection-enhanced drug delivery in three brain tumor patients treated with Taxol *(41)*. This was the first report of the application of DWMRI for noninvasive monitoring of CEDD into brain tumors. In this report, the authors showed that DWMRI enables the observation of early changes in water diffusion in tissues, and, therefore, the extent and effect of the convection wave. In addition, DWMRI revealed that the three patients in this study had different diffusion characteristics suggesting that this technique might enable the distinction between variable response rates of different patients.

4.2. Microchip Drug Delivery

A novel and potentially powerful method of complex drug delivery involves the use of newly developed microchips *(54)* (Fig. 7). This technology depends on a solid-state silicon microchip that can provide controlled release of a single or multiple chemical substances on demand. The release mechanism is based on the electrochemical dissolution of a thin anode membrane covering multiple microreservoirs. The reservoirs can be filled with solids, liquids, or gels, and the release profile can be tailored either sequentially or simultaneously from a single device. A microbattery, multiplexing circuitry, and memory can be integrated onto the device, allowing it be mounted on a tip of small probe, implanted in the brain or spine, or swallowed. With proper selection of a biocompatible device material, this "pharmacy-on-a-chip" may be used to deliver up to 1000 different drugs on a variety of time schedules.

5. CONCLUSION

The delivery of drugs to tumors of the central nervous system has been a challenging area of research for many years. The two major obstacles, overcoming the physiological barriers of the brain and achieving high drug concentrations within the tumor bed, have prompted an intensive search for alternative routes of drug delivery. Within the confines of these limitations, biodegradable polymers have allowed a new approach for delivering pharmaceutical agents to the brain. Gliadel®, a BCNU impregnated polymer, represents the first successful drug developed as a result of this technology. In clinical trials, it has been shown to be safe and effective against malignant brain tumors. As a result

Table 1
Preclinical Studies With Various Polymer/Drug Formulations for the Treatment of Brain Tumors

Polymer/drug formulation	Mechanism of drug's antineoplastic activity	Extension in median survival in 9L or F98 glioma model	Refs.
pCPP:SA (20:80)/3.8% BCNU	DNA alkylation	127%	58
pCPP:SA (20:80)/20% BCNU	DNA alkylation	>1,200%	58
pCPP:SA (20:80)/20% taxol	Inhibition of microtubule depolymerization	215%	66
pCPP:SA (20:80)/50% camptothecin	Inhibition of the DNA-replicating enzyme topoisomerase 1	306%	68
pCPP:SA (20:80)/5% adriamycin	Intercalation with DNA leading to strand scission and double-stranded cross-breaks	137%	67
pCPP:SA (20:80)/5% carboplatin	Binding to DNA leading to interstrand cross-links	Untested in 9L or F98 model	45
pCPP:SA (20:80)/1.25 D₃ analogs	Upregulation of cell-cycle control proteins and inhibition of angiogenesis	Untested in 9L or F98 model	46
pCPP:SA (20:80)/IUdR	Radiosensitization via incorporation into replicating DNA	Untested in 9L or F98 model	71
pCPP:SA (20:80)/50% minocycline	Inhibition of tumor angiogenesis	Testing in progress	
EVAc/50% minocycline	Inhibition of tumor angiogenesis	331% (in combination with IPBCNU)	69
FAD:SA (50:50)/5-FU	Interferes with DNA synthesis	Untested in 9L or F98 model	13
FAD:SA (50:50)/5% carboplatin	Binding to DNA leading to interstrand cross-links	150%	46
FAD:SA (50:50)/1% methotrexate	Antimetabolite	140%	15
FAD:SA (50:50)/20% 4-HC	DNA alkylation	121%	59
FAD:SA (50:50)/20% 4-HC and BSO	DNA alkylation and inhibition of glutathione synthesis	200%	59
Polymer microspheres/ cytokine IL-2	Promotion of antitumoral immune response	100%	25

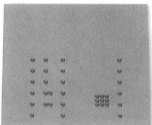
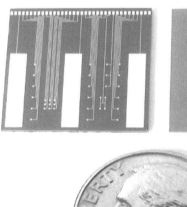
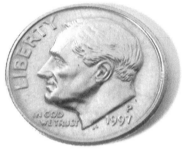

Fig. 7. Microchip with dime caption. Front (left) and back views of a new microchip for the controlled release of chemicals. The dots between the three large bars (cathodes) on the front are the caps (anodes) covering the reservoirs that hold chemicals. An electrical voltage applied between a reservoir cap and a cathode causes a reaction that dissolves the cap, releasing the chemical. The back view shows the larger openings for each reservoir through which chemicals are deposited (these openings are sealed by a waterproof material after the reservoirs are filled). (Photo by Paul Horwitz, Atlantic Photo Service, Inc.)

of Gliadel®, numerous clinical trials involving other new drug-polymer combinations are currently under way. Moreover, recent advances in biotechnology are leading the way in the development of new approaches. The application of local and controlled drug delivery to the central nervous system has represented an advance in the field of neuro-oncology in that it allows for the rational application of therapeutic agents.

ACKNOWLEDGMENTS

The reserach presented in this work has been supported in part by the National Cooperative Drug Discovery Group (UO1-CA52857 and AI 47739) of the National Cancer Institute (NCI-NIH), Bethesda, Maryland. Dr. Lesniak is a neurosurgical fellow whose research is supported by a grant from the American Brain Tumor Association, Chicago, IL. James Frazier is supported by a grant from the Howard Hughes Medical Institute, Bethesda, Maryland.

REFERENCES

1. Abbott N.J., Romero I.A. 1996. Transporting therapeutics across the blood-brain barrier. *Mol. Med. Today* **3:**106–113.
2. Barker F.G., Chang S.M., Gutin P.H., Malec M.K., McDermott M.W., Prados M.D., Wilson C.B. 1998. Survival and functional status after resection of recurrent glioblastoma multiforme. *Neurosurgery* **42:**709–723.
3. Bobo R.H., Laske D.W., Akbasak A., Morrison P.F., Dedrick R.L., Oldfield E.H. 1994. Convection-enhanced delivery of macromolecules in the brain. *Proc. Natl. Acad. Sci. USA* **91:**2076–2080.
4. Brem H., Tamargo R.H., Olivi A., Pinn M., Weingart J.D., Wharam M., Epstein J.I. 1994. Biodegradable polymers for controlled delivery of chemotherapy with and without radiation therapy in the monkey brain. *J. Neurosurg.* **80:**283–290.
5. Brem H., Mahaley M.S. Jr., Vick N.A., Black K.L., Schold S.C. Jr., Burger P.C., et al. 1991. Interstitial chemotherapy with drug polymer implants for the treatment of recurrent gliomas. *J. Neurosurg.* **74:**441–446.

6. Brem H., Piantadosi S., Burger P.C., Walker M., Selker R., Vick N.A., et al. 1995. Placebo-controlled trial of safety and efficacy of intraoperative controlled delivery of biodegradable polymers of chemotherapy for recurrent gliomas. *Lancet* **345:**1008–1012.

7. Brem H., Ewend M.G., Piantadosi S., Greenhoot J., Burger P.C., Sisti M. 1995. The safety of interstitial chemotherapy with BCNU-loaded polymer in the treatment of newly diagnosed malignant gliomas. *Phase I trial. J. Neurooncol.* **26:** 111–123.

8. Brem H., Langer R. 1996. Polymer-based drug delivery to the brain. *Sci. Med.* **3:**52–61.

9. Cahan M.A., Walter K.A., Colvin O.M., Brem H. 1994. Cytotoxicity of taxol in vitro against human and rat malignant brain tumors. *Cancer Chemother. Pharmacol.* **33:**441–444.

10. Calabresi P., Parks R.E. 1985. Chemotherapy of neoplastic diseases, in *The Pharmacological Basis of Therapeutics,* 7 ed. (Gilman, A.G., Goodman L.S., Rall T.W., Murad F. eds), MacMillan, New York, pp.1240–1306.

11. Chandler W.F., Greenberg H.S., Ensminger W.D., Diaz R.F., Junck L.R., Hood T.W., et al. 1988. Use of implantable pump systems for intraarterial, intraventricular, and intratumoral treatment of malignant brain tumors. *Ann. N. Y. Acad. Sci.* **531:**206–212.

12. Chasin M. 1990. Polyanhydrides as drug delivery systems, in *Biodegradable Polymers as Drug Delivery Systems* (Chasin M., Langer R., eds.), Marcel Dekker, New York, pp. 43–70.

13. Choti M.A., Saenz J., Yang X., Brem H. 1995. Intrahepatic FUdR delivered from biodegradable polymer in experimental liver metastases from colorectal carcinoma. *Proc. of A.A.C.R.* **36:**309.

14. Damascelli B., Marchiano A., Frigerio L.F., Salvetti M., Spreafico C., Garbagnati F., et al. 1991. Flexibility and efficacy of automatic continuous fluorodeoxyuridine infusion in metastases from a renal cell carcinoma. *Cancer* **68:**995–998.

15. Dang W., Colvin O.M., Brem H., Saltzman W.M. 1994. Covalent coupling of methotrexate to dextran enhances the penetrations of cytotoxicity into tissue-like matrix. *Cancer Res.* **54:**1729–1735.

16. Diemath H.E. 1987. Lokale anwendung von zytostatika nach exstripation von glioblastomen. *Wien. Klin. Wochenshr.* **99:**674–676.

17. Domb A., Bogdansky S., Olivi A., Judy K., Dureza C., Lenartz D., et al. 1991. Controlled delivery of water soluble and hydrolytically unstable anti-cancer drugs for polymeric implants. *Polymer Preprints* **32:**219–220.

18. Elliott P.J., Hayward N.J., Dean R.L., Blunt D.G., Bartus R.T. 1996. Intravenous RMP-7 selectively increases uptake of carboplatin in experimental brain tumors. *Cancer Res.* **56:**3998–4005.

19. Fung L.K., Ewend M.G., Sills A., Sipos E.P., Thompson R., Watts M., et al. 1998. Pharmacokinetics of interstitial delivery of carmustine, 4-hydroperoxycyclophosphamide, and paclitaxl from a biodegraable polymer implant in the monkey brain. *Cancer Res.* **58:**672–684.

20. Gabizon A. 1994. Liposomal anthracyclines. *Hematol. Oncol. Clin. North Am.* **8:**431–450.

21. Golumbek P.T., Azhari R., Jaffe E.M., Levistky H.I., Lazenby A., Leong K., Pardoll D.M. 1993. Controlled release, biodegradable cytokine depots: new approach in cancer vaccine design. *Cancer Res.* **53:**5841–5844.

22. Green S.B., Byar D.P., Walker D.P., Pistenmaa D.A., Alexander E. Jr, Batzdorf U., et al. 1983. Comparisons of carmustine, procarbazine, and high-dose methylprednisolone as additions to surgery and radiotherapy for the treatment of malignant glioma. *Cancer Treat. Rep.* **67:**121–132.

23. Gref R., Minamitake Y., Peracchia M.T., Trubetskoy V., Torchilin V., Langer R. 1994. Biodegradable long-circulating polymeric nanospheres. *Science* **263:**1600–1603.

24. Grossman S.A., Reinhard C., Colvin O.M., Chasin M., Brundrett R., Tamargo R.J., Brem H. 1992. The intracerebral distribution of BCNU delivered by surgically implanted biodegradable polymers. *J. Neurosurg.* **76:**640–647.

25. Hanes J., Sills A.K., Zhao Z. 2001. Controlled local delivery of interleukin-2 by biodegradable polymers protects animals from experimental brain tumors and liver tumors. *Pharm. Res.* **18:**899–906.

26. Heruth K.T. 1988. Medtronic SynchroMed drug administration system. *Ann. N.Y. Acad. Sci.* **531:**72–75.

27. Itoh Y. 1980. Treatment of malignant brain tumors by local injection of adriamycin. *Nippon Ika Daigaku Zasshi* **47:** 527–537.

28. Judy K., Olivi A., Buahin K.G., Domb A., Epstein J.I., Colvin O.M., Brem H. 1995. Effectiveness of controlled release of a cyclophosphamide derivative with polymers against rat glioma. *J. Neurosurg.* **82:**481–6.

29. Kornblith P.L., Walker M. 1988. Chemotherapy for malignant gliomas. *J. Neurosurg.* **68:**1–17.

30. Kubo O., Himuro H., Inoue N., Tajika Y., Tajika T., Tohyama T., et al. 1986. Treatment of malignant brain tumors with slowly releasing anticancer drug-polymer composites. *No Shinkei Geka* **14:**1189–1195.

31. Langer R., Folkman J. 1976. Polymers for the sustained release of proteins and other macromolecules. *Nature* **263:**797–800.

32. Laske D.W., Morrison P.F., Lieberman D.M., Corthesy M.E., Reynold J.C., Stewart-Henney P.A., et al. 1997. Chronic interstitial infusion of protein to primate brain: determination of drug distribution and clearance with single-photon emission computerized tomography imaging. *J. Neurosurg.* **87:**586–594.

33. Legler J.M., Gloeckler Ries L.A., Smith M.A., Warren J.L., Heineman E.F., Kaplan R.S., Linet M.S. 1999. Brain and other central nervous system cancers: recent trends in incidence and mortality. *J. Natl. Cancer Inst.* **91:**1382–1390.

34. Leong K.W., Brott B.C., Langer R. 1985. Bioerodible polyanhydrides as drug-carrier matrices. I. Characterization, degradation, and release characteristics. *J. Biomed. Mater. Res.* **19:**941–955.

35. Leong K.W., D'Amore P.D., Marletta M., Langer R. 1986. Bioerodible polyanhydrides as drug-carrier matrices. II. Biocompatibility and chemical reactivity. *J. Biomed. Mater. Res.* **20:**51–64.

36. Lieberman D.M., Laske D.W., Morrison P.F., Bankiewicz K.S., Oldfield E.H. 1995. Convection-enhanced distribution of large molecules in gray matter during interstitial drug infusion. *J. Neurosurg.* **82:**1021–1029.

37. Lin S.Y., Cheng L.F., Lui W.Y., Chen C.F., Han S.H. 1989. Tumoricidal effect of controlled-release polymeric needle devices containing adriamycin hydrochloride in tumor-bearing mice. *Biomater. Artif. Cells Artif. Org.* **17:**189–203.

38. Lonser R.R., Corthesy M.E., Morrison P.F., Gogate N., Oldfield E.H. 1999. Convection-enhanced selective excitotoxic ablation of the neurons of the globus pallidus internus for treatment of parkinsonism in honhuman primates. *J. Neurosurg.* **91:**294–302.

39. Loo T.L., Dion R.L., Dixon R.L., Rall D.P. 1966. The antitumor agent, 1,3-bis(2-chloroethyl)-1-nitrosourea. *J. Pharm. Sci.* **55:**492–497.

40. Lord P., Allami H., Davis M., Diaz R., Heck P., Fischell R. 1988. MiniMed Technologies Programmable Implantable Infusion System. *Ann. N.Y. Acad. Sci.* **531:**66–71.

41. Mardor Y., Roth Y., Lidar Z., Jonas T., Pfeffer R., Maier S.E, et al. 2001. Monitoring response to convection-enhanced taxol delivery in brain tumor patients using diffusion-weighted magnetic resonance imaging. *Cancer Res.* **61:**4971–4973.

42. Menei P., Benoit J.P., Boisdron-Celle M., Fournier D., Mercier P., Guy G. 1994. Drug targeting into the central nervous system by stereotactic implantation of biodegradable microspheres. *Neurosurgery* **34:**1058–1064.

43. Menei P., Boisdron-Celle M., Croue A., Guy G., Benoit J.P. 1996. Effect of stereotactic implantation of biodegradable 5-fluorouracil-loaded microspheres in healthy and C6 glioma-bearing rats. *Neurosurgery* **39:**117–124.

44. Mohan D.S., Suh J.H., Phan J.L., Kupelian P.A., Cohen B.H., Barnett G.H. 1998. Outcome in elderly patients undergoing definitive surgery and radiation therapy for supratentorial glioblastoma multiforme at a tertiary institution. *Int. J. Rad. Oncol. Biol. Phys.* **42:**981–987.

45. Olivi A., Gilbert M., Duncan K.L., Corden B., Lenartz D., Brem H. 1993. Direct delivery of platinum-based antineoplastics to the central nervous system: A toxicity and ultrastructural study. *Cancer Chemother. Pharmacol.* **31:** 449–454.

46. Olivi A., Ewend M.G., Utsuki T., Tyler B., Domb A.J., Brat D.J., Brem H. 1996. Interstitial delivery of carboplatin via biodegradable polymers is effective against experimental glioma in the rat. *Cancer Chemother. Pharmacol.* **39:**90–96.

47. Pardridge W.M. 1999. Vector-mediated drug delivery to the brain. *Adv. Drug Deliv. Rev.* **36:**299–321.

48. Prokai L., Prokai-Tatrai K., Bodor N. 2000. Targeting drugs to the brain by redox chemical delivery systems. *Med. Res. Rev.* **20:**367–416.

49. Rama B., Mandel T., Jansen J., Dingeldein E., Mennel H.D. 1987. The intraneoplastic chemotherapy in a rat brain tumor model utilizing methotrexate-polymethylmethacrylate-pellets. *Acta Neurochir (Wien)* **87:**70–75.

50. Reinhard C.S., Randomsky M.L., Saltzman W.M., Hilton J., Brem H. 1991. Polymeric controlled release of dexamethasone in normal rat brain. *J. Contr. Rel.* **16:**331–340.

51. Rowinsky E.K., Burke P.J., Karp J.E., Tucker R.W., Ettinger D.S., Donehower R.S. 1989. Phase I and pharmacodynamic study of taxol in refractory acute leukemias. *Cancer Res.* **49:**4640–4647.

52. Rubin R.C., Ommaya A.K., Henderson E.S., Bering E.A., Rall D.P. 1966. Cerebrospinal fluid perfusion for central nervous system neoplasms. *Neurology* **16:**680–692.

53. Sanovich E., Bartus R.T., Friden P.M., Dean R.L., Le H.Q., Brightman M.W.. 1995. Pathway across blood-brain barrier opened by the bradykinin RMP-7. *Brain Res.* **705:**125–35.

54. Santini J.T., Cima M.J., Langer R. 1999. A controlled-release microchip. *Nature* **397:**335–338.

55. Shapiro W.R., Green S.B., Burger P.C., Selker R.G., VanGilder J.C., Robertson J.T, et al. 1992. A randomized comparison of intra-arterial versus intravenous BCNU, with or without intravenous 5-fluorouracial, for newly diagnosed patients with malignant glioma. *J. Neurosurg.* **76:**772–781.

56. Shimura T., Nakazawa S., Ikeda Y., Node Y. 1992. Cyst formation following local chemotherapy of malignant brain tumor: A clinicopathological study of two cases. *No Shinkei Geka* **20:**1179–1183.

57. Sills A.K., Tamargo R.J., Brem H. 1990. Reduction of peritumoral brain edema by intracranial polymer implant. *Surg. Forum* **41:**516–518.

58. Sipos E.P., Tyler B., Piantadosi S., Burger P.C., Brem H. 1997. Optimizing interstitial delivery of BCNU from controlled release polymers for the treatment of brain tumors. *Cancer Chemother. Pharmacol.* **39:**383–389.

59. Sipos E.P., Witham T.F., Ratan R., Baraban J., Li K.W., Piantadosi S., Brem H. 2001. L-buthionine sulfoximine potentiates the antitumor effect of 4-hydroperoxycyclophosphamide when administered locally in a rat glioma model. *Neurosurg.* **48:**392–400.

60. Tamargo R.J., Myseros J.S., Epstein J.I., Yang M.B., Chasin M., Brem H. 1993. Interstitial chemotherapy of the 9L gliosarcoma: controlled release polymers for drug delivery in the brain. *Cancer Res.* **53:**329–333.

61. Tamargo R.J., Sills A.J., Reinhard C.S., Pinn M.L., Long D.M., Brem H. 1991. Interstitial delivery of dexamethasone in the brain for the reduction of peritumoral edema. *J. Neurosurg.* **74:**956–961.

62. Tamargo R.J., Bok R.A., Brem H. 1991. Angiogenesis inhibition by minocycline. *Cancer Res.* **51:**675–675.

63. Uldry P.A., Teta D., Regli L. 1991. Necrose cerebrate focalize secondaire a une chimiotherapie intraventriculaire au methotrexate. *Neurochirurgie* **37:**72–74.

64. Valtonen S., Timonen U., Toivanen P., Kalimo H., Kivipelto L., Heiskanen O., et al. 1997. Interstitial chemotherapy with carmustine-loaded polymers for high-grade gliomas: a randomized double-blind study. *Neurosurg.* **41**:44–48.

65. Walker M.D., Green S.B., Byar D.P., Alexander E. Jr., Batzdorf U., W.H. Brooks, et al. 1980. Randomized comparisons of radiotherapy and nitrosoureas for the treatment of malignant glioma after surgery. *N. Engl. J. Med.* **303**:1323–1329.

66. Walter K., Cahan M., Gur A., Tyler B., Hilton J., Colvin O.M, et al. 1994. Interstitial taxol delivered from a biodegradable polymer implant against experimental malignant glioma. *Cancer Res.* **54**:2207–2212.

67. Watts M.C., Lesniak M.S., Burke M., Samdani A., Tyler B., Brem H. 1997. Controlled release of adriamycin in the treatment of malignant glioma. Presented at the American Association of Neurological Surgeons Annual Meeting, Denver, CO, April.

68. Weingart J., Thompson R., Tyler B., Colvin O.M., Brem H. 1995. Local delivery of the topoisomerase I inhibitor camptothecin prolongs survival in the rat intracranial 9L gliosarcoma model. *Int. J. Cancer* **62**:605–609.

69. Weingart J., Sipos E.P., Brem H. 1995. The role of minocycline in the treatment of intracranial 9L glioma. *J. Neurosurg.* **82**:635–640.

70. Weiss S.R., Raskind R. 1969. Treatment of malignant brain tumors by local methotrexate: A preliminary report. *Int. Surg.* **51**:149–155.

70a. Westphal M., Hilt D.C., Bortey E., et al. 2003. A phase III trial of local chemotherapy with biodegradable carmustine (BCNU) wafers (Gliadel wafers) in patients with primary glioma. *Neurooncol.* **5**:79–88.

71. Williams J.A., Sills A., Zhao., Suh K.W., Tyler B., DiMeco F., et al. 1997. Implantable biodegradable polymers for IUdR radiosensitization of experimental human malignant glioma. *J. Neurooncol.* **32**:181–192.

72. Williams P.C., Henner W.D., Roman-Goldstein S., Dahlborg S.A., Brummett R.E., Tableman M., et al. 1995. Toxicity and efficacy of carboplatin and etoposide in conjuction with disruption of the blood-brain barrier in the treatment of intracranial neoplasms. *Neurosurgery* **37**:17–28.

73. Wu M.P., Tamada J.A., Brem H., Langer R.. 1994. In vivo versus in vitro degradation of controlled release polymers for intracranial surgical therapy. *J. Biomed. Mater. Res.* **28**:387–295.

74. Yang M.B., Tamargo R.J., Brem H. 1989. Controlled delivery of 1,3-bis(2-chloroethyl)-1-nitrosourea from ethylene-vinyl acetate copolymer. *Cancer Res.* **49**:5103–5107.

75. Zeller W.J., Bauer S., Remmele T., Wowra B., Sturm V., Stricker H. 1990. Interstitial chemotherapy of experimental gliomas. *Cancer Treat. Rev.* **17**:183–189.

19

Rational Design and Development of Targeted Brain Tumor Therapeutics

Francis Ali-Osman, Henry S. Friedman, Gamil R. Antoun,
David Reardon, Darell D. Bigner, and John K. Buolamwini

1. INTRODUCTION

The majority of agents currently used to treat patients with tumors of the central nervous system (CNS) are cytotoxins, developed initially for their ability to kill cells directly. Subsequent drugs were derived by an analog strategy in which relatively small chemical modifications were made to the parent drug to either increase its potency or decrease its systemic toxicity, often with little to no change in the drug's mechanism of action. This approach has yielded chemotherapeutic agents, notably DNA damaging agents, such as 2-chloroethylnitrosoureas (CENUs), nitrogen mustard-type drugs, and the platinum analogs that have been the mainstay of brain tumor chemotherapy to date.

In the last two decades, however, largely as the result of the advances in our understanding of the molecular nature of cancer and of the mechanisms underlying tumor response and/or resistance to therapy, coupled with the sequencing of the human genome and the exciting developments in genomic technology, anticancer drug development has entered a new era that is driven by the rational targeting of molecular alterations and defects in the cancer cell. The drug discovery paradigms and strategies required in the rational discovery and development of targeted anticancer therapeutics are different from those used in the past to discover cytotoxic anticancer drugs. In this chapter, we will provide a brief overview of these strategies and discuss some of the molecular targets that are being, or have the potential to be exploited for treating tumors of the CNS.

2. STRUCTURE-BASED RATIONAL DRUG DISCOVERY FOR BRAIN TUMORS

The rapid and explosive increase in knowledge of the cellular and molecular biology of cancer and the advances in the science and technology of structural and functional genomics have led to the unraveling of a plethora of molecular and cellular defects and other abnormalities in tumors that provide novel targets for the rational development of novel therapeutics for cancer, including brain tumors *(24,25,38,71,117)*. The exploitation of these advances to develop new anticancer therapies requires the integration of multiple disciplines. Figure 1 shows an integrated scheme of the different components of rational drug discovery of targeted anticancer agents. The most critical part of this process is the identification and credentialing of the molecular defect or cellular pathway to be targeted. Frequently, the target is a protein that is mutated, abnormally expressed, or otherwise altered in the tumor relative to normal tissues and is critical to the genesis, progression, survival, and/or response of the tumor to therapy. Identification of such targets has received a major boost by the

From: *Contemporary Cancer Research: Brain Tumors*
Edited by: F. Ali-Osman © Humana Press Inc., Totowa, NJ

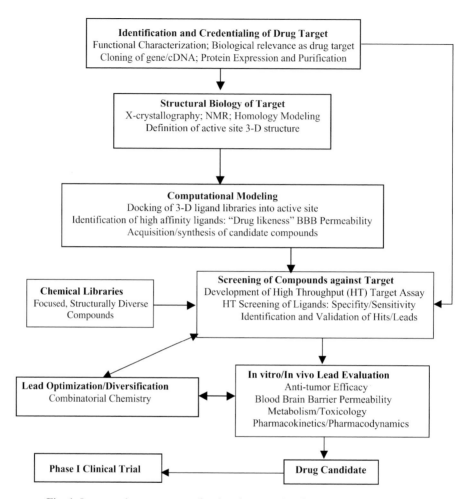

Fig. 1. Integrated components of rational targeted anti-cancer drug discovery.

advances in high throughput technologies, functional genomics and proteomics, and the new knowl-edge being generated by molecular profiling of CNS tumors *(29,36,113,121,139,146)*. Another important step in the rational anticancer drug discovery process is the use of computer modeling and related strategies to examine the potential of a molecule/ligand to bind to the target, a process that requires knowledge of the three-dimensional (3-D) structure of the target *(97)* and the availability of 3-D libraries of molecules and chemical fragments. The goal is to identify compounds with the potential to bind to the target with high affinity and specificity. For this, the 3-D structure of a target is obtained primarily by X-ray crystallography, high-field magnetic resonance (NMR) spectroscopy, or homology modeling. Where the target is novel and its structure not yet elucidated, the use of crystallography and NMR spectroscopy to accomplish this can be an expensive undertaking. Homol-ogy modeling, on the other hand, despite its limitations, provides a much less expensive alternative with which to obtain 3-D structural approximations that provide a starting point for such structural analyses. Using this technique, initial 3-D models of proteins and other macromolecules can be obtained based on homologous structures, and is thus a cost-effective approach with which to exploit the large numbers of potential new drug targets that are being uncovered by high-throughput genomic and proteomic strategies. Molecules identified by the computational modeling approach are subjected to experimental testing for biological activity and the results used to create a pharmacophore for further development. In addition to the computational approach, a frequently used and highly effective strategy is to screen libraries of structurally highly diverse compounds, consisting of tens or even hundreds of thousands of compounds, for their ability to bind to the target, or to modify or inhibit its activity and/or function in a therapeutically desirable manner. Such high volume compound screening requires high-throughput technologies, including, one for assaying target inhibition and or binding. Hits identified from the high-throughput screening are examined more extensively for biological activity and specificity. A set of criteria, based on physico-chemical properties and theoretical predictions are used to define "drug-likeness," *(3,4,89,99,100,115,165,177)* and together with the degree of target inhibitory activity and specificity, are used to rank candidates with the highest potential for pharmacological activity. Drug-likeness is generally based on chemical properties of the compounds that include the number of hydrogen bonds, molecular weight, formal charge, number of rotatable bonds, and the presence of pharmacophoric groups, such as, amines, amidines, carboxylic groups, and guanidines. These reductionist criteria have been very useful in the prioritization of compounds with physiological effects.

A major challenge unique to the design of drugs for treating CNS malignancies is that the compounds have the ability to cross the blood–brain barrier *(50,52)*. This is best defined by the water/octanol partition coefficient, Log P, of the molecule. Theoretical Log P values can be computed from the structures of the inhibitors and those of the lead candidates are then confirmed experimentally. Lead active compounds from the high throughput screenings that meet the criteria of drug-likeness and blood–brain barrier permeability are then further optimized by structural diversification, primarily by combinatorial chemistry, on the lead scaffolds. The resulting combinatorial libraries are subjected to additional round(s) of screening, target validation, and biological testing. Lead candidates from this process are then identified for evaluation for preclinical antitumor activity in vivo and, subsequently, for toxicological, pharmacokinetic and pharmacodynamic evaluation. If successful this process will yield a drug candidate for clinical phase I/II trials.

3. THERAPEUTIC TARGETS FOR BRAIN TUMOR

An ultimate goal of the new paradigms for therapeutic exploitation of targets for cancer treatment is to develop agents whose actions are highly cancer selective and nontoxic to normal cells and tissues. In some cases, the targeted therapies are designed to enhance the efficacy of classical cytotoxics or overcome tumor resistance to them. In this context, a number of molecular targets have been shown to be relevant and targetable for brain tumor therapy. Many of the targets with a potential to provide new therapeutic directions for brain tumors are involved in multiple cellular processes and pathways critical to the genesis and progression of CNS tumor, or mediate their response to therapy. Table 1 summarizes some of these targets. A selected number of these therapeutic targets and the pathways and/or phenotypes they are involved in are discussed later to provide an overview of the progress and challenges of the future in developing targeted therapeutics for CNS tumors.

3.1. Drug Resistance-Related Therapeutic Targets

Many of the agents in current clinical use in brain tumor therapy induce damage to the cellular genome as their primary mode of action. The DNA lesions, in turn, trigger cellular responses that ultimately lead to cell death. In addition, the cellular genome is constantly undergoing modifications from endogenous physiological processes, such as oxidations and from exogenous xenobiotics, including, chemotherapeutic agents. These lesions are substrates for a variety of DNA repair processes, and their efficient repair preserves genomic integrity, or in the case of tumors, is a primary cause of drug resistance and therapeutic failure. Impairment or inhibition of the DNA repair pathway restores the vulnerability of the genome to DNA damaging agents and, consequently, DNA repair pathways and the complex spectrum of genes and proteins involved in them represent potential targets for developing novel anticancer therapeutics.

Table 1
Examples of Some Potential Targets for the Rational Development of Brain Tumor Therapeutics

Tumor suppressor and related target: p53, p10, p16

Oncogenes and related targets: Epidermal growth factor receptor (EGFR), Platelet-derived growth factor (PDGF), Platelet derived growth factor receptor (PDGFR), Transforming growth factor (TGF), mdm2, Ras, Myc, Myb

Cell signaling/cell-cycle control: Protein kinase A (PKA), Protein kinase B (PKB, Akt), Protein kinase (PKC), Tumor necrosis factor (TNF)-α, Insulin growth factor (IGF), Insulin growth factor-binding protein (IGFBP), Phosphoinositol 3-phosphate kinase (PI3-kinase), Farnesyltransferase (FT), Isoprenylcysteine methyltransferase (Icmt), Nuclear factor-κ B (NF-κ B), Mitogen-activated protein kinase (MAPK), MAPK kinases (MAPKK), Fibroblast growth factor (FGF) and FGF-receptors, (FGFR), Jak/Stat proteins

DNA repair and related targets: O^6-methylguanine DNA methyltransferase (MGMT), DNA polymerases, Topoisomerases I and II, PolyADP ribosyltransferase (PARP), Apurinic/apyrimidinic endonuclease (APE), Mammalian target of rapamycin (m-Tor), Nucleotide excision repair (NER)

Cell survival/cell death: Trail, Fas/Fas ligand, IAP (inducers of apoptosis proteins), Bcl2, Bclx, Bax, Bad, Caspases

Invasion/migration: Matrix metalloprotenaises (MMPs), Tissue inhibitor of metalloprotenaises (TIMP), Urokinase plasminogen activator (uPA), uPA receptor, Cathepsins

Angiogenesis: Vascular endothelial growth factor (VEGF), VEGF-receptors (Flk-1/VEGFR-1, Flt-1/VEGFR-2); Endothelins

Metabolism/drug disposition: Glutathione S-transferases, Metallothionines, Cytochromes P450, γ-glutamylcysteine synthase (γ-GCS), Cyclooxygenase 2 (COX 2), Phospholipases

Drug transport: Multidrug resistance-associated proteins (MRPs), p-Glycoprotein (MDR1), glucose transporters, Ion channels and amino acid transporters

Miscellaneous targets: Histone deacetylase, Ubiquitin/proteasome, Retinoic Acid receptors, Integrins

Despite the categorizations, many of these targets/phenotypes are inter-related and are frequently regulated by common cellular pathways.

In addition to DNA repair, a major mechanism of drug resistance of CNS and other tumors is the ability of the tumor cells to metabolically inactivate the anticancer agents and/or their active intermediates. Two major families of proteins involved in this critical pathway are the cytochromes P450 and the glutathione S-transferases. The former is involved in Phase I, and the latter in Phase II metabolism. The cytochrome P450 proteins are diverse, highly polymorphic proteins that metabolize many agents used in CNS tumor therapy. Despite their attractiveness as drug targets, direct inhibitors of cytochrome P450 proteins are only in the early stages of development as anticancer agents. In this section, therefore we will focus on the glutathione S-transferases. Examples of these drug-resistance-related therapeutic targets for brain tumors are described below.

3.1.1. O^6-Methylguanine DNA Methyltransferase

The 2-chloroethylnitrosoureas, temozolomide, and other methylating agents are among the clinically active agents often used in first-line brain tumor therapy. Although these drugs induce multiple lesions in DNA, a considerable body of evidence has established the O^6-methylguanine DNA adduct as the major cytotoxic lesion. This lesion is repaired by the protein, O^6-methylguanine DNA methyltransferase (MGMT), and when this occurs efficiently, leads to tumor drug resistance. MGMT, a suicide enzyme, encoded on chromosome 10, removes the alkyl group from alkylated O^6-guanine

DNA onto the sulfhydryl in its active site, thereby regenerating the guanine and restoring the integrity of the DNA. This methyl excision repair (MER) phenotype, mediated by MGMT, is a major mechanism of resistance of brain tumors to alkylating agents that produce O^6-guanine DNA lesions *(2,16,86,91,107)*. Extensive clinical and preclinical studies have shown a strong correlation between MGMT over-expression and the response of brain tumors, primarily, malignant gliomas and primitive neuroectodermal tumors (PNETs), to chemotherapy with the CENUs, and temozolomide. As a result, this repair pathway and the MGMT protein was among the first to be exploited for targeted therapy of brain tumors *(110)*. The approaches to targeting MGMT have been multiple and include the use of (a) antisense oligonucleotides and ribozymes to down-regulate expression, (b) methylating agents to saturate the active site, and (c) small molecule inhibitors of MGMT. Of these, the most successful has been a class of alkylated guanine analogs with high affinity to the MGMT active site, the lead agent being O^6-benzylguanine *(43–45,90,91,128,166)*. In clinical trials, O^6-benzylguanine has shown efficacy in potentiating tumor response to CENUs *(59)*, temozolomide *(171)*, and cyclophosphamide *(60)*. Despite its initial promise, the targeting of the MGMT protein with O^6-benzylguanine to enhance tumor response to chemotherapy has been limited by two major factors. The first is the high bone marrow toxicity of the combination, whereas the second relates to the lack of response of mismatch repair deficient tumors to this modulation.

3.1.2. Base Excision Repair

There is now considerable evidence that whereas repair of the O^6-alkylguanine lesion is an established mechanism of resistance to methylators and other alkylating agents used in brain tumor therapy, other mechanisms of resistance to these agents exist that are unrelated to the O^6-alkylguanine DNA adducts. An interesting aspect of agents that induce O^6-alkylguanine lesions is that this lesion is only a small percentage (<2%) of the adducts that they generate in DNA. Indeed, N^3 and N^7-alkylated purines and pyrimidines, together, constitute approx 80% of the lesions induced by methylating, ethylating, and chloroethylatylating agents in DNA. These adducts, however, do not result in cytotoxicity because they are readily repaired by the base excision repair (BER) pathway. One of the first steps of BER is the hydrolysis of the *N*-glycosidic bond linking the alkylated bases to the DNA phosphodiester backbone, resulting in abasic sites in the DNA. In addition to alkylating anticancer agents and related chemical agents, abasic sites are also generated in cells through endogenous mechanisms and after DNA damage by both ionizing or ultraviolet (UV) radiation, base oxidations, and other chemical alterations. These abasic sites are recognized by the multifunctional protein, apurinic/apyrimidinic endonulease 1 (APE1) and following binding, APE1 hydrolyzes the phosphodiester backbone immediately 5' of the site, introducing a strand break that is then repaired by the BER protein complex. In addition to its function in BER, APE1 is also a redox factor (ref-1) and regulates cellular response to oxidative stress by regulating the activity of a variety of transcription factors, including, AP-1 binding factors, p53, and Nf-kB *(87,176)*. Current therapeutic strategies targeting BER include the development of small molecule specific inhibitors of APE1, the rationale being that by inhibiting APE1, the process of repair of abasic sites resulting from the *N*-alkyl adducts will be blocked, leading to an accumulation of these lesions in the cellular genome, which ultimately leads to cell death. It was recently demonstrated that, in a paired series, over 90% of human malignant gliomas had elevated APE-1 activities relative to normal brain tissues *(12)*. This, together with the observation that APE-1 activity correlates with resistance to BCNU in glioblastoma cells, supports the therapeutic targeting of BER and, specifically, APE-1, in gliomas and other tumors *(103)*. To date, the best studied APE-1 inhibitor is methoxyamine *(105,159)*. The mechanism of action of methoxyamine is uniquely different from other protein inhibitors in that, rather than interacting with the APE-1 protein directly, it reacts chemically with the abasic site created as part of BER. The resulting methoxyamine-abasic site is not recognized by APE-1. Liu et al. *(104)* have shown that the antitumor efficacy of 1,3-*bis*(2-cloroethyl)-1-nitrosourea (BCNU) is significantly enhanced by methoxyamine in colon tumor xenografts. There is a need to extend these studies to malignant gliomas.

3.1.3. Poly(ADP-Ribose) Polymerase

Poly(ADP-ribose) polymerases (PARPs) are chromatin-bound zinc finger proteins that play a key role in multiple cellular processes, including DNA replication, cell survival, apoptosis, DNA repair, and DNA damage and stress response *(102,151)*. The primary enzyme of this class is PARP-1, a DNA damage sensor and signaling protein. PARP-1 is activated by DNA damage, particularly single- and double-strand breaks, redox stress, and following treatment of cells with alkylating agents *(39,102,137)*. Upon activation, PARP-1 binds to DNA strand breaks and catalyzes the cleavage of ADP-ribose residues from NAD^+, and polymerizes these unto nuclear acceptor proteins, including histones, topoisomerase I and II, and laminin transcription factors, as well as PARP itself. Accumulating evidence supports a role for PARP in the cellular processing of alkylator-induced DNA damage and in the apoptotic response of cells to this damage *(40)*. One of the deleterious consequences of oxidative stress and excessive DNA damage in cells is the depletion of NAD^+ and ATP, resulting from the high levels of ADP-ribosylation. Similarly, the strand breaks induced by BCNU and other carbamoylating nitrosoureas used in brain tumor therapy have been shown to induce significant NAD^+ and, subsequently, ATP depletion. Immunohistochemical studies have shown PARP-1 to be overexpressed in primary glioblastomas *(174)*, and PARP inhibition with 3-aminobenzamide has been shown to significantly sensitize human glioblastoma to BCNU *(102,173)*. In addition, in mismatch repair deficient cells treated with the methylating triazene, temozolomide, the inability to repair O^6-methylguanine thymine mispairings in the genome results in DNA strand breaks that then trigger ADP-ribosylation and apoptosis. These and other studies together establish PARP as a valid therapeutic target in gliomas, and other tumors and significant efforts are ongoing to develop PARP inhibitors as anticancer therapeutics *(152,160,164)*. Several novel classes of PARP-1 inhibitors are currently being evaluated against glioblastoma, primarily for their ability to enhance the efficacy of chemotherapeutic agents, such as temozolomide. These inhibitors include AG 14361 *(37)*, the nicotinic amidoximine derivative, BGP-15 *(137)* and GP15427. Recently, it was shown that treatment of temozolomide-resistant cells with AG14361 restored temozolomide sensitivity *(37)*. The results of these preclinical studies have been very positive and phase I/II clinical trials are ongoing in recurrent glioblastomas at Duke University.

3.1.4. Glutathione and Glutathione S-Transferase

Glutathione *S*-transferases (GSTs) are homo- and heterodimeric proteins encoded by a family of genes with limited structural homologies and different chromosomal localizations *(109)*. GSTs are enzymes of phase II metabolism, in which they catalyze the *S*-conjugation of the tripeptide glutathione (GSH) with electrophiles *(32)*, including many mutagens, carcinogens, and anticancer agents. To date, eight classes of human soluble GSTs, namely α, κ, μ, ω, π, σ, τ, and ζ have been described. Of these, GSTP1 (GST-pi) is the most significantly overexpressed in human tumors, even though the corresponding normal tissues have low or no expression of the protein. A major advance in understanding the role of the GSTP1 gene in cancer was the isolation of full-length cDNAs of polymorphic variants of the gene from λ gt 11 cDNA libraries created from human malignant glioma cell lines *(6)*. These allelic variants resulted from nucleotide transitions that altered codons 104 and 113 from Ile to Val and Ala to Val, respectively. These transitions also significantly altered both the architecture of the active, electrophile-binding (H) site and the binding to and enzymatic function of the encoded proteins toward anticancer agents and several known carcinogens *(6,21–23,79,80,85,88,179)*. Crystal structures of the three variant peptides have been elucidated *(88,140)*. Figure 2 shows the space-filling secondary structures of the three variant GSTP1 peptides showing spatial differences in the architecture of the active site regions of the allelic proteins. As would be expected, the structural differences between the different proteins have major implications on the structure-based development of GSTP1-targeted therapeutics.

Evidence credentialing the GSTP1 protein as a target for the rational development of novel therapeutics for CNS has accumulated over the last decade from several independent laboratories

hGSTP1a   **hGSTP1b**   **hGSTP1c**

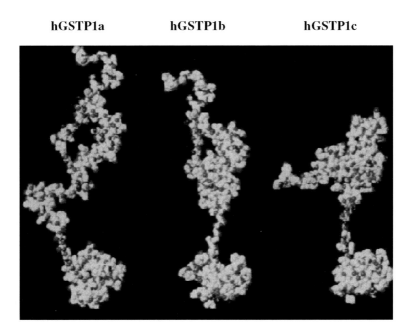

Fig. 2. Space-filling secondary structures of GSTP1a, GSTP1b and GSTP1c allelic peptides. The latter two were derived by homology modeling on the crystal structure of GSTP1a. Note the significant differences in the regions (upper end of structures) of the electrophile-binding site of the peptides, with a more open form in hGSTP1a than in the other two peptides.

(161,170). First, a consistently strong correlation has been observed between the level of GSTP1 expression and the degree of anaplasia in malignant gliomas and tumor grade, with the highest levels present in glioblastoma multiforme and the least in low-grade gliomas *(7,73)*. In retrospective clinical trials, our laboratory showed that high GSTP1 protein expression and its nuclear localization correlates with poor clinical outcome in glioma and medulloblastoma patients*)*. In addition, several anticancer agents including, cyclophosphamide and its analogues ifosphamide and 4-hydroxy-ifosphamide, melphalan, cisplatin/carboplatin, thiotepa, and the 2-chloroethyl-nitrosoureas that have shown clinical efficacy in the treatment of brain tumors undergo inactivation, following GSTP1-catalyzed conjugation with GSH *(42,43,68,84,85,127,153)*. The resulting metabolites are less cytotoxic and are excreted by the ATP-dependent multidrug resistance-associated protein 1 (MRP1) transport protein. Furthermore, GSTP1 gene transfer and/or transfections into both normal and tumor cells induces cellular resistance to some of these agents and inhibition of the GSTP1 protein and/or its downregulation with antisense oligodeoxynucleotides, and cDNAs induces apoptosis and sensitizes tumors to several anticancer agents *(92)*.

A relatively recent but critically important function of the GSTP1 protein is its role as a major intracellular inhibitor of the downstream signaling target, *jun*-N-terminal kinase (JNK)*)*. Thus, the GSTP1 protein protects cells against JNK-mediated apoptosis GSTP1, and regulates cell signaling in response to stress, cell proliferation, and apoptosis *(145)*. Recently, we showed that this provides a survival advantage to GSTP1-overexpressing brain tumor cells *(106)*. A related finding is that the Ser/Thr kinase, protein kinase A (PKA) and PKC (often over-expressed in tumors) phosphorylate the GSTP1 protein, thereby increasing its metabolic function leading to increased drug resistance. Together, these signaling functions of the GSTP1 protein further validate the GSTP1 protein as a therapeutic target. The fact that crystal structures and 3-D architectures of all three GSTP1 proteins have been resolved *(41,122)* and the critical amino acid residues in the GSTP1 active site identified, facilitate structure-based drug design of GSTP1-targeted drugs. The absence/low expression of GSTP1 in the normal brain and most normal tissues suggests that these new GSTP1-targeted agents are likely to have a high therapeutic index. Some of the efforts to target the GSTP1 protein in cancer therapy are summarized below.

3.1.4.1. ETHACRYNIC ACID

Ethacrynic acid (EA) [2,3-dichloro-4-(2-methylenebutyryl)-phenoxy]acetic acid, is a clinically active diuretic, and is both a specific substrate and an inhibitor of the GSTP1 protein. It is the first agent to be evaluated clinically for therapeutic inhibition of GSTP1. In initial in vitro studies EA increased tumor cell sensitivity to alkylating agents, *(27,72,116,129,142,160a)* and in nude mice it increased growth delay in colon cancer xenografts, albeit with increased bone marrow toxicity *(161)*. Clinical trials in advanced cancers, subsequently demonstrated the ability of EA to inhibit GSTP1 activity in patients and to increase tumor sensitivity to the alkylating agents, chlorambucil and thiotepa *(124,128a)*. Despite these promising early clinical results, the clinical use of EA as a GSTP1 inhibitor has been discontinued because of the severe diuresis and electrolyte imbalance it induces at the high doses required for inhibiting GSTP1 in tissues.

3.1.4.2. STRUCTURAL ANALOGS OF GLUTATHIONE

These compounds, designed to maintain high affinity to the GSTP1 G-site are in the early stages of developments as therapeutic inhibitors of GSTP1. Generally, the analogs are obtained by systematic chemical modifications of the three main GSH residues, namely, the glycyl, cysteinyl, and γ-glutamyl residues.

3.1.4.3. PHOSPHONOGLUTATHIONYL ANALOGS

This class of GSTP1 inhibitors results from replacing the cysteinyl group of GSH with a phosphono group *(98)*. The compounds are readily taken up by cells and inhibit GSTP1 and other GSTs with distinct and different specificities. Although active in vitro, this class of GSTP1 inhibitors are yet to show any antiploriferative activities or ability to enhance tumor sensitivity to anticancer agents.

3.1.4.4. PEPTIDOMIMETIC TRIPEPTIDE GLUTATHIONEANALOGS

This recently developed class of GSTP1 inhibitors are produced by replacing the peptide bonds in GSH with isosteres, such as "reduced" amides, urethane, and methylene bridges *(26)*. In some cases, conjugates of these compounds were created with GST substrates, such as ethacrynic acid. The compounds are in the very early stages of evaluation and some have shown significant GST inhibitory activity and are stable to the action of gamma-glutamyltranspeptidase, a GSH metabolizing enzyme. As with the phosphono-GSH compounds, these peptidomimetics are yet to be evaluated for their antitumor activity.

3.1.4.5. TERRAPIN/TELIK (TER/TLK) COMPOUNDS

TER/TLK compounds are the most active new class of GSTP1 inhibitors generated to date, The rationally designed compounds target the glutathione-binding site (G-site) of the GSTP1 protein. One of the developmentally advanced of these inhibitors, TLK199, γ-glutamyl, *S*-benzyl-phenyl-ylglycyl diethyl ester, is rapidly hydrolyzed to its monoethyl ester and then to its active metabolite *(63)*. A unique additional property of TLK199 is that it stimulates maturation and proliferation of bone marrow progenitor cells, presumably through its effect on the redox state of the marrow. TLK199 is in phase I/II clinical trial as a treatment for myelodysplastic syndrome. Another GSTP1-targeted therapeutic strategy that exploits the GSTP1 overexpression in tumors is to develop prodrugs that are activated by GSTP1. This has resulted in TLK 286, a glutathionylconjugate of nitrogen mustard that, upon cleavage by GSTP1, releases active mustard *(162a)*. In a recent phase I clinical trial in advanced refractory solid malignancies, TLK 286 was well tolerated with minimal systemic toxicity *(144)*, and is undergoing further clinical evaluation in a number of malignancies (www.telik.com).

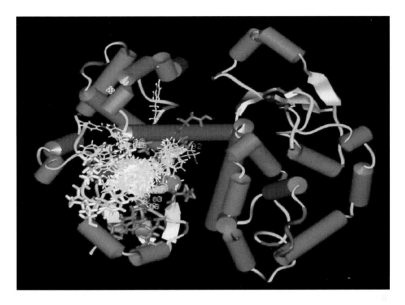

Fig. 3. Structure-based rational design of GSTP1-targeted anticancer therapeutics. The three-dimensional structure of the human GSTP1 protein is shown with chemical ligands docked into the H-site (Ali-Osman and Brolamwini, unpublished data).

3.1.4.6. NOVEL THERAPEUTIC STRATEGIES TARGETING THE GSTP1 ELECTROPHILE BINDING SITE

The majority of small molecule GSTP1 inhibitors being developed to date target the G-(GSH-binding) site of the GSTP1 protein. An alternative approach that is being pursued in our laboratory, is to target the H-(electrophile-binding) site of the GSTP1 protein. This is the site to which anticancer agents bind in the process of their metabolism by GSTP1. Inhibitors that bind to this site are likely to be less affected by high tumor GSH concentrations. Our strategy involves molecular docking of 3-D chemical libraries to the GSTP1H-site, using both nonenergy based and force-field (energy-based) methods *(14)*. X-ray crystallographic coordinates of GSTP1 in complex with inhibitors are used to model the H-site cavity, which is then used for virtual screening of a database of 3-D molecular structures to identify potential ligands that bind to the GSTP1 active site with high affinity and specificity (Fig. 3). The ligands serve as potential lead compounds for the development of GST-selective inhibitors and cancer therapeutic agents, which are then optimized by structure-based design and diversification by combinatorial chemistry approaches.

3.2. Cell Signaling As Therapeutic Target

Defects and/or abnormalities in the structure, function, and/or expression of many of the proteins involved in cell signaling and cellular response to stress and other external stimuli, such as growth factors, are a common feature of neoplastic biology. Many of the proteins involved in these processes are encoded by oncogenes and tumor suppressor genes, many of which are abnormal in CNS tumors. Consequently, these proteins are attractive targets for rational targeted anticancer drug discovery and targeting *(53,119)*. Examples of cell-signaling related targets relevant to CNS tumors are described later.

3.2.1. Epidermal Growth Factor

Abnormalities in epidermal growth factor (EGF)/epidermal growth factor receptor (EGFR) signaling are among the most common in human CNS tumors, particularly malignant gliomas *(150)*. EGFR (erB-1, HER-1) is a receptor tyrosine kinase of the erB family, many members of which are also dysregulated in CNS tumors. Structurally, EGFR comprises of an extracellular ligand-binding domain, a transmembrane domain, an intracellular domain, and a C-terminal domain. The tyrosine kinase activity resides in the intracellular domain, whereas the C-terminus contains the auto-phophosphorylation sites of the protein. Following activation by a ligand, such as EGF or TGF-α, EGFR homodimerizes or forms heterodimers with another tyrosine kinase of the erbB family. This dimerization then activates the tyrosine autophosphorylation by the intracellular domain and subsequent transduction of signaling to downstream effectors, such as the PI3K/PDK1/Akt, the JAK/STAT, and the Ras/Raf/MEK/MAPK (Erk) pathways *(81)*. EGFR can also be activated ligand-independently by stimuli, such as stress, cytokines, and hormones. The resistance of glioma cells to both BCNU and radiation therapy has been linked to abnormal EGFR signaling through a ras-dependent mechanism *(30)*. Other erbB proteins whose overexpression has been observed in CNS tumors, include HER-2 and Her-4, the increase of which has been associated with increased metastatic potential and with poor prognosis in medulloblastomas *(65)*. The therapeutic targeting of HER-2 is particularly interesting as it has been shown to signal through the PI3 kinase/AKT pathway and is, thus associated with protection of the cells against apoptosis *(82,180)*.

More than half of glioblastomas examined have been shown to harbor amplification of the EGFR gene, and in almost half of these the amplified gene is the EGFRvIII mutant, in which exons 2–7 are lost *(10)*. EGFRvIII is unique in that the mutation results in loss of a large part of the extracellular ligand-binding domain, leading to a protein that is constitutively and ligand-independently active *(10)*. The abnormal and constitutive kinase activity of EGFRvIII has been shown to be associated with gliomagenesis, increased malignant phenotype, and increased drug resistance. The EGFRvII is thus a unique therapeutic target for brain tumors *(96)*.

The high frequency of EGFR abnormalities and the association of these with the malignant phenotype summarized above have made EGFR an attractive target for rational development of antiglioma therapeutics. The main strategies being used to target both wild-type and the mutant EGFR involve antibodies *(149)* and small molecules. The former approach has been discussed in depth in the section of this book on immunotherapy. Thus, the discussion here will focus on the small molecule anti-EGFR strategies. Targeting the kinase domain of EGFR has yielded several active agents that are in various stages of clinical evaluation. The observation that HER-2 can be depleted by inhibitors of the heat shock protein HSP90, provides another strategy in which indirect inhibitors of HER-2 function, such as geldanamycin and its analogs *(112,118)* are being developed. In phase I and II clinical trials, these EGFR tyrosine kinase inhibitors (TKIs) have shown activity against a wide variety of tumors.

Currently, early clinical trials with small molecule inhibitors of EGFR tyrosine kinase are ongoing in CNS tumors, such as Iressa (ZD1839), a selective inhibitor of EGFR tyrosine kinase activity in a multi-institutional phase I/II trial in progressive and recurrent malignant gliomas and meningiomas. This follows preclinical studies in mice demonstrating efficacy of ZD1839 in glioblastoma xenografts *(75)*. Other ongoing clinical trials include a phase I evaluation of the combination of ZD1839 with temozolomide in malignant gliomas, and a phase I/II combination of ZD1839 with radiation therapy in previously untreated glioblastoma multiforme. ZD1839 functions, in part, by suppressing EGFR phosphorylation in EGFR overexpressing cells. It enhances apoptotic induction, possibly through downstream induction of the pro-apoptotic Bad protein. Nude mice studies with human glioblastoma xenografts bearing the EGFRvIII mutant were unresponsive to ZD1839, suggesting that the regulation of the tyrosine domain in the wild-type and mutant EGFR form may be different *(75)*. The dependence of ZD1839 antitumor activity on EGFR expression, however, remains unclear. The results of a large body of preclinical studies, however, suggest that the effects of ZD1839 is likely to involve multiple pathways. Of interest in this context is that the in vivo effects of EGFR inhibition include the inhibition of tumor angiogenesis and invasion.

Another specific inhibitor of EGFR is the quinazoline OSI-774, Tarceva, erlotinib, and CP-358 *(119,120)*. OSI-774 induces apoptosis and cell-cycle inhibition (primarily G1) resulting in growth arrest. Its action in blocking EGFR phosphorylation may be related to its ability to mimic ATP. Treatment of animals with OSI-774 has been shown to result in decreased phosphorylation of Akt and Erk, indicating that inhibition of these critical signaling targets may contribute to the antitumor action of this inhibitor. Of interest is the observation that OSI-774 inhibits the invasiveness of EGFRvIII-expressing human glioblastoma cells. A clinical phase I trial is ongoing with OSI-774 alone and in combination with temozolomide in highly malignant gliomas.

3.2.2. Platelet-Derived Growth Factor Receptor

The platelet-derived growth factor (PDGF) is involved in multiple cellular functions, including cell proliferation, cytoskeletal integrity, chemotaxis, and angiogenesis *(76,81,94,130,131,172)*. PDGF is frequently dysregulated in gliomas and other CNS tumors. Four chains, A, B, C, and D, exist for the human PDGF, the first two being the best characterized. The four chains are modified post-translationally by disulfide linkages to yield homo- and hetero-dimers, the active form of PDGF. Activated PDGF functions through binding to its receptor, PDGFR. PDGFR is a transmembrane glycoprotein tyrosine kinase with multiple domains, including a ligand-binding extracellular domain and an internal tyrosine kinase domain. Similar to PGF, PDGFR forms homo- and hetero-dimers with its two, α and β, subunits. Following binding of the dimeric (activated) PDGF ligand to the extra-celllular domain of PDGF, a domain rearrangement is induced resulting in the autophosphorylation of tyrosine residues of the tyrosine kinase domain. This creates attachment sites for signaling molecules with the Src homology, SH-2, domains, including Src, Grb2, GTPases, PI3-kinase, Jaks, Stats and PLC-γ.

The overexpression of PDGF and PDGFR *(55,172)* in human gliomas and other cancers, has led to efforts to develop anticancer therapeutics that target this pathway. The most productive of these efforts have been those with antibodies and small molecules that target PDGFR directly, as well as its downstream signaling pathways. These efforts have yielded several selective small molecule inhibitors of PDGFR, including, the 2-phenylaminopyrimidines, the 3-arylsubstituted quinoxalines and quinolines (Fry, 1996). An early small molecule PDGFR inhibitor, SU101, an isoxazole derivative, has been examined in phase I, II, and III clinical trials. The trials demonstrated efficacy but was associated with severe systemic toxicities of SU101.

The most active PDGFR tyrosine kinase inhibitor to date is imatinib mesylate or Gleevec (STI1571 or CGP57148). STI1571 is an orally available 2-phenylaminopyrimidine with inhibitory activity against the Abl kinase, c-kit, and PDGFR tyrosine kinases. It was developed initially as a specific treatment for chronic myelogenous leukemia *(46,123)*, because the 9:22 chromosomal translocation (Philadelphia chromosome) that characterizes this disease results in a truncated Abl and truncated Bcr fusion gene encoding the chimeric p210BCR-ABL protein that is constitutively and ligand-independently activated in CML cells. Because of its inhibitory activity against other tyrosine kinases, however, STI1571 is now being evaluated for treating other human tumors, including those of the CNS. A number of clinical trial are ongoing to evaluate the efficacy of STI1571 against brain tumors. These include a phase I/II trial in recurrent malignant gliomas in combination with radiation in high- and low-grade gliomas.

3.2.3. Serine/Threonine Kinases

Serine/threonine kinases are a family of proteins that phosphorylate serine and/or threonine residues present in specific motifs in a wide variety of proteins. Such phosphorylation leads to functional activation, inactivation, and/or alteration of the stability of the proteins. These kinases include the cAMP-dependent protein kinase A (PKA), protein kinase B (PKB or Akt) and protein kinase C (PKC). PKCs, which are activated by phorbol esters, various hormones, and transmitters are the most widely studied class of Ser/Thr kinases in human CNS cancers. The more than 12 PKC isoforms known to date are grouped into conventional or calcium (α, βI, βII, γ), atypical (δ, ε, τ and η) and novel (λ, ζ) differ with respect to their specific activators *(9)*. PKCs are involved in many processes critical to both normal and neoplastic cells, including synaptic transmission, cell-cycle control, ion flux across membranes, cell survival and cell death, oncogenenesis, tumor progression, and metastasis. In brain tumors, overactivation of various PKC-dependent pathways are associated with increased cellular proliferation, decreased apoptosis, and increased drug resistance in malignant gliomas *(9,17,28,31)*. Reports on PKC expression in human malignant gliomas have, however, been conflicting with some showing higher levels and others similar or lower levels compared to normal astrocytes *(178)*. Despite these disparate observations, the majority of reports have shown consistently, both in vitro and in vivo, that the inhibition of the PKC pathway induces significant growth inhibition and sensitizes gliomas to chemotherapeutic agents, making the targeting of PKC an attractive strategy and valid for pursuing novel agents for CNS tumor therapy *(9,38,135,168,169)*. An important aspect of activated PKC of therapeutic relevance is its association with increase invasion and angiogenesis. Thus, treatment of glioblastoma cells with the PKC inhibitor, hypericin, was shown to significantly inhibit the motility and invasiveness of these cells. Such observations open up possibilities of targeting PKC as an anti-invasive and antimetastatic therapeutic strategy in gliomas.

One of the early PKC-directed anticancer therapies involved the use of tamoxifen, a hormonal agent active in breast cancer with PKC inhibitory activity. Following in vitro studies showing suppression of the growth of glioma cells by tamoxifen *(130,131)*, clinical trials with tamoxifen in malignant glioma were conducted in which impressive patient response rates were observed *(16,33,35,132)*. Significant toxicity and the lack of durable responses, however, have limited the more extensive use of this strategy in malignant gliomas. Overall, the strategies for therapeutic targeting of PKC pursued to date can be classified based on the site of the PKC protein, namely the catalytic or the catalytic (ATP-binding) domain that the agents interact with. Thus, the indolocarbazoles, such as staurosporine and its derivatives, e.g., 7-OH-staurosporine or UCN-01, bind to the ATP-binding site. Staurosporine, unlike its more specific derivative UCN-01, is not highly specific for PKC and inhibits other kinases, notably PKA, phosphorylase kinase, and EGFR *(78,148)*. Subsequent staurosporine derivatives have shown much higher specificity. Another PKC inhibitor that is selective for the PKC-β isoform is the bisindolylmaleimide, LY333531. PKC-β inhibition with this and other agents has been shown, not only to have direct antitumor activity, but also to overcome drug resistance and to block angiogenesis in human glioblastoma xenografts models *(159a)*. In addition to the small molecule approach, an antisense oligonucleotide targeted to the PKC-α isoform has been evaluated clinically in patients with high grade astrocytomas, but showed no activity *(8)*. The availability of X-ray crystal structure of PKC-δ in complex with a phorbol ester has stimulated efforts at structure-based design and rational development of novel PKC inhibitors *(135,168,169)*. Despite its power and potential, no clinically active PKC-directed therapeutics has yet been developed with this approach.

Akt (PKB), another serine/threonine kinase of therapeutic relevance in CNS tumors, is implicated in the oncogenic process in many human cancers *(13)* and is aberrantly expressed in brain tumors. In gliomas, Akt dysregulation has been associated with an aggressive histology and poor patient survival *(51)*. Akt is phosphorylated and activated by phosphoinositol-3-kinase (PI3-K), a downstream target of various growth factors and scr-like kinases. The phosphorylated Akt regulates the activities of multiple downstream signaling targets. This includes down-regulation of the pro-apoptotic Bad and up-regulation of mTOR, both of which lead to a suppression of apoptosis and enhancement of tumor cell survival. The tumor suppressor, p10, frequently mutated and inactivated in malignant gliomas, regulates Akt by its ability to dephosphorylate PI3-K. The p10/PI3-K/Akt/ pathway has thus been a target in anticancer drug development, and a number of agents targeting different steps in the pathway are being actively developed. One of these in clinical trial is CCI-779, a rapamycin analogue that inhibits the downstream Akt target, mTOR. Following xenografts studies showing its activity against glioblastomas and medulloblastoma, CCI-779 is now in phase I/II clinical trials in recurrent glioblastoma.

3.3. Invasion/Migration

Tumors of the CNS, in particular malignant gliomas, have an inherent propensity to migrate locally and to diffusely invade the normal brain, a property that is a major obstacle to successful therapy of these tumors (reviewed in other sections of this volume). It is now well-established that the migratory phenotype of malignant gliomas is inter-related with the high proliferative and angiogenic properties of these tumors, and that these three phenotypes are regulated, in part, by common pathways. Invasion of brain tumor cells into the normal brain results from an enhanced activity of both proteases and migratory proteins, and is highly linked to the brain microenvironment. The tumor invasive phenotype is driven, primarily, by three main molecular regulators, namely the Zinc-dependent matrix metalloproteinases (MMPs), the plasminogen activators (PAs), their receptors (PARs) and inhibitors (PAIs), and the lysomal cystein peptidases or cathepsins. Human malignant gliomas express high levels of MMPs (in particular, the gelatinases, MMP2 and MMP9, urokinase PAs [uPAs] and cathepsin) *(95,138)*. All the components of the tumor invasive process are potential anticancer therapeutic targets. The most actively pursued, however, have been inhibitors of the MMPs, the common strategy being to develop agents that bind to the critical Zinc at the MMP active site. This approach has yielded a number of agents, including Marimastat (BB-251), an MMP inhibitor that functions by chelating the MMP active site Zn^{2+}. In clinical phase I and II trials, Marimastat demonstrated some activity against recurrent malignant gliomas. Other MMP inhibitors that have been evaluated clinically for activity against malignant gliomas are Metastat (COL-3, CMT-3, Collagenex) and Prinomastat (AG3340). Although all these MMP inhibitors, alone and in combination with chemotherapy, have shown some therapeutic efficacy clinically they are associated with significant toxicity, in part, a result of the relatively low specificity of their chelating action. Thus, there is a continuing need for MMP inhibitors with higher target specificity.

The uPA/uPAR system has also been a target for novel anticancer drug discovery *(47,49,138)*. uPA is a serine protease formed initially as high molecular weight uPA (HMWuPA). uPA is cleaved into an amino terminal fragment (ATF), and the low molecular weight uPA (LMWuPA) is involved in tumor metastasis and angiogenesis *(136,175)*. Both uPA and uPAR cooperate with MMPs, especially MMP-9, to cause tumor cell intravasation *(92a)*. uPA has been targeted in tumors both using antisense oligonucleotides, as well as small molecule inhibitors. Both have shown in vitro and in vivo antitumor activity. The amiloride-analog uPA inhibitors, such as B623, have been shown to block tumor invasion in vivo *(134)*. Recently, in malignant gliomas the downregulation of both uPAR and uPA by antisense sequences delivered in a bicistronic single adenoviral vector showed a markedly decreased invasive activity of glioblastoma cells in both an in vitro matrigel invasion assay and in tumor xenografts *(139)*, thus demonstrating the therapeutic potential of targeting the simultaneous targeting of both uPA and uPAR.

3.4. Oncogenes and Related Genes

The activation of oncogenes and the loss of function and/or reduced expression of tumor suppressor genes, such as p53, p10, and retinoblastoma (Rb)are common characteristics of CNS tumors *(150)*. A number of these oncogenes, including EGFR and PDGFR, have been discussed earlier because of their role in specific pathways. Others, such as ras and MDM2 will be discussed in this section.

MDM2 is an oncogene that functions by binding the tumor suppressor p53, thereby targeting p53 for proteolytic degradation via the ubiquitin/proteasome pathway *(93,133)*. The resulting phenotype is equivalent to one in which the p53 gene is functionally inactivated by mutation. The MDM2 protein is significantly overexpressed in brain and other tumors *(114,125)*. As a result, the MDM2 protein has been a target for novel anticancer drug discovery. Efforts to develop MDM2-targeted therapeutics have included peptides *(15,62)*, small molecule inhibitors *(155)*, and antisense oligonucleotides *(167)*. However, to date direct inhibitors of MDM2 have not been evaluated in human brain tumors, although indirect inhibitors such as proteasome inhibitors that affect both p53 and

MDM2 levels have been examined for their antiglioma activity. Some of these might benefit brain cancer treatment.

Amplification and overexpression of the myc oncogene family, especially C-myc and N-myc have been observed in gliomas and medulloblastomas *(11,20,77,108,162)*. One-third of all neuroblastomas (NBL) show amplification of N-myc, which correlates with poor prognosis *(18,19)*. Insulin-like growth factor I receptor has also been shown to be constitutively activated in medulloblastomas *(167)*. Thus, Myc is an appropriate target for novel cancer therapeutics.

An interesting potential therapeutic target for primitive neuroectodermal tumors (PNETs) is the sonic hedgehog (Shh)-Gli signaling pathway that is implicated in the early stages of several cancers, including basal cell carcinoma *(126)*, rhamdomyosarcoma, and medulloblastoma *(154,156)*. Small molecule inhibitors of this pathway and of smoothened, a key molecular downstream target in the pathway, are likely to offer novel treatment opportunities for medulloblastoma and other tumors. Such compounds include cyclopamine *(83,157)* and Cur41414 *(34,58)*.

Recently, hypoxia-inducible factor 1 (HIF-1), a redox-sensitive transcription factor, has been shown to be important in tumor progression and angiogenesis. Its overexpression was correlated with treatment failure and mortality in brain, breast, cervical, esophageal, oropharyngeal, and ovarian cancers *(147)*. Activating mutations in the β-catenin gene has been observed in medulloblastomas, resulting in a significant increase in transcription activity of a variety of genes, including cyclin D1, c-myc, and T-cell factor *(181)*. Both HIF-1 and beta-catenin thus offer potential targets for novel anticancer therapeutics.

The ras family of oncogenes (H-Ras, K-Ras and N-Ras) are G-proteins that cycle between an inactive GDP-bound and an activated GTP-bound form. In many human tumors the ras proto-oncogenes are often activated by a single mutation, and the activated ras plays a major role in the malignant transformation and subsequent progression of these tumors, notably adenocarcinomas of the pancreas, colon, and lung. However, unlike other solid tumors, to date, a growing body of evidence indicates that ras mutations are uncommon in CNS tumors *(69)*. Despite the absence of mutations in the ras gene, the ras pathway and its downstream effectors are frequently activated in brain tumors, particularly astrocytomas. Thus, high levels of ras-GTP have been observed in gliomas lacking ras mutations *(54)*. The ras activation occurs, putatively, through upstream growth factor effectors such as EGFR that can activate the ras protein in the absence of mutations. Following its activation, the transforming activity of the ras protein requires it to undergo post-translational farnesylation in a reaction catalyzed by the enzyme, farnesyltransferase (FT) in which the isoprenoid, farnersyl, is attached via a thioether bridge to the cystein residues in the CAAX motif in ras. Several approaches have been pursued in the therapeutic targeting of the ras pathway in cancer, including targeting raf, MEK, and both FT and geranylgeranyl transferase. Because of the requirement of FT-catalyzed farnesylation for ras oncogenic function, FT inhibitors have been a particularly active focus of these efforts. This has resulted in a number of FT inhibitors (FTIs), some of which have been evaluated clinically against brain tumors. These include R115777 (tipifarnib, Zarnestra), a methylquinolone, and SCH66336 (lonafarnib, Sarasar), a halogenated pyperidinyl derivative *(66,163)*. Both of these have been in phase I/II clinical trials against glioblastoma multiforme, following demonstration of anti-proliferative activity, alone and in combination with chemotherapeutic agents and/or radiation in glioblastoma cell lines.

3.5. Angiogenesis

Inhibition of angiogenesis is an attractive therapeutic strategy in CNS tumors, particularly malignant gliomas, in which increased vascular endothelial proliferation is a hallmark of tumor progression and poor clinical outcome *(1)*. The approaches to targeting tumor angiogenesis have been multiple and are generally directed at the vascular endothelial growth factors (VEGF) or their receptor tyrosine kinases, VEGFR-1 (flt-1), VEGFR-2 (flk-1), and VEGFR-3. VEGFR-1 and VEGFR-2 are involved directly in angiogenesis *(70,134,143)*, whereas VEGFR-3 has been demonstrated to be more involved in maintaining the integrity of the endothelial lining during angiogenesis. Several approaches have been pursued to develop anticancer agents that target the different steps of angiogenesis. The most concerted efforts have, however, been directed at VEGFR-1 and VEGFR-2, both of which have been successfully targeted to produce first generation angiogenesis inhibitors. In addition, regulators of angiogenesis, such as basic fibroblast growth factor receptor (bFGFR) and PDGFR-β *(56,94)* have been targeted to inhibit tumor angiogenesis. Interestingly, the resulting agents not only inhibit tumor angiogenesis, but also enhance the tumor-killing effect of radiation *(48,64,101)*. Thus, indoline-2-one (SU5416), that targets VEGFR2 and PDGFR-b kinase activity *(57,111),* has been shown in xenografts of glioblastomas to induce tumor cell death associated with a significant reduction in vascularity *(158)* and has been in clinical trials against various human cancers, including lung and acute myeloid leukemia. A VEGFR-2 inhibitor in clinical trial is CGP-7978, which alone and in combination with chemotherapy has shown modest efficacy against malignant gliomas.

Despite early enthusiasm for many of these anti-angiogenic agents, the phase I and II trials have shown the majority to have significant dose-limiting toxicities, and clinical phase III trials have yet to demonstrate significant increases in overall survival with them. As we better understand the complex biology of the angiogenic process and characterize the critical molecular components, such knowledge is likely to facilitate the design of more effective and less toxic targeted therapies.

4. CONCLUSION AND FUTURE PERSPECTIVES

Despite advances in neurosurgical techniques, radiation therapy, and a large number of clinical trials with chemotherapy and, more recently, with other modalities, including biological, immuno- and gene therapy, therapeutic outcome in malignant tumors of the CNS remains abysmal with few long term survivors. Therefore, there is an urgent need for novel, more effective, and less toxic therapeutics and therapeutic strategies for these devastating tumors. The significant advances that have been made in the last two decades in our understanding of the molecular events underlying the genesis of these tumors and of the genes and proteins that drive the malignant growth process, and the therapeutic response in them provide unique opportunities for the rational development of novel and more effective therapeutics and therapeutic strategies for them. The sequencing of the human genome and the tremendous developments in structural and functional genomics, combined with the rapid evolution of high throughput technologies, provide unparalleled opportunities for a new era in which therapeutics can be developed that are targeted to the molecular and cellular defects and alterations in CNS tumors. This chapter has examined some of the approaches used to date to achieve this and provided some examples of progress in efforts to develop targeted therapeutics for brain tumors. Many of these efforts are in their early stages and, while the clinical trials have not yielded highly effective agents, they have provided important insights into the limitations of the approaches taken and future strategies as to how to improve upon them. One of the obvious lessons from the results of these efforts so far is that whereas the new therapies are target-directed, many of the approaches taken to develop the therapeutics have not been highly rational and have drawn heavily from classical medicinal chemistry and established preclinical and clinical drug evaluation methodologies, which often are inadequate for target-directed therapeutics. This, in part, accounts for the poor tumor selectivity and the high level of systemic toxicity of the new therapeutics.

A major current obstacle to rational targeted drug discovery for CNS tumors, and indeed for human tumors in general, remains the identification and validation of the molecular defects or abnormality to be targeted, as well as the limited availability of appropriate cellular systems and animal models that recapitulate the biology of the human disease and reflect the molecular defect(s). In this regard, transgenic and knock-out/knock-in animals provide appropriate models for credentialing the target for its biological and disease relevance, and for testing the potential efficacy of the novel therapeutics in the whole animal context of the interactions involved in disease progression and in the mediation of therapeutic outcome. The challenge, however, in generating animal models of human CNS tumors lies in the extreme intra- and inter-tumoral heterogeneity of these tumors and in identifying the specific molecular defect or genes to be targeted in creating the animals. Part of the problem is that when a specific gene is knocked in or out in isolation in the normal animal the change can be embryonically lethal, or else the defect is compensated for in such a way that the resulting phenotype is not consistent with that of the human tumor. This problem can be addressed, in part, by employing conditional expression systems such as the CRE/LoxP strategy to create knockout animals. Specific promoters can then be used to drive these genes spatially and temporally in the CNS. In addition to animal models, cell-based systems, if adequately developed, could also provide a simple, less expensive but versatile tool in the discovery of novel antitumor agents for the CNS. The advantage of such systems is that the cells are of human origin and can be derived from both normal CNS elements and/or specific tumors, and can be engineered to harbor the genetic defect or abnormality that is being targeted. They can be evaluated as xenografts or in complex in vitro systems, such as multicellular spheroids that simulate the cellular interactions and heterogeneity in the tumors.

The identification of appropriate therapeutic targets is being facilitated by the information being generated from high-throughput genotyping, molecular profiling, tissue arrays, and other high-throughput technologies that are providing the initial indication of many of the genes that are lost, altered, or abnormally expressed in CNS tumors. The rational application of the massive amount of data generated by these analyses to identify and credential specific targets for therapeutic development, however, remains a major bioinformatics and biological challenge for the future.

Even after a target or molecular defect has been identified and its disease relevance validated, the task of developing therapeutics against it for clinical use is a challenging one and requires a multidisciplinary team approach that brings together experts in molecular pharmacology, structural biology, medicinal chemistry, computational sciences, clinical trials, and bioinformatics/biostatistics. The quest for targeted anticancer drugs thus provides unique opportunities for synergistic interactions between academia and industry in which the initial stages of target identification and credentialing, lead identification, validation, and optimization are concentrated in the academic center and the later stage preclinical and clinical development are more suited for the infrastructure and expertise of industry. The National Institutes of Health, notably the National Cancer Institute (NCI), and the National Institute for Neurological Diseases and Stroke (NINDS), as well as other governmental agencies such as the Food and Drug Administration and many private organizations, including the American Association for Cancer Research, the American Cancer Society, the Pediatric Brain Tumor Foundation of the United States, and the Brain Tumor Society are critical partners in this endeavor with respect to brain tumors. The NCI and the NINDS, with their multiple funding mechanisms for basic and clinical research and their infrastructural resources in the form of compound and tissue repositories, have played and continue to play a critical and central role in these efforts. Another challenge in the development of targeted anticancer therapeutics is in the design of clinical trials to evaluate these agents. This requires new criteria for optimizing dosage and monitoring efficacy which are different from those used to develop the cytotoxic anticancer agents currently in clinical use. Clinical protocol design to evaluate these agents will have to incorporate new requirements, such as tissue sampling for determination of the therapeutic target (or its surrogate) and for pharmacokinetic and pharmacodynamic monitoring. Appropriate biomarkers for predicting response will also have to be included as the current endpoints, such as minimum tolerated dose (MTD), time to tumor progression, and survival times, etc., that are hallmarks of current methods are inadequate. The heterogeneity and multiplicity of molecular defects in CNS tumors, however, suggest that future effective therapies will involve the rational combination of multiple-targeted therapeutics, as well as current modalities, particularly chemotherapy and radiation therapy. Despite the unique challenges of developing these novel therapies, they offer significant potential benefits over current treatments and are likely to be more active with greatly reduced systemic toxicities. They provide hope for a significant improvement in the management and overall prognosis of patients with malignant brain tumors.

ACKNOWLEDGMENTS

Supported by grants RO1 CA91438, RO1 CA79644, P20 CA096890 and P30 CA14236 from the National Cancer Institute, National Institute of Health (USA).

REFERENCES

1. Abdollahi A., Lipson K.E., Sckell A., Zieher H., Klenke F., Poerschke D., et al. 2003. Combined therapy with direct and indirect angiogenesis inhibition results in enhanced antiangiogenic and antitumor effects. *Cancer Res.* **63**:8890–8898.

2. Aida T., Cheitlin R.A., Bodell W.J. 1987. Inhibition of O6-alkylguanine-DNA-alkyltransferase activity potentiates cytotoxicity and induction of SCEs in human glioma cells resistant to 1,3-bis(2-chloroethyl)-1-nitrosourea. *Carcinogenesis* **8**:1219–23.

3. Ajay A., Walters W.P., Murcko M.A. 1998. Can we learn to distinguish between "drug-like" and "nondrug-like" molecules? *J. Med. Chem.* **41**:3314–3324.

4. Ajay A., Bemis G.W., Murcko M.A. 1999. Designing libraries with CNS activity. *J. Med. Chem.* **42**:4942–4951.

5. Ali-Osman F., Stein D.E., Renwick A. 1990. Glutathione content and glutathione-S-transferase expression in 1,3-bis(2-chloroethyl)-nitrosourea-resistant human malignant astrocytoma cell lines. *Cancer Res.* **50**:6976–6980.

6. Ali-Osman F., Akande O., Antoun G., Mao J-X., Buolamwini J. 1997. Molecular cloning, characterization and expression in Escherichia coli of full-length cDNAs of three human glutathione S-transferase-pi gene variants. *J. Biol. Chem.* **272**:10,004–10,012.

7. Ali-Osman F., Brunner J.M., Kutluk T.M., Hess, K. 1997. Prognostic significance of glutathione S-transferase π expression and subcellular localization in human gliomas. *Clin. Cancer Res. Clin. Cancer Res.* **3**:2253–2261.

8. Alvi J.B., Grossman S.A., Supko K., Carson K., Priet R., Dorr A., Holmlund J. 2000. Efficacy, toxicity and pharmacology of an antisense oligonucleotide directed against protein kinase C alpha (ISI-3521) delivered as a 21 day continuous intravenous infusion in patients with recurrent high grade astrocytomas (HGA)). *Proc. Am. Assoc. Clin. Oncol.*

9. Battaini F. 2001. Protein kinase C isoforms as therapeutic targets in nervous system disease states. *Pharmacol. Res.* **44**:353–361.

10. Batra S.K., Castelino-Prabhu S., Wikstrand C.J., Zhu X., Humphrey P.A., Friedman H.S., Bigner D.D. 1995 Growth factor ligand-independent, unregulated, cell-transforming potential of a naturally occurring human mutant EGFRvIII gene. *Cell Growth Differ.* **6**:1251–1259.

11. Bigner S.H., Friedman H.S., Vogelstein B., Oakes W.J., Bigner D. D. 1990. Amplification of the c-myc gene in human medulloblastoma cell lines and xenografts. *Cancer Res.* **50**:2347–2350.

12. Bobola M.S., Blank A., Berger M.S., Stevens B.A., Silber J.R. 2001. Apurinic/apyrimidinic endonuclease activity is elevated in human adult gliomas. *Clin. Cancer Res.* **7**:3510–3518.

13. Blume-Jensen P., Hunter T. 2001. Oncogenic kinase signalling. *Nature* **411**:355–356.

14. Bohm H.J. 1992. LUDI: rule-based automatic design of new substituents for enzyme inhibitor leads. *J. Comput. Aided Mol. Des.* **6**:593–606.

15. Bottger A., Bottger V., Garcia-Echeverria C., Chene P., Hochkeppel H.-K., Sampson W., et al. 1997. Design of a synthetic MDM2-binding mini protein that activates the p53 response in vivo. *Curr. Biol.* **7**:860–869

16. Brandes A.A., Basso U., Pasetto L.M., Ermani M. 2001. New strategy developments in brain tumor therapy. *Curr. Pharmaceut. Design* **7**:1553–1580

17. Bredel M., Pollack I.F. 1997. The role of protein kinase C (PKC) in the evolution and proliferation of malignant gliomas, and the application of PKC inhibition as a novel approach to anti-glioma therapy. *Acta Neurochir (Wien)*. **139**:1000–1013.

18. Brodeur G.M. 1994. Molecular pathology of human neuroblastomas. *Sem. Diagn. Pathol.* **11**:118–125.

19. Brodeur G.M. 1995. Molecular basis for heterogeneity in human neuroblastomas. *Eur. J. Cancer* **31**:505–510.

20. Bruggers C.S., Tai K. F., Murdock T., Sivak L., Le K., Perkins S.L., et al. 1998. Expression of the C–myc protein in childhood medulloblastoma. *J. Pediatr. Hematol. Oncol.* **20**:18–25.

21. Buolamwini J.K., Ali-Osman F. 1999. Flexible docking of 4-hydroxyifosfamide in the putative H-site of allelo-polymorphic human glutathione S-transferase pi (GST-p) proteins. *Proc. Am. Assoc. Cancer Res.* **40**:674.

22. Buolamwini J. K., Ali-Osman F. 2000. Dynamic docking dtudy of 1-chloro-2,4-dinitrobenzene (CDNB) binding at the putative H-site of human glutathione S-transferase Pi (GST-p) polymorphic proteins, in *Biologically Active Natural Products: Pharmaceuticals* (Cutler H., Cutler S.J., eds.), CRC Press, Boca Raton, FL, pp. 197–207.

23. Buolamwini J.K., Ali-Osman F. 2000. A docking study of the binding of thiotepa in the putative H-site pocket of human glutathione S-transferase pi allelo-polymorphs. *Proc. Am. Assoc. Cancer Res.* **41**:282.

24. Buolamwini J.K. 2001. *Novel Molecular Targets for Cancer Drug Discovery In The Molecular Basis of Human Cancer* (Coleman W.B., Tsongalis G.J., eds.), Humana Press, Totowa, NJ, pp. 521–540.

26. Burg D., Filippov D.V., Hermanns R., van der Marel G.A., van Boom J.H., Mulder G.J. 2002. Peptidomimetic glutathione analogues as novel gamma-GT stable GST inhibitors. *Bioorg. Med. Chem.* **10**:195–205.

27. Caffrey P.B., Zhu M., Zhang Y., Chinen N., Frenkel G.D. 1999. Rapid development of glutathione-S-transferase-dependent drug resistance in vitro and its prevention by ethacrynic acid. *Cancer Lett.* **136**:47–52.

28. Capronigro F., French R.C., Kaye S.B. 1997. Protein kinase C: a worthwhile target for anticancer drugs?. *Anti-Cancer Drugs* **8**:26–33.

29. Caskey L.S., Fuller G.N., Bruner J.M., Yung W.K., Sawaya R.E., Holland E.C., Zhang W. 2000. Toward a molecular classification of the gliomas: histopathology, molecular genetics, and gene expression profiling. *Histol. Histopathol.* **15**:971–981.

30. Chakravarti A., Chakladar A., Delaney M.A., Latham D.E., Loeffier J.S. 2002. The epidermal growth factor receptor pathway mediates resistance to sequential administration of radiation and chemotherapy in primary human glioblastoma cells in a RAS-dependent manner. *Cancer Res.* **62**:4307–4315.

31. Chakrabarty S., Huang S. 1996 Modulation of chemosensitivity in human colon carcinoma cells by downregulating protein kinase C alpha expression. *J. Exp. Ther. Oncol.* **1**:218–221.

32. Chasseaud L.F. 1979. The role of glutathione and glutathione-S-transferases in the metabolism of chemical carcinogens and other electrophilic agents. *Adv. Cancer Res.* **28**:175–274.

33. Chen T.C., Su S., Fry D., Liebes L. 2003. Combination therapy with irinotecan and protein kinase C inhibitors in malignant glioma. *Cancer* **97**:2363–2373.

34. Chen J.K., Taipale J., Young K.E., Maiti T., Beachy P.A. 2002. Small molecule modulation of Smoothened activity. *Pro. Natl. Acad. Sci. USA* **99**:14,071–14,076

35. Couldwell W.T., Hinton D.R., Surnock A.A., DeGiorgio C.M., Weiner L.P., Apuzzo M.L., et al. 1996. Treatment of recurrent malignant gliomas with chronic oral high-dose tamoxifen. *Clin. Cancer Res.* **2**:619–622.

36. Costello J.F., Plass C., Arap W., Chapman V.M., Held W.A., Berger M.D.1997. Cyclin-dependent kinase 6 (CDK6) amplification in human gliomas identified by using two-dimensional separation of genomic DNA. *Cancer Res.* **57**: 1250–1254.

37. Curtin N.J., Wang L.Z., Yiakouvaki A., Kyle S., Arris C.A., Canan-Koch S., et al. 2004. Novel poly(ADP-ribose) polymerase-1 inhibitor, AG14361, restores sensitivity to temozolomide in mismatch repair-deficient cells. *Clin. Cancer Res.* **10**:881–889.

38. da Rocha A.B., Mans D.R., Regner A., Schwartsmann G. 2002 Targeting protein kinase C: new therapeutic opportunities against high-grade malignant gliomas? *Oncologist* **7**:17–33.

39. Dantzer F., Schreiber V., Niedergang C., Trucco C., Flatter E., De La Rubia G., et al. 1999. Involvement of poly(ADP-ribose) polymerase in base excision repair. *Biochimie.* **81**:69–75.

40. de Murcia J.M., Niedergang C., Trucco C., Ricoul M., Dutrillaux B., Mark M., et al. 1997.. Requirement of poly(ADP-ribose) polymerase in recovery from DNA damage in mice and in cells. *Proc. Natl. Acad. Sci. USA* **94**:7303–7307.

41. Dirr H., Reinemer P., Huber R.1994. Refined crystal structure of porcine class Pi glutathione S-transferase (pGST P1-1) at 2.1 A resolution. *J. Mol. Biol.* **243**:72–92.

42. Dirven H., van Ommen B., Bladderen P. 1994. Involvement of human glutathione S-transferase isoenzymes in the conjugation of cyclophosphamide metabolites with glutathione. *Cancer Res.* **54**:6215–6220.

43. Dirven H.A., Megens L., Oudshoorn M.J., Dingemanse M.A., van Ommen B., van Bladeren P.J. 1995. Glutathione conjugation of the cytostatic drug ifosfamide and the role of human glutathione S-transferases. *Chem. Res. Toxicol.* **8**: 979–986.

44. Dolan M.E., Stine L., Mitchell R.B., Moschel R.C., Pegg A.E. 1990. Modulation of mammalian O6-alkylguanine-DNA alkyltransferase in vivo by O6-benzylguanine and its effect on the sensitivity of a human glioma tumor to 1-(2-chloroethyl)-3-(4-methylcyclohexyl)-1-nitrosourea. *Cancer Commun.* **2**:371–377.

45. Dolan M.E., Pegg A.E. 1997. O6-benzylguanine and its role in chemotherapy. *Clin. Cancer Res.* **3**:837–847.

46. Druker B.J. 2002. STI571 (GleevecTM) as a paradigm for cancer therapy. *Trend Mol. Med.* **8**:S14–S18.

47. Edwards D.R., Murphy G. 1998. Proteases - invasion and more. *Nature* **394**:527–528.

48. Edwards E., Geng L., Tan J., Onishko H., Donnelly E., Hallahan D. E. 2002. Phosphatidylinositol 3- kinase/Aktsignaling in the response of vascular endothelium to ionizing radiation. *Cancer Res.* **62**:4671–4677.

49. Engelhard H., Narang C., Homer R., Duncan H. 1996. Urokinase antisense oligonucleotides as a novel therapeutic agent for malignant glioma: in vitro and in vivo studies of uptake, effects and toxicity. *Biochem. Biophys. Res. Commun.* **227**:400–405.

50. Engkvist O., Wrede P., Rester U. 2003. Prediction of CNS activity of compound libraries using substructure analysis. *J. Chem. Inf. Comput. Sci.* **43**:155–160.

51. Ermoian R.P., Furniss C. S., Lamborn, K. R., Basila, D., Berger, M. S.,Gottschalk, et al. 2002. Dysregulation of PTEN and protein kinase B is associated with glioma histology and patient survival. *Clin. Cancer Res.* **8**:1100–1106.

52. Feher M., Sourial E., Schmidt J.M.2000. A simple model for the prediction of blood-brain partitioning. *Int. J. Pharm.* **201**:239–247.

53. Feldkamp M.M., Lau N., Guha A. 1997. Signal transduction pathways and their relevance in human astrocytomas. *J. Neurooncol.* **35**:223–248.

54. Feldkamp M.M., Lala P., Lau N., Roncari L., Guha A. 1999. Expression of activated epidermal growth factor receptors, Ras-guanosine triphosphate, and mitogen-activated protein kinase in human glioblastoma multiforme specimens. *Neurosurgery* **45**:1442–1453.

55. Fleming T.P., Saxena A., Clark W.C., Robertson J.T., Oldfield E.H., Aaronson S.A., Ali I.U. 1992. Amplification and/ or overexpression of platelet-derived growth factor receptors and epidermal growth factor receptor in human glial tumors. *Cancer Res.* **52:**4550–4553.

56. Folkman J., Klagsbrun M. 1987. Angiogenic factors. *Science* **235:**442–447

57. Fong T.A., Shawver L.K., Sun L., Tang C., App H., Powell J.T., et al. 1999. SU5416 is a potent and selective inhibitor of the vascular endothelial growth factor receptor (Flk-1/KDR) that inhibits tyrosine kinase catalysis, tumor vascular-ization, and growth of multiple tumor types. *Cancer Res.* **59:**99–106.

58. Frank-Kamenetsky M., Zhang X.M., Bottega S., Guicherit O., Wichterle H., Dudek H., et al. 2002. Small-molecule modulators of Hedgehog signaling: identification and characterization of Smoothened agonists and antagonists. *J. Biol.* **1:**10.

59. Friedman H.S., Kokkinakis D.M., Pluda J., Friedman A.H., Cokgor I., Haglund M.M., et al. 1998. Phase I trial of O6-benzylguanine for patients undergoing surgery for malignant glioma. *J. Clin. Oncol.* **16:**3570–3575.

60. Friedman H.S., Pegg A.E., Johnson S.P., Loktionova N.A., Dolan M.E., Modrich P., et al. 1999. Modulation of cyclo-phosphamide activity by O6-alkylguanine-DNA alkyltransferase. *Cancer Chemother. Pharmacol.* **43:**80–85.

61. Fry D.W. 1996. Recent advances in tyrosine kinase inhibitors. *Ann. Rep. Med. Chem.* **31:**151–160.

62. Garcia-Echeverria C., Chene P., Blommers M.J.J., Furet, P. 2000. Discovery of potent antagonists of the interaction between human double minute 2 and tumor suppressor p53. *J. Med. Chem.* **43:**3205–3208.

63. Gate L., Tew K.D. 2001. Glutathione S-transferases as emerging therapeutic targets. *Expert Opin. Ther. Targets.* **5:** 477–489.

64. Geng L., Donnelly E., McMahon G., Lin P.C., Sierra-Rivera E., Oshinka H., Hallahan D.E. 2001. Inhibition of vascular endothelial growth factor receptor signaling leads to reversal of tumor resistance to radiotherapy. *Cancer Res.* **61:**2413–2419.

65. Gilbertson R.J., Perry R.H., Kelly P.J., Pearson A.D., Lunec J. 1997. Prognostic significance of HER2 and HER4 coexpression in childhood medulloblastoma. *Cancer Res.* **57:**3272–3280.

66. Glass T.L., Liu T.J., Yung W.K. 2000. Inhibition of cell growth in human glioblastoma cell lines by farnesyltransferase inhibitor SCH66336. *Neuro-oncol.* **2:**151–158.

67. Gondi C.S., Lakka S.S., Yanamandra N., Siddique K., Dinh D.H., Olivero W.C., et al. 2003. Expression of antisense uPAR and antisense uPA from a bicistronic adenoviral construct inhibits glioma cell invasion, tumor growth, and angiogenesis. *Oncogene* **22:**5967–5975.

68. Goto S., Iida T., Cho S., Oka M., Kohno S., Kondo T. 1999. Overexpression of glutathione S-transferase π enhances the adduct formation of cisplatin with glutathione in human cancer cells. *Free Rad Res.* **31:**549–558.

69. Guha A., Feldkamp M.M., Lau N., Boss G., Pawson A. 1997. Proliferation of human malignant astrocytomas is depen-dent on Ras activation. *Oncogene* **15:**2755–2765.

70. Hanahan D. 1997. Signaling vascular morphogenesis and maintenance. *Science* **277:**48–50.

71. Hanash S.M., Bobek M.P., Rickman D.S., Williams T., Rouillard J.M., Kuick R., Puravs E. 2002. Integrating cancer genomics and proteomics in the post-genome era. *Proteomics* **2:**69–75.

72. Hansson J., Berhane K., Castro V.M., Jungnelius U., Mannervik B., Ringborg U. 1991. Sensitization of human mela-noma cells to the cytotoxic effect of melphalan by the glutathione transferase inhibitor ethacrynic acid. *Cancer Res.* **51:** 94–98.

73. Hara A., Yamada H., Sakai N., Hirayama H., Tanaka T., Mori H.1990. Immunohistochemical demonstration of the placental form of glutathione S-transferase, a detoxifying enzyme in human gliomas. *Cancer* **66:**2563–2568.

74. Hayes J.D., Pulford D.J. 1995. The glutathione S-transferare supergene family: Regulation of GST and the contribution of the isoenzymes to cancer chemoprotection and drug resistance. *Crit. Rev. Biochem. Mol. Biol.* **30:**445–600.

75. Heimberger A.B., Learn C.A., Archer G.E., McLendon R.E., Chewning T.A., Tuck F.L., et al. 2002. Brain tumors in mice are susceptible to blockade of epidermal growth factor receptor (EGFR) with the oral, specific, EGFR-tyrosine kinase inhibitor ZD1839 (iressa). *Clin. Cancer Res.* **8:**3496–3502.

76. Heldin C.-H., Ostman A., Ronnstrand L. 1998. Signal transduction via platelet-derived growth factor receptors. *Biochem. Biophys. Acta* **1378:**F79-F113.

77. Herms J., Neidt I., et al. 2000. C-myc expression in medulloblastoma and its prognostic value. *Int. J. Cancer* **20:**18–25.

78. Hofmann J. 2002. Modulation of protein kinase C in antitumor treatment. *Rev. Physiol. Biochem. Pharmacol.* **142:**1–96.

79. Hu X., Xia H., Srivastava S.K., Herzog C., Awasthi Y.C., Ji X., Zimniak P., Singh, S.V. 1997. Activity of four allelic forms of glutathione S-transferase P1-1 hGSTP1-1 for diol epoxides of polycyclic aromatic hydrocarbons. *Biochem. Biophys. Res. Comm.* **238:**397–402.

80. Hu X., Ji X., Srivastava S.K., Xia H, Awasthi S., Nanduri B., Awasthi Y.C., et al. 1997. Mechanism of differential catalytic efficiency of two polymorphic forms of human glutathione S-transferase P1-1 in the glutathione conjugation of carcinogenic diol epoxide of chryses. *Arch. Biochem. Biophys.* **345:**32–38.

81. Hubbard S.R., Till J.H. 2000. Protein tyrosine kinase structure and function. *Ann. Rev. Biochem.* **69:**373–398.

82. Hudziak R.M., Lewis G.D., Shalaby M.R., Eessalu T.E., Aggarwal B.B., Ullrich A., Shepard H.M. 1988. Amplified expression of the HER2/ERBB2 oncogene induces resistance to tumor necrosis factor alpha in NIH 3T3 cells. *Proc. Natl. Acad. Sci. USA* **85:**5102–5106.

83. Incardona J.P., Gaffield W., Kapur R.P., Roelink H. 1998. The teratogenic Veratrum alkaloid cyclopamine inhibits sonic hedgehog signal transduction. *Development* **125**:3553–3562.

84. Ishikawa T., Ali-Osman F. 1994. Glutathione conjugation and ATP-dependent export of anticancer drugs, in *Drug Transport in Antimicrobial and Anticancer Drugs* (Georgopapadakou N.H., ed.), Marcel Dekker,Inc., New York, pp. 577–612.

85. Ishimoto T.M., Ali-Osman F. 2002. Allelic variants of the human glutathione S-transferase P1 gene confer differential cytoprotection against anticancer agents in escherichia coli. *Pharmacogenetics* **12**:543–553.

86. Jaeckle K.A., Eyre H.J., Townsend J.J., Schulman S., Knudson H.M., Belanich M., et al. 1998. Correlation of tumor O6 methylguanine-DNA methyltransferase levels with survival of malignant astrocytoma patients treated with bis-chloroethylnitrosourea: a Southwest Oncology Group study. *J. Clin. Oncol.* **16**:3310–3315.

87. Jayaraman L., Murthy K.G., Zhu C., Curran T., Xanthoudakis S., Prives C. 1997. Identification of redox/repair protein Ref-1 as a potent activator of p53. *Genes Dev.* **11**:558–570.

88. Ji, X., Tordova M., O'Donnel R., Parsons J.F., Hayden J.B., Gilliland G.L., Zimniak P. 1997. Structure and function of the xenobiotic substrate-binding site in a class π glutathione S-transferase. *Biochemistry* **36**:9690–9702.

89. Jorgensen W.L., Duffy E.M. 2002. Prediction of drug solubility from structure. *Adv. Drug Deliv. Rev.* **54**:355–366.

90. Kanzawa T., Bedwell J., Kondo Y., Kondo S., Germano I.M. 2003. Inhibition of DNA repair for sensitizing resistant glioma cells to temozolomide. *J. Neurosurg.* **99**:1047–1052.

91. Keir S.T., Dolan M.E., Pegg A.E., Lawless A., Moschel R.C., Bigner D.D., Friedman H.S. 2000. O6-benzylguanine-mediated enhancement of nitrosourea activity in Mer- central nervous system tumor xenografts—implications for clinical trials. *Cancer Chemother. Pharmacol.* **45**:437–440.

92. Keller C., Ali-Osman F.1998. Translational inhibition of messenger RNA of the human pi class glutathione S-transferase by antisense oligodeoxyribonucleotides in *Glutathione and Glutathione Linked Enzymes in Cancer and Other Diseases*, (Ali-Osman F., Tew K.D., Strange R., eds.) Elsevier, pp. 307–323.

92a. Kim J., Yu W., Kovalski K., Ossowski L. 1998. Requirement for specific proteases in cancer cell intravasation as revealed by a novel semiquantitative PCR-based assay. *Cell* **94**:353–362.

93. Kitagawa H., Tani E., Ikemoto H., Ozaki I., Nakano A., Omura S. 1999. Proteasome inhibitors induce mitochondria-independent apoptosis in human glioma cells. *FEBS Lett.* **443**:181–186.

94. Kolibaba K.S., Druker B.J. 1997. Protein tyrosine kinases and cancer. *Biochim. Biophys. Acta* **1333**:F217–F248.

95. Konduri S., Lakka S.S., Tasiou A., Yanamandra N., Gondi C.S., Dinh D.H., et al. 2001. Elevated levels of cathepsin B in human glioblastoma cell lines. *Int. J. Oncol.* **19**:519–524.

96. Kuan C.T., Wikstrand C.J., Bigner D.D. 2001. EGF mutant receptor vIII as a molecular target in cancer therapy. *Endocr. Relat. Cancer.* **8**:83–96.

97. Kuntz I.D. 1992. Structure-based strategies for drug design and discovery. science **257**:1078–1082.

98. Kunze T., Heps S. 2000. Phosphono analogs of glutathione: inhibition of glutathione transferases, metabolic stability, and uptake by cancer cells. *Biochem. Pharmacol.* **59**:973–981.

99. Lipinski C.A., Lombardo F., Dominy B.W., Feeney P.J. 2001. Experimental and computational approaches to estimate solubility and permeability in drug discovery and development settings. *Adv. Drug Deliv. Rev.* **46**:3–26.

100. Lipinski C.A. 2000. Drug-like properties and the causes of poor solubility and poor permeability. *J. Pharmacol. Toxicol. Methods* **44**:235–49.

101. Lin P., Sankar S., Shan S., Dewhirst M.W., Polverini P.J., Quinn T.Q., Peters K.G. 1998. Inhibition of tumor growth by targeting tumor endothelium using a soluble vascular endothelial growth factor receptor. *Cell Growth Differ.* **9**:49–58.

102. Lindahl T., Satoh M.S., Poirier G.G., Klungland A. 1995. Post-translational modification of poly(ADP-ribose) polymerase induced by DNA strand breaks. *Trends Biochem. Sci.* **20**:405.

103. Liu L., Nakatsuru Y., Gerson S.L. 2002. Base excision repair as a therapeutic target in colon cancer. *Clin. Cancer Res.* **8**:2985–2991.

104. Liu L., Yan L., Donze J.R., Gerson S.L. 2003.Blockage of abasic site repair enhances antitumor efficacy of 1,3-bis-(2-chloroethyl)-1-nitrosourea in colon tumor xenografts. *Mol. Cancer Ther.* **2**:1061–1066.

105. Liuzzi M., Talpaert-Borle M. 1985. A new approach to the study of the base-excision repair pathway using methoxyamine. *J. Biol. Chem.* **260**:5252–5258.

106. Lo H.-W., Ali-Osman F. 2001. The human glutathione S-transferase P1 protein is a phosphorylation target of Ser/Thr protein kinases: A novel mechanism in signaling related drug resistance. *Proc. Am. Assoc. Cancer Res.* **42**:672.

107. Ludlum D.B., Mehta J.R., Tong W.P. 1986. Prevention of 1-(3-deoxycytidyl),2-(1-deoxyguanosinyl)ethane cross-link formation in DNA by rat liver O6-alkylguanine-DNA alkyltransferase. *Cancer Res.* **46**:3353–3357.

108. MacGregor D.N., Ziff E.B. 1990. Elevated c-myc expression in childhood medulloblastomas. *Pediatr. Res.* **28**:63–68.

109. Mannervik B., Awasthi Y.C., Board P.G., Hayes J.D., Illo C.D., Ketterer B., et al. 1992. Nomenclature for human glutathione transferases. *Biochem. J.* **282**:305–306.

110. McElhinney R.S., McMurry T.B., Margison G.P. 2003. O6-alkylguanine-DNA alkyltransferase inactivation in cancer chemotherapy. *Mini. Rev. Med. Chem.* **3**:471–485.

111. Mendel D.B., Laird A.D., Xin X., Louie S.G., Christensen J.G., Li, G., et al. In vivo antitumor activity of SU11248, a novel tyrosine kinase inhibitor targeting VEGF and PDGF receptors: Determination of a pharmacokinetic/pharmacodynamic relationship. *Clin. Cancer Res.* **9**:327–337.

112. Miller P., DiOrio C., Moyer M., Schnur R.C., Bruskin A., Cullen W., Moyer J.D. 1994. Depletion of the erbB-2 gene product p185 by the benzoquinone ansamycins. *Cancer Res.* **54:**2724–2730.

113. Mischel P.S., Nelson S.F., Cloughesy T.F. 2003. Molecular analysis of glioblastoma: pathway profiling and its implications for patient therapy. *Cancer Biol. Ther.* **2:**242–247.

114. Momand J., Jung D., Wilczynski S., Niland J. 1998. The MDM2 gene amplification database. *Nucleic Acids Res.* **26:**3453–3459.

115. Muegge I. 2003. Selection criteria for drug-like compounds. *Med. Res. Rev.* **23:**302–321.

116. Nagourney R.A., Messenger J.C., Kern D.H., Weisenthal L.M. 1990. Enhancement of anthracycline and alkylator cytotoxicity by ethacrynic acid in primary cultures of human tissues. *Cancer Chemother. Pharmacol.* **26:**318–322.

117. Neamati N., Barchi Jr, J.J. 2002. New paradigms in drug design and discovery. *Curr. Topic. Med. Chem.* **2:**211–227.

118. Neckers L. 2002. Hsp90 inhibitors as novel cancer chemotherapeutic agents. *Trend. Mol. Med.* **8:**S55–S61.

119. Newton H.B. 2003. Molecular neuro-oncology and development of targeted therapeutic strategies for brain tumors. Part 1: Growth factor and Ras signaling pathways. *Expert Rev. Anticancer Ther.* **3:**595–614.

120. Norman P. 2001. OSI-774 OSI Pharmaceuticals. *Curr. Opin. Investig. Drugs.* **2:**298–304.

121. Nutt C.L., Mani D.R., Betensky R.A., Tamayo P., Cairncross J.G., Ladd C., et al. 2003. Gene expression-based classification of malignant gliomas correlates better with survival than histological classification. *Cancer Res.* **63:**1602–1607.

122. Oakley A.J., Bello M.L., Battistoni A., Ricci G,. Rossjohn J., Villar H.O., Parker M.W. 1997. The structures of human glutathione transferase P1-1 in complex with glutathione and various inhibitors at high resolution. *J. Mol. Biol.* **274:**84–100.

123. O'Dwyer M.E., Druker B.J. 2001. The role of the tyrosine kinase inhibitor STI571 in the treatment of cancer. *Curr. Cancer Drug Targets* **1:**49–57.

124. O'Dwyer P.J., LaCreta F., Nash S., Tinsley P.W., Schilder R., Clapper M.L., et al. 1991. Phase I study of thiotepa in combination with the glutathione transferase inhibitor ethacrynic acid. *Cancer Res.* **51:**6059–6065.

125. Oliner J.D., Kinzler K.W., Meltzer P.S., George P.L., Vogelstein B. 1992. Amplification of a gene encoding a p53-associated protein in human sarcomas. *Nature* **358:**80–83

126. Oro A.E., Higgins K.M., Hu Z., Bonifas J.M., Epstein E.H., Scott M.P. 1997. Basal cell carcinomas in mice overexpressing sonic hedgehog. *Science* **276:**817–821.

127. Pandya U., Srivastava S.K., Singhal S.S., Pal A., Awasthi S., Zimniak P., et al. 2000. Activity of allelic variants of pi class human glutathione S-transferase toward chlorambucil. *Biochem. Biophys. Res. Commun.* **278:**258–262.

128. Pegg A.E., Boosalis M., Samson L., Moschel R.C., Byers T.L., Swenn K., Dolan M.E. 1993. Mechanism of inactivation of human O6-alkylguanine-DNA alkyltransferase by O6-benzylguanine. *Biochemistry* **32:**11998–2006.

128a. Petrini M., Conte A., Caracciolo F., Sabbatini A., Grassi B., Ronca G. 1993. Reversing of chlorambucil resistance by ethacrynic acid in a B-CLL patient. *Br. J. Haematol.* **85:**409–410.

128b. Pickett C.B., Lu A.Y. 1989. Glutathione S-transferases: gene structure, regulation, and biological function. *Annu. Rev. Biochem.* **58:**743–764.

129. Ploemen J.H., van Ommen B., Bogaards J.J., van Bladeren P.J. 1993. Ethacrynic acid and its glutathione conjugate as inhibitors of glutathione S-transferases. *Xenobiotica* **23:**913–923.

130. Pollack I.F., Randall M.S., Kristofik M.P., Kelly R.H., Selker R.G., Vertosick F.T. 1990. Response of malignant glioma cell lines to epidermal growth factor and platelet-derived growth factor in a serum-free medium. *J. Neurosurg.* **73:**106–112.

131. Pollack I.F., Randall M.S., Kristofik M.P., Kelly R.H., Selker R.G., Vertosick F.T. 1990. Response of malignant glioma cell lines to epidermal growth factor and platelet-derived growth factor in a serum-free medium. *J. Neurosurg.* **73:**106–112.

132. Pollack IF, DaRosso RC, Robertson PL, Jakacki RL, Mirro JR Jr, Blatt J, et al. 1997. A phase I study of high-dose tamoxifen for the treatment of refractory malignant gliomas of childhood. *Clin. Cancer Res.* **3:**1109–1115.

133. Pomerantz, J., Shreiber-Argus, N., Liegeois, N.J., Silverman A., Alland, L., Chin, L., et al. 1998. The Ink4a tumor suprssor gene product, p19[Arf] interacts with MDM2 and neutralizes MDM2's inhibition of p53. *Cell* **92:**713–723.

134. Powell D., Skotnicki J., Upeslacis J. 1997. Angiogenesis inhibitors. *Ann. Rep. Med. Chem.* **32:**161–170

135. Qiao L., Wang S., George C., Lewin L.E., Blumberg P.M., Kozikowski A.P. 1998. Structure-based design of a new class of protein kinase C modulators. *J. Am. Chem. Soc.* **120:**6629–6630.

136. Rabbani S.A. 1998. Metalloproteases and urokinase in angiogenesis and tumor progression. *In Vivo* **12:**135–142.

137. Racz I., Tory K., Gallyas F. Jr., Berente Z., Osz E., Jaszlits L., Bernath S., et al. 2002. BGP-15 - a novel poly(ADP-ribose) polymerase inhibitor - protects against nephrotoxicity of cisplatin without compromising its antitumor activity. *Biochem. Pharmacol.* **63:**1099–1111.

138. Rao R.D., Uhm J.H., Krishnan S., James C.D. 2003. Genetic and signaling pathway alterations in glioblastoma: relevance to novel targeted therapies. *Front Biosci.* **8:**270–280.

139. Rao J.S. 2003. Expression of antisense uPAR and antisense uPA from a bicistronic adenoviral construct inhibits glioma cell invasion, tumor growth, and angiogenesis. *Oncogene* **22:**5967–5975.

140. Reinemer P., Dirr H.W., Ladenstein R., Schaffer J., Gallay O., Huber R. 1991. The three dimensional structure of class pi glutathione S-transferase in complex with glutathione sulfonate at 2.3 A resolution. *EMBO J.* **10:**1997–2005.

141. Reuning U., Sperl S., Kopitz C., Kessler H., Kruger A., Schmitt M., Magdolen V. 2003.Urokinase-type plasminogen activator (uPA) and its receptor (uPAR): development of antagonists of uPA/uPAR interaction and their effects in vitro and in vivo. *Curr. Pharm.* **9:**1529–1543.

142. Rhodes T., Twentyman P.R. 1992. A study of ethacrynic acid as a potential modifier of melphalan and cisplatin sensitivity in human lung cancer parental and drug-resistant cell lines. *Br. J. Cancer* **65:**684–690.

143. Risau W. 1997. Mechanisms of Angiogenesis. *Nature* **386:**671–674.

144. Rosen L.S., Brown J., Laxa B., Boulos L., Reiswig L., Henner W.D., et al. 2003. Phase I study of TLK286 (glutathione S-transferase P1-1 activated glutathione analogue) in advanced refractory solid malignancies. *Clin. Cancer Res.* **9:**1628–1638.

145. Ruscoe J.E., Rosario L.A., Wang T., Gate L., Arifoglu P., Wolf C.R., Henderson C.J., Ronai Z., Tew K.D. 2001. Pharmacologic or genetic manipulation of glutathione S-transferase P1-1 (GSTpi) influences cell proliferation pathways. *J. Pharmacol. Exp. Ther.* **298:**339–345.

146. Sallinen S.L., Sallinen P.K., Haapasalo H.K., Helin H.J., Helen P.T., Schraml P., et al. 2000. Identification of differentially expressed genes in human gliomas by DNA microarray and tissue chip techniques. *Cancer Res.* **60:**6617–6622.

147. Semenza G.L. 2002. HIF-1 and Tumor progression: pathophysiology and therapeutics. *Trend. Mol. Med.* **8:**S62–S67.

148. Senderowicz A.M. 2003. Small-molecule cyclin-dependent kinase modulators. *Oncogene* **22:**6609–6620.

149. Shak S. (1999) Overview of the trastuzumab (herceptin) anti-HER2 monoclonal antibody clinical programme in HER-2 overexpressing metastatic breast bancer. Herceptin Multinational Investigator Study Group. *Semin. Oncol.* **26:**71–77.

150. Shapiro J.R., Coons S.W. 1998. Genetics of adult malignant gliomas. *BNI Quarterly* **14:**27–42.

151. Simbulan-Rosenthal C.M., Rosenthal D.S., Iyer S., Boulares A.H., Smulson M.E. 1998. Transient poly(ADP-ribosyl)ation of nuclear proteins and role of poly(ADP-ribose) polymerase in the early stages of apoptosis. *J. Biol. Chem.* **273:** 13,703–13,712.

152. Southan G.J., Szabo C. 2003. Poly(ADP-ribose) polymerase inhibitors. *Curr. Med. Chem***10:**321–340.

153. Srivastava S.K., Singhal S.S., Hu X., Awasthi Y.C., Zimniak P., Singh S.V. 199. Differential catalytic efficiency of allelic variants of human glutathione S-transferase pi in catalyzing the glutathione conjugation of thiotepa. *Arch. Biochem. Biophys.* **366:**89–94.

154. Stecca B., Altaba A.R. 2002. The therapeutic potential of modulators of the Hedgehog-Gli signaling pathway. *J. Biol.* **1:**9.1–9.4.

155. Stoll R., Renner C., Hansen S., Palme S., Klein C., Belling A., et al. 2001. Chalcone derivatives antagonize interactions between the human oncoprotein MDM2 and p53. *Biochemistry* **40:**336–344.

156. Taipale J., Beachy P.A. 2001. The Hedgehog and wnt signalling pathways in cancer. *Nature* **411:**349–354.

157. Taipale J., Chen J.K., Cooper M.K., Wang B., Mann R.K., Melinkovic L., et al. 2000. Effects of oncogenic mutations in Smoothened and Patched can be reversed by cyclopamine. *Nature* **406:**1005–1009.

158. Takamoto T., Sasaki M., Kuno T., Tamaki N. 2001. Flk-1 specific kinase inhibitor (SU5416) inhibited the growth of GS-9L glioma in rat brain and prolonged the survival. *Kobe J. Med. Sci.* **47:**181–191.

159. Taverna P., Liu L., Hwang H.S., Hanson A.J., Kinsella T.J., Gerson S.L. 2001. Methoxyamine potentiates DNA single strand breaks and double strand breaks induced by temozolomide in colon cancer cells. *Mutat. Res.* **485:**269–281.

159a. Teicher B.A., Menon K., Alvarez E., Shih C., Faul M.M. 2002. Antiangiogenic and antitumor effects of a protein kinase Cbeta inhibitor in human breast cancer and ovarian cancer xenografts. *Invest New Drugs* **20:**241–251.

160. Tentori L., Portarena I., Graziani G. 2002. Potential clinical applications of poly(ADP-ribose) polymerase (PARP) inhibitors. *Pharmacol. Res.* **45:**73–85.

160a. Tew K.D., Bomber A.M., Hoffman S.J. 1988. Ethacrynic acid and piriprost as enhancers of cytotoxicity in drug resistant and sensitive cell lines. *Cancer Res.* **48:**3622–3625

161. Tew K.D., Dutta S., Schultz M. 1997. Inhibitors of glutathione S-transferases as therapeutic agents. *Adv. Drug Deliv. Rev.* **26:**91–104.

162. Tomlinson F.H., Jenkins R.B., Scheithauer B.W., Keelan PA, Ritland S., Parisi J.E., et al. 1994. Aggressive meduloblastoma with high-level N-myc amplification. *Mayo Clinic Proc.* **69:** 359–365.

162a. Townsend D., Tew K. 2003. Cancer drugs, genetic variation and the glutathione-S-transferase gene family. *Am. J. Pharmacogenomics* **3:**157–172.

163. Tremont-Lukats I.W., Gilbert M.R. 2003. Advances in molecular therapies in patients with brain tumors. *Cancer Control* **10:**125–137.

164. Virag L., Szabo C. 2002. Therapeutic potential of poly(ADP-ribose) polymerase inhibitors. *Pharmacol. Rev.* **54:** 375–429.

165. Walters W.P., Murcko M.A. 2002. Prediction of "drug-likeness." *Adv. Drug Deliv. Rev.* **54:**255–271.

166. Wan Y., Wu D., Gao H., Lu H. 2000. Potentiation of BCNU anticancer activity by O6-benzylguanine: a study in vitro and in vivo. *J. Environ. Pathol. Toxicol. Oncol.* **19:**69–75.

167. Wang J.Y., Del Valle L., Gordon J., Rubini M., Romano G., Croul S., et al. 2001. Activation of the IGF-IR system contributes to malignant growth of human and mouse medulloblastomas. *Oncogene* **20:**3857–3868.

168. Wang S., Milne G.W.A., Nicklaus M.C., Marquez V.E., Lee J., Blumberg P.M. 1994. Protein kinase C. modeling of the binding site and prediction of binding constants. *J. Med. Chem.* **37:**1326–1338.

169. Wang S., Zaharevitz D.W., Sharma R., Marquez V.E., Milne G.W.A., Lewin N.E., et al. 1994. Discovery of novel, structurally diverse protein kinase C agonists through computer 3D-database pharmacophore search. molecular modeling mtudies. *J. Med. Chem.* **37:**4479–4489.

170. Waxman D.J. 1990. Glutathione S-transferases: role in alkylating agent resistance and possible target for modulation chemotherapy: a review. *Cancer Res.* **50:**6449–6454.

171. Wedge S.R., Newlands E.S. 1996. O6-benzylguanine enhances the sensitivity of a glioma xenograft with low O6-alkylguanine-DNA alkyltransferase activity to temozolomide and BCNU. *Br. J. Cancer.* **73:**1049–1052.

172. Westermark B., Heldin C.H., Nister M. 1995. Platelet-derived growth factor in human glioma. *Glia.* **15:**257–263.

173. Winter S., Weller M. 2000. Poly(ADP-ribose) polymerase-independent potentiation of nitrosourea cytotoxicity by 3-aminobenzamide in human malignant glioma cells. *Eur. J. Pharmacol.* **398:**177–183.

174. Wharton S.B., McNelis U., Bell H.S., Whittle I.R. 2000. Expression of poly(ADP-ribose) polymerase and distribution of poly(ADP-ribosyl)ation in glioblastoma and in a glioma multicellular tumour spheroid model. *Neuropathol. Appl. Neurobiol.* **26:**528–535.

175. Weidle U.H., Konig, B. 1998. Urokinase Receptor Antagonists: novel agents for the treatment of cancer. *Exp. Opin. Invest. Drugs* **7:**391–440.

176. Xanthoudakis S., Smeyne R.J., Wallace J.D., Curran T. 1996. The redox/DNA repair protein, Ref-1, is essential for early embryonic development in mice. *Proc. Natl. Acad. Sci. USA* **93:**8919–8923.

177. Xu J Stevenson J. 2000. Drug-like index: a new approach to measure drug-like compounds and their diversity. *J. Chem. Inf. Comput. Sci.* **40:**1177–1187.

178. Zellner A., Fetell M.R., Bruce J.N., De Vivo D.C., O'Driscoll K.R. 1998. Disparity in expression of protein kinase C alpha in human glioma versus glioma-derived primary cell lines: therapeutic implications. *Clin. Cancer Res.* **4:** 1797–1802.

178a. Taylor M.D., Liu L., Raffel C., Hui C.C., Mainprize T.G., Zhang X., et al. 2002. Mutations in SUFU predispose to medulloblastoma. *Nat Genet.* **31:**306–310.

178b. Zhang W., Law R.E., Hinton D.R., Couldwell W.T. 1997. Inhibition of human malignant glioma cell motility and invasion in vitro by hypericin, a potent protein kinase C inhibitor. *Cancer Letters* **120:**31–38.

179. Zhou B.P., Hung M.C. 2002. Novel targets of Akt, p21(Cipl/WAF1), and MDM2. *Semin. Oncol.* **29:**62–70.

180. Zimniak P., Nanduri B., Pikuba S., Bandorowicz-Pikuba J., Singhal S.S., Srivastava, S.K., et al. 1994. Naturally occurring human glutathione S-transferase GSTP1-1 isoforms with isoleucine and valine in position 104 differ in enzymic properties. *Eur. J. Biochem.* **224:**893–899.

181. Zurawel R.H., Chiappa S.A., Allen C., Raffel C. 1998. Sporadic medulloblastomas contain oncogenic beta-catenin mutations. *Cancer Res.* **58:**896–899.

Index